Anesthesiology and Critical Care Morning Report: Beyond the Pearls

Anesthesiology and Critical Care Morning Report

Beyond the Pearls

Series Editors

RAJ DASGUPTA, MD, FACP, FCCP, FAASM

Associate Professor of Clinical Medicine
Department of Medicine Division of Pulmonary Critical Care and Sleep Medicine
Keck School of Medicine of the University of Southern California, Los Angeles
California, United States

Associate Program Director
Sleep Medicine Fellowship
Keck School of Medicine of the University of California, Los Angeles
California, United States

Assistant Program Director
Internal Medicine Residency
Keck School of Medicine of the University of California, Los Angeles
California, United States

R. MICHELLE KOOLAEE, DO

Assistant Professor of Medicine
Division of Rheumatology
University of Southern California
Los Angeles
California, United States

Presbyterian Intercommunity Health Medical Group
Attending Rheumatologist Whittier
California, United States

Volume Editors

PAUL NEIL FRANK, MD

PATRICK CHAN, MD

RAJ DASGUPTA, MD, FACP, FCCP, FAASM

ELSEVIER

Elsevier
1600 John F. Kennedy Blvd.
Ste 1800
Philadelphia, PA 19103-2899

ANESTHESIOLOGY AND CRITICAL CARE MORNING REPORT:
BEYOND THE PEARLS

ISBN: 978-0-323-84776-6

Notice

Practitioners and researchers must always rely on their own experience and knowledge in evaluating and using any information, methods, compounds or experiments described herein. Because of rapid advances in the medical sciences, in particular, independent verification of diagnoses and drug dosages should be made. To the fullest extent of the law, no responsibility is assumed by Elsevier, authors, editors or contributors for any injury and/or damage to persons or property as a matter of products liability, negligence or otherwise, or from any use or operation of any methods, products, instructions, or ideas contained in the material herein.

Content Strategist: James Merritt
Content Development Specialist: Ranjana Sharma
Content Development Manager: Somodatta Roy Choudhury
Publishing Services Manager: Shereen Jameel
Project Manager: Haritha Dharmarajan
Design Direction: Bridget Hoette

Printed in India

Last digit is the print number: 9   8   7   6   5   4   3   2   1

Working together
to grow libraries in
developing countries

www.elsevier.com • www.bookaid.org

Volume Editors

Dr. Paul Frank: Michelle, you are my rock and my biggest supporter. I am so grateful to have such a wonderful wife. Noah, you are my inspiration and my mini-me. It is a joy to watch you grow and to teach you everything I know. Max, I love you and cannot wait to meet you.

Dr. Patrick Chan: To Shirley, to my brother, to my sister, and to my parents – without your support, I would not be who I am today."

Series Editors

Dr. Koolaee and I would like to dedicate this book to all healthcare, frontline, and essential workers for their courage, strength, compassion, and patience throughout this COVID-19 pandemic. We thank them for their perseverance and strength during moments of grief, loneliness, and depression. It truly is amazing how much hardship, anger, and sadness that so many have gone through these past years; and yet through all of this, they are still here to help with a positive attitude and hope for a better and safer life for everyone. We are honored to dedicate this book to them as a symbol that their hard work and sacrifice is paying off.

CONTRIBUTORS

David C. Asseff, MD
Cardiac Anesthesiologist, Anesthesia
and Perioperative Care, Veterans
Administration, Palo Alto, California,
United States

Braden Barnett, MD
Clinical Assistant Professor of Medicine,
Division of Endocrinology, Department of
Medicine, Keck School of Medicine of the
University of Southern California,
Los Angeles, California, United States

Nora Bedrossian, MD
Fellow Physician, Division of Endocrinology,
University of Southern California,
Los Angeles, California, United States

Christian Bohringer, MBBS
Professor of Clinical Anesthesiology,
Anesthesia, UC Davis, Sacramento,
California, United States

Ian Brooks, MD
Doctor, Anesthesiology, UC Davis,
Sacramento, California, United States

Sophie Mestman Cannon, MD
Fellow Physician, Division of Endocrinology,
University of Southern California,
Los Angeles, California, United States

Benjamin N. Cantrill, DO
Fellow Physician, Division of Pulmonary,
Critical Care and Sleep Medicine,
University of Southern California,
Los Angeles, California, United States

Patrick Chan, MD
Fellow Physician, Division of Pulmonary,
Critical Care and Sleep Medicine,
University of Southern California,
Los Angeles, California, United States

Juliann Cho, MD
Resident Physician, Department of
Anesthesiology, University of California,
Davis, Sacramento, California,
United States

Joon Choi, MD
Fellow Physician, Division of Pulmonary,
Critical Care and Sleep Medicine,
University of Southern California,
Los Angeles, California, United States

Ammar Quresh Dahodwala, MD
Resident Physician, Department of Internal
Medicine + Pediatrics, LAC+USC
Medical Center/University of Southern
California,
Los Angeles, California, United States

Raj Dasgupta, MD, FACP, FCCP, FAASM
Associate Professor of Clinical Medicine,
Department of Medicine Division of
Pulmonary, Critical Care and Sleep
Medicine, Keck School of Medicine of
the University of Southern California,
Los Angeles, California, United States
Associate Program Director, Sleep Medicine
Fellowship, Keck School of Medicine of
the University of California,
Los Angeles, California, United States
Assistant Program Director, Internal
Medicine Residency, Keck School of
Medicine of the University of California,
Los Angeles, California, United States

Dominic Engracia, MD
Fellow, Division of Pulmonary, Critical
Care and Sleep Medicine,
University of Southern California,
Los Angeles, California, United States

Reihaneh Forghany, MD
Dr. Reihaneh Forghany, Anesthesiology,
UC Davis Medical Center, Sacramento
California, United States

Paul Neil Frank, MD
Assistant Professor, Department of
    Anesthesiology and Pain Medicine,
    University of California, Davis,
    Sacramento, California, United States

Elizabeth C. Fung, BS, MSPH
Medical Student, School of Medicine,
    University of California Davis, Sacramento,
    California, United States

Tyler Gouvea, DO
Physician, Anesthesiology, Mercy General
    Hospital, Sacramento, California,
    United States

Anne Grzegorczyk, MD
Fellow, Division of Pulmonary, Critical
    Care and Sleep Medicine,
    University of Southern California,
    Los Angeles, California, United States

Thomas Leland Hughes, MD, PharmD
Associate Clinical Professor, Anesthesiology
    and Pain Medicine, University of
    California Davis, Sacramento, California,
    United States

Stefano Azelio Iantorno, MD, PhD
Resident Physician, Department of Internal
    Medicine, University of Southern
    California, Los Angeles, California,
    United States

Ryan Jones, MD
Department of Anesthesiology and Pain
    Medicine, University of California Davis,
    Sacramento, California, United States

Michael J. Jung, MD, MBA
Assistant Clinical Professor, Department of
    Anesthesiology and Pain Medicine,
    UC Davis Medical Center, Sacramento,
    California, United States

Bahar Kasimi, MD
Resident, Anesthesiology, UC Davis Medical
    Center, Sacramento, California,
    United States

Justine Ko, MD, MPH
Resident Physician, Department of Internal
    Medicine, University of Southern
    California, Los Angeles, California,
    United States

Harsha Koneru, MD
Resident, Department of Anesthesiology and
    Pain Medicine, University of California
    Davis, Sacramento, California,
    United States

Moses Koo, MD
Resident Physician, Department of
    Internal Medicine,
    University of Southern California,
    Los Angeles, California, United States

R. Michelle Koolaee, DO
Assistant Professor of Medicine, Division
    of Rheumatology, University of Southern
    California, Los Angeles, California,
    United States
Presbyterian Intercommunity Health Medical
    Group, Attending Rheumatologist,
    Whittier, California, United States

Robert Scott Kriss, DO
Associate Clinical Professor, Department
    of Anesthesiology and Pain Medicine,
    University of California, Davis Children's
    Hospital, Sacramento, California,
    United States

Gene Kurosawa, MD
Assistant Professor, Department of
    Anesthesiology, Loma Linda University
    Health, Loma Linda, California,
    United States

Quintin Kuse, BS
Medical Student, Anesthesiology,
    UC Davis, Sacramento, California,
    United States

Sean X. T. Lam, MD
Resident, Department of Anesthesiology and
    Pain Medicine, University of California,
    Davis, Sacramento, California,
    United States

David Li, MD, BA
Assistant Professor, Anesthesiology and Pain
Medicine, UC Davis Medical Center,
Sacramento, California, United States

Nathan Lim, MD
Fellow Physician, Division of Rheumatology,
University of Southern California,
Los Angeles, California, United States

Deanna Lo, MD
Clinical Assistant Professor, Medicine,
LAC+USC Medical Center, Los Angeles,
California, United States

Curtis Y. Maehara, MD
Resident Physician, Department of Internal
Medicine, University of Southern
California, Los Angeles, California,
United States

Shane P. McGuire, DO
Resident Physician, Anesthesiology and Pain
Management, University of California,
Davis, Sacramento, California,
United States

Michelle Elyse Meshman, MD
Volunteer Clinical Faculty, Department of
Psychiatry and Behavioral Sciences,
University of California, Davis,
Sacramento, California, United States

Benjamin Morey, MD
Anesthesiologist, Anesthesiology, St Cloud
Hospital, St Cloud, Minnesota,
United States

Mark R. Murphy, DO
Fellow Physician, Department of
Anesthesiology and Pain Medicine-
Pediatric Anesthesiology, University
of California Davis School of
Medicine, Sacramento, California,
United States

Lee Huynh Nguyen, MD
Resident Physician, Department of
Anesthesiology, Perioperative and
Pain Medicine, Stanford University
Medical Center, Stanford, California,
United States

Ashil Panchal, MD
Hospital Medicine Physician, Department of
Internal Medicine, LAC+USC Medical
Center, Los Angeles, California,
United States

Mike Priem, MD
Anesthesiologist, Department of
Anesthesiology and Pain Medicine,
University of California Davis, Sacramento,
California, United States

Rastko Rakocevic, MD, MSc
Fellow Physician, Division of Pulmonary,
Critical Care and Sleep Medicine,
University of Southern California,
Los Angeles, California, United States

Niroop R. Ravula, MBBS, FRCA
Associate Clinical Professor, Anesthesiology
and Pain Medicine, University of
California Davis, Sacramento, California,
United States

Nancy Suliman Saied, MD
Anesthesia Resident, Department of
Anesthesia and Pain Medicine, University
of California, Davis, Sacramento,
California, United States

Michelle Schiltz, CRNA
Department of Anesthesiology and Pain
Medicine, University of California Davis,
Sacramento, California, United States

Stuart Schroff, MD
Assistant Professor, Department of Radiology,
University of Southern California,
Los Angeles, California, United States

Alice Seol, MD
Resident Physician, Department of
Anesthesiology and Acute Pain Medicine,
The University of California, Davis,
Sacramento, California, United States
Fellow Physician, Department of
Anesthesiology, Stanford, Stanford,
California, United States

Abigail Susan Smith, MD, TS-C
Resident Physician, Department of
Anesthesiology, University of California
Davis, Sacramento, California,
United States

Justin Wayne Tiulim, MD
Fellow Physician, Division of Hematology
and Oncology, University of Southern
California, Los Angeles, California,
United States

Jeff Tully, MD
Associate Physician, Department of
Anesthesiology, UC San Diego Health,
La Jolla, California, United States

Ara Vartanyan, MD
Resident Physician, Department of
Internal Medicine, University of
Southern California, Los Angeles,
United States

Nicole Shirakawa Wei, MD
Assistant Professor, Department of
Anesthesiology and Pain Medicine,
University of California Davis, Sacramento,
California, United States

Aaron M. Yim, MD
Resident Physician, Department of
Anesthesiology, Los Angeles County
and University of Southern California
Medical Center, Los Angeles,
California, United States

Liye Billy Zhang, MD
Anesthesiologist, Anesthesiology, University
of California Davis, Sacramento,
California, United States

I am humbled and honored to have been asked by the editors of this valuable publication to present the foreword. Dr. Paul Frank is one of the best anesthesiologists of his generation. He was our chief resident, our fellow, my personal anesthesiologist. There is no greater endorsement.

For generations, physicians in training have benefitted from the experience of others by review of challenging cases. Case presentations are one of the cornerstones of clinical training in medicine. This treatise honors that tradition in the best possible way. Presentations are laid out in a formal, organized manner. The presentations are similar in format to cases which are presented for the American Board of Anesthesiology oral examination as well the Medically Challenging Cases at the American Society of Anesthesiologists Annual Meeting. Learning to organize the thought process in this manner is an essential skill for those who aspire to train and practice Anesthesiology.

Now in the twilight of a career which has spanned parts of five decades, I have been fortunate to be the beneficiary of numerous sentinel innovations (development of ET CO_2 monitoring, pulse oximetry, and revolutionary airway devices) in anesthesiology which have made patient care safer, with better outcomes and higher expectations. To you, the successors of my profession, I hope you will find this work valuable in the development of your own journey in anesthesiology, a specialty which has given my professional life so much meaning. Dare to advocate for and advance this great medical specialty!

Yours truly,

Robert T. Naruse, MD, FAS

It is with great pleasure that we present to you our seventh book in the Morning Report: Beyond the Pearls series, *Anesthesiology and Critical Care Morning Report: Beyond the Pearls*. Writing the "perfect" case-based review text has been a dream of mine ever since I was a first-year medical student. Dr. Koolaee and I envisioned a text that integrates a United States Medical Licensing Examination (USMLE) Steps 1, 2, and 3 focus with up-to-date, evidence-based clinical medicine. We wanted the platform of the text to be drawn from a traditional theme that many of us are familiar with from residency, the "morning report" format. This book is written for a wide audience, from medical students to attending physicians practicing Anesthesiology and Critical Care Medicine. The cases have been carefully chosen, and each case was written and reviewed by Anesthesiologist or Pulmonary and Critical Care specialist. The cases in the book cover scenarios and questions frequently encountered on the USMLE, shelf exams, wards, and board exams, integrating both basic science and clinical pearls.

We sincerely thank the many contributors who have helped to create this text. Their insightful work will be a valuable tool for medical students and physicians to gain an in-depth understanding of Anesthesiology and Critical Care Medicine. It should be noted that while a variety of clinical cases in Anesthesiology and Critical Care were selected for this book, it is not meant to substitute a comprehensive reference.

Dr. Koolaee and I would like to thank our volume editors Dr. Paul Frank and Dr. Patrick Chan for all their hard work and dedication to this book. It was truly a pleasure to work with everyone associated with the book, and we look forward to our next project together.

CONTENTS

VIDEO CONTENTS

Preoperative Evaluation

The foundation of an anesthetic plan begins with a preoperative evaluation. In some centers, a preoperative evaluation begins in the preanesthesia clinic days or weeks before surgery. In other centers, the preoperative evaluation occurs entirely in the preoperative area just prior to surgery. The goal of the preoperative evaluation is to enhance patient safety by ensuring that the patient can tolerate the planned procedure and anesthetic and to minimize the risk posed by the patient's comorbidities.

The evaluation should start with an understanding of the planned procedure and indication for the procedure. Especially in complex patients, understanding the procedure helps the anesthesiologist weigh the operative and anesthetic risks against the patient's condition and expected outcome. For example, a patient with heart failure and kidney disease may not tolerate a long operation with a large volume of expected blood loss.

HISTORY

The anesthesiologist should inquire about the patient's medical conditions. For each medical problem, the onset, frequency and character of symptoms, and treatment should be elucidated. Depending on the diagnosis, other information may be relevant. For example, if a patient has asthma, when were they first diagnosed? How often do they have attacks? Have they ever been hospitalized or intubated? Are they taking oral steroids or inhaled medications? Have they had pulmonary function tests? All of this information tells the anesthesiologist what to expect intraoperatively and ultimately deliver safer care.

Past surgical history is also critically important. The type and location of the prior surgical procedure may directly affect anesthetic management. For instance, a patient who has undergone a cervical spine fusion may have reduced neck mobility, which may increase the difficulty of laryngoscopy and intubation. A patient who has had a tracheostomy may have a narrow trachea. The prior surgical procedure may also give important clues about the patient's past medical history that the patient overlooked. Did the patient have a coronary artery bypass graft (CABG)? They probably have coronary artery disease even if they didn't mention it.

Discussion of the patient's surgical history is an ideal time to discuss anesthetic history. Has the patient had anesthesia before? Were they told of any complications? Maybe a prior anesthesiologist told them they have a small airway or developed an "anesthetic fever." These clues should prompt the anesthesiologist to ask follow-up questions regarding a history of difficult airway or malignant hyperthermia.

The anesthesiologist should obtain a complete list of the medications that the patient is taking and when they last took each medication. A complete medication list will include the dose and frequency of both prescription and over-the-counter drugs. Some drugs require particular attention. For example, anticoagulants (e.g., warfarin) and antiplatelet agents (e.g., clopidogrel) should prompt a discussion of the indication for the medication. A plan should also be developed between the anesthesiologist, surgeon, patient, and prescribing physician regarding the perioperative management of these agents.

A social history will cover at least the frequency and duration of smoking, alcohol consumption, and recreational drug use. Smoking history is usually expressed as pack-years, calculated by

$$(\text{packs per day}) \times (\text{number of years the patient has smoked})$$

For example, a patient who has smoked 2 packs of cigarettes per day for the last 10 years is a 20-pack-year smoker. It is also important to know when the patient last smoked and advise them to stop smoking prior to surgery. Alcohol consumption is measured in drinks per week, but it is important to note that this refers to a "standard drink":

- 12 fluid ounces of beer
- 5 fluid ounces of wine
- 1.5 fluid ounces of distilled spirits (e.g., vodka, whiskey)

Recreational drugs include any drug that is not prescribed to the patient by a doctor and used in the way prescribed. This entails both street drugs (e.g., heroin) as well as prescription drugs that may have been prescribed to a relative or prescribed to the patient but are used in greater quantity or frequency than prescribed. It is important to ask how much they use and how frequently they use these drugs.

Alcohol abuse and recreational drug use can significantly elevate perioperative risks. Frequent alcohol use that abruptly stops when the patient is admitted to the hospital predisposes the patient to hallucinations and seizures, known as delirium tremens. Frequent methamphetamine use can cause myocardial injury and arrhythmia. In patients who chronically abuse heroin or other opiates, postoperative pain control can prove challenging, as the patient has developed a tolerance and may require higher than expected doses of opioids. If a patient is actively intoxicated on the day of surgery, postponing the elective operation should be strongly considered.

Another important element of the preoperative evaluation is the patient's functional capacity or exercise tolerance. Patients are generally asked how far they can walk on level ground or how many flights of stairs they can climb. Exercise tolerance is expressed as metabolic equivalents (METs). One metabolic equivalent is equivalent to oxygen consumption of 3.5 cc/kg/min. This represents oxygen consumption at rest. More strenuous activity is assigned a higher number of METs. For example, raking leaves is considered 4 METs, and cross-country skiing is considered 11 METs. Adequate exercise tolerance is generally considered to be 4 METs. It should be noted, however, that patients' subjective assessment of their own exercise tolerance is poorly correlated with their ability to achieve 4 METs on formal exercise testing.

Whenever possible, review prior anesthetic records. The anesthetic record will contain valuable information like an airway note—was the patient intubated easily?—as well as what drugs were used. Perhaps the patient reports a history of postoperative nausea after a prior anesthetic. A review of the record of that anesthetic may help identify the culprit agent. The anesthetic record will also help the anesthesiologist determine whether the patient has tolerated a particular type of anesthesia, such as sedation without an airway, in the past.

PHYSICAL EXAM

A focused physical examination provides practical and objective data that will affect the anesthetic plan. Vital signs, including heart rate, blood pressure, respiratory rate, oxygen saturation, and temperature, provide a snapshot of the patient's baseline physiologic state. Is the patient tachycardic? Hypotensive? Febrile? For an elective case, the answers to these questions may result in postponement. For an urgent case, the answers to these questions may result in an urgent case becoming an emergent case.

Body size measurements—height, total body weight (TBW, the number read off the scale), ideal body weight (IBW, calculated based on height and gender), and body mass index (BMI, weight in kg divided by the square of height in meters)—are crucial for anesthetic planning. Most drugs are dosed based on the patient's body weight. Some are dosed on IBW and some on TBW. For those who require single-lung ventilation (see Case 21), patient height determines double-lumen endotracheal tube size.

TABLE 1 ■ Obesity Classification Based on Body Mass Index

Body Mass Index (BMI) (kg/m²)	Range
<18.5	Underweight
18.5–25	Normal
25–30	Overweight
30–35	Obese (class 1)
35–40	Obese (class 2)
BMI > 40	Obese (class 3)

BMI helps determine whether the patient's weight is appropriate for their height, or whether the patient may be under- or overweight. For example, say two patients each weigh 85 kg (187 lb). One patient is 2 m (6 feet, 6 inches) tall, and the another patient is 1.5 m (5 feet) tall. The BMI of the first patient is 21.3 kg/m², whereas the BMI of the second patient is 38 kg/m². The first patient is of normal body habitus, and the second patient is obese. Obesity has implications for all aspects of the anesthetic plan, including drug dosing, airway management, ventilation strategy, and postoperative pain control (see Case 14). Table 1 shows the criteria for obesity based on BMI.

The preoperative airway exam allows the anesthesiologist to identify patient anatomical factors that may contribute to difficult bag mask ventilation and/or difficult laryngoscopy. Factors that contribute to difficult bag mask ventilation include the following:

- thick facial hair
- edentulous (no teeth)
- large tongue
- excess soft tissue of face and neck (as in obesity).

Factors that contribute to difficult laryngoscopy include the following:

- long upper incisors
- prominent overbite (upper incisors very anterior relative to lower incisors)
- inability to protrude mandible enough to bite upper lip with lower teeth
- less than 3 cm between upper and lower incisors (small mouth opening)
- inability to visualize uvula with mouth open and tongue protruded (Mallampati 3 or 4)
- high or narrow palate
- thyromental distance less than 3 cm (distance from chin to thyroid cartilage)
- short, thick neck
- limited range of motion on neck flexion and extension (inability to look up or down, common in patients who have had cervical spine fusion)
- evidence of radiation or prior surgery (including tracheostomy).

One common way to describe airways is the Mallampati classification. To determine the patient's Mallampati classification, ask the patient to open his or her mouth and protrude his or her tongue. The classification is based on how much of the uvula is visible. Fig. 1 and Table 2 show the criteria for Mallampati classification.

Based on the findings of the preoperative airway examination, it may be necessary to have specialized airway equipment or extra personnel in the room for induction and intubation. The anesthesiologist may also determine that the patient requires awake intubation.

A cardiopulmonary examination is a customary part of the preoperative evaluation. Auscultation of the heart may reveal arrhythmias or murmurs that require additional workup prior to surgery. For example, a harsh systolic murmur at the right upper sternal border may indicate aortic stenosis. This patient should undergo echocardiogram, and if the findings are severe enough, it may be

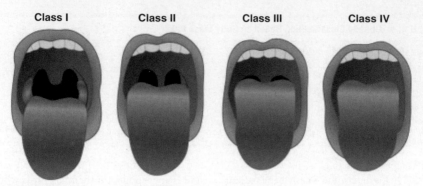

Fig. 1 Mallampati classification. The patient is asked to open his or her mouth and protrude his or her tongue, without saying "ahh," for this assessment. (Reproduced from Wijeysundera, D. N., & Finlayson, E. [2020]. Preoperative evaluation. In M. A. Gropper, R. D. Miller, N. H. Cohen, L. I. Eriksson, L. A. Fleisher, K. Leslie, et al. (Eds.), *Miller's Anesthesia* [Vol. 31, 9th Ed., pp. 918–998.e12]. Philadelphia, PA: Elsevier. Fig. 31.3.)

TABLE 2 ■ **Mallampati Classification Criteria**

Class	View
Class I	Entire uvula visible
Class II	Soft palate, fauces, and only part of the uvula visible
Class III	Soft palate and only the base of the uvula visible
Class IV	Only hard palate visible, none of the uvula visible

necessary to replace the valve prior to surgery. Of course, in urgent or emergent operations, it is not feasible to delay for additional workup. In this case, additional monitoring or subspecialized personnel may be required to provide a safe anesthetic. Auscultation of the lungs may reveal crackles or wheezes, which may suggest respiratory pathology, such as pulmonary edema or reactive airway disease. It may be necessary to request additional workup for any unanticipated and unexplained findings on physical examination.

Based on the information gathered in the preoperative interview and examination, as well as a review of the patient's chart, the anesthesiologist will assign the patient a classification with the American Society of Anesthesiology (ASA) physical status schema. This is a rough estimation of the patient's overall state of health. Table 3 shows the criteria for each ASA classification.

Airway Management

One of the primary responsibilities of the anesthesiologist is to maintain adequate oxygenation and ventilation. Depending on the procedure and type of anesthetic, this will require varying amounts of intervention.

Anesthesia care almost always entails some amount of sedation. One of the well-described effects of sedation is respiratory depression. The profundity of respiratory depression depends on the depth of sedation. Some procedures, such as colonoscopy, can be performed with relatively light sedation. Patients usually breathe spontaneously during this type of procedure. Other procedures, such as a bowel resection, require general anesthesia with endotracheal intubation and mechanical ventilation. Regardless of the depth of anesthesia, airway management means ensuring adequate ventilation and oxygenation.

TABLE 3 ■ Criteria for Each American Society of Anesthesiology Classification Based on the Patient's Overall State of Health

American Society of Anesthesiology (ASA) Physical Status	Definition	Example
ASA I	Healthy patient with no medical problems who does not smoke	• No past medical history • Does not smoke • Drinks little or no alcohol
ASA II	Patient with mild systemic disease without functional limitation	• Well-controlled diabetes or hypertension • Current daily smoker
ASA III	Patient with significant systemic disease causing functional limitation	• Poorly controlled diabetes or hypertension • Morbid obesity • Permanent pacemaker • End-stage renal disease on dialysis • History of coronary artery disease • History of heart attack or stroke more than 3 months ago
ASA IV	Patient with severe systemic disease that is a constant threat to life	• Heart attack or stroke within the last 3 months • Severe cardiac valve dysfunction • Severely reduced left ventricular ejection fraction • Septic shock
ASA V	Patient moribund (on the verge of death); not expected to survive without the operation	• Ruptured aortic aneurysm • Massive trauma • Intracranial bleed with mass effect
ASA VI	Brain dead patient donating organs	• Already declared brain dead

In cases where only sedation is necessary, the patient will receive a hypnotic agent that will depress consciousness. Apnea in these cases may be central (e.g., from excessive sedation) or obstructive (e.g., from the tongue falling back and blocking the oropharynx). The anesthesiologist must be prepared to handle both eventualities. In the case of central apnea, it may be necessary to reduce the dose of anesthetic drug and/or ventilate the patient with positive pressure via ventilator mask until the resumption of adequate spontaneous ventilation. Fig. 2 shows proper positioning of the anesthesiologist's hand and mask over the patient's face for positive pressure ventilation. It is important to avoid compressing the submental soft tissue with the fingers of the left hand, as this can create or worsen upper airway obstruction.

Upper airway obstruction is a common cause of apnea in patients receiving sedation. Patients who are overweight or obese are at increased risk of obstruction, as are patients with obstructive sleep apnea (OSA), large tongues, and excess soft tissue of the face and neck. If the obstruction is transient, a simple chin tilt or jaw thrust may suffice. Try placing a pillow or blanket under the patient's shoulders to extend his or her neck and relieve the airway obstruction. If the obstruction persists, an oropharyngeal airway, also called an oral airway, will help alleviate obstruction. An oropharyngeal airway stents open the airway by relieving the obstruction caused by the base of the tongue against the posterior wall of the oropharynx. A nasopharyngeal airway, also known as

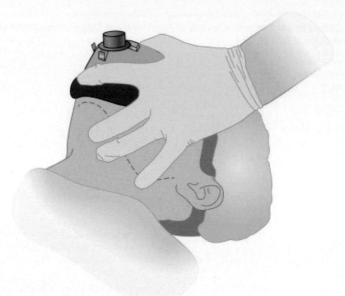

Fig. 2   One-handed mask ventilation. The thumb and index finger of the left hand should form the shape of a "C" around the mask. The third and fourth fingers of the left hand should be on the patient's mandible—and not on the submental soft tissue. The fifth finger of the left hand should be around the ramus of the mandible and elevating the jaw toward the mask to relieve obstruction. The right hand should be squeezing the Ambu bag (or ventilator bag). (Reproduced from Miller Fig. 44.12.)

a nasal trumpet, stents open the airway in a manner like that of an oropharyngeal airway, but the nasopharyngeal airway is placed through the nostril. Nasopharyngeal airway placement carries a risk of nosebleed. Many adults take antiplatelet or anticoagulant medications, and nasopharyngeal airway placement in these patients is not recommended.

The laryngeal mask airway (LMA) is an airway device that can help relieve airway obstruction, support spontaneous or assisted ventilation, and facilitate administration of inhaled anesthetic gas. Other advantages of LMA placement include relative ease of placement and less invasiveness compared to endotracheal intubation. Additionally, muscle relaxant is not required for LMA placement.

The LMA is inserted through the mouth and rests in the pharynx, overlying the larynx. There are many strategies for placement of an LMA. Whichever placement method is used, it is important to ensure an adequate seal in the pharynx. The LMA allows free communication between the larynx and the esophagus. *Therefore, there is a risk of gastric aspiration.* There is also a risk of gastric insufflation with positive pressure ventilation. For this reason, positive pressure should be kept as low as possible. Additionally, the LMA is large relative to the size of the mouth and pharynx, and upper airway trauma may occur with multiple placement attempts. Finally, there is a risk of dislodgement of the LMA, resulting in poor ventilation and airway obstruction.

An endotracheal tube with the cuff inflated below the vocal cords is a definitive airway. It protects the lungs from gastric aspiration, allows for positive pressure ventilation, facilitates administration of inhaled anesthetic gas, and is relatively unlikely to become dislodged. Endotracheal tubes are most commonly placed through the mouth and into the trachea, although they can also be placed through the nose if orotracheal intubation is not possible.

Prior to endotracheal intubation, all necessary supplies should be gathered and arranged in a way that is easily accessible. Necessary supplies include the following:

- patient monitor (at least pulse oximeter, 3-lead electrocardiogram, and blood pressure cuff)
- endotracheal tube with stylet
- 10 mL syringe
- laryngoscope handle and blade
- suction catheter
- oxygen source
- Ambu bag and ventilator mask
- tape (or other way to secure the tube after placement)
- carbon dioxide (CO_2) detector, known as capnogram (either free standing or within the ventilator)
- induction drugs, muscle relaxant
- emergency medications
- other specialized equipment if necessary, based on airway examination and prior intubation records.

Once all supplies have been gathered, attach the patient to the monitor. This should include at least pulse oximetry, noninvasive blood pressure, and cardiac rhythm strip. Stand at the head of the bed. Ensure working intravenous (IV) access. If the patient is on a hospital bed (as opposed to an operating room table), remove the headboard to allow easier access to the patient. Reposition the patient so that his or her head is close to the head of the bed. Adjust the bed height so that the patient's head is at the level of anesthesiologist's upper abdomen.

The steps for endotracheal intubation vary depending on whether the intubation is elective or emergent. Elective intubations generally occur in the operating room before a planned operation. For elective intubations, a minimum duration of time should have passed since the patient's last oral intake. These minimum guidelines are established to increase the likelihood that the patient's stomach is empty, thereby reducing the risk of gastric aspiration. This minimum duration of time since last oral intake, known as *nil per os* (NPO, *nothing per mouth* in Latin) guidelines, are:

- 2 hours since last clear liquids (e.g., black coffee without cream, apple juice)
- 4 hours since last breast milk
- 6 hours since last light meal (e.g., toast)
- 8 hours since last heavy meal (e.g., hamburger)

Certain patients are never considered to meet NPO guidelines because of their physiology or disease state. These patients do not meet criteria for elective intubation regardless of how much time has passed since their last oral intake. These patients include the following:

- obstetric patients beyond 12 weeks' gestation
- patients with bowel obstruction or acute intraabdominal inflammation
- patients with gastric motility disorder or severe gastroesophageal reflux disease (GERD)
- trauma and other patients whose last oral intake time is unknown
- patients actively nauseated or vomiting

Most patients presenting for elective surgery are candidates for elective intubation and have abstained from oral intake for the appropriate amount of time. For an elective intubation, the steps are as follows:

1. Turn on the oxygen supply and place the ventilator mask over the patient's mouth and nose. Ask the patient to breathe normally. As the patient breathes oxygen from the mask, the air (only 21% oxygen) in the patient's lungs is replaced with pure oxygen (100% oxygen). Continue preoxygenating for 3 minutes, or until the end-expiratory oxygen concentration is at least 80%.

2. Administer the induction agent. This is frequently a hypnotic drug such as propofol. The patient will become apneic, and his or her eyes will close. You may consider taping the

patient's eyes closed; however, some anesthesiologists prefer to wait to tape the eyes closed until after the endotracheal tube is secured in place.

3. Squeeze the Ambu bag to ensure that you can mask-ventilate the patient. Look for chest rise, fogging of the ventilator mask, and the presence of CO_2 detected on capnogram. If these signs are present, you are successfully ventilating the patient. If you cannot ventilatcve the patient, consider placing an oral airway, repositioning your mask on the patient's face, or repositioning the patient. If you still cannot ventilate the patient, call for help. The classic teaching here is that if you cannot ventilate the patient, do not give muscle relaxant. However, muscle relaxants generally make mask ventilation easier.

4. Administer the muscle relaxant and continue mask ventilating the patient. Depending on which muscle relaxant was administered, the dose of muscle relaxant administered, and other patient factors, you may need to continue mask ventilating the patient for 45 seconds to 3 minutes until the patient is fully relaxed.

5. Stop squeezing the Ambu bag and remove the mask from the patient's face. Extend the patient's neck and open their jaw using the thumb and middle finger on your right hand.

6. With the laryngoscope in your left hand, carefully insert the laryngoscope blade on the right side of the patient's mouth and sweep the tongue to the left. Most of the force here is directed toward the patient's feet, with a small amount of force in the upward direction. *Be careful not to "lever" the laryngoscope blade against the patient's upper lip or teeth.* The vocal cords should be visible.

7. Maintain your view of the vocal cords with the laryngoscope in your left hand. With your right hand, place the endotracheal tube at the level of the vocal cords. Ask an assistant to remove the stylet from the tube. Advance the tube until the cuff disappears past the vocal cords.

8. Inflate the cuff. Attach the breathing circuit to the tube and ventilate. Look for CO_2 on capnogram.

9. Auscultate the lungs to ensure breath sounds are present bilaterally. If breath sounds can only be heard on one side, the tube may be too deep and may be in the main bronchus of one side. In this case, the tube should be withdrawn slightly until bilateral breath sounds are appreciated. If breath sounds are not heard on either side, the tube may be in the esophagus. In this case, remove the tube and attempt intubation again.

10. Attach the endotracheal tube to the ventilator circuit.

In the emergent setting, or in any setting where the patient does not meet minimum NPO criteria, the above steps are accelerated. This accelerated pattern is called a rapid sequence intubation (RSI). The goal of a rapid sequence intubation is to prevent gastric aspiration. The steps in RSI are as follows:

1. If the patient is breathing on his or her own, turn on the oxygen supply and place the ventilator mask over the patient's mouth and nose. If not, proceed to induction.

2. Consider asking an assistant to use their thumb and index finger to apply posteriorly directed pressure to the patient's cricoid ring. This is called cricoid pressure, and it may help reduce the risk of passive gastric aspiration (see Case 13).

3. Administer the induction agent followed immediately by the muscle relaxant.

4. Do not mask-ventilate the patient. Wait for the muscle relaxant to take effect. Based on common dosing of muscle relaxant in RSI settings, this will take 45–90 seconds.

5. Perform laryngoscopy as mentioned above, and insert the endotracheal tube.

6. Once the cuff is inflated beyond the vocal cords and CO_2 has been confirmed on capnogram, your assistant may release cricoid pressure if they have been applying it.

7. Listen for breath sounds as mentioned above.

8. Attach the endotracheal tube to the ventilator circuit.

Anesthetic Gases

Maintenance of anesthesia, particularly with an endotracheal tube or LMA in place, is frequently accomplished with inhaled anesthetic gases, also known as volatile anesthetics. Anesthetic gases are primarily halogenated ethers (e.g., sevoflurane, desflurane) or inorganic compounds (e.g., nitrous oxide [N_2O]). The mechanism of these molecules is complex and incompletely understood. They exert their effects in the central nervous system (CNS), including the brain and the spinal cord. Possible mechanisms include potentiation of inhibitory gaba-aminobutyric acid type A ($GABA_A$) receptors and glycine receptors, inhibition of excitatory nicotinic acetylcholine and glutamate receptors, as well as interactions with many other receptors.

As the name implies, inhaled anesthetic gases enter the body via inhalation. An understanding of the pharmacology of inhaled anesthetic gases requires an understanding of the underlying physics of these compounds, as well as some relevant vocabulary.

- Partial pressure: This is the amount of pressure of a mixture of gases attributable to one particular gas. According to Dalton's law, the partial pressure of each gas in a mixture of gases is proportional to the fraction of molecules of mixture represented by one particular compound. For example, consider a closed container at a pressure of 500 mm Hg with a total of 1000 molecules of gas: 750 molecules of nitrogen, and 250 molecules of oxygen. The concentration of nitrogen is

$$\frac{750 \; molecules \; nitrogen}{1000 \; molecules \; total} = 0.75 = 75\%$$

and the concentration of oxygen is

$$\frac{250 \; molecules \; oxygen}{1000 \; molecules \; total} = 0.25 = 25\%$$

The partial pressure of nitrogen is

$$500 \; mm \; Hg \times 0.75 = 375 \; mm \; Hg$$

and the partial pressure of nitrogen is

$$500 \; mm \; Hg \times 0.25 = 125 \; mm \; Hg$$

Notice that the sum of the partial pressures of the two gases in the mixture is equal to the total pressure in the container.

- Minimum alveolar concentration (MAC): Half of patients with at least this concentration (known as 1 MAC) of inhaled anesthesia gas in their alveolar air spaces would not move in response to a painful stimulus, such as a surgical incision. This is a measure of potency of a gas and is expressed as a percentage of ambient pressure. It should be noted, however, that this percentage assumes that the patient is at sea level, where atmospheric pressure is 760 mm Hg. *The measurement of the dose of anesthetic gas that correlates with its effect is partial pressure, not percentage of ambient pressure.* For example, the MAC of sevoflurane is 2.2%. To calculate the corresponding partial pressure, multiply this pressure by the MAC of sevoflurane expressed as a decimal

$$760 \; mm \; Hg \times 0.022 = 16.7 \; mm \; Hg$$

In other words, the partial pressure of sevoflurane necessary to achieve 1 MAC is 16.7 mm Hg. This partial pressure does not change with ambient pressure, although the MAC expressed as a concentration does change with ambient pressure. For example, in Denver, CO, where ambient pressure is 615 mm Hg, the concentration of sevoflurane necessary to achieve 1 MAC in Denver, CO is

$$16.7 \text{ mm Hg} / 615 \text{ mm Hg} = 0.027 = 2.7\%$$

Notice that while the concentration of anesthetic gas corresponding to 1 MAC has changed in Denver, the partial pressure has not. Remember, the CNS responds to the alveolar *partial pressure* of inhaled anesthetic gas, not the alveolar *concentration* of anesthetic gas.

- Vapor pressure: Volatile liquids, such as inhaled anesthetic gases, tend to vaporize, whereby molecules at the surface of the liquid enter the gaseous phase. The partial pressure of vapor from the volatile liquid is known as the vapor pressure. Vapor pressure is an intrinsic property of a compound and *is therefore unique to each compound*. Vapor pressure increases with temperature but is not affected by ambient pressure.
- Blood:gas partition coefficient: This is a measurement of the relative solubility of an inhaled anesthetic gas in blood versus gas. Essentially, in a closed container containing blood, air, and some amount of anesthetic gas, this represents how much of the gas dissolves in the blood and how much remains in the gaseous phase. As discussed above, alveolar partial pressure of an anesthetic gas is effectively the dose of anesthetic gas. When a patient inhales anesthetic gas, some of that gas remains in the alveoli, where it contributes to alveolar partial pressure of the gas, while the rest of the gas dissolves in the blood, where it does not contribute to alveolar partial pressure of the gas. The goal of anesthesia is to put CNS cells to sleep, not red blood cells. In establishing anesthesia with inhaled anesthetic gas starting with an alveolar partial pressure of zero, as in an inhaled induction, inhaled anesthetic gases that have higher blood:gas partition coefficient diffuse across respiratory epithelium and dissolve in blood more than they remain in the alveoli. Therefore, it will take longer to achieve 1 MAC of anesthetic gas using an agent with a higher blood:gas partition coefficient. At the end of anesthesia, agents with a higher blood:gas partition coefficient will diffuse out of the blood and into the alveoli more slowly. This will maintain a higher alveolar partial pressure of gas for a longer period of time, resulting in a slower emergence from anesthesia than if an agent with a lower blood:gas partition coefficient had been used.

Inhaled anesthetic gas is delivered via the breathing circuit of the anesthesia machine. The most common type of breathing circuit used with anesthesia machines is called a circle system. A circle system contains the following components:

- Fresh gas inlet: This allows flow of air, oxygen, and/or nitrous oxide from pipeline supply or storage cylinders into the breathing circuit. Most anesthetic vaporizers also attach upstream of the fresh gas inlet.
- One-way valves: This is an inspiratory valve proximal to the patient, and an expiratory valve distal to the patient. These valves prevent backward flow of gas in the circuit.
- Corrugated tubing: This includes one inspiratory limb, and one expiratory limb.
- Y connector: This connects inspiratory and expiratory corrugated tubing to the patient (via endotracheal tube, LMA, or ventilator mask). Dead space calculation begins at the Y connector.
- Pop-off valve: This is also called an adjustable pressure-limiting (APL) valve. It allows for release of excess pressure within the circuit when the patient is being manually ventilated.
- Reservoir bag: This allows for manual ventilation of the patient and assessment of lung compliance (accomplished by squeezing the bag).
- CO_2 absorbent: These are chemicals, usually constituted as small beads, that react with CO_2 and remove it from the breathing circuit before the gas in the circuit returns to the

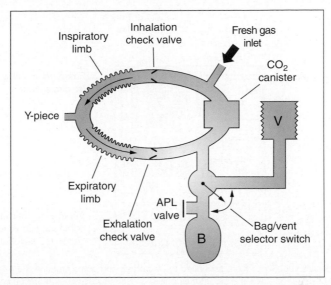

Fig. 3 Circle system. The reservoir bag is squeezed by the anesthesiologist during manual ventilation, or air is moved by the ventilator bellows during mechanical ventilation, and gas flows through the CO_2 absorber, fresh gas is added, and the gas mixture flows through the inspiratory valve, through the inspiratory corrugated tubing, past the Y connector, and into the patient's lungs (via endotracheal tube, LMA, or ventilator mask). Exhaled gas flows from the patient's lungs to the expiratory corrugated tubing and through the expiratory check valve. (Roth P. [2018]. *Anesthesia delivery systems*. In M. C. Pardo, & R. D. Miller [Eds.], Basics of anesthesia. [7th ed., pp. 220–238]. Philadelphia, PA: Elsevier. Fig 15.9.)

inspiratory limb. Ideally, these compounds do not react with anesthetic gas. There are many brands of absorbent with varying reagents, but most involve calcium hydroxide, $Ca(OH)_2$, as well as other compounds containing the hydroxide (OH^-) moiety.

Fig. 3 shows a circle system with the basic components labeled.

The final major component of inhaled anesthetic delivery systems is the vaporizer, which outputs an adjustable concentration of inhaled anesthetic gas. One common type of vaporizer is the variable bypass vaporizer. There are two pathways for fresh gas flow through the vaporizer, one of which leads to a chamber that contains liquid anesthetic gas (known as the vaporizing chamber), and the other does not. By the laws of physics, the chamber containing liquid anesthetic gas also contains vaporized anesthetic gas. Remember, any liquid has some vapor pressure based on molecules at the surface entering the gaseous phase. Depending on the desired concentration of anesthetic gas input by the anesthesiologist, a variable amount of fresh gas will be directed through the chamber containing liquid and vaporized anesthetic gas, and the rest of the fresh gas will bypass the vaporizing chamber, hence the name variable bypass vaporizer. The fresh gas directed through the chamber containing anesthetic gas will take up the vaporized anesthetic gas and rejoin the fresh gas that bypassed the chamber containing anesthetic gas. This mixture is then delivered to the patient. Fig. 4 shows the basic functional structure of the variable bypass vaporizer.

Variable bypass vaporizers are named as such because, as the anesthesiologist adjusts the concentration control dial, a variable amount of fresh gas will bypass the vaporizing chamber. With a higher dialed concentration of anesthetic gas, less fresh gas will bypass the vaporizing chamber. Because vapor pressure is a property unique to each liquid, including each inhaled anesthetic gas, each vaporizer is *specific to one anesthetic agent*. So a variable bypass vaporizer designed for sevoflurane should not be filled with isoflurane or halothane, for example. It should also be noted that,

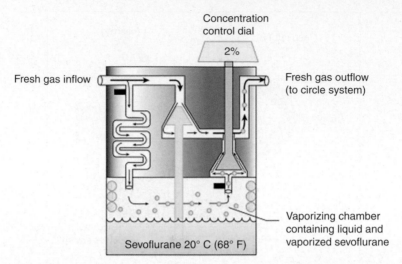

Concentration control dial

2%

Fresh gas inflow

Fresh gas outflow
(to circle system)

Vaporizing chamber
containing liquid and
vaporized sevoflurane

Sevoflurane 20° C (68° F)

Fig. 4 Variable bypass vaporizer. Fresh gas enters the vaporizer, and some amount of the fresh gas flow is directed into the chamber containing liquid and vaporized anesthetic gas, where it becomes saturated with anesthetic gas vapor before rejoining the fresh gas flow that did not flow through the vaporizing chamber. (Modified from Bokoch, M. P., & Weston, S. D. [2020]. In M. A. Gropper, R. D. Miller, N. H. Cohen, L. I. Eriksson, L. A. Fleisher, K. Leslie, et al. (Eds.), *Inhaled Anesthetics: Delivery Systems* [Vol. 22, 9th Ed., pp. 572–637.e6]. Philadelphia, PA: Elsevier. Fig. 22.21.)

since vapor pressure varies with temperature, variable bypass vaporizers have been designed to compensate for temperature and deliver a predictable amount of anesthetic gas over a wide range of ambient temperatures.

Neuromuscular Blockers

Motor neurons release acetylcholine, which binds ligand-gated sodium channels on the muscle fibers at the neuromuscular junction. These channels are called nicotinic ion channels. Binding of acetylcholine induces a conformational change in the ligand-gated ion channel, facilitating an influx of positively charged sodium ions (i.e., cations) that leads to the depolarization, and contraction, of the muscle fiber. Neuromuscular blockers (also known as paralytics, muscle relaxants, and neuromuscular blocking agents) inhibit the normal functioning of the neuromuscular junction.

There are two types of neuromuscular blockers: depolarizing neuromuscular blockers and nondepolarizing neuromuscular blockers. The only depolarizing neuromuscular blocker used clinically is succinylcholine. It binds to and activates nicotinic acetylcholine receptors, causing the muscle fiber to depolarize. While the succinylcholine molecule activates the nicotinic acetylcholine receptor, the muscle fiber remains depolarized after contraction, and it cannot contract again. Meanwhile, nondepolarizing neuromuscular blockers work by competitively inhibiting the effect of acetylcholine on the nicotinic acetylcholine receptor. As the name implies, nondepolarizing neuromuscular blockers do not activate the nicotinic acetylcholine receptor and therefore do not depolarize the muscle fiber.

The degree of neuromuscular blockade, and the necessity of an additional dose of neuromuscular blocker, is monitored clinically by a device called a twitch monitor (there are newer modalities, but twitch monitoring is still widely used). A twitch monitor is a small, battery-powered device with two electrodes attached. These electrodes are placed close to one another on the patient over some nerve distribution, commonly the ulnar nerve or facial nerve. The muscle innervated by the stimulated nerve will twitch in response to an electrical impulse. The strength and duration of the contraction are indicators of the degree of neuromuscular blockade in effect. A pattern of four electrical impulses of 10–80 milliamps, one every 500 milliseconds, is delivered, and the strength of muscle contraction is observed. This is called train of four monitoring. The patient may show zero, one, two, three, or four twitches in response to train of four monitoring.

After administration of succinylcholine, the patient will have no twitches in response to train of four stimulation. If the patient has any twitches, they will have four twitches of equal strength. In most patients, the drug will wear off in a matter of minutes. As the drug wears off, the strength of the twitches will return to baseline strength.

After administration of a nondepolarizing neuromuscular blocker, the patient will have no twitches on train of four stimulations. As the drug wears off, they will first have only one twitch, then two twitches with the first stronger than the second, then three twitches of decreasing strength, then four twitches of decreasing strength, and finally four strong twitches at baseline strength. Fig. 5 shows the twitch responses on train of four monitoring over time after administration of both types of neuromuscular blockers.

Advice for Your First Week in the Operating Room

Your first few days in the operating room as an anesthesiologist-in-training can be intimidating—lots of equipment and monitors, different drugs and concentrations to keep track of, a surgeon breathing down your neck, and an environment that demands efficiency and accuracy. Here are a few tips to help you succeed.

1. Know your patient. This is true in any field of medicine but particularly so in anesthesiology. Make sure you read your patient's chart. Know what operation they are having and why. Do they have any major comorbidities like heart disease or diabetes? Know those too. Know their allergies, home medications, BMI, and lab results. If they have a history of major anesthetic complications like malignant hyperthermia or difficult airway, it is important to know that as well. It is a good idea to write down this information, not only as a memory aide, but also to help you organize your thoughts. On the morning of surgery, your attending or resident will want to discuss the case with you. The more you know about your patient, the better. You may even know something your attending or resident does not.

2. Demonstrate a strong fund of knowledge. Know your physiology—what is the baroreceptor reflex? How is blood flow to the brain regulated? What is septic shock? Have a basic understanding of common anesthetic drugs—hypnotics like propofol, neuromuscular blockers, and inhaled anesthetic gases. Know what those drugs do and when they are used.

3. Have an assessment and plan. It doesn't have to be an answer that would pass the oral boards, but it shows that you've put some thought into it. An assessment and plan should consist of the following:

   - patient's ASA status
   - type of anesthesia (e.g., general with endotracheal intubation, general with LMA, regional anesthesia, sedation, local, etc.)
   - types of intravascular access (e.g., peripheral IV, central venous catheter)
   - plans for special monitoring (e.g., arterial catheter, bladder catheter, 5-lead ECG)
   - plan for premedication (e.g., midazolam in the preoperative holding area)
   - plan for induction of anesthesia and airway management (e.g., RSI)
   - plan for maintenance of anesthesia (e.g., inhaled anesthesia gas, IV anesthesia)
   - plan for intraoperative and postoperative pain control (e.g., regional block, opioids).

4. Link your fund of knowledge with your knowledge of the patient. If the patient has diabetes, plan for a preoperative glucose check. If the patient has end-stage renal disease,

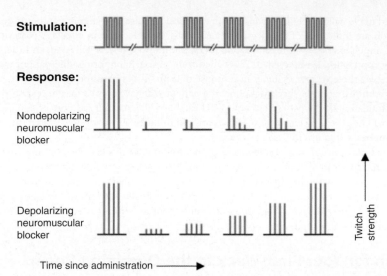

Fig. 5 Twitch strength on train of four stimulations after administration of depolarizing and nondepolarizing neuromuscular blockers. Notice that, after administration of a depolarizing neuromuscular blocker, all four twitches are of the same strength. This is not the case after administration of a nondepolarizing neuromuscular blocker. (Modified from Claudius, C., & Fuchs-Buder, T. [2020]. Neuromuscular monitoring. In M. A. Gropper, R. D. Miller, N. H. Cohen, L. I. Eriksson, L. A. Fleisher, K. Leslie, et al. (Eds.), *Miller's Anesthesia* [Vol. 43, 9th Ed., pp. 1354–1372.e4]. Philadelphia, PA: Elsevier. Fig. 43.5.)

plan for a potassium check and avoid drugs that are cleared by the kidneys. These small things will demonstrate that you understand the anesthetic implications of your patient's comorbidities.

5. Watch procedural videos. Understand the steps of laryngoscopy and endotracheal intubation. Understand the steps of arterial line placement. The more comfort you demonstrate with procedures, the more the attending will let you do, and the more smoothly the procedure will go.

6. Be vigilant. This is sage advice for all anesthesiologists. Pay attention to the patient monitor. Check the ventilator regularly. Make sure that the bag of IV fluid does not run out, and that the IV fluids do not run in too fast. Keep a close eye on the surgical field. Check the suction canisters for blood loss and the Foley bag for urine output. These habits will serve you well throughout your career.

7. Be enthusiastic. The more interested you are in what's happening, the more you'll learn.

References

Apfelbaum, J. L., Hagberg, C. A., Caplan, R. A., Blitt, C. D., Connis, R. T., Nickinovich, D. G., et al. (2013). Practice guidelines for management of the difficult airway: An updated report by the American Society of Anesthesiologists Task Force on Management of the Difficult Airway. *Anesthesiology*, *118*(2), 251–270.

ASA Physical Status Classification System. ASA Physical Status Classification System | American Society of Anesthesiologists (ASA), www.asahq.org/standards-and-guidelines/asa-physical-status-classification-system. (accessed November 10, 2021).

Defining Adult Overweight and Obesity. Centers for Disease Control and Prevention. 17 September 2020, www.cdc.gov/obesity/adult/defining.html.

Forman, S. A., Ishizawa, Y. (2020). Inhaled anesthetic uptake, distribution, metabolism, and toxicity. In M. A. Gropper, R. D. Miller, N. H. Cohen, L. I. Eriksson, L. A. Fleisher, K. Leslie, et al. (Eds.), *Miller's Anesthesia* (Vol. 20, 9th ed., pp. 509–539.e6). Philadelphia, PA: Elsevier.

Perouansky, M., Pearce, R. A., Hemmings, H. C., & Franks, N. P. (2020). Inhaled anesthetics: Mechanism of action. In M. A. Gropper, R. D. Miller, N. H. Cohen, L. I. Eriksson, L. A. Fleisher, K. Leslie, et al. (Eds.), *Miller's Anesthesia* (Vol. 19, 9th ed., pp. 487–508.e6). Philadelphia, PA: Elsevier.

What Is a Standard Drink? *National Institute on Alcohol Abuse and Alcoholism.* Department of Health and Human Services. Retrieved from: www.niaaa.nih.gov/alcohols-effects-health/overview-alcohol-consumption/what-standard-drink. (accessed November 08, 2021).

Wijeysundera, D. N., & Finlayson, E. (2020). Preoperative evaluation. In M. A. Gropper, R. D. Miller, N. H. Cohen, L. I. Eriksson, L. A. Fleisher, K. Leslie, et al. (Eds.), *Miller's Anesthesia* (Vol. 31, 9th ed., pp. 918–998.e12). Philadelphia, PA: Elsevier.

Regional

Michael J. Jung

A 62-Year-Old Man Scheduled for Right Shoulder Replacement for Osteoarthritis

Paul Neil Frank ■ Shane P. McGuire ■ Michael J. Jung

A 62-year-old man is scheduled for right shoulder replacement for osteoarthritis. He takes apixaban for atrial fibrillation, and his last dose was 3 days ago. This morning vital signs are blood pressure 142/57 mm Hg, pulse 72/min, respirations 16/min, oxygen saturation 95% on room air, and temperature 37°C.

STEP 1 PEARL

Apixaban is an oral anticoagulant that works by inhibiting activated factor X (Xa). Rivaroxaban is another factor Xa inhibitor. Low-molecular-weight heparin bound to antithrombin (AT), as well as fondaparinux bound to AT, also inhibit factor Xa. Fig. 1.1 illustrates the mechanism of action of common anticoagulants.

What are the anesthetic options for this patient?

This patient could have a safe operation under general anesthesia. Postoperative pain, which is usually significant, could be managed with oral and parenteral (i.e., intravenous [IV], intramuscular) opioid and nonopioid analgesics. If the patient were to receive a regional anesthetic (i.e., nerve block), the operation could safely be performed under general anesthesia or sedation with much less postoperative pain.

What regional nerve block is most appropriate?

The interscalene brachial plexus block targets the trunks of the brachial plexus (see Case 4) where the brachial plexus courses between the anterior scalene muscle (ASM) and middle scalene muscle (MSM). Fig. 1.2 shows the anatomic relationships between the ASM, MSM, and brachial plexus.

The superior trunk (C5, C6 nerve roots) and middle trunk (C7 nerve root) will be well-anesthetized by the interscalene nerve block, but the inferior trunk (C8, T1 nerve roots) is often spared. Fig. 1.3 shows the dermatomes corresponding to the cervical nerve roots. Therefore the interscalene block will cover the territory of the shoulder but may not adequately anesthetize the distribution of the ulnar nerve in the forearm and hand.

The interscalene block can be performed as a single injection of local anesthetic (sometimes with adjunctive medications such as steroids or epinephrine), or a catheter can be left in place for continuous infusion of local anesthetic.

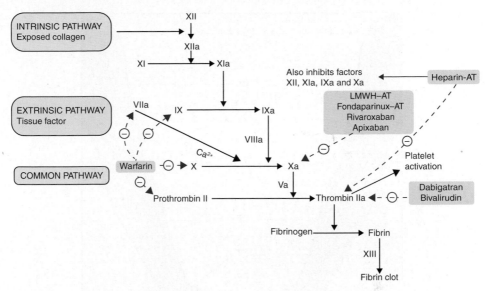

Fig. 1.1 The coagulation cascade begins with the intrinsic and extrinsic pathways, activated by exposed subendothelial collagen and tissue factor, respectively. There are a multitude of anticoagulant medications used clinically. Each of these anticoagulants acts as an inhibitor in the coagulation cascade. (Waller, D. G., & Sampson, A. P. [2018]. Haemostasis. In: *Medical pharmacology and therapeutics* [Chapter 11, pp. 175–190]. Philadelphia, PA: Elsevier. Fig. 11.3.)

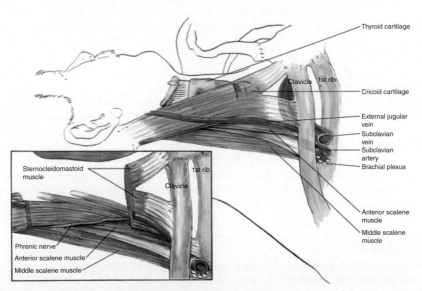

Fig. 1.2 The brachial plexus courses between the anterior and middle scalene muscles, then over the first rib with the subclavian artery *(SCA)*. *ASM,* Anterior scalene muscle; *MSM,* middle scalene muscle. (Farag, E., Brown, D. L. [2021]. Interscalene Block. In E. Farag, L. Mounir-Soliman, D. L. Brown [Eds.], *Brown's Atlas of Anesthesia* [6th ed, pp. 33–44]. Philadelphia, PA: Elsevier. Fig. 5.2.)

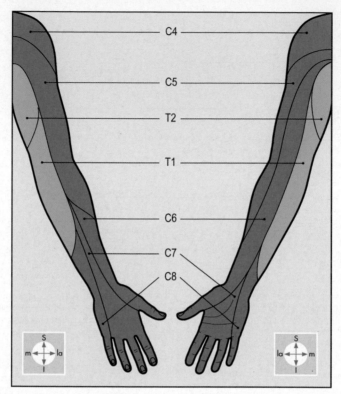

Fig. 1.3   Dermatomes of the upper extremity. *I*, Inferior; *la*, lateral; *m*, medial; *S*, superior. (Gosling, J. A., Humpherson, J. R., Whitmore, I., & William, P. L. T. [1986]. Upper limb. In: *Human anatomy: Color atlas and textbook* [Chapter 3, pp. 71–133]. Philadelphia, PA: Elsevier. Fig. 3.6.)

How should the patient be positioned for this block?

The patient should be in the supine position with the head of the bed slightly elevated. The patient's head should be turned to the contralateral side (i.e., away from the side where the block will be placed).

How is the block performed?

Fig. 1.4 shows proper ultrasound probe placement and the ultrasonographic view of a common approach to the interscalene block. The needle is inserted laterally and advances medially toward the nerve roots. This approach is considered to be "in plane" because the entire length of the needle is visible on ultrasound. The ultrasound probe and the needle are parallel to one another.

STEP 1 PEARL

Each peripheral nerve consists of multiple neurons. The axon of each neuron is encased in its own endoneurium. Axons are bundled into fascicles, each of which is surrounded by a perineurium. Finally, groups of fascicles are wrapped in an epineurium. This microanatomy is shown in Fig. 1.5.

What are the contraindications to an interscalene block?

The interscalene block anesthetizes the phrenic nerve, resulting in paralysis of the ipsilateral hemi-diaphragm. This weakens respiratory effort. Although this is well-tolerated by healthy patients,

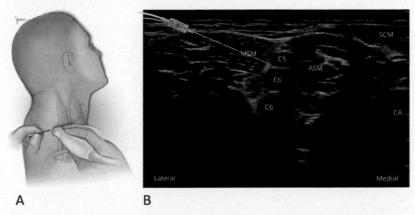

A   B

Fig. 1.4 (A) Ultrasound probe and needle placement for in-plane, lateral to medial approach. (B) Ultrasonographic view of the brachial plexus at the level of the interscalene groove. The sternocleidomastoid muscle *(SCM)* and carotid artery *(CA)* are medial, and the *C5, C6,* and *C7* nerve roots course between anterior scalene muscle *(ASM)* and middle scalene muscle *(MSM)*. Local anesthetic should be deposited in the region shaded blue. (Farag, E., Brown, D. L. [2021]. Interscalene Block. In E. Farag, L. Mounir-Soliman, D. L. Brown [Eds.], *Brown's Atlas of Anesthesia* [6th ed, pp. 33–44]. Philadelphia, PA: Elsevier. Modified from Fig. 5.13.)

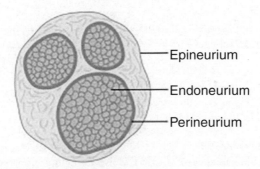

Fig. 1.5 Cross-section of a peripheral nerve showing each axon wrapped in an individual endoneurium, groups of axons wrapped in perineurium (known as fascicles), and groups of fascicles wrapped in an epineurium. (Lirk, P., & Berde, C. B. [2019]. Local anesthetics. In: *Miller's anesthesia* [Chapter 29, pp. 865–890.e4]. Philadelphia, PA: Elsevier. Modified from Fig. 29.4.)

individuals with respiratory diseases such as chronic obstructive pulmonary disease (COPD) may become dyspneic and/or hypoxic with this block.

In addition, patients on anticoagulation are at greater risk of hematoma and nerve damage following peripheral nerve blocks. The American Society of Regional Anesthesia (ASRA) publishes guidelines listing the minimum wait time between the last dose of anticoagulant and neuraxial anesthesia or deep peripheral nerve block. This patient is taking apixaban, and his last dose was 3 days ago. The ASRA guidelines recommend abstaining from apixaban for at least 72 hours prior to neuraxial anesthesia or deep peripheral nerve block.

During the injection, the patient complains of numbness around his mouth and the taste of metal, and then he seizes.

What's going on?

This is concerning for local anesthetic systemic toxicity (LAST) caused by intravascular injection of local anesthetic. Since the seizure happened immediately during injection, this was likely caused by injection into the carotid or vertebral artery. This is a rare but known complication of interscalene block.

LAST can occur when an excessive amount of local anesthetic enters systemic circulation. Recalling that the primary mechanism of action of local anesthetics is through sodium channel blockade, it is no surprise that central nervous system (CNS) and cardiovascular systems, both of which rely heavily on sodium channels for normal functioning, can be affected. The CNS is more sensitive to local anesthetic toxicity and therefore initial symptoms often present as lightheadedness, dizziness, circumoral numbness, tinnitus, and restlessness and can ultimately progress to tonic-clonic seizures.

Cardiovascular effects occur after CNS effects and can include vasodilation or vasoconstriction, PR interval prolongation, and QRS complex widening, leading to cardiac arrhythmias including ventricular fibrillation.

What should you do?

Immediately stop the injection. Call for help. Support the patient's breathing with 100% oxygen and mask ventilation if necessary. The seizure can be treated with a benzodiazepine. The patient may require emergent intubation. Continue close hemodynamic monitoring—LAST can progress to cardiovascular collapse. Administer intralipid. If intralipid is ineffective, the patient may need emergent cardiopulmonary bypass.

What is intralipid?

Intralipid is a fat emulsion that traps local anesthetic. By sequestering the molecules of local anesthetic, it can help treat LAST. Begin with an IV bolus of 1.5 mL/kg and an infusion of 0.25 mL/kg/min.

Propofol is a lipid emulsion. Would it be helpful here?

Although propofol is a fat emulsion, the concentration of lipid is low and the propofol itself may act as a cardiac depressant. Therefore it is not recommended.

How could this have been prevented?

No single measure can eliminate the risk of LAST. However, multiple measures have proven helpful. Ultrasound guidance should be used whenever possible. Use the lowest dose of local anesthetic that will achieve the desired block. Any time local anesthetic is injected, it is important to ensure the injection is not intravascular. Aspirate on the syringe to ensure there is no blood return prior to starting injection and again every 5 mL of injection. Pause the injection every 5 mL for up to 30 seconds to monitor for untoward side effects.

Can LAST only be caused by intravascular injection?

No. LAST can also be caused by injection at the intended site. In these instances, large doses of local anesthetic deposited in the soft tissues seep into the blood stream. Plasma levels of local anesthetic rise, and eventually the patient develops LAST. LAST develops more slowly in these cases than when it is caused by intravascular injection. The rate and magnitude of the rise of plasma levels of local anesthetics depend on the site of injection (sites that are more vascularized have more systemic absorption), the local anesthetic used, the dose, and whether a vasoconstrictor was added.

What sites of injection have the most systemic absorption of local anesthetic?

From greatest to least systemic absorption: intercostal > caudal > epidural > brachial plexus > sciatic = femoral > subcutaneous infiltration.

TABLE 1.1 ■ **The Maximum Safe Dose Differs With Each Local Anesthetic**

Local Anesthetic	Maximum Safe Dose
Lidocaine without epinephrine	5 mg/kg
Lidocaine with epinephrine	7 mg/kg
Bupivacaine	2.5 mg/kg
Ropivacaine	3 mg/kg
Chloroprocaine	12 mg/kg

Addition of a vasoconstrictor such as epinephrine will increase the maximum safe dose for some local anesthetic agents.

What are the maximum safe doses of local anesthetic?
The maximum safe dose is unique to each anesthetic. Table 1.1 shows the maximum safe dose for commonly used local anesthetics.

Why would epinephrine be added to a local anesthetic?
Epinephrine is an agonist at α- and β-adrenergic receptors. The effect of its α agonism is to cause vasoconstriction. Vasoconstriction in the area of the local anesthetic injection prolongs the effect of the local anesthetic by reducing blood flow that will absorb the local anesthetic away from the target site and into systemic circulation. In addition, α_2 agonism may have some adjuvant analgesic effects.

Addition of epinephrine to a local anesthetic will also help identify inadvertent intravascular injection. β Agonism will cause tachycardia. If the anesthesiologist were to unknowingly inject a solution containing epinephrine directly into the patient's blood stream, the patient would develop tachycardia and palpitations. These clues should alert the anesthesiologist to possible intravascular needle tip placement.

The patient stabilizes and surgery is rescheduled. When the patient returns, you plan to perform an interscalene block with 1% lidocaine with epinephrine.

The patient weighs 60 kg. What is the maximum safe volume of local anesthetic that can be used?
Notice that the maximum safe doses for each anesthetic listed in Table 1.1 are expressed in milligrams of local anesthetic per kilogram of body weight. The key here is to convert the maximum dose expressed in mg/kg to a maximum dose in mg, and then to convert the maximum dose in mg to a maximum volume of solution. In a patient who weighs 60 kg, the maximum dose of lidocaine with epinephrine (from Table 1.1) is

$$7 \text{ mg/kg} \times 60 \text{ kg} = 420 \text{ mg}$$

To calculate a volume of solution, the concentration of the solution, expressed as a percentage, should be converted to mg/mL. That conversion is given by

$$1\% \text{ solution} = 10 \text{ mg/mL}$$

Therefore 1% lidocaine contains 10 mg of lidocaine per milliliter of solution.
Now that we have a maximum dose in milligrams and a concentration of solution in mg/mL, we can calculate a maximum volume of solution. Conversion to a volume of local anesthetic solution is given by

$$\text{volume} \times 10 \text{ mg/mL} = 420 \text{ mg}$$

$$\text{volume} = \frac{420 \text{ mg}}{10 \text{ mg/mL}}$$

$$\text{volume} = 42 \text{ mL}$$

Therefore the maximum safe volume of 1% lidocaine with epinephrine this patient can receive is 42 mL. It should be noted that this is significantly more than would be administered for an interscalene block.

The vial of local anesthetic says it contains epinephrine 1:200,000. What is the concentration of epinephrine?
This is an expression of the dilution of 1 g of epinephrine. The conversion of this ratio 1:*x* to concentration in micrograms per milliliter (μg/mL) is given by

$$\text{concentration} = 1,000,000/x$$

Simply put, divide 1 million by the number after the "1:" to calculate the concentration in μg/mL. For this 1:200,000 solution, the concentration of epinephrine is

$$1,000,000/200,000 = 5 \text{ μg/mL}$$

Similarly, a 1:100,000 solution of epinephrine would have an epinephrine concentration of

$$1,000,000/100,000 = 10 \text{ μg/mL}$$

The interscalene block is uneventful. Twenty minutes later, you notice the patient's eyes look strange (Fig. 1.6). His eyes looked normal when you first met him this morning.

What's going on?
These findings are consistent with Horner syndrome, a blockade of sympathetic innervation of the ipsilateral face and neck. This is a benign and self-resolving complication of interscalene block. Local anesthetic injected near the ASM can block the cervical ganglion, which provides sympathetic innervation to the face.

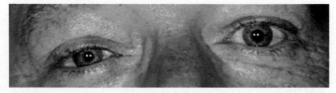

Fig. 1.6 Right-sided miosis, conjunctival hyperemia, ptosis, and elevation of the lower eyelid. (Reede, D. L., Garcon, E., Smoker, W. R. K., & Kardon, R. [2008]. Horner's syndrome: Clinical and radiographic evaluation. *Neuroimaging Clinics of North America*, *18*(2), 369–385. Fig. 2.)

STEP 1 PEARL

Sympathetic nerves to the face and eyes course from the superior cervical ganglion along the carotid plexus (Fig. 1.7). There are several important targets of sympathetic fibers in the eye and surrounding structures:
- Müller muscle, which arises from the deep surface of the levator palpebrae superioris muscle, is responsible for elevation of the upper eyelid when the eye is open. Muscle in the inferior eyelid responsible for retraction of the lower eyelid when the eye is open is also called Müller muscle. Loss of sympathetic stimulation causes drooping of the upper eyelid and elevation of the lower eyelid.
- Dilator iridis muscle is responsible for pupillary dilation. Loss of sympathetic innervation causes unopposed action of sphincter pupillae (innervated by the parasympathetic nervous system) and miosis (i.e., pupillary constriction).
- Vascular smooth muscle of the conjunctiva. Loss of sympathetic innervation results in vasodilation and conjunctival hyperemia.

What if the patient were to develop severe hypotension and bradycardia during surgery after interscalene block?

This may be caused by the Bezold-Jarisch reflex. In the case of a patient having shoulder surgery in the sitting position after an interscalene block, it is hypothesized that the decreased venous return to the heart stimulates intracardiac mechanoreceptors that cause a significant decrease in sympathetic tone and increase in parasympathetic tone.

It should be noted that there is some debate as to whether hypotension and bradycardia in this context are truly attributable to this mechanism.

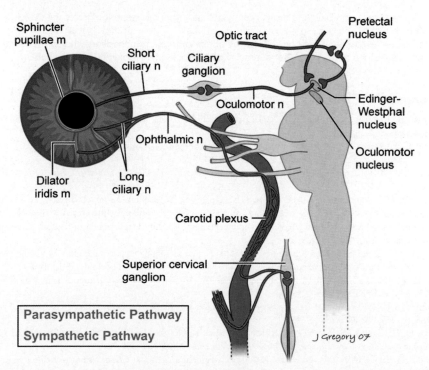

Fig. 1.7 Courses of sympathetic and parasympathetic nerves to the eye. *n*, nerve; *m*, muscle. (Reede, D. L., Garcon, E., Smoker, W. R. K., & Kardon, R. [2008]. "Horner's syndrome: Clinical and radiographic evaluation." *Neuroimaging Clinics of North America*, *18*[2], 369–385. Fig. 4.)

What if the patient were to develop paralysis, respiratory arrest, bilateral mydriasis, hypotension, and bradycardia after interscalene block?
These findings are suggestive of inadvertent intrathecal injection of local anesthetic. This is a rare but known complication of interscalene block and results in total anesthesia of the body and brain stem. This requires rapid recognition and supportive management such as intubation for mechanical ventilation and hemodynamic support until symptoms resolve.

The patient tolerates the operation with moderate sedation. Postoperatively, the patient complains of a hoarse voice.

What's going on?
This is likely caused by blockade of the recurrent laryngeal nerve by spread of local anesthetic. This is yet another known and self-limited complication of interscalene block. The right recurrent laryngeal nerve is more susceptible to blockade than the left side.

BEYOND THE PEARLS

- The anticoagulant effect of apixaban can be measured by anti–factor Xa assay calibrated for apixaban.
- For all regional nerve blocks, it is important to inject local anesthetic *surrounding* but not *into* nerve bundles.
- Accidental intravascular injection of a local anesthetic with added epinephrine or other vasopressor can cause ischemia to areas with little collateral circulation, such as the toes, fingers, and penis.
- Administration of β-blocking drugs prophylactically may decrease the risk of the Bezold-Jarisch reflex.
- Interscalene block can be complicated by pneumothorax from inadvertent pleural puncture, but this may be more likely after supraclavicular block given proximity to the pleura.

References

Berde, C. B., Koka, A., & Drasner, K. (2007). Local anesthetics. *Basics of Anesthesia, 10,* 139–155. Philadelphia, PA: Elsevier.

Crystal, G. J., Assaad, S. I., & Heerdt, P. M. Cardiovascular physiology: Integrative function. In: *Pharmacology and physiology for anesthesia* (Chapter 24, pp. 473–519).

Fletcher, A. (2019). Action potential: Generation and propagation. *Anesthesia and Intensive Care Medicine, 20*(4), 243–247.

Horlocker, T. T., Vandermeulen, E., Kopp, S. L., Gogarten, W., Leffert, L. R., & Benzon, H. T. (2018). Regional anesthesia in the patient receiving antithrombotic or thrombolytic therapy: American Society of Regional Anesthesia and Pain Medicine Evidence-Based Guidelines (fourth edition). *Regional Anesthesia and Pain Medicine, 43,* 263–309.

Johnson, R. L., Kopp, S. L., Jens, K., & Gray, A. T. (2019). Peripheral nerve blocks and ultrasound guidance for regional anesthesia. *Miller's anesthesia* (Chapter 46, pp. 1450-1479.e3). Philadelphia, PA: Elsevier.

Lirk, P., & Berde, C. B. (2019). Local anesthetics. In: *Miller's anesthesia* (Chapter 29, pp. 865-890.e4). Philadelphia, PA: Elsevier.

Malamed, S. F. (2013). Clinical action of specific agents. In: *Handbook of local anesthesia* (Chapter 4, pp. 57-84). Philadelphia, PA: Elsevier.

Reede, D. L., Garcon, E., Smoker, W. R. K., & Kardon, R. (2008). Horner's syndrome: Clinical and radiographic evaluation. *Neuroimaging Clinics of North America, 18*(2), 369–385.

Steckelberg, R. C., Mihm, F., & Derby, R. (2019). Regional anesthesia. *Global Reconstructive Surgery, 1*(4), 23–33.

Ultrasound-Guided Interscalene Brachial Plexus Block. *New York School of Regional Anesthesia.* https://www.nysora.com/techniques/upper-extremity/intescalene/ultrasound-guided-interscalene-brachial-plexus-block (accessed December 24, 2020).

A 75-Year-Old Woman With Rheumatoid Arthritis and Limited Neck Range of Motion

Liye Billy Zhang ■ Elizabeth C. Fung ■ Paul Neil Frank ■ Michael J. Jung

A 75-year-old woman with rheumatoid arthritis (RA) and limited neck range of motion requiring a video laryngoscopic intubation in the past is scheduled for a total knee arthroplasty.

What are the anesthetic options for this patient?
The two main anesthetic options in this patient are (1) general anesthesia with or without regional nerve block or (2) neuraxial anesthesia with or without regional nerve block. An epidural may be used instead of a spinal.

What are the advantages of spinal anesthesia over general anesthesia?
Spinal anesthesia has a number of advantages that make it an appealing choice for lower extremity surgeries. The main advantages are avoidance of the risks of general anesthesia. In this patient with a challenging airway, spinal anesthesia provides exquisite analgesia while allowing the patient to breathe spontaneously and obviating the need for airway instrumentation. By avoiding airway manipulation, the risk of aspiration during induction and extubation is eliminated (of course, the patient may aspirate at any point during the anesthetic, especially without an endotracheal tube in place). By avoiding paralytics, the risk of the dreaded "paralyzed-and-aware" scenario is eliminated. If the patient is kept awake, the anesthesiologist can assess neurologic status intraoperatively, thus reducing the risk of an unwitnessed stroke.

In addition, spinal anesthesia is associated with decreased rates of mortality, deep vein thrombosis, blood transfusion, and pulmonary complications compared with general anesthesia.

What are the particular concerns for a patient with rheumatoid arthritis (RA)?
Patients with RA may have limited jaw and neck range of motion, reduced mouth opening, and atlantoaxial instability. Atlantoaxial instability is caused by degradation and weakness of the transverse ligament. This increases the risk of atlantoaxial subluxation, which is characterized by separation of the odontoid process from the anterior arch of the atlas (Fig. 2.1). This can result in pressure on the spinal cord when the neck is manipulated, leading to spinal cord injury.

STEP 1, 2 PEARL

Rheumatoid arthritis is a systemic, inflammatory autoimmune disorder that causes synovial inflammation and progressive joint damage. Common clinical findings include joint pain and stiffness in the morning lasting more than 1 hour that improves with activity, joint tenderness, soft tissue swelling of the joint, and effusions. Joint involvement is symmetric and generally

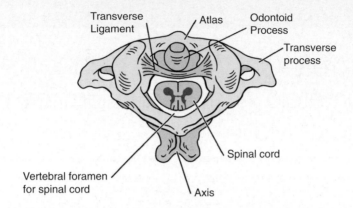

Fig. 2.1 Normal relationship between the C1 ("atlas") and C2 ("axis") vertebrae and the spinal cord. Ordinarily, the transverse ligament holds the odontoid process of C2 against the anterior arch of C1. Degradation of the transverse ligament allows for increased movement of C1 relative to C2 and increases the risk of subluxation and compression of the spinal cord. (Magee, D., & Manske, R. C. [2021]. Cervical spine. In *Orthopedic Physical Assessment* [pp. 164–242.e6]. Philadelphia, PA: Elsevier. Modified from Fig. 3.63.)

involves the metacarpophalangeal interphalangeal joints, proximal interphalangeal joints, and wrist. Systemic symptoms (e.g., elevated temperature, weight loss, and fatigue) and extra-articular manifestations (e.g., pulmonary fibrosis, rheumatoid nodules, anemia of chronic disease) are also common.

STEP 1, 2 PEARL

Initial evaluation of rheumatoid arthritis typically includes x-rays of joints and serologic studies for rheumatoid factor, anti-cyclic citrullinated peptide antibodies, erythrocyte sedimentation rate, and C-reactive protein.

STEP 2 PEARL

Early in the disease, rheumatoid arthritis most commonly affects the cervical spine rather than the thoracic and lumbar spine. Cervical involvement most often manifests as atlantoaxial instability, a potentially life-threatening complication. Degradation of the transverse ligament causes excessive mobility between C1 and C2 and leads to spinal cord compression. Clinical features of atlantoaxial subluxation include neck pain and stiffness at rest, back pain, urinary incontinence, ataxia, peripheral paresthesias, and signs of upper motor neuron injury such as hyperreflexia, positive Babinski sign, and progressive spastic quadriparesis. These neurologic deficits typically develop later in the disease course. However, atlantoaxial subluxation can be acutely worsened during endotracheal intubation and result in acute onset of neurologic symptoms. In addition to RA, Down syndrome and juvenile idiopathic arthritis are also associated with atlantoaxial instability.

What are the risks of spinal anesthesia?

Although spinal anesthesia appears to be an ideal choice of anesthetic in many cases for lower extremity surgeries, it is not without risk. Table 2.1 lists possible complications of spinal anesthesia.

In our patient, RA may affect the lumbar or thoracic spine and may obliterate typical landmarks due to deformities or contractures. In addition, if the operation lasts longer than expected and the subarachnoid (i.e., spinal) block wears off, it may be challenging to convert to a general endotracheal anesthetic in this patient with RA.

TABLE 2.1 ■ Complications of Spinal Anesthesia

Minor	Moderate	Major
• Mild hypotension • Nausea/Vomiting • Urinary retention • Shivering	• Postdural puncture headache • Failed spinal requiring conversion to general anesthesia	• Infection • Spinal hematoma • Spinal cord ischemia • Total spinal anesthesia • Death

TABLE 2.2 ■ Contraindications to Spinal Anesthesia

Absolute Contraindications	Relative Contraindications
• Skin or soft tissue infection at injection site • Hypovolemia • History of allergic reaction to local anesthetic • Elevated intracranial pressure • Patient refusal	• Sepsis • Fixed cardiac output states (e.g., aortic stenosis) • Coagulopathy • Demyelinating neurological disease (e.g., multiple sclerosis) • Previous spinal surgery

What are the contraindications to spinal anesthesia?
Table 2.2 lists the absolute and relative contraindications to spinal anesthesia.

What are the techniques of for placement of spinal anesthesia?
There are two approaches to placement of spinal anesthesia: midline and paramedian (Fig. 2.2). The midline approach is more commonly used. Always start with a sterile prep and drape.

For the midline approach,

1. Palpate the posterior superior iliac spine (Fig. 2.3) bilaterally. This is generally the level of L4 to L5.
2. Palpate the desired interspace (this is usually about the level of the posterior superior iliac spines), noting the position of the spinous processes.
3. Inject local anesthetic (usually 1% or 2% lidocaine), making a skin wheal at the midline.
4. Place the introducer needle with a 10 to 20 degrees cephalad angle.
5. Place the spinal needle through the introducer, making note of the changes of resistance that you feel along the way.
    a. The spinal needle should pass through the subcutaneous tissue, supraspinous ligament, interspinous ligament, ligamentum flavum, epidural space, dura mater, and subarachnoid mater. Oftentimes the most obvious "pops" are felt at the ligamentum flavum and dura mater (Fig. 2.4).
6. Once the second "pop" is felt, remove the stylet from the spinal needle and check for flow of cerebrospinal fluid (CSF).
    a. It is important to hold the spinal needle firmly with the fingers of the nondominant hand and brace the back of this hand on the patient's back to ensure that the spinal needle does not move. A fraction of a millimeter may be all that it takes for the tip of the spinal needle to exit the subarachnoid space.
7. Attach your local anesthetic syringe to the spinal needle and aspirate to confirm CSF flow. You may see a "swirl" of fluid as CSF mixes with the local anesthetic (generally with hyperbaric local anesthetic).
8. Slowly inject your local anesthetic. You may choose to aspirate midway during your injection to again confirm flow of CSF.

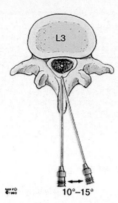

Fig. 2.2 Axial diagram of the lumbar spine comparing the angle of approach with midline and paramedian spinal placement. (Nathan, N., & Wong, C. A. [2020]. Spinal, epidural, and caudal anesthesia: Anatomy, physiology, and technique. In D. H. Chestnut, C. A. Wong, L. C. Tsen, W. D. N. Kee, Y. Beilin, J. M. Mhyre, et al. (Eds.), *Chestnut's Obstetric Anesthesia* [Chapter 12, pp. 238–270]. Philadelphia, PA: Elsevier. Modified from Fig. 12.10.)

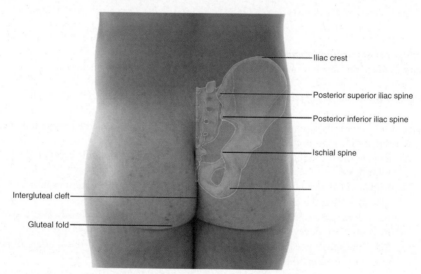

Fig. 2.3 Surface anatomy of the lower back illustrating the position of prominent structure of the pelvic bones, including the iliac crest and posterior superior iliac spine. (Drake, R. L., Vogl, A. W., & Mitchell, A. W. M. [2021]. Pelvis and perineum. In *Gray's Atlas of Anatomy* [Vol. 5, pp. 213–292].)

    9. Remove the spinal needle and introducer together from the patient's back.

    10. Position the patient, check for sensory level, and adjust table position as necessary.

The paramedian approach is typically reserved for difficult spinals, as in the case of ligamentous calcifications, abnormal anatomy, or inability to properly position the patient. For the paramedian approach

    1. Palpate the spinous processes to determine your level of injection.

    2. Inject local anesthetic approximately 1 cm lateral to the level of the inferior spinous process.

    3. Insert the introducer in a cephalad and medial angulation (approximately 10 to 15 degrees cephalad and 10 to 15 degrees medially).

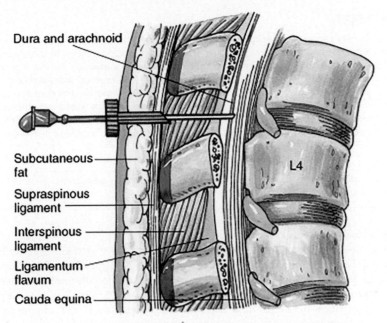

Fig. 2.4 Midsagittal section of the lumbar spine showing the subcutaneous tissue, supraspinous ligament, interspinous ligament, and ligamentum flavum, dura mater, and arachnoid mater. (Brown, D. L. [2021]. Spinal block. In *Brown's Atlas of Regional Anesthesia* [Vol. *40*, 6th ed., pp. 249–260]. Modified from Fig. 40.8.)

4. Pass the spinal needle through the introducer.
   a. Using small movements, insert the needle until you encounter bone, then retract and angle slightly cephalad, advance until you encounter bone again, then repeat until you enter the interspace. This is sometimes referred to as "walking off" bone.
   b. The spinal needle will pass through subcutaneous tissues, ligamentum flavum, dura mater, subdural space, and subarachnoid mater to reach the subarachnoid space.
   c. You may only feel a "pop" while going through the ligamentum flavum.
5. Remove the stylet from the spinal needle, and check for flow of CSF.
6. Attach your local anesthetic syringe to the spinal needle, and aspirate to confirm CSF flow. You may see a "swirl" of fluid as CSF mixes with the local anesthetic.
7. Slowly inject your local anesthetic. You may choose to aspirate midway during your injection to again confirm flow of CSF.
8. Remove spinal needle and introducer together from the patient's back.
9. Position the patient, check for sensory level, and adjust table position as necessary.

What are the options for lower extremity nerve blocks in this patient?
Peripheral nerve blocks have been shown to decrease hospital length of stay and rehabilitation, decrease opioid requirements, and improve postoperative pain control. A femoral or sciatic nerve block would provide adequate coverage for the surgical site; however, these blocks will cause a dense motor blockade that will prevent early ambulation postoperatively.

A continuous adductor canal block via indwelling catheter would provide comparable analgesia while avoiding the dense motor blockade of a femoral or combined femoral and sciatic blocks. This allows the patient to regain functional mobility faster as well as decreases the chance of a fall, which could be a potentially devastating postoperative complication.

STEP 1, 2 PEARL

The femoral nerve arises from spinal nerves L2–L4. It provides sensory innervation to the anterior thigh and medial leg below the knee. It provides motor innervation to the quadriceps, iliacus, pectineus, and sartorius muscles. The femoral nerve is classically injured in pelvic fractures and manifests as weakness with leg extension and decreased patellar reflex.

The sciatic nerve arises from spinal nerves L4–S3 and branches into the common peroneal nerve (L4–S2) and the tibial nerve (L4–S3). The sciatic nerve supplies sensory innervation to the posterior thigh and the leg below the knee (except the medial calf). It supplies motor innervation to the posterior compartment of the thigh and all of the leg below the knee.

After discussion with the surgeon and the patient, you plan for a preoperative placement of an adductor canal catheter in addition to a spinal anesthetic.

How is an adductor canal block placed?

The patient should be in the supine position with the operative leg externally rotated. Place the ultrasound probe on the medial aspect of the patient's midthigh (Fig. 2.5). The femoral artery will be your major landmark. Move the ultrasound probe medially or laterally until the femoral artery is visualized. After injecting local anesthetic into the skin, insert the needle in-plane, aspirate on the syringe (to confirm the needle tip is not intravascular; see Case 1), and advance toward the femoral artery. Position the needle tip adjacent to the saphenous nerve, and inject 1 mL of local anesthetic to visualize spread. If appropriate spread is seen, deposit local anesthetic in the space, directing the needle as needed to ensure appropriate spread in the adductor canal space.

The adductor canal catheter and spinal placement are uneventful. A sterile tourniquet is placed over the patient's thigh. The surgeon asks you to inflate the tourniquet.

How much pressure should be applied to the tourniquet?

Tourniquet pressures are typically 200 to 250 mm Hg when on the arm and 250 to 300 mm Hg when on the leg. Alternatively, the tourniquet may be pressurized based on the patient's blood pressure. In this case, the tourniquet is inflated 100 mm Hg greater than systolic blood pressure for procedures on the arm and 100 to 150 mm Hg greater than systolic pressure for procedures on the leg.

The surgeon wants to let the intern get some experience operating.

How long can the tourniquet remain inflated?

There are no strict guidelines regarding tourniquet time; however, recommendations state that tourniquet time should be no more than 3 hours. After 2 to 2.5 hours of tourniquet inflation, release the tourniquet for 10 minutes at a time every hour, or you risk ischemic damage to the limb.

You deflate the tourniquet 110 minutes after it was inflated.

What changes do you expect?

While the tourniquet is inflated, the limb distal to the tourniquet does not receive blood flow. Ischemic metabolites (e.g., lactate, adenosine diphosphate) accumulate in the ischemic tissue. When the tourniquet is deflated, these metabolites are released into the systemic circulation as the previously ischemic vascular beds are reperfused, causing decreased preload, afterload, cardiac contractility, and mean arterial pressure. You should also expect an increase in end-tidal carbon dioxide, a transient decrease in core body temperature, and increases in potassium and lactate.

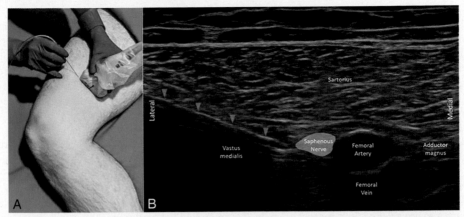

Fig. 2.5 (A) Proper ultrasound probe for the adductor canal block. (Ghassemi, J. [2019]. Adductor Canal block. In *Atlas of Ultrasound-Guided Regional Anesthesia* [Vol. *42*, pp. 169–173]. Modified from Fig. 42.2.) (B) Corresponding ultrasonographic image showing appropriate needle placement (identified with blue arrows) for injection of local anesthetic for adductor canal block. Relevant anatomy is labeled. (Courtesy Michael Jung, MD. Department of Anesthesiology and Pain Medicine. UC Davis Medical Center.)

STEP 1, 2 PEARL

Reperfusion injury is the exacerbation of cellular injury and death caused by reintroduction of blood flow into a previously ischemic environment. Reperfusion of blood and oxygen into the ischemic tissue causes free radical generation, mitochondrial damage, and disruption of cellular architecture. Complications of reperfusion injury include acidosis, rhabdomyolysis, disseminated intravascular coagulation (DIC), edema, and compartment syndrome (see Case 16). Reperfusion injury can also be a result of arterial thrombosis, crush injuries, or thrombolytic therapy.

STEP 2 PEARL

One complication of reperfusion injury is compartment syndrome, which occurs due to interstitial edema and intracellular swelling. Compartment syndrome occurs when the pressure within a fascial compartment approaches the blood pressure, thereby limiting blood flow to muscles and nerves. Acute compartment syndrome is a surgical emergency, and a fasciotomy should be performed within 6 hours of onset to reduce the chance of tissue necrosis. Acute compartment syndrome classically presents with pain out of proportion to injury, pain on passive stretch of the affected limb, rapidly increasing swelling, paresthesias or numbness, and motor weakness.

The surgeon needs to finish hammering in the prosthesis. You smell a pungent glue-like odor. As he is hammering, the blood pressure drops to 52/34 mm hg and the oxygen saturation drops from 99% to 60%.

What's going on?

This is concerning for bone cement implantation syndrome (BCIS), which may also be called cement embolism. When cement is used, a seal is created. Subsequent insertion of the prosthesis then causes high intramedullary canal pressures, which may then force intramedullary fat into the systemic circulation. This can travel to the lungs. This embolic load can present similarly to pulmonary embolism, causing systemic hypotension, pulmonary hypertension, hypoxemia, cardiogenic shock, right ventricular failure, and even cardiac arrest.

What should you do?
Treatment is supportive. Intubate the patient if definitive airway control has not been established, ventilate with 100% FiO_2, turn off all anesthetic agents, support hemodynamics with vasopressors, inotropes, and judicious fluid administration, place large-bore intravenous access, and place an arterial line for continuous blood pressure monitoring. Echocardiographic evaluation of the heart may assist in diagnosis and guiding management.

Transthoracic echocardiogram (TTE) shows akinesis (i.e., no Movement) of the free wall of the right ventricle (RV) but normal motion of the RV apex. What's going on?
This constellation of findings is called McConnell sign. This is consistent with acute right heart strain, as may be seen with BCIS or pulmonary embolism.

What other findings would you expect on TTE?
TTE findings of BCIS would present similarly to those of pulmonary embolism. You would expect to see signs of right ventricular strain. Common findings are listed in Table 2.3.

The patient's hemodynamics improve with initiation of an epinephrine infusion.

Should you extubate the patient at the end of surgery?
In this patient with likely pulmonary emboli, pulmonary hypertension, pulmonary edema, and right heart strain, receiving inotropes, the safer choice is to leave him intubated and transfer him to the intensive care unit.

BEYOND THE PEARLS

- The midline and paramedian approaches can also be used for epidural catheter placement, although your Touhy needle would target (and not advance beyond) the epidural space.
- In addition to rheumatoid arthritis, Down syndrome, achondroplasia, osteogenesis imperfecta, neurofibromatosis, and systemic lupus erythematosus are associated with atlantoaxial instability.
- The femoral nerve arises from branches of the L2–L4 spinal nerves. It provides sensation to the anterior thigh and medial calf (as the saphenous nerve for the medial calf). The femoral nerve also provides motor innervation to the muscles of the anterior thigh (e.g., quadriceps).
- The sciatic nerve is the largest nerve in the body and arises from branches of the L4 to S3 spinal nerves. The sciatic nerve bifurcates into the tibial and common fibular nerves around the level of the knee. The sciatic nerve provides sensation to the posterior thigh and the leg below the knee (as the tibial and common fibular nerves below the knee) except the medial calf (which is innervated by the saphenous nerve, a branch of the femoral nerve).

TABLE 2.3 ■ **Echocardiographic Signs of Right Ventricular Strain**

Finding	Description	Image
Dilated right ventricle (RV)	Visualized in the apical 4-chamber view, the RV should normally be approximately two thirds the size of the left ventricle (LV). A dilated RV would look similar or greater in size compared to the LV.	Fig. 2.6
Interventricular septal flattening	In the short axis view, the interventricular septum appears flattened, turning the normal "O" shape of the LV into a "D."	Fig. 2.7
Tricuspid regurgitation	RV pressure and/or volume overload can cause tricuspid regurgitation.	Fig. 2.8

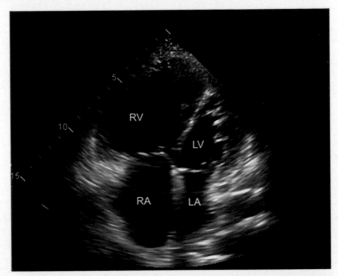

Fig. 2.6 Apical four-chamber view on transthoracic echocardiogram showing a dilated right ventricle *(RV)* and right atrium *(RA)*. *LA*, Left atrium; *LV*, left ventricle. (King, C., May, C. W., Williams, J., & Shlobin, O. A. [2014]. Management of right heart failure in the critically ill. *Critical Care Clinics, 30*[3], 475–498. Modified from Fig. 2.)

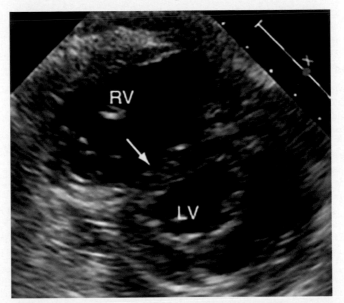

Fig. 2.7 Parasternal short-axis view on transthoracic echocardiogram shows an enlarged right ventricle *(RV)* with flattening of the interventricular septum. The white arrow shows deviation of the septum toward the left ventricle (LV). (Roldan, C. A. [2017]. Echocardiographic findings in systemic diseases characterized by immune-mediated injury. *Practice of Clinical Echocardiography*, 692–723. Modified from Fig. 35.18.)

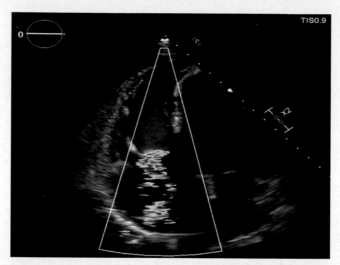

Fig. 2.8 Apical four-chamber view on transthoracic echocardiogram showing severe tricuspid regurgitation. (Harb, S. C., Spilias, N., Griffin, B. P., Svensson, L. G., Klatte, R. S., Bakaeen, F. G., et al. [2020]. Surgical repair for primary tricuspid valve disease: Individualized surgical planning with 3-dimensional printing. *JACC Case Reports, 2*[14], 2217–2222. Modified from Fig. 2.)

- The sciatic nerve also provides motor innervation to the posterior compartment of the thigh (e.g., hamstring) and all of the leg below the knee (as the tibial and common fibular nerves and their branches).

References

Agarwal, D., Mohta, M., Tyagi, A., & Sethi, A. K. (2010). Subdural block and the anaesthetist. *Anaesthesia and Intensive Care, 38*(1), 20–26.

Davis, J. J., Bond, T. S., & Swenson, J. D. (2009). Adductor canal block: More than just the saphenous nerve? *Regional Anesthesia and Pain Medicine, 34*(6), 618–619.

Donaldson, A. J., Thomson, H. E., Harper, N. J., & Kenny, N. W. (2009). Bone cement implantation syndrome. *British Journal of Anaesthesia, 102*(1), 12–22.

Fields, J. M., Davis, J., Girson, L., Au, A., Potts, J., Morgan, C. J., Vetter, I., & Riesenberg, L. A. (2017). Transthoracic echocardiography for diagnosing pulmonary embolism: A systematic review and meta-analysis. *Journal of the American Society of Echocardiography, 30*(7), 714–723.e4.

Greene, N. M., & Brull, S. J. (1981). *Physiology of spinal anesthesia* (4th ed.). Philadelphia, PA: Williams & Wilkins.

Kam, P. C., Kavanagh, R., & Yoong, F. F. (2001). The arterial tourniquet: Pathophysiological consequences and anaesthetic implications. *Anaesthesia, 56*(6), 534–545. https://doi.org/10.1046/j.1365-2044.2001.01982.xKumar.

Railton, K., C., & Tawfic, Q. (2016). Tourniquet application during anesthesia: "What we need to know?" *Journal of Anaesthesiology Clinical Pharmacology, 32*(4), 424–430. https://doi.org/10.4103/0970-9185.168174.

Lambert, D. H. (1989). Complications of spinal anesthesia. *International Anesthesiology Clinics, 27*(1), 51–55.

Samanta, R., Shoukrey, K., & Griffiths, R. (2011). Rheumatoid arthritis and anaesthesia. *Anaesthesia, 66*(12), 1146–1159. https://doi.org/10.1111/j.1365-2044.2011.06890.x.

Saranteas, T., Anagnostis, G., Paraskeuopoulos, T., Koulalis, D., Kokkalis, Z., Nakou, M., et al. (2011). Anatomy and clinical implications of the ultrasound-guided subsartorial saphenous nerve block. *Regional Anesthesia and Pain Medicine, 36*(4), 399–402.

Wildsmith, J. A. (2000). Management of hypotension during spinal anesthesia. *Regional Anesthesia and Pain Medicine, 25*(3), 322.

A 92-Year-Old Man With History of Aortic Stenosis

Ryan Jones ■ Paul Neil Frank ■ Michael J. Jung

A 92-year-old man with history of aortic stenosis (AS) sustained a fracture of his right hip as a result of a ground-level fall. He thinks he tripped and fell but is not certain. He takes carvedilol daily. He has good exercise tolerance, saying he uses the exercise bicycle 30 min/day without difficulty. Vital signs show blood pressure 164/85 mm Hg, pulse 65/min, respirations 10/min, oxygen saturation 97% on 2 L/min nasal cannula, and temperature 35.9°C. On physical exam he is breathing comfortably. There is a harsh systolic murmur on auscultation of the chest. Lungs sounds are clear.

What are the possible causes of the fall for this patient? How might they affect your anesthetic management?

Etiologies of a ground-level fall can be divided into mechanical and nonmechanical mechanisms. Mechanical falls are caused by external forces or objects that lead to slipping or tripping. These types of falls are more common in the elderly because they often have impaired vision, balance, stability, and coordination compared with younger individuals. A nonmechanical fall is due to a patient factor such as a stroke, seizure, arrhythmia, heart attack, drug reaction, orthostasis, cardiac valvular lesion, pulmonary embolism, or hypoglycemia. It is important to obtain a detailed history and thoroughly work up an elderly patient after a fall to understand the reason for the fall. The reason for the fall can affect anesthetic management and can identify factors that may be optimized prior to surgery.

What physiologic changes occur with normal aging?

Table 3.1 shows common physiologic changes associated with normal aging.

The patient is having a lot of pain. What regional anesthetic options can you offer him?

Several types of anesthesia can be used in this patient to provide adequate perioperative analgesia. Aside from pharmacologic agents, epidural and regional anesthesia are both techniques that can be used for hip fracture patients. In particular, a femoral nerve block or fascia iliaca nerve block would be helpful regional anesthetic options for this patient.

What nerves are anesthetized by a femoral nerve block? What territory does this block cover?

The femoral nerve block anesthetizes the branches of the femoral nerve, including the anterior femoral cutaneous nerves and the saphenous nerve. This provides anesthesia to the anterior thigh and medial calf.

What are the functions of the femoral nerve? What nerve roots contribute to it?

The femoral nerve is derived from the anterior rami of the L2, L3, and L4 spinal nerves. It provides motor innervation to the muscles of the anterior thigh and sensation to the anterior thigh and medial leg below the knee.

TABLE 3.1 ■ Physiologic Changes Associated With Normal Aging

Neurologic
- Decreased executive function, processing speed, memory, and maintenance of circadian rhythm.
- Increased sensitivity to anesthetic agents. Minimum alveolar concentration (MAC) of anesthetic gas decreases by 6% per decade of age beyond age 40 years.
- Elevated risk of postoperative cognitive dysfunction and delirium.
- Impairment in hearing, vision, and balance.

Cardiovascular
- Calcification and stiffening of blood vessels lead to widened pulse pressure and increased afterload.
- Although systolic cardiac function is usually preserved, diastolic dysfunction becomes more common. These patients are more dependent on adequate preload and the atrial contraction to maintain stroke volume.
- Lower maximum heart rate.
- Decreased sensitivity to β-adrenergic receptor stimulation.
- Attenuated baroreceptor reflex.

Respiratory
- Attenuated responses to hypoxia and hypercapnia.
- Weakened diaphragm and degeneration of joints of chest wall (e.g., costovertebral joints) cause increased work of breathing.
- Emphysematous changes lead to increased closing capacity.
- Weakened pharyngeal muscles and decreased mucociliary transport increase the risk of aspiration and pneumonia.

Renal
- Decreased glomerular filtration rate. This slows the metabolism and elimination of drugs.
- Blunted responses to aldosterone, vasopressin, and renin decrease the ability to adjust to changes in volume or acid-base status.

Hepatic/Gastrointestinal
- Although synthetic function is preserved, hepatic blood flow is decreased, resulting in slower metabolism of drugs.
- Decreased incidence of postoperative nausea and vomiting (PONV).

Musculoskeletal
- Muscle mass decreases by 1% per year, but strength decreases by 3% per year.
- Decreased subcutaneous fat makes temperature regulation more difficult.

What nerves are anesthetized by a fascia iliaca nerve block? What territory does it cover?
The fascia iliaca nerve block anesthetizes the femoral nerve and the lateral femoral cutaneous nerve. This provides analgesia to the anterior and lateral thigh.

What is the function of the lateral femoral cutaneous nerve? What nerve roots contribute to it?
The lateral femoral cutaneous nerve, also known as the lateral cutaneous nerve of the thigh, is a sensory branch of the lumbar plexus that is derived from the L2 and L3 spinal nerves.

Describe the anatomy relevant to a fascia iliaca nerve block.
The fascia iliaca lies on the anterior surface of the iliacus muscle. It is bound superolaterally by the iliac crest and merges medially with the fascia overlying the psoas muscle. Both the femoral and lateral cutaneous nerves of the thigh lie under the fascia iliaca (see Fig. 3.1).

The surgeon is not as familiar with the fascia iliaca nerve block and asks if the patient can be up and walking without assistance right after surgery.

Both the femoral nerve block and fascia iliaca nerve block are likely to cause quadriceps muscle weakness, which can make early mobilization difficult. Patients should be advised

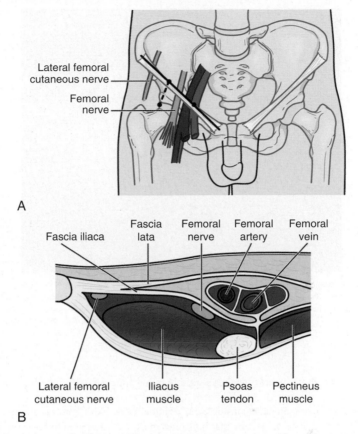

Fig. 3.1 (A) Coronal anatomic diagram of the lateral femoral cutaneous and femoral nerves as they course from the pelvis to the thigh. (B) Axial anatomic diagram showing lateral femoral cutaneous and femoral nerves coursing deep to fascia iliaca and above the iliacus muscle. (Kelly, J. J., & Younga, J. [2018]. Regional anesthesia of the thorax and extremities. In J. R. Roberts, C. B. Custalow & T. W. Thomsen [Eds.], *Roberts and Hedges' clinical procedures in emergency medicine and acute care* [7th ed., Chapter 31, pp. 560–587.e1] Fig. 31.16.)

of this temporary leg weakness, and they should be monitored and assisted with movement when the block is in effect.

How is a fascia iliaca block performed?

Position the patient supine. Place the ultrasound probe at the level of the inguinal crease oriented parallel to the inguinal crease. Immediately lateral and deep to the femoral artery and vein is the iliacus muscle. It is covered by a hyperechoic fascia, which can be seen separating the muscle from the subcutaneous soft tissue (see Fig. 3.2). The hyperechoic femoral nerve should be seen between the iliopsoas muscle and the fascia iliaca, lateral to the femoral artery. The fascia lata (superficial in the subcutaneous layer) is more superficial and may have more than one layer.

This block is typically performed distal to the inguinal ligament with a 5- to 7-cm needle and a linear transducer in the long axis approach from lateral to medial. It is important to identify the femoral artery, femoral vein, femoral nerve, iliopsoas muscles, and fascia lata on ultrasound. Classically, two "pops" can be felt as the needle advances through the fascia lata and the fascia iliaca, respectively. The local anesthetic is deposited just deep to the fascia iliaca. An alternative

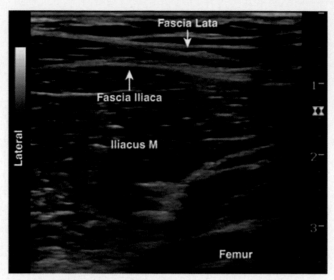

Fig. 3.2 Ultrasonographic image of the anterior thigh showing the fascia lata, fascia iliaca, and the iliacus muscle. The lateral femoral cutaneous and femoral nerves course deep to the fascia iliaca. (From Shastri, U., Kwofie, K., Salviz, E., & Xu, D. [2022]. Lower extremity nerve blocks. In H. T. Benzon, J. P. Rathmell, C. L. We, D. C. Turk, C. E. Argoff, R. W. Hurley et al. [Eds.], *Practical management of pain* [pp. 732–744.e2]. Philadelphia, PA: Elsevier. Modified from Fig. 54.11.)

approach to the fascia iliaca nerve block is a suprainguinal approach with the ultrasound probe in a sagittal position.

The fascia iliaca nerve block is considered a "volume block," so it requires a larger volume of lower concentration of local anesthetic that infiltrates more area compared to other blocks. It relies on a volume of 20–40 mL of local anesthetic to accomplish the block.

What is the pathophysiology of aortic stenosis?

Aortic stenosis (AS) is a common cardiac valvular lesion, particularly in the elderly. Endothelial dysfunction, lipid deposition, and oxidative stress lead to fibrosis and calcification of the leaflets of the aortic valve, ultimately resulting in reduced opening of the valve during systole. This is analogous to the pathologic processes that lead to atherosclerosis.

The hemodynamic consequences of AS arise from the decreased aortic valve orifice, which increases the resistance to the ejection of blood from the left ventricle into the aortic root (i.e., increased afterload). The left ventricle must generate increased pressure during systole to overcome this resistance.

Over time, this leads to thickening (i.e., hypertrophy) of the left ventricle, which can also lead to diastolic dysfunction.

You are about to review the report from the patient's transthoracic echocardiogram from last week.

What do you want to know?

You want to know the severity of the patient's AS. You also want to know about the patient's left and right ventricular function and whether there are any other significant valvular lesions.

TABLE 3.2 ■ **Although There Are Many Ways to Describe the Severity of Aortic Stenosis, Three of the Most Common are Valve Area, Mean Gradient, and Peak Velocity**

	Valve Area (cm²)	Mean Gradient (mm Hg)	Peak Velocity (m/s)
Mild	>1.5	<20	<3
Moderate	1–1.5	20–40	3–4
Severe	<1	>40	>4

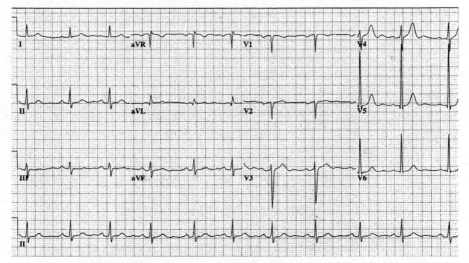

Fig. 3.3   Electrocardiogram (ECG) showing normal sinus rhythm and left ventricular hypertrophy (notice tall QRS complexes in leads V5). (Ofman, P., Cook, R. J., Navaravong L, Levine, R. A., Peralta, A., Gaziano, J. M., et al. [2012]. T-wave inversion and diastolic dysfunction in patients with electrocardiographic left ventricular hypertrophy. *Journal of Electrocardiology, 45*[6], 764–769. Fig. 1.)

The echocardiogram report shows normal biventricular function. There is significant concentric left ventricular hypertrophy. The aortic valve area is 0.7 Cm², and the mean gradient across the aortic valve is 50 mm Hg.

What does that mean?
This patient meets criteria for severe AS. The criteria for grading the severity of AS are listed in Table 3.2.

You order a 12-lead electrocardiogram (ECG). The result is shown in Fig. 3.3.

How do you interpret this?
This ECG is notable for left ventricular hypertrophy, which is an expected finding in patients with AS. The left ventricular myocardium is constantly working hard (i.e., exercising) to generate enough systolic pressure to eject against the stenotic aortic valve. Over time, this muscle hypertrophies.

After a discussion with the patient and cardiologist, the decision is made to proceed with repair of the hip fracture prior to any intervention for the aortic valve. The surgeon asks if the case can be done under spinal anesthesia.

Spinal anesthesia is not the best option in patients with AS. Patients with AS have a thick myocardium that requires a high perfusion pressure during diastole, when the left ventricle is perfused. Spinal anesthesia causes rapid and profound loss of vascular tone at and below the level of the spinal injection. This reduces the pressure driving blood through the coronary arteries during diastole. In addition, patients with AS require adequate preload to fill the thick noncompliant ventricle. Loss of vascular tone from a spinal anesthetic will reduce venous return to the heart.

Slowly dosing an epidural catheter may be a safer option for neuraxial anesthesia, resulting in less rapid and less profound drop in vascular tone, and this may be better tolerated.

You plan for preoperative fascia iliaca block and then general anesthesia with endotracheal intubation.

How will you induce anesthesia?

Important anesthetic considerations in patients with AS include maintaining normal sinus rhythm, avoiding bradycardia or tachycardia, avoiding hypotension, and optimizing intravascular fluid to maintain left ventricular filling.

It is advisable to place an arterial line prior to the start of induction to allow for continuous blood pressure monitoring. Induction can be accomplished using opioids, benzodiazepines, and traditional hypnotic agents such as propofol, etomidate, or barbiturates. Regardless of the specific induction agent or agents that are used, the key is to go slowly. Start with small doses of induction agents and allow time for them to circulate because patients with cardiac disease may have slower cardiac output.

After administration of fentanyl 100 mcg and propofol 50 mg, the patient's blood pressure is 70/40 mm Hg.

What should you do?

Hypotension is not well tolerated in patients with severe AS. Remember, modern anesthetic drugs drop blood pressure by causing vasodilation. Therefore hypotension should be treated judiciously with a vasopressor such as phenylephrine or norepinephrine. A bolus of fluid to increase intravascular volume will also be helpful.

The patient's blood pressure normalizes, and the operation proceeds uneventfully. In the recovery room, the patient is agitated and confused.

What should you do?

Postoperative delirium is a well-known complication of anesthesia in elderly patients. Common etiologies include uncontrolled pain, hypoxia, infection, electrolyte abnormalities (including hypoglycemia), urinary retention, constipation, and medication side effects.

Management of postoperative delirium entails frequent verbal reorientation, allowing patients to wear their glasses and/or hearing aids, and correcting any of the possible etiologies listed above.

It is also important to maintain a calm environment and limit lines, tubes, drains, and restraints as much as possible. If pharmacologic treatment is necessary, a low dose of haloperidol or an atypical antipsychotic (e.g., risperidone, quetiapine) should be used.

What medications may have contributed to this patient's delirium?
Anticholinergic drugs (e.g., diphenhydramine, scopolamine), benzodiazepines, and meperidine may contribute to postoperative cognitive dysfunction. Opioid analgesics should be used in the lowest possible dose.

BEYOND THE PEARLS

- The normal aortic valve has three cusps. Patients born with an aortic valve with only two cusps are said to have a bicuspid aortic valve (BAV), and they are at increased risk of developing AS and aortic insufficiency.
- Cardiopulmonary resuscitation (CPR) may be less successful in patients with AS due to inability to create stroke volume across stenosis aortic valve during chest compressions.
- In AS, prognosis is determined by symptoms. Findings that portend a survival of 5 years or less include angina, syncope, and congestive heart failure.
- Even in asymptomatic patients, aortic valve replacement may be performed for risk reduction prior to high-risk noncardiac surgery.
- Postoperative delirium can occur up to 5 days after surgery.
- Risk factors for postoperative delirium include age greater than 65 years, preoperative cognitive impairment, severe comorbidities, hearing or vision impairment, and infection.
- Some elderly patients have do-not-resuscitate orders or have designated a surrogate decision-maker. The patient's wishes should be clarified with the patient and family, surgeon, and anesthesiologist prior to surgery.

References

Bavry, A. A., & Arnaoutakis, G. J. (2021). Perspective to 2020 American College of Cardiology/American Heart Association (ACC/AHA) guideline for the management of patients with valvular heart disease. *Circulation, 143,* 407–409.

Berger, A., Acker, L., & Deiner, S. (2019). Geriatric anesthesia. In R. D. Miller (Ed.), *Miller's anesthesia* (9th ed., pp. 2102–2114). Philadelphia, PA: Churchill Livingstone, Elsevier.

A 40-Year-Old Female With a Past Medical History of Well-Controlled Type 2 Diabetes Mellitus

Shane McGuire ■ Michael J. Jung ■ Paul Neil Frank

A 40-year-old female with a past medical history of well-controlled type 2 diabetes mellitus and obesity (body mass index of 32 kg/m²) presents for left-sided carpal tunnel release. Approximately 8 months ago, she started experiencing pain in her left hand, mostly the first 3 digits, that would intermittently wake her up from sleep. Nerve conduction studies were performed, and the diagnosis of carpal tunnel syndrome was confirmed. Nonsurgical management, including splinting and steroid injections, failed, and she will now undergo surgical intervention. In the preoperative holding area, her vital signs are blood pressure 134/78 mm Hg, pulse 82/min, respiration rate 10/min, oxygen saturation 99% on room air, temperature 36.3°C.

What is the carpal tunnel?

The carpal tunnel is located on the volar surface of the wrist and is formed by the flexor retinaculum and the carpal bones (Fig. 4.1). The flexor retinaculum is composed of three parts: fascia continuous with the volar antebrachial fascia, the transverse carpal ligament proper, and the fibrous structure between the thenar and hypothenar eminences.

What structures course through the carpal tunnel?

The nine flexor tendons of the forearm muscles as well as the median nerve course through the carpal tunnel.

What is carpal tunnel syndrome?

Carpal tunnel syndrome is a form of entrapment or compressive neuropathy. Entrapment or compression of the median nerve within the carpal tunnel results in the characteristic pain, numbness, and/or tingling within the first three digits and the lateral side of the fourth digit (see Fig. 4.2).

The cause of carpal tunnel syndrome is multifactorial and can include tenosynovial proliferation, arthritic deformity, and fluid collection or edema. Risk factors include diabetes, hypothyroidism, trauma, and rheumatoid arthritis. Flexion and extension of the wrist can increase the compressive pressure on the median nerve in the carpal tunnel.

STEP 1 PEARL

Maneuvers/tests used to clinically diagnose carpal tunnel syndrome include:
- Tinel test: tapping over carpal tunnel irritates the compressed median nerve, reproducing pain and paresthesia in the median nerve distribution.
- Phalen maneuver: patient places dorsum of hands together ("reverse prayer"), which causes wrist flexion and, when held for 30–60 seconds, can reproduce symptoms.

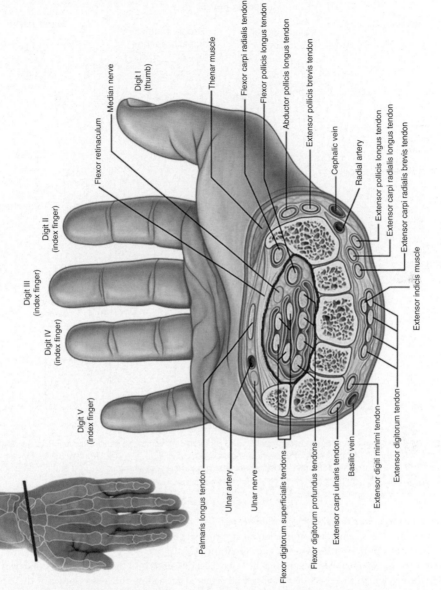

Fig. 4.1 Transverse section of wrist showing the carpal tunnel (outlined in *red*) containing the flexor tendons of the forearm and the median nerve. (Drake, R. L., Vogl, A. W. & Mitchell, A. W. M. [2021]. Upper limb. In *Gray's Atlas of Anatomy* [3rd ed.] Modified. Pages 385–476. Philadelphia, PA: Elsevier.)

- Carpal compression test: operator places thumbs over patient's carpal tunnel and applies firm and constant pressure for approximately 30 seconds, which reproduces symptoms in median nerve distribution.
- Hand elevation test: patient raises both hands above head and holds for 2 minutes; reproduction of pain or paresthesia in median nerve distribution is a positive test.

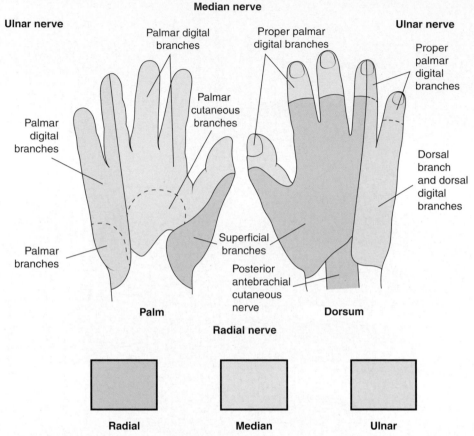

Fig. 4.2 Sensory distribution of the ulnar, median, and radial nerves within the hand. (Reavey, P. L. & Rafijah, G. [2017]. Anatomy & examination of the hand, wrist, forearm, and elbow. In T. E. Trumble, G. M. Rayan, J. E. Budoff, M. E. Baratz & D. J. Slutsky [Eds.], *Principles of hand surgery and therapy* [3rd ed.]. Philadelphia, PA: Elsevier. Figure E1.39.)

What is the origin and course of the median nerve?

The median nerve originates from the lateral and medial cords of the brachial plexus and receives contribution from nerve roots C6–T1 and sometimes C5.

After the median nerve leaves the brachial plexus, it descends into the arm accompanied by the axillary artery, which then becomes the brachial artery after passing the lower border of the teres major muscle. As shown in Fig. 4.3, the median nerve continues distally, coursing in the medial aspect of the upper arm as it passes through the cubital fossa.

Once in the forearm, the nerve passes between the two heads of the pronator teres muscle, then courses between the flexor digitorum profundus and flexor digitorum superficialis before entering the carpal tunnel to reach the hand.

What is the brachial plexus? Why is it important to an anesthesiologist?

The brachial plexus is a collection of nerves originating in ventral rami of C5–T1 nerve roots. These roots come together to form trunks as they pass between the anterior and middle scalene muscles. After entering the axilla under the clavicle, the trunks separate to create divisions and

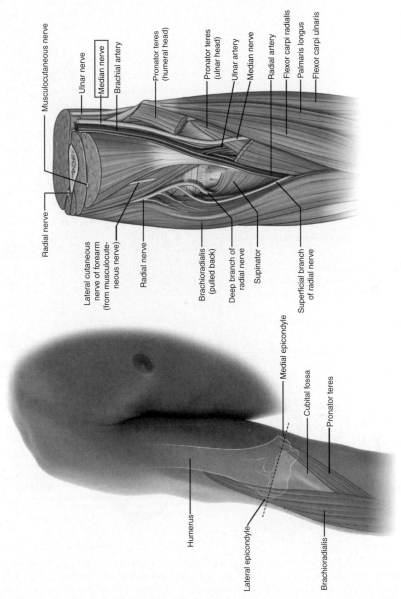

Fig. 4.3 Course of the median nerve through the upper extremity. Care must be taken when placing an intravenous catheter into the cubital fossa as injury to the median nerve can occur. (*Gray's atlas of anatomy* [3rd ed.]. Upper limb, cubital fossa. Modified. Pages 385–476.)

then recombine again to create cords adjacent to the axillary artery. The cords of the brachial plexus then divide into the terminal branches (musculocutaneous, axillary, radial, median, and ulnar nerves) that provide motor and sensory function to the arm. Fig. 4.4 illustrates the path taken by the nerves of the upper extremity from their origin in the cervical and thoracic spine. Knowledge of this anatomic pathway allows the anesthesiologist to selectively anesthetize specific parts of the upper extremity using targeted injections of local anesthetics (see Case 1).

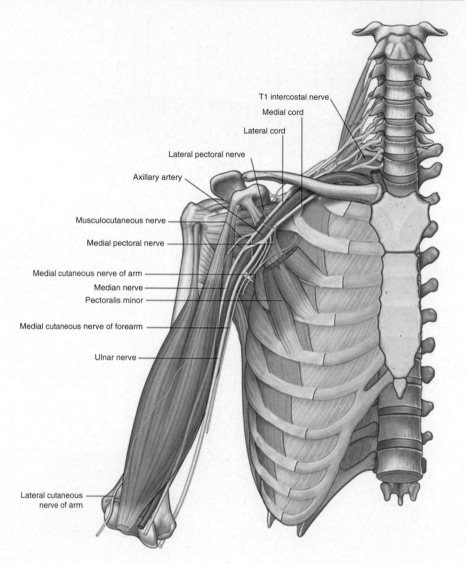

Fig. 4.4 The nerves of the upper extremity originate in the cervical and thoracic spine as the brachial plexus, passing deep to the clavicle and into the axilla as they extend distally towards the hand. (Drake, R. L., Vogl, A. W. & Mitchell, A. W. M. [2021]. Upper limb. In *Gray's atlas of anatomy* [3rd ed., pp. 385–476.]. Philadelphia, PA: Elsevier.)

STEP 1 PEARL

The sections of the brachial plexus are roots, trunks, divisions, cords, and branches oriented in a medial (i.e., proximal) to lateral (i.e., distal) fashion (see Fig. 4.5).

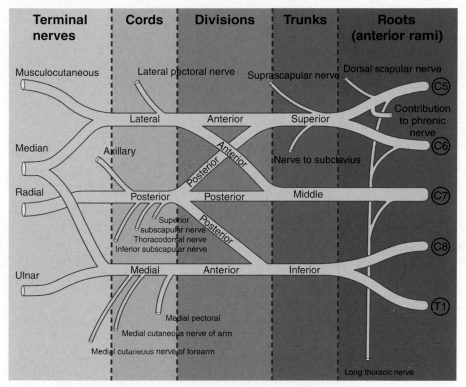

Fig. 4.5 Diagram of the brachial plexus and its associated roots, trunks, divisions, cords, and terminal branches. (Drake, R. L., Vogl, A. W. & Mitchell, A. W. M. [2021]. Upper limb. In *Gray's atlas of anatomy* [3rd ed., pp. 385–476]. Philadelphia, PA: Elsevier.)

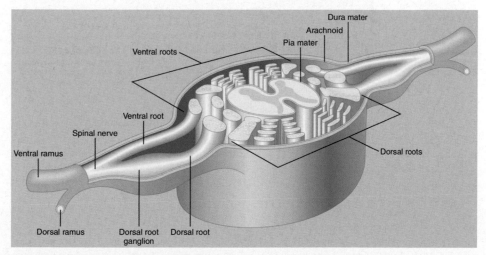

Fig. 4.6 The spinal cord and nerve roots which ultimately divide into ventral and dorsal rami. (*Miller's basics of anesthesia* [6th ed.]. Figure 17-10, page. 258.)

STEP 1 PEARL

Each nerve root is composed of a ventral and dorsal component. Motor neurons are carried through the ventral root, while sensory neurons are carried in the dorsal root. These roots combine to form spinal nerves which branch into ventral and dorsal rami (see Fig. 4.6). The ventral rami supply motor and sensory function to the anterolateral aspect of the body, while the dorsal rami supply the posterior regions of the body.

STEP 1 PEARL

Although there are only seven cervical vertebrae, there are eight nerve roots (C1–C8). In the cervical spine, the nerve roots exit *above* the corresponding vertebrae (e.g., the C2 nerve root exits the spine above the C2 vertebra). There is no C8 vertebra, and the C8 nerve root exits below the C7 vertebra. In the thoracic spine and below, all nerve roots will exit the spinal cord *below* their corresponding vertebrae.

What is the function of the median nerve?

In the forearm, the median nerve provides motor innervation to most of the muscles responsible for forearm flexion and pronation as well as the muscles responsible for wrist flexion and abduction. Some of the tendons of these flexor muscles continue into the hand and assist with finger flexion, particularly of the first three digits. The median nerve also provides most of the sensation on the palmar aspect of the hand (first three digits and the lateral side of the fourth, see Fig. 4.2).

STEP 1 PEARL

The last branch of the median nerve is the palmar cutaneous branch, which arises proximal to, and travels over, the flexor retinaculum to provide sensation to the thenar eminence. This branch does not travel through the carpal tunnel. This means that the thenar eminence will be spared the symptoms of carpal tunnel syndrome.

What is a carpal tunnel release?

Carpal tunnel release is the most commonly performed procedure in hand surgery. The procedure consists of the transection of the carpal ligament and may be performed either open or endoscopically. The procedure may be performed with a tourniquet in place and lasts approximately 30–90 minutes.

What are the anesthetic options for this patient?

Given the relatively localized incision site and short duration of the procedure, one option for carpal tunnel release is simply local anesthetic injected at the surgical site, although this will not prevent or treat pain from the tourniquet. Other options include intravenous regional anesthesia (IVRA; i.e., Bier block), particularly for procedures less than 60 minutes, and peripheral nerve blocks for longer procedures. In the event that a patient is not able to tolerate any of these techniques, general anesthesia is always an option.

What is a Bier block and how is it performed?

A Bier block entails intravenous injection of relatively large volumes of local anesthetic (commonly 50 mL of 0.5% lidocaine or 30 mL if using a forearm cuff) into the involved extremity after it has been exsanguinated and a tourniquet inflated. This technique provides anesthesia to the entire limb distal to the tourniquet and is an alternative to performing a nerve block. It is believed that local anesthetic reaches the nerves through the vascular beds, including the vasa nervorum and valveless venules, as well as diffusion through the tissues.

To perform a Bier block
1. Place intravenous access distal in the extremity (i.e., the dorsal hand). This intravenous catheter will be used for injection of local anesthetic, but it will not be used for anything else. Therefore you must place another intravenous catheter somewhere else not on the operative extremity.
2. Place one or two tourniquets proximally (usually over the biceps), but do not inflate yet.
3. Elevate the arm to allow passive blood flow out of the arm.
4. Wrap an Esmarch bandage tightly in a spiral fashion around the extremity, starting distally and advancing proximally (i.e., starting at the hand and moving toward the shoulder).
5. Inflate the proximal tourniquet (i.e., the one closer to the shoulder) to 250–275 mm Hg, approximately 100 mm Hg greater than the patient's systolic blood pressure.
6. Administer local anesthetic via the intravenous catheter in the distal extremity, and then remove that intravenous catheter.

How do local anesthetics work?
Local anesthetics inhibit neuronal firing by blocking voltage-gated sodium channels on neurons. These molecules are weak bases that can be positively charged or neutral, depending on the pKa of the local anesthetic and the pH of the environment (see Fig. 4.7). In the neutral state, they diffuse across the hydrophobic neuronal membrane. Once inside the neuron, the charged form reversibly binds to the intracellular surface of the sodium channel.

STEP 1 PEARL

At rest, the neuron maintains a voltage difference of −60 to −90 mV relative to the extracellular environment. Potassium ion channels in the cell membrane are open in the resting state, whereas sodium ion channels are not. Sodium/potassium pumps in the cell membrane, known as Na^+/K^+-ATPase, pump sodium out of the cell and take potassium into the cell. Because the potassium channels are open at rest, potassium passively flows back across the membrane out of the cell. The net effect is to create both concentration and electrical gradients that would drive sodium from outside the cell into the cell.

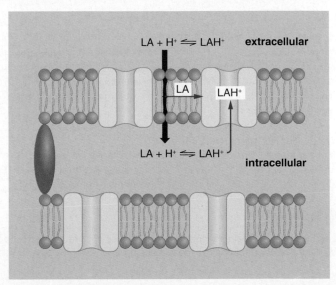

Fig. 4.7 Only the uncharged form of the local anesthetic can diffuse across the nerve sheath and membrane. Once intracellular, it will become charged. It is the charged form of the local anesthetic that will then block the sodium channel and prevent propagation of an action potential. *LA*, Local anesthetic. (*Miller basics of anesthesia* [6th ed.]. Modified from Fig 11-4.)

When an action potential raises the membrane voltage to +20 mV (i.e., the threshold potential), voltage-gated sodium channels in the cell membrane open, thereby allowing extracellular sodium to enter the cell. This changes the membrane potential from negative at baseline to positive during depolarization. These voltage-gated sodium channels then become temporarily inactivated and close quickly, and intracellular potassium leaves the cell via passive diffusion. This reestablishes the negative membrane potential.

Three minutes after your Bier block is placed, the surgeon is called away to an emergent procedure.

Because the case is canceled, can you deflate the tourniquet now?

No, release of the tourniquet so soon after injection of a large amount of local anesthetic can lead to local anesthetic systemic toxicity (LAST; see shoulder replacement chapter).

Too much local anesthetic can be detrimental to a patient, and in this case, early release of the tourniquet would likely lead to toxic amounts of the local anesthetic being released into systemic circulation.

What do you do because surgery has been canceled within minutes of application of the Bier block?

Local anesthetic serum levels peak 2–5 minutes after a tourniquet has been deflated. Keep the tourniquet inflated for at least 20 minutes after injection of local anesthetic. This may be enough time for some local anesthetic to leave the intravascular space. After 20 minutes, the local anesthetic can be "leaked" back into the circulation by deflating and then immediately reinflating the tourniquet, and then deflating one last time after 1 minute after the reinflation. If 40 minutes has elapsed since injection of local anesthetic, the tourniquet can be safely deflated without need for "leaking."

The surgery is rescheduled for tomorrow. The next day, a Bier block is applied and the surgery proceeds. After 45 minutes, the patient complains of severe pain in her left upper arm.

What's going on?

The tourniquet can be extremely painful. This type of pain is relatively resistant to local anesthesia, and even intravenous opiates may not successfully relieve the pain. It is hypothesized that the pain signals from the stimulus of the tourniquet are carried by unmyelinated, slow-conduction C fibers. Inflate the distal tourniquet and deflate the proximal tourniquet (this is why two tourniquets should be placed prior to Bier block). In cases in which tourniquet pain persists, conversion to a general anesthetic may be necessary.

Can anything else be done to prevent tourniquet pain?

Regional block of the intercostobrachial nerve preoperatively may be helpful. The tourniquet will usually be positioned across the C5, T1, and T2 dermatomes (see Fig. 4.8). The T2 dermatome (and occasionally the T1 dermatome) is supplied by the intercostobrachial nerve.

BEYOND THE PEARLS

- Care must be taken when placing an intravenous catheter into the cubital fossa because there is increased risk of damaging the median nerve, which courses superficially through the fossa.

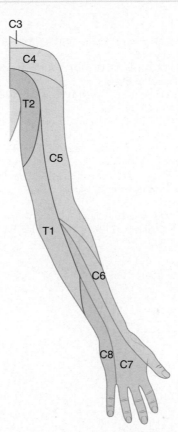

Fig. 4.8 Dermatomes of the upper limb. (*Gray's anatomy for students* [4th ed.]. Figure 7.15. Pages 671–821.)

- There are 2 chemical groups of local anesthetics: aminoesters and aminoamides. Aminoesters are metabolized by plasma esterases, whereas aminoamides are metabolized by the liver. Aminoester local anesthetics are more likely to cause allergic reactions than aminoamide local anesthetics. Patients who are allergic to one class of local anesthetic can safely receive the other.
- Preservatives such as methylparaben used with local anesthetics can cause allergic reactions.
- Local anesthetics bind sodium channels in the open and inactivated states more avidly than they bind sodium channels in the resting state.
- In an acidic environment (i.e., where the pH is low), the local anesthetic will remain in its positively charged form, so it will not diffuse across the neural cell membrane as readily. Therefore local anesthetics are less effective when injected into acidic environments, such as injection over an abscess prior to incision and drainage. Bicarbonate, a base, may be added to a solution of local anesthetic to increase its effectiveness by raising the pH of solution, thereby increasing the fraction of molecules that exist in the neutral form.
- The "thumbs up" sign with the left hand, looks like a 6 and is an easy way to remember that the C6 dermatome covers the thumb.

References

Collins, A., & Gray A. (2011). Peripheral nerve blocks. In R. D. Miller (Ed.), *Basics of anesthesia* (6th ed., pp. 287–298). Philadelphia, PA: Elsevier.

Drake. (2018). Head and neck. In R. L. Drake, A. W. Vogl & A. W. M. Mitchell (Eds.), *Gray's basic anatomy* (2nd ed., pp. 413–596). Philadelphia, PA: Elsevier.

Drake. (2020). Upper limb. In R. L. Drake, A. W. Vogl & A. W. M. Mitchell (Eds.), *Gray's anatomy for students* (4th ed., pp. 671–821). Philadelphia, PA: Elsevier.

Drasner, K. Local anesthetics. In R. D. Miller (Ed.), *Basics of anesthesia* (6th ed., pp. 130–141). Philadelphia, PA: Elsevier.

Drasner, K., & Larson, M. (2011). Spinal and epidural anesthesia. In R. D. Miller (Ed.), *Basics of anesthesia* (6th ed., pp. 257–258). Philadelphia, PA: Elsevier.

Fox, P. M., Curtin, C., Hentz, V. R., & Vokach-Brodsky, L. (2019). Hand surgery. In R. A. Jaffe, C. A. Schmiesing & B. Golianu (Eds.), *Anesthesiologist's manual of surgical procedures* (6th ed., pp. 1027–1058). Philadelphia, PA: Wolters Kluwer.

Pasternak, J., & Lanier, W. (2017). Diseases of the autonomic and peripheral nervous systems. In *Stoelting's anesthesia and co-existing disease* (7th ed., pp. 315–325). Philadelphia, PA: Elsevier.

Pediatrics

A 5-Year-Old Boy Undergoing Repair of a Hydrocele

Paul Neil Frank ■ Elizabeth C. Fung ■ Robert Scott Kriss

A 5-year-old boy is undergoing repair of a hydrocele. He is otherwise healthy.

What are the anesthetic options for this patient?
This patient could have general anesthesia with endotracheal intubation or laryngeal mask airway (LMA). A caudal block or other regional block would be useful for controlling pain, reducing the depth of anesthesia required intraoperatively, and reducing the use of pain medication postoperatively.

STEP 1, 2 PEARL

A hydrocele is an accumulation of fluid in the tunica vaginalis that surrounds the testis. Hydroceles can be classified as either communicating or noncommunicating. A communicating hydrocele is caused by persistent drainage of peritoneal fluid through a patent processus vaginalis. A congenital hydrocele (as seen in this patient) is a communicating hydrocele caused by failure of the processus vaginalis to close during development (see Fig. 5.1). A noncommunicating hydrocele does not have a connection with the peritoneal cavity and is secondary to an underlying cause such as trauma, infection, testicular torsion, or a tumor. Clinically, hydroceles present as a fluctuant, painless swelling of the scrotum. Hydroceles will transilluminate (i.e., shine a light through it, and it will light up), which is an important distinguishing factor from testicular tumors and varicoceles.

STEP 2 PEARL

Incomplete closure of the processus vaginalis predisposes patients to hydroceles and indirect inguinal hernias (see Fig. 5.1).

STEP 2 PEARL

Congenital hydroceles usually resolve by 6 months of age. If spontaneous resolution of the hydrocele does not occur by 1 year of age, then surgical intervention can be considered.

STEP 2 PEARL

In addition to hydrocele, varicocele is also on the differential diagnosis of painless scrotal swelling. Varicocele is caused by dilation of the pampiniform venous plexus. The left testicle is more commonly affected than the right because the right testicular vein drains into the inferior vena cava, whereas left testicular vein drains into the left renal vein, which has higher pressure than the inferior vena cava.

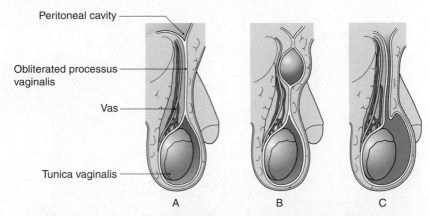

Fig. 5.1 Sagittal sections of the male inguinal region. (A) Normal anatomy with obliterated processus vaginalis, (B) noncommunicating hydrocele, and (C) communicating hydrocele. (Modified from Rader, C., & Campbell, J. [2021]. Inguinal hernias and hydroceles. *Pediatric Gastrointestinal and Liver Disease, 52*, 555–558.e1. Fig 52.1.)

If you intubate this patient, what size endotracheal tube (ETT) is appropriate?
The formula for cuffed ETT size in pediatric patients is:

$$ETT\ size = [(age\ in\ years)/4] + 3.5$$

For this patient,

$$ETT\ size = 5/4 + 3.5 = size\ 4.5\ or\ 5.0\ mm\ cuffed\ ETT\ would\ be\ appropriate$$

What is a caudal block?
A caudal block is an epidural block that anesthetizes the lowest dermatomal levels for procedures below the umbilicus. The caudal block is preferred because of its high historical frequency and unparalleled safety. The child is typically placed in the lateral decubitus position (see Fig. 5.2), and the needle is placed through the sacral hiatus and the sacrococcygeal ligament into the sacral-epidural space (see Fig. 5.3). Once aspiration of the syringe is negative for cerebrospinal fluid (CSF) and blood, a test dose should be administered prior to injection of the entire dose of local anesthetic Ultrasound confirmation is becoming common (see Fig. 5.4).

What are the potential complications of a caudal block? What are the contraindications?
The risks and contraindications are the same as for epidural anesthesia. Risks include cardiac arrest from intravenous (IV), intrathecal, or intraosseous injection, hematoma, neural injury, and infection. Patients should be off anticoagulation and should not have infection or sacral dimpling (because this may indicate neural tube defect) in the area where the block will be performed. Of course the parent/guardian must consent to the procedure. Sacral catheters are an option for certain surgeries, and careful dressing is necessary because fecal contamination is more likely.

What other regional anesthesia options are available for surgeries below the umbilicus?
Ilioinguinal, iliohypogastric, scrotal, or transversus abdominis plane (TAP) blocks may also be helpful.

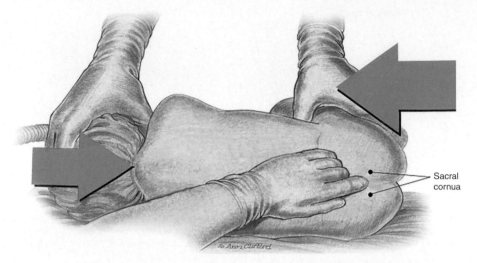

Sacral
cornua

Fig. 5.2   Patient positioning for placement of a caudal block. (Brown DL. [2021]. Caudal Block. In E. Farag, L. Mounir-Soliman, & D. L. Brown [Eds.], *Brown's atlas of regional anesthesia*. 42. 273–278. Philadelphia, PA: Elsevier. Fig 42.4.)

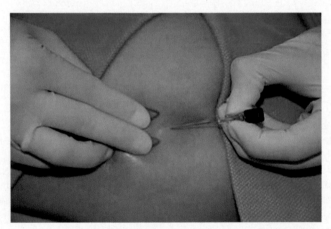

Fig. 5.3   The block needle or catheter is placed between the sacral cornua until a loss of resistance is felt. (Modified from Siddiqui A. [2007]. Caudal blockade in children. *Techniques in Regional Anesthesia and Pain Management, 11*(4), 203–207. Fig. 1.)

Shortly after the caudal injection, the patient becomes apneic.

What's going on?

This is concerning for high spinal or total spinal, a rare but potentially lethal complication of epidural anesthesia where local anesthetic is inadvertently injected into the intrathecal space. In children, apnea is often the first sign of total spinal, whereas adults will develop bradycardia and hypotension prior to apnea.

The patient requires intubation and mechanical ventilation. Treat bradycardia with atropine. Hypotension can be managed with fluids and vasopressors. He should be admitted to the intensive care unit for supportive care until the total spinal wears off.

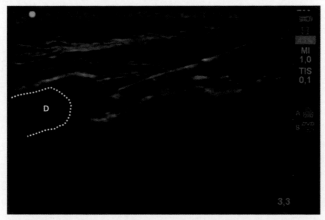

Fig. 5.4 Longitudinal ultrasonographic view of the sacral hiatus showing proper needle position. The distal end of the dural sac (D) is outlined. (Domingo-Rufes, T., Bong, D. A., Mayoral, V., et al. [2013]. Ultrasound-guided pain interventions in the pelvis and the sacral spine. *Techniques in Regional Anesthesia and Pain Management*. *17*[3], 107–130. Fig 19.)

STEP 2 PEARL

Although more common in children, high or total spinal anesthesia is one of the most common serious complications of obstetric anesthesia. High or total spinal anesthesia occurs when the anesthetic spreads cephalad and causes depression of the electrical activity of the brain stem and spinal cord. Early signs include ascending sympathetic, sensory, and motor block as well as hypotension, bradycardia, and apnea. Diaphragmatic paralysis and cardiopulmonary arrest may result.

The patient stabilizes and the case is rescheduled for the next week.

How will you induce this patient?

Placing an IV catheter in an awake and uncooperative 5-year-old will be challenging or impossible. The best option here is an inhaled induction following an effective preoperative preparation to reduce patient anxiety. This avoids the placement of an IV catheter in an awake patient.

Premedication with oral midazolam (0.5–1 mg/kg) 15–20 minutes prior to moving to the operating room (OR) is a common strategy. Evidence shows similar results with appropriate distraction techniques (i.e., electronics). Consultation with child life colleagues can be invaluable; parental presence should be considered. Planning and flexibility are key to a successful pediatric induction.

What are the best agents for inhaled induction?

An ideal agent for inhaled induction is one that is odorless, is nonirritating, provides cardiovascular stability, and will induce anesthesia very quickly. An agent with all of these characteristics does not exist, but sevoflurane is our best option. It is least irritating to the lungs, is least pungent, and results in stable hemodynamics with limited exposure at 8% inhaled concentration compared with other inhaled agents. It is often combined with nitrous oxide (N_2O), which allows for a fast inhaled induction. Thus sevoflurane with or without N_2O is a common method of inhaled induction following adequate anxiolysis to allow the child to enter the OR with minimal discomfort.

Why isn't N_2O used by itself for induction?

The minimum alveolar concentration (MAC) of N_2O is 104% in adults; a pediatric value is not known. In other words, assuming the anesthetic is occurring in a facility at or around sea level, an adult patient would have to breathe more than 100% N_2O, which would leave no room for oxygen, in order to achieve 1 MAC of anesthesia.

What is MAC?

MAC is the minimum alveolar concentration of an anesthetic gas such that 50% of patients receiving that concentration of gas do not move in response to a noxious stimulus (i.e., surgical incision). MAC varies with age. It is effectively a measure of the potency of an anesthetic gas: more potent gasses have lower MAC, and vice versa.

Unlike the MAC of desflurane or isoflurane, the MAC of sevoflurane does not decrease substantially with age—the MAC of sevoflurane is 3.3% at 6 months of age and 2.5% for older infants and children. Desflurane is rarely used in pediatric anesthesia because of increased airway reactivity and perceived emergence delirium.

MAC is expressed as a percentage of atmospheric pressure at sea level minus water vapor pressure (at sea level):

$$760 \text{ mm Hg} - 47 \text{ mm Hg} = 713 \text{ mm Hg}$$

However, what determines the depth of anesthesia is the partial pressure of a gas expressed in mm Hg, and not the concentration of gas expressed as a percentage. For example, the MAC of desflurane in older children is 6.6%, so the partial pressure of desflurane in the patient's lungs to achieve one MAC is

$$713 \text{ mm Hg} \times 0.066 = 47 \text{ mm Hg}$$

Considering N_2O, the MAC of 104% means that a partial pressure of

$$713 \times 1.04 = 742 \text{ mm Hg}$$

is required to achieve 1 MAC of N_2O.

Why does N_2O work quickly?

When N_2O is used, it is administered in concentrations up to 70%, with the other 30% oxygen, corresponding to an FiO_2 of 0.3. Although this is not enough to achieve 1 MAC of N_2O, this high delivered concentration causes the alveolar concentration of the gas to rise quickly, which allows for a faster inhaled induction. This is called the concentration effect.

STEP 2 PEARL

N_2O can be neurotoxic, especially in those who receive N_2O chronically and those who use it acutely but are deficient in vitamin B12. Vitamin B12 is a necessary coenzyme of methionine synthase. Nitrous oxide inactivates B12 by converting it from the active monovalent form to the inactive bivalent form. This subsequently inhibits methionine synthase, leading to the neurotoxic effects of nitrous oxide.

During induction, the patient, who had been calm, begins flailing. He is tachycardic and breathing irregularly. His eyes are dysconjugate.

What's going on? What should you do?

This is the excitement or hyperreflexic phase of anesthesia, sometimes known as "stage 2" and can be exaggerated with a gradual increase in the inspired concentration of sevoflurane on inhaled induction. Continue supporting the patient's breathing with gentle jaw support and minimal positive pressure if necessary. As the alveolar concentration of anesthesia gas increases, so will the depth of anesthesia. Increase the inspired concentration of sevoflurane as rapidly as possible to minimize the excitement phase and maintain the highest sevoflurane concentration tolerated until an IV catheter can be inserted. Loss of eyelash reflex and establishment of an IV catheter typically signals an appropriate depth of anesthesia for the surgeon and nurses to begin positioning, prepping, and draping patient for surgery.

The risk of laryngospasm is highest during the excitement phase. Avoid manipulating the airway (e.g., suctioning, laryngoscopy, extubation, or nonessential contact) during this time.

The patient stops flailing, eyelash reflex is absent, an IV catheter is inserted, and vital signs are stable. An LMA is placed. The operation is uncomplicated. As the patient is waking up, you remove the LMA and place the ventilator mask over his face. There is no misting in the mask, and no end-tidal CO_2 on the ventilator, although the patient is making significant respiratory effort.

What's going on?
Ventilation is inadequate, likely due to upper airway obstruction from laryngospasm. This may have been triggered by removal of the LMA when the patient was still emerging, neither asleep nor awake (i.e., during stage 2). Call for assistance, increase the FiO_2 to 1.0, and apply gentle positive pressure (<20 cm H_2O) with the adjustable pressure-limiting (APL) valve of the breathing circuit. If the laryngospasm persists, try deepening the anesthetic with sevoflurane or an IV bolus of propofol.

What are the major components of an anesthesia breathing circuit?
The circle system is the most common anesthesia breathing circuit (see Fig. 5.5). It is designed to prevent rebreathing of exhaled carbon dioxide. Table 5.1 lists the major components of the anesthesia breathing circuit.

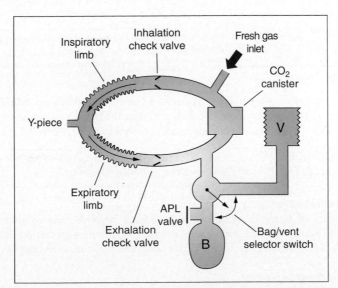

Fig. 5.5 The circle system showing the relative position of all major components. *APL*, adjustable pressure-limiting valve; *B*, reservoir bag; *V*, ventilator. (Roth P. [2018]. Anesthesia delivery systems. In M. C. Pardo, & R. D. Miller [Eds.], *Basics of anesthesia*. [7th ed., pp. 220–238]. Philadelphia, PA: Elsevier. Fig 15.9.)

TABLE 5.1 ■ The Components of the Circle System Each Play a Role in Maintaining Safe Ventilation

Component	Function
Fresh gas inlet	Fresh gas (usually a mixture of oxygen and air, sometimes with N_2O) enters the breathing circuit from the wall pipeline supply or E cylinders.
Unidirectional valves	One valve is in the inspiratory limb of the circuit, and one valve is in the expiratory limb of the circuit. These valves prevent rebreathing of exhaled gas. These also allow for positive pressure ventilation. Proper function of these valves ensures that the only dead space in the breathing circuit is distal to the Y connector.
Corrugated tubing	One length of tubing is in the inspiratory limb of the circuit, and one length of tubing is in the expiratory limb of the circuit. This tubing connects the anesthesia machine to the patient. This tubing is large caliber (i.e., low-resistance) and unlikely to kink.
Y connector	A connector between the patient (via endotracheal tube [ETT], laryngeal mask airway [LMA], or ventilator mask) and the inspiratory and expiratory limbs of the breathing circuit.
Adjustable pressure-limiting (APL) valve	The circle system can facilitate either mechanical or manual ventilation. In mechanical ventilation, the ventilator generates positive pressure during inhalation and releases that pressure during exhalation. In manual ventilation (or spontaneous ventilation), the APL valve controls the positive pressure that is generated in the circuit. When a patient is breathing spontaneously, the APL valve should be open to allow for easy exhalation. When the anesthesiologist is manually ventilating the patient by squeezing the reservoir bag, the APL valve should be adjusted to increase the positive pressure within the circuit.
Reservoir bag	This distensible bladder maintains a reservoir of fresh gas to satisfy the patient's spontaneous inspiratory flow rate. It also acts as a buffer to maintain a safe pressure in the breathing circuit <60 cm H_2O, even when the APL valve is closed.
CO_2 absorbent	Removes exhaled CO_2 from circuit before gas reaches inspiratory limb. Commonly based on calcium hydroxide.

After 45 seconds, there is still no fogging of the facemask. The oxygen saturation drops to 72%, and the heart rate drops from 110/min to 60/min.

Now what?

Once the patient becomes bradycardic, ventilation must be reestablished quickly to prevent hypoxic cardiac arrest. Administer succinylcholine to relax the muscles of the larynx and atropine to treat the bradycardia. Chest compressions are infrequently required to circulate the medications.

The laryngospasm resolves with succinylcholine. The patient wakes up uneventfully, but the pulse oximeter is reading SpO_2 88%, and he is coughing up pink frothy fluid.

What is the likely cause?

Given the history of recent laryngospasm, this is likely negative pressure pulmonary edema (NPPE). NPPE results when the patient tries to inhale against an upper airway obstruction and fluid extravasates into the lungs. In this case, that obstruction was caused by laryngospasm.

How should you treat this patient?

The treatment of NPPE is mainly supportive. Provide supplemental oxygen. Patients may benefit from continuous positive airway pressure (CPAP) or noninvasive positive pressure ventilation

(NIPPV). If the oxygen saturation continues to decrease or if work of breathing is significantly elevated, it may be necessary to intubate the patient. Some sources also suggest giving a dose of diuretic to these patients. This may be helpful if the patient is volume overloaded.

At the very least, this patient should be monitored closely in the recovery area for 6–12 hours.

The patient's mother asks if he can have a prescription for codeine for pain at home.

Is that a good choice for this patient?

Codeine is not a good choice for this patient. Codeine is a prodrug of morphine, meaning codeine must be metabolized into morphine to have an effect. There is significant genetic variability in the hepatic enzyme responsible for this metabolism, CYP 2D6. Therefore the peak effect, in terms of both analgesia *and respiratory depression*, depends on how quickly CYP 2D6 generates morphine from codeine.

Patients are generally categorized into three groups depending on the efficacy and speed of their CYP 2D6:

- Poor metabolizer: Codeine is not converted to morphine to a significant degree, or it is converted to morphine very slowly. These patients do not get an analgesic effect from codeine.
- Intermediate metabolizer: Codeine is converted to morphine such that the patient does get an analgesic effect and possibly some mild respiratory depression.
- Extensive or rapid metabolizers: Codeine is rapidly converted to morphine, as the name implies. This is analogous to giving an excessive dose of morphine to the patient. There is an analgesic effect but also significant respiratory depression, just as if a patient had received an overdose of morphine.

STEP 2 PEARL

Standard urine drug screen will detect natural opioids such as morphine, heroin, and codeine. However, a standard drug screen will not detect semisynthetic opioids (e.g., oxycodone, hydrocodone, hydromorphone) or synthetic opioids (e.g., tramadol, fentanyl, methadone).

BEYOND THE PEARLS

- Unrepaired hydrocele increases the risk of inguinal hernia.
- If the patient develops laryngospasm during inhaled induction, before an IV line has been placed, succinylcholine and atropine can be given intramuscularly. The full intramuscular dose of succinylcholine is 4 mg/kg, although a lower dose can frequently be used.
- Have succinylcholine and atropine in a syringe with a 22-gauge intramuscular needle ready to treat laryngospasm whenever caring for the child, as laryngospasm is common in children.
- The pink frothy fluid sometimes seen in NPPE is from extravasation of fluid from the pulmonary capillaries into the alveolar air spaces.

References

Hawksworth, D. J., Khera, M., & Herati, A. S. (2021). Surgery of the scrotum and seminal vesicles. In A. W. Partin, R. R. Dmochowski, L. R. Kavoussi, & C. A. Peters (Eds.), *Campbell-Walsh-Wein Urology* (12th ed. Chapter 83). Philadelphia, PA: Elsevier.

Roth, P. (2018). Anesthesia delivery systems. In M. C. Pardo, & R. D. Miller (Eds.), *Basics of Anesthesia*. (7th ed., pp. 220–238). Philadelphia, PA: Elsevier.

A 4-Year-Old Girl With Obstructive Sleep Apnea

Jeff Tully ■ Mark Murphy

A 4-year-old girl presents for a tonsillectomy and adenoidectomy (T+A) for obstructive sleep apnea (OSA) secondary to tonsillar hypertrophy. Her mother reports that the child had a heart murmur at birth and underwent open heart surgery at 6 months of age but cannot remember additional particulars, although all of her recent checkups with the cardiologist have been fine. The child is otherwise growing and developing appropriately, although her mother also mentions that 2 weeks ago the child had several days of rhinorrhea and a dry, nonproductive cough.

What are indications for pediatric T + A?

Tonsillectomy and/or adenoidectomy are one of the most common surgical procedures performed in children. Patients will usually present with a diagnosis of sleep disordered breathing such as OSA, recurrent tonsillitis, hypertrophy of the tonsils or adenoids, or some combination thereof. If the child is receiving treatment for sleep apnea, they may have a polysomnogram, which can provide additional information including the degree to which their oxygen level drops during sleep and how frequently episodes occur. This can give an indication as to the severity of the disease and the need for close postoperative monitoring. Less commonly, T+A may be performed in the setting of tonsillar asymmetry or abnormal growth to rule out a malignancy.

What else would you like to know about this patient?

The preoperative evaluation of a child is similar to that of the adult patient, with a few notable exceptions. A comprehensive review of the child's medical history is critical, as is an understanding of the child's current state of health. Information is almost never obtained directly from the child but instead from caregivers who may have varying degrees of medical literacy.

For most children, prenatal and birth histories join medical and surgical histories as key histories to review. With increasing advances in neonatology and maternal fetal medicine, premature infants of decreasing gestational age are surviving with increasingly positive outcomes. It is important to remember that, although a child may present for surgery at an age of, for example, 6 months, if they were born at 28 weeks' gestational age, that child has an adjusted age of 3 months (24 weeks of age minus 12 weeks of missed gestation). As many physiologic capabilities, including respiratory centers in the brain, liver metabolism, and renal function, progressively develop with age, it is important for the anesthesiologist to tailor the anesthetic appropriately.

Although most healthy children will not have the extensive problem lists or polypharmacy that characterize many adult patients, some pediatric patients will have complex care needs as a result of congenital or acquired disease. The parents or other caregivers of these children are often very involved with their medical care and are highly knowledgeable resources. Additional useful information may be found in notes from primary care providers. "Well child" exams detail important clinical, development, and social information at regular intervals as a child ages.

Family history is another key element of the preoperative work-up. Although a pediatric patient may have never had surgery or exposure to anesthesia before, it is critical to evaluate whether a condition such as malignant hyperthermia or congenital muscular dystrophy runs in the family so as to avoid a devastating intraoperative discovery. Parents may likewise report less significant reactions such as minor allergies or significant emergence delirium occurring in siblings or other family members.

Upon further review of the medical record and discussion with the child's mother, the child had a membranous ventricular septal defect (VSD) that was surgically repaired at 1 year of age. Since the operation, she has had no residual symptoms, and she no longer needs to see a cardiologist.

What information is important in a patient with congenital heart disease?
There is a wide spectrum of congenital heart disease with varying severity, treatments, and outcomes (see Case 8). Understanding the congenital defect, the surgical procedure(s) performed, and the resulting anatomy and physiology—whether fully corrected or still abnormal—is highly important. Documentation from the child's cardiologist and surgeon, related studies and imaging, and assessment from the parent as to the child's growth and function are all important.

STEP 1 PEARL

Fetal cardiac cells are derived embryologically from the mesoderm.

STEP 2, 3 PEARL

Administration of oxygen to some patients with unrepaired cyanotic congenital heart disease can be disastrous. Oxygen-induced pulmonary vasodilation can cause increased pulmonary blood flow, tipping the careful balance between pulmonary and systemic circulation and leading to acute right ventricular (or in the case of single ventricle physiology, ventricular) failure. Some patients with congenital heart disease may have baseline oxygen saturations between 75% and 85%. When in doubt, always check with the pediatric cardiologist when considering oxygen administration.

Does this child need antibiotics for endocarditis prophylaxis?
Certain surgical procedures (i.e., dental work, oral surgery, and surgery involving the gastrointestinal tract) may cause transient introduction of body flora into the bloodstream. This may increase the risk of developing endocarditis in some patients with congenital heart disease. The American Heart Association guidelines recommend antibiotic prophylaxis for the following patients:
- Patients with cyanotic congenital heart disease that has not been fully corrected.
- Patients who have undergone repair using prosthetic material or device within the past 6 months.
- Patients who have undergone repair of congenital heart disease with residual anatomic or physiologic abnormalities.

Given our patient's history of a VSD repair occurring more than 6 months ago with no residual issues requiring cardiology follow-up, she does not meet the criteria for antibiotic prophylaxis.

Given her recent upper respiratory infection (URI), is it safe for this child to undergo anesthesia?
Respiratory infections are common in the pediatric population, particularly in younger children and toddlers. Although lower respiratory tract infections resulting in pneumonia or bronchitis often result in children becoming sick enough to require medical attention, most parents will be

familiar with the otherwise playful and happy child afflicted by mild rhinorrhea or intermittent cough. The anesthesiologist caring for children scheduled for elective surgery will often be presented with the dilemma of the patient who recently demonstrated symptoms of URI but who otherwise appears healthy. The anesthesiologist must weigh the disruption and cost of rescheduling a surgery against the concern for perioperative respiratory complications, including laryngospasm, bronchospasm, or aspiration. The literature suggests that, although children with recent URIs are at increased risk for such manifestations of airway reactivity, many such episodes are largely transient and can be anticipated and managed without impacting overall clinical outcomes when compared with children without URI symptoms.

Therefore many providers will choose to proceed with such cases provided the child is not actively febrile or dyspneic, but management continues to rely on individual judgment and experience.

STEP 1, 2 PEARL

Most URIs in children are caused by viruses, with rhinovirus being the most common pathogen, followed by influenza, respiratory syncytial virus (RSV), enteroviruses, and adenoviruses. Bacterial infections are less common. Group A streptococcus are the most common cause of bacterial pharyngitis and tonsillitis, with *Streptococcus pyogenes* being the predominant agent in this group.

The patient's mother wishes to accompany the patient to the operating room "to make sure she's not scared when she goes to sleep."

How will you respond?
It is natural for parents to be nervous for and protective of their children, particularly because the perioperative process may be entirely new to them. Parents may request to accompany the child to the operating room for induction of anesthesia. Parental presence at induction of anesthesia (PPIA) is a special situation for the perioperative team and requires consensus and a plan.

Research has demonstrated that PPIA can reduce the incidence of the postoperative sequelae in anxious children (i.e., emergence delirium, increased postoperative pain) *but only if the parent participating is a calming presence.* Anxious children going to sleep in the presence of equally anxious parents have been shown to have greater incidence of delirium and other issues than anxious children without parents in the room. While the potential benefits of this technique are well established, the appropriateness of PPIA in a given situation remains in the judgment of the anesthesiologist. Prior to PPIA, it is important to clearly discuss with parents the process that will occur and the expectations for them, particularly when they will leave their child in the care of the operating room team, which is usually immediately following a successful inhalational induction.

What about the patient's anxiety?
An unfamiliar environment, abundance of strangers, disruption of normal routine, and potentially unpleasant or painful experiences such as the administration of oral premedication (i.e., midazolam) or the starting of a peripheral intravenous (IV) catheter can be upsetting to children across the spectrum of age and development. Preoperative anxiety in the pediatric patient has been shown to be associated with increased rates of emergence delirium and elevated postoperative pain scores, among other negative outcomes. Prevention and treatment of anxiety in the pediatric patient are key goals for the anesthesiologist and perioperative team.

Many institutions, particularly those caring predominantly or exclusively to children, have pediatric developmental experts, known as child life specialists, who are dedicated to normalizing and improving the experience of the hospitalized child. Child life specialists can be invaluable in the perioperative environment, explaining procedures or protocols in age-appropriate language, assisting and distracting during painful experiences, and helping the child achieve some degree of autonomy or choice during the surgical period ("do you want to have a red cast or a blue cast?"), and are particularly skilled at minimizing anxiety.

The surgeon asks if you are planning an awake or deep extubation.

What is your response?

Emergence is a key consideration in an anesthetic for any surgery that involves manipulation of the airway or pharyngeal tissues. There are risks and benefits involved with both awake and deep extubations, and consideration of these factors are important in developing an anesthetic plan.

Awake extubation allows the anesthesiologist to be confident that the patient has metabolized or exhaled most of the anesthetic agent and has demonstrated restoration of both respiratory drive and airway protective reflexes. However, significant coughing or bucking, which may accompany awake extubation, will be problematic in the setting of recently cauterized tissue, increasing the risk of stimulating a laryngospasm or bronchospasm with fresh bleeding or secretions. The awake child can be fussy, disoriented, or even delirious coming out of the operating room and into the postanesthesia care unit (PACU).

Deep extubation can be performed in the child with spontaneous respiration or in a patient who requires additional support up to and including manual ventilation. The latter situation is considered to be more dangerous, as any difficulties with ventilation may result in precipitous oxygen desaturation requiring emergency airway management. With a spontaneously breathing child, the presence of a deep plane of anesthesia is thought to decrease the risk of airway reactivity resulting in laryngospasm with the removal of the endotracheal tube.

While deep extubation allows for the removal of a sedated, comfortable-appearing child from the operating room, there are a number of additional considerations one must keep in mind when performing a deep extubation. The deeply sedated child, although spontaneously breathing, may require additional intervention and manipulation to avoid airway obstruction (i.e., oral airway placement, jaw thrust) arising from decreased pharyngeal muscle tone. In the case of volatile anesthetics in particular, patients will still progress through a period of emergence in which airway protective reflexes are not fully recovered but airway reactivity is increased (so-called stage 2 of anesthesia see Case 5). Deep extubations result in this period occurring not in the operating room in the presence of airway management equipment and an anesthesia machine but rather in the PACU, where nurses may have varying degrees of comfort with managing a child in respiratory distress.

The decision between an awake and deep extubation should be made with the consideration of the aforementioned factors, as well as patient characteristics, including the amount of sedatives, narcotics, and anesthetics received during a case, underlying respiratory dynamics including the presence of OSA, original ease of securing the airway, as well as the clinician's practice style.

What is a deep extubation?

A deep extubation entails removing the endotracheal tube while the patient is still *fully anesthetized*. Several criteria must be met to safely perform a deep extubation:

- Neuromuscular blockade must be fully reversed.
- The intubation must have been easy. For example, a patient who required an awake fiberoptic intubation is not a candidate for a deep extubation.
- The patient must not be at increased risk of aspiration of gastric contents. For example, a patient who is not appropriately *nil per os* (NPO) prior to surgery, such as a trauma patient, would not be a candidate for a deep extubation.
- The patient must be breathing spontaneously at a normal physiologic rate and tidal volume (at least 4 mL/kg of ideal body weight).

- The patient must be fully anesthetized with at least 1 MAC of anesthesia. A patient breathing only 0.5 MAC of anesthetic gas who is already starting to move is not a candidate for deep extubation. There is a risk of laryngospasm when manipulating the airway or extubating a patient who has already begun to emerge from anesthesia.
- The patient must be hemodynamically stable and oxygenating well.

You meet the child's mother in the PACU after getting the patient settled. The mother asks how long the patient will need to recover before they can go home.

What do you tell her?
Children undergoing tonsillectomy for recurrent pharyngitis can often be discharged after several hours in the PACU, provided they meet discharge criteria including the ability to eat or drink, as well as adequate pain control. If the surgery was performed for tonsillar hypertrophy or OSA, further monitoring to ensure absence of significant obstruction or oxygen desaturation in the postoperative period is warranted. In patients with severe sleep apnea at high risk for respiratory compromise, an overnight stay in the pediatric intensive care unit may be warranted.

The following morning, near the end of your 24-hour call, you are paged urgently for an emergency case. You are surprised to see your tonsillectomy patient in the emergency room, having returned vomiting bright red blood.

Tonsillar rebleeds in the hours to days following tonsillectomy present a true emergency situation and can have catastrophic outcomes. They can cause airway obstruction and hypoxia. Bleeds beginning in the first 24 hours following the surgery are referred to as primary posttonsillectomy hemorrhage, and those occurring after 24 hours are referred to as secondary posttonsillectomy hemorrhage. Patients with chronic tonsillitis and history of using aspirin, as well as those with coagulopathies such as hemophilia are at increased risk of this serious complication. Blood loss can be significant, and ongoing bleeding in the setting of swollen upper airway tissue can render endotracheal intubation difficult. Large-bore IV access, dedicated suction (some clinicians prefer two Yankauers), and direct and video laryngoscopes are essential. Rapid sequence intubation is required, as these patients will be at high risk for aspiration due to ongoing bleeding and the presence of blood in the stomach, which itself is a risk factor for vomiting and subsequent aspiration. Perioperative management of a tonsillar rebleed will involve resuscitation, correcting potentially significant hypovolemia and anemia.

BEYOND THE PEARLS

- Tonsillectomies are quick cases. Experienced surgeons can be done in less than 20 minutes, and a private practice line up may include a dozen or more of these cases a day. Such speed may influence how the anesthetic is performed, favoring techniques that do not require reversal agents or long emergence periods.
- Intranasal administration is an effective route of premedication for the child who is uncooperative with IV placement or oral medications. Although fentanyl and midazolam are options for this technique, the potential for sedative-induced airway obstruction in this patient population makes them less attractive candidates (midazolam in particular "burns" when given intranasally). Dexmedetomidine (1–2 mcg/kg) is an effective and

safe choice but has a time to onset of 45–60 minutes, so plan the preoperative workflow accordingly.

- Throat packs and/or mouth gags are commonly used by surgeons to reduce passage of blood into the trachea or stomach. *It is critical to ensure that packs or gags have been removed prior to leaving the operating room.* Serious consequences including death from airway obstruction have been reported as a result of retained throat packs.
- Make sure your endotracheal tube is of adequate length! Oral RAE tubes (specialized endotracheal tubes with a pre-formed bend that can improve surgical access for facial, oral, and nasal surgery) in particular may extend a shorter distance past the vocal cords relative to their standard counterparts given their curvature. Subsequent manipulation of the head and neck by the surgeon may result in herniation of the cuff out of the trachea and displacement of the tube.
- While a laryngeal mask airway (LMA) may be used as an alternative to an endotracheal tube, it may be associated with less-than-ideal operating conditions and does not provide a definitive secure airway.
- *Be careful with aggressive suctioning during emergence and the immediate postoperative period. Always suction in the midline.*
- Avoid red-colored foods and juice in the PACU. You do not want to be wondering whether the red-colored vomitus your patient just had is the result of an innocent red ice pop or an ominous sign of ongoing bleeding.

References

Doyle, D. J. (2015). Anesthesia for ear, nose, and throat surgery. *Miller's anesthesia* (8th ed., pp. 2523–2549). Philadelphia, PA: Elsevier Saunders.

Greeley, W. J. (2015). Anesthesia for pediatric cardiac surgery. *Miller's anesthesia* (8th ed., pp. 2799–2853). Philadelphia, PA: Elsevier Saunders.

Hannallah, R. S., Brown, K. A., & Verghese, S. T. (2019). Otorhinolaryngologic procedures. *A practice of anesthesia for infants and children* (pp. 754–789). Philadelphia, PA: Elsevier.

Tao, J., & Kurup, V. (2018). Obstructive respiratory diseases. In *Stoelting's anesthesia and co-existing disease* (pp. 15–32). Philadelphia, PA: Elsevier.

Truong, M. T., Messner, A. H., Mireles, S. A., Wang, E. Y., & Hammer, G. B. (2020). Pediatric otolaryngology. In: *Anesthesiologist's manual of surgical procedures* (pp.1345–1347). Philadelphia, PA: Wolters Kluwer.

An 8-Year-Old Boy With a History of Asthma

Mark Murphy ■ Jeff Tully

An 8-year-old boy with a history of asthma presents for an outpatient strabismus correction surgery.

What is strabismus? How is it corrected?

Strabismus, or malalignment of the eyes when focusing on an object, is one of the most common ophthalmic conditions in children requiring corrective surgery. The surgery involves realigning the divergent visual axes by altering the extraocular muscles (EOMs). There are seven EOMs, including the four recti muscles (medial, lateral, superior, and inferior rectus) and the two oblique muscles (superior and inferior oblique). The levator palpebrae superioris (see Case 1) muscle is a standalone EOM. Fig. 7.1 shows the anatomic relationships of the EOMs. Fig. 7.2 shows the eye movements associated with each EOM.

STEP 1 PEARL

Table 7.1 shows cranial nerve innervation of the eye

What are the preoperative considerations in strabismus surgery?

Strabismus is often idiopathic but may manifest with other systemic diseases or syndromes. The anesthesiologist should review the child's birth history; any previous anesthesia history or records; identify any syndromes, myopathies, or neurological problems; and review the child's respiratory and cardiac history. Associated neurological conditions include cerebral palsy, myelomeningocele, hydrocephalus, neurofibromatosis, and seizure disorders. Some of the syndromes and chromosomal abnormalities associated with strabismus include Down syndrome, Apert syndrome, cri du chat syndrome, Crouzon syndrome, Goldenhar syndrome, Marfan syndrome, Turner syndrome, Strickler syndrome, Moebius Sequence, myotonic dystrophy, and homocystinuria.

The parents deny a family history of any problems with anesthesia. What is malignant hyperthermia (MH)? Should you be concerned about the possibility of MH in this patient?

MH is a life-threatening hypermetabolic disorder of skeletal muscle that is triggered by inhalation agents or the depolarizing muscle relaxant succinylcholine. There are multiple gene mutations associated with MH, but the classic mutation is of the ryanodine receptor (RYR1) gene. This mutation causes dysregulation of intracellular calcium leading to an increased need for adenosine triphosphate (ATP) to drive the calcium across the sarcoplasmic reticulum, resulting in hypermetabolism and sustained muscle contraction.

It was once believed that patients undergoing strabismus surgery had a higher risk of MH, but this is no longer the case. Strabismus is not considered a risk factor for MH. Children with

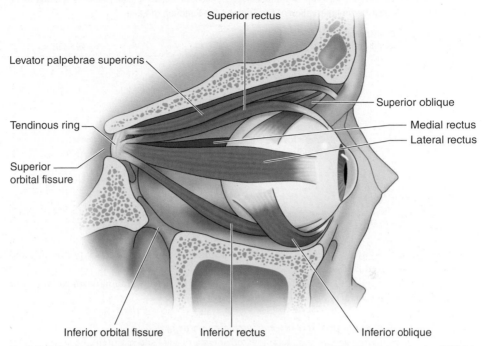

Fig. 7.1 Lateral view of the orbit showing the anatomic relationships of the extraocular muscles (EOMs). (Drake, R. L., Vogl, A. W., & Mitchell, A. W. M. [2021]. Head and Neck. In *Gray's atlas of anatomy* [Vol. 8, 3rd ed., pp. 477–610]. Philadelphia, PA: Elsevier. Modified.)

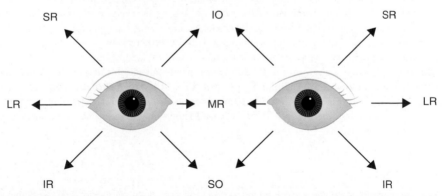

Fig. 7.2 Direction of eye movement associated with each extraocular muscle (EOM). *IO*, Inferior oblique; *IR*, inferior rectus; *LR*, lateral rectus; *MR*, medial rectus; *SO*, superior oblique; *SR*, superior rectus. (Huff, J. S., & Austin, E. W. [2016]. Neuro-ophthalmology in emergency medicine. *Emerg Med Clin North Am*. *34*(4),967–986.)

strabismus are routinely anesthetized with inhalational agents without any apparent increase in the incidence of MH.

What are the signs of MH?
One of the earliest signs of MH is hypercarbia or increased end-tidal carbon dioxide ($EtCO_2$) that persists even with increased minute ventilation. Other signs include tachycardia, tachypnea (not always noticeable under general anesthesia), hypoxia, hypertension, generalized muscle rigidity,

TABLE 7.1 ■ Cranial Nerve Innervation of the Eye and the Function of Each

Name	Cranial Nerve Number	Function	Modality
Optic	II	**Vision**	Sensory
Oculomotor	III	**Eye movement** (superior rectus, inferior rectus, medial rectus, inferior oblique EOMs), eyelid opening (levator palpebrae superioris), pupillary constriction, lens accommodation	Motor
Trochlear	IV	**Eye movement** (superior oblique EOM)	Motor
Abducens	VI	**Eye movement** (lateral rectus EOM)	Motor
Facial	VII	Eyelid closing, facial expressions and taste sensation of the anterior two thirds of the tongue, lacrimation, salivation	Motor/Sensory

EOM, Extraocular muscle.

skin mottling, rhabdomyolysis, and acidosis (mixed respiratory and metabolic) Hyperthermia and hyperkalemia are often late signs.

Masseter muscle rigidity or spasm after administration of succinylcholine is an early sign of MH and indicates high susceptibility for further progression.

What should you do if you suspect MH intraoperatively or postoperatively?
Discontinue all triggering agents (e.g., halogenated anesthetic gas) and maintain intravenous (IV) anesthetics and nondepolarizing muscle relaxation. Increase the fresh gas flow in the breathing circuit to at least 10 L/min, and hyperventilate with fraction inspired oxygen of 100% (1.0 FiO$_2$).

The mainstay pharmacologic treatment is dantrolene, which prevents the release of calcium from the sarcoplasmic reticulum. Administer dantrolene (2.5 mg/kg IV every 5–10 minutes, up to four doses, until symptoms subside). Administer bicarbonate to treat metabolic acidosis and to alkalinize the urine to protect the kidney from myoglobinuria. Treat hyperthermia by cooling the patient (e.g., cold IV fluids, filling body cavities with sterile ice fluids) until the temperature reaches 38°C.

Monitor for cardiac arrhythmia and treat as appropriate (although calcium channel blockers should be avoided). Check arterial blood gases (see Case 30) and electrolytes frequently. Treat hyperkalemia as appropriate (see Case 31). Monitor coagulation studies and treat as appropriate.

These patients should be monitored for at least 24 hours in the intensive care unit once the acute symptoms resolve.

STEP 1 PEARL

There are many intricate steps involved in the contraction of skeletal muscle. First, an action potential causes release of acetylcholine from vesicles in the presynaptic axon into the neuromuscular junction. Acetylcholine binds and activates nicotinic ligand-gated ion channels on the postsynaptic motor end plate (i.e., the muscle). These ion channels open, allowing sodium to flow into and depolarize the motor end plate. T-tubules transmit this depolarization to dihydropyridine receptors on the sarcoplasmic reticulum; this in turn stimulates ryanodine receptors to release calcium from the sarcoplasmic reticulum. This calcium binds troponin C, creating a conformation change in tropomyosin that allows the myosin head to interact with actin; this is known as cross bridging. Myosin releases a molecule of adenosine diphosphate (ADP, cleaved from ATP) and moves along the actin filament, thereby causing muscle contraction. This cycle continues as long as calcium ions are present.

What is asthma? What should we consider preoperatively given the patient's history of asthma?
Asthma is a chronic inflammatory state of the lungs and a major cause of childhood illness of the industrialized world. This disorder involves mast cells, eosinophils, neutrophils, and activated T-helper cells and results in reactive inflammatory disease of the small airway, leading to airflow obstruction. Asthma signs and symptoms include breathlessness, chest tightness, wheezing, coughing, night awakenings, and tachypnea, and an acute attack may progress to bronchospasm, hypoxia/hypoxemia, and respiratory failure.

Asthma is classified based on severity and control. Severity is classified as intermittent or persistent, and persistent is further divided into mild, moderate, or severe. Control refers to the response a patient has to both prophylactic and rescue therapies and can be described as well controlled, not well controlled, or very poorly controlled. Familiarity with this classification can help guide physicians for management.

Often, looking at the child's prescribed medications gives the anesthesiologist an idea of the asthma severity. Quick-relief medications for intermittent asthma include inhaled anticholinergic agents (e.g., ipratropium) or short-acting β agonists (e.g., albuterol). As the severity increases to persistent, inhaled glucocorticoids are the foundation of long-term asthma management alongside long-acting β agonists. Alternative asthma medications include leukotriene modifiers, cromolyn, or theophylline. In severe cases or in the setting of acute exacerbation, a child may be placed on oral glucocorticoids.

> **STEP 2, 3 PEARL**
>
> Morphine has been shown to cause histamine release, leading to bronchospasm, and is therefore not recommended in patients with asthma.
> Aspirin-exacerbated respiratory disease (AERD), or Samter triad is a rare chronic condition of asthma, nasal polyps, and aspirin or non-steroidal anti-inflammatory drugs (NSAID) sensitivity. These people will develop upper and lower respiratory symptoms after taking aspirin or NSAIDs.

Ask about the history of the patient's asthma by identifying any symptoms, recent exacerbations, and the child's current medication use. Take special note when children appear to have worsening symptoms or increased inhaler use without any new escalation of their prescribed medications. Determine if the child has had any previous emergency room visits or hospitalizations or if they have ever required intubation for asthma exacerbations.

All asthma medications should be continued on the day of surgery, and clinicians may administer an albuterol metered dose inhaler treatment preoperatively. Children with severe asthma or a recent exacerbation taking oral glucocorticoids should be considered for stress-dose glucocorticoids prior to surgical incision. Anticholinergic agents such as glycopyrrolate or atropine can decrease airway secretions and airway vagal responses, although their use comes with tachycardia. Anxiolytics and sedatives are helpful to calm the child and ultimately decrease the work of breathing prior to surgery. Oral or IV midazolam is a common preoperative anxiolytic. Centrally acting α agonists (e.g., clonidine, dexmedetomidine) have sedative properties and have been shown to blunt bronchoconstriction when given prior to intubation. Regardless of the agent or agents that are used, the patient should be deeply anesthetized prior to manipulation of the airway to avoid bronchospasm.

> **STEP 2, 3 PEARL**
>
> An awake patient experiencing an asthma exacerbation will often hyperventilate, resulting in a decreased CO_2 and respiratory alkalosis. If the patient becomes fatigued, they may progress to CO_2 retention leading to respiratory acidosis, a sign of impending respiratory failure which may require intubation.

How will you induce anesthesia in this patient?

An inhalation induction with sevoflurane will often be performed for strabismus surgery, although an IV induction with propofol is an alternate option; however, this requires placing a peripheral IV line in an awake child. Desflurane is not recommended for inhalation due to its pungency and airway irritability, and use of this agent may lead to a laryngospasm or bronchospasm.

Will you use a laryngeal mask airway or endotracheal tube? How will you decide?

Discussion with the surgeon can help decide the use of a laryngeal mask airway (LMA) or an endotracheal tube (ETT) for general anesthesia. LMAs are less invasive, decrease the risk of airway trauma, and do not require muscle relaxation, and patients are usually kept spontaneously breathing. In contrast, an endotracheal intubation is a more stimulating procedure involving laryngoscopy and frequently requiring muscle relaxation. Endotracheal intubation is associated with an increased risk of bronchospasm relative to using an LMA or face mask. It should be noted that an LMA does not protect the airway from aspiration and may have a poor seal, leading to inadequate ventilation. An ETT is a more secure airway in preventing aspiration and may be more desirable for some physicians in strabismus surgery.

Access to the airway should be considered as well because the operating table is usually turned 90 or 180 degrees away from the anesthesiologist. In addition, the ophthalmologist may request muscle relaxation to directly manipulate the EOMs to evaluate for muscle palsies or restriction.

Is ketamine an appropriate medication for this case?

Ketamine has amnestic, analgesic, hypnotic, and varying degrees of anesthetic properties, making it a valuable drug in the field of anesthesia. It works mainly by noncompetitive antagonism of the N-methyl D-aspartic acid (NMDA) receptor. It may be helpful in this case because it also causes bronchodilation and has been traditionally used for induction in patients with severe asthma.

However, there are some downfalls to using ketamine in this case. Ketamine causes copious secretions that may in turn exacerbate an irritable airway and result in laryngospasm. Therefore an antisialagogue (e.g., glycopyrrolate) may be given preoperatively. When used with older children, ketamine may elicit hallucinations or bad dreams, but this is reduced with concurrent administration of a benzodiazepine. Some studies have shown postoperative vomiting in up to 33% of children undergoing surgery with its use. There is no clear consensus on ketamine and its effect on intraocular pressure (IOP), but some studies have shown an increase in IOP. Ketamine also produces nystagmus or blepharospasm, which may be undesirable for the ophthalmologist during strabismus surgery.

Is succinylcholine an appropriate drug for this case?

Succinylcholine is relatively contraindicated in strabismus surgery if the patient is undergoing forced duction testing because the EOMs may remain contracted for at least 15 minutes after it is given. As mentioned previously, strabismus is no longer considered a risk factor for MH, and provided the child does not have a history of any myopathy or neuromuscular disorder precluding them from receiving succinylcholine, use of this medication would not be considered dangerous.

Despite the fact that succinylcholine has shown to elevate IOP, it remains an option for rapid sequence inductions. The rise in IOP from succinylcholine is inconsequential in relation to the possible rise caused by coughing and gagging during laryngoscopy and intubation. In an elective strabismus surgery, it would rarely be indicated, although there is no absolute contraindication to its use.

The ophthalmologist requests muscle relaxation for a forced duction test, so you decide to intubate the child for the procedure. Induction and intubation are uneventful. When the ophthalmologist manipulates the eye, the patient's heart rate drops to 42/min.

What's going on? What should you do?

This is very likely the oculocardiac reflex (OCR). The reflex is common in strabismus surgery and is elicited by traction of the EOMs or pressure on the eye. The afferent limb (i.e., from the periphery to the brain) of the reflex includes the trigeminal nerve (cranial nerve VI), and the efferent limb (i.e., from the brain to the periphery) is the vagus nerve (cranial nerve X). The reflex can cause a range of arrhythmias, including sinus bradycardia, atrioventricular block, ventricular bigeminy, ventricular tachycardia, or even asystole.

Quickly notify the surgeon and ask them to stop manipulating the eye. If bradycardia persists, administer atropine (10 to 20 mcg/kg) or glycopyrrolate (10 to 20 mcg/kg). Empiric prophylactic administration of these agents prior to strabismus surgery has been debated, with many anesthesiologists administering an anticholinergic prior to the surgeon manipulating the EOMs. Some studies have also showed that ketamine may counteract the vagal stimulation caused by the OCR. Epinephrine (1 to 10 mcg/kg) is rarely required but should be available should the reflex persist or progress.

The operation is uneventful. You decide to wake the child up fully for extubation. After adequately reversing your muscle relaxant, you begin to titrate down the sevoflurane. Suddenly the child begins to cough and desaturate. The capnogram is shown in Fig. 7.3A. You administer propofol to deepen the anesthetic, but he continues to desaturate. On auscultation of the child's chest there is audible bilateral wheezing.

What's going on? What can you do?

This is most consistent with bronchospasm, although less likely etiologies include: secretions, a mucous plug, herniation of the ETT cuff, main stem intubation, inadequate anesthesia depth, aspiration, pneumothorax, pulmonary embolism, acute pulmonary edema, or anaphylaxis. Intraoperative bronchospasm is characterized by bilateral expiratory wheezes, increased peak inspiratory pressure and airway pressures, increased and slow up-sloped $EtCO_2$, and hypoxemia.

Treat the bronchospasm by increasing FiO_2 to 100% and increase the anesthetic depth with volatile agent and/or propofol. Administer 2 to 10 puffs of albuterol to the inspiratory limb of the circuit. Consider administering IV ketamine 1 to 2 mg/kg. If the bronchospasm is severe,

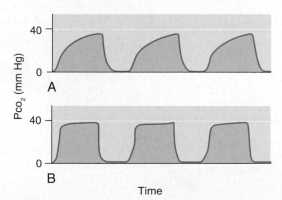

Fig. 7.3 (A) Capnogram showing a steep upslope of the end-tidal carbon dioxide ($EtCO_2$) waveform consistent with air trapping as in bronchospasm. (B) For comparison, a normal capnogram with a plateau appearance of the $EtCO_2$ waveform. (Kaczka, D. W., Chitilian, H. V., & Vidal Melo, M. F. [2020]. Respiratory monitoring. In M. A. Gropper, R. D. Miller, N. H. Cohen, L. I. Eriksson, L. A. Fleisher, K. Leslie, et al. (Eds.), *Miller's anesthesia* [Vol. 41, 9th ed., pp. 1298–1339]. Philadelphia, PA: Elsevier. Modified from Fig 41.11.)

administer IV epinephrine 1 to 2 mcg/kg. If refractory, administer magnesium sulfate 50 to 75 mg/kg over 20 minutes. In addition, despite their delayed action, consider IV glucocorticoids.

The patient's ventilatory status stabilizes with a deeper plane of anesthesia and four puffs of albuterol down the ETT.

Should this child be extubated awake or deep?

If feasible, deep extubation would be preferred in an asthmatic child to prevent airway irritation and potential reflexive bronchoconstriction or bronchospasm (see Case 6). In general, deep extubation in ophthalmologic surgery will help to minimize the risk of coughing and gagging, leading to increased IOP or intracranial pressure.

Should this child receive medication to prevent postoperative nausea and vomiting (ponv)?

Yes. Strabismus surgery in children has one of the highest incidences of PONV, at 45% to 85%. IV hydration (20 to 30 mL/kg) of a balanced salt solution (lactated Ringer's or Plasmalyte) decreases this risk of PONV. Other medications shown to reduce this incidence include preoperative benzodiazepines, propofol, clonidine, dexmedetomidine, serotonin 5-HT3 5-HT3 receptor blockers (e.g., ondansetron), dexamethasone, and metoclopramide.

Avoid opioids if possible, or use only short-acting opioids (e.g., remifentanil, fentanyl). Avoid nitrous oxide (N_2O).

If the anesthesiologist is very concerned about PONV, total IV anesthesia (i.e., avoid anesthetic gas) with propofol may reduce the risk.

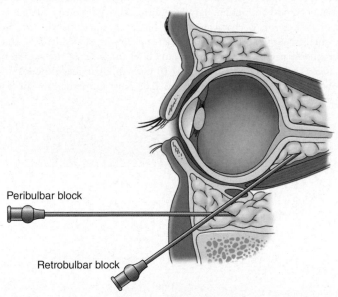

Fig. 7.4   Proper needle placement for peribulbar or retrobulbar block. (Fang, Z., Liew, E. C., & Keyes, M. A. [2020]. Anesthesia for ophthalmic surgery. In M. A. Gropper, R. D. Miller, N. H. Cohen, L. I. Eriksson, L. A. Fleisher, K. Leslie, et al. (Eds.), *Miller's anesthesia* [Vol. 69, 9th ed., pp. 2194–2209]. Philadelphia, PA: Elsevier. Fig 69.2.)

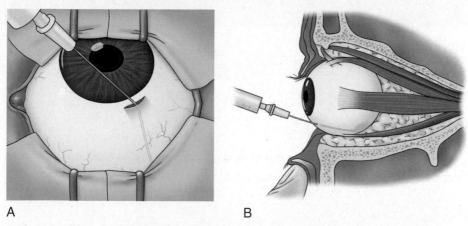

A   B

Fig. 7.5 Proper cannula placement for a sub-Tenon block. (A) The cannula is inserted into the sub-Tenon space and (B) advanced until the tip is posterior to the equator of the eye. (Gupta, M., & Rhee, D. J. Ophthalmic anesthesia. *Glaucoma* 76, 734–748. Fig 76-5.)

BEYOND THE PEARLS

- A child may have intermittent strabismus or crossed eyes before 2 months of age. If it lasts beyond 2 months of age and is persistent, then an ophthalmology consult is necessary.
- Strabismus is categorized by the direction of misalignment or turn: downward turn (hypotropia), upward turn (hypertropia), outward turn (exotropia), and inward turn (esotropia).
- Stroke is the leading cause of new-onset strabismus in adults.
- Adult strabismus surgery often involves a regional anesthesia technique with a retrobulbar, peribulbar, or a sub-Tenon block (see Figs. 7.4 and 7.5). A regional technique has been shown to blunt the OCR and has decreased the incidence of PONV in strabismus surgery as well.
- β-Blockers should be avoided in asthmatics and patients with chronic obstructive pulmonary disease (COPD). They block the vital β_2 receptors which keep airways patent by dilation of the bronchi. Note that the first-line treatment used for an asthma attack is albuterol, a short-acting β_2 agonist.

References

Tobin, J. R., & Weaver, R. G. (2019). Ophthalmology. In C. J. Cote, J. Lerman, & B. J. Anderson (Eds.), *A practice of anesthesia for infants and children* (6th ed., Chapter 34, pp. 790-803). Philadelphia, PA: Elsevier.

Ricketts, K., & Nischal, K. (2022). Anesthesia for Ophthalmic Surgery. In P. J. Davis, & F. P. Cladis (Eds.), *Smith's anesthesia for infants and children* (10th ed., Chapter 37, pp. 1001–1023). Philadelphia, PA: Elsevier.

A 9-Week-Old Boy Born at 32 Weeks' Gestation Presenting With Inguinal Hernia

Niroop R. Ravula ■ Lee Huynh Nguyen ■ Abigail Susan Smith

A 9-week-old boy born at 32 weeks' gestation presents for inguinal hernia repair. Mom reports an otherwise healthy pregnancy and uneventful delivery. He weighs 3050 g.

What is the cutoff for prematurity?
Babies born prior to 37 weeks' gestation are considered premature. The degree of prematurity correlates with increased mortality. For example, infants born at 37–38 weeks' gestation have mortality rates nearly double of those born at 38–39 weeks. Subcategories of prematurity include extremely preterm (<28 weeks), very preterm (28–32 weeks) and moderate to late preterm (32–37 weeks). The classifications for the length of gestation are shown in Fig. 8.1.

How is postconceptual age (PCA) defined? What is this infant's PCA?
PCA is the duration of gestation (in weeks) plus the number of weeks since birth. Since this baby's gestational period was 32 weeks, and he was born 9 weeks ago, his PCA is 41 weeks.

What are the anesthetic options for the case?
Inguinal hernia repair can be performed under regional anesthesia with the patient awake, or it can be performed under general anesthesia with or without regional anesthesia.

What are the advantages and disadvantages for the anesthetic options above?
Advantages of regional anesthesia include avoidance of risks of endotracheal intubation, extubation, and reduction in postoperative apnea (especially with spinal anesthesia), as well as enhanced pain control in the early postoperative period.

Disadvantages of regional anesthesia include risk of block failure, total spinal anesthesia (also known as high spinal), accidental intravascular injection (see Case 1), inadequate duration of surgical anesthesia, infection, and agitation necessitating intraoperative sedation.

Advantages of general anesthesia with endotracheal intubation include a secure airway, a completely still patient, and muscle relaxation.

What are the risk factors for postoperative apnea after anesthesia?
Risk factors for postoperative apnea include prematurity, young PCA, and anemia. Postoperative apnea can occur in patients without a history of apnea. Postoperative apnea will usually develop in the first 2 hours after anesthesia, although it may present up to 12 hours postoperatively.

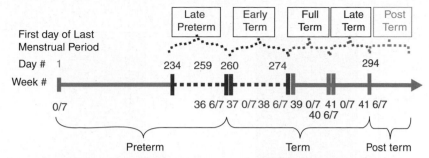

Fig. 8.1 Classification of the duration of gestation. (From Stewart, D. L., Barfield, W. D., Committee on Fetus and Newborn. [2019, November]. Updates on an at-risk population: Late-preterm and early-term infants. *Pediatrics, 144*[5], e20192760, Fig. 1. https://doi.org/10.1542/peds.2019-2760.)

Is there a risk of postoperative apnea after regional anesthesia?
Yes. The main difference between general and regional anesthesia is the timing of the apnea. After general anesthesia, apnea is most common within the first 30 minutes after emergence. Although the exact timing of postoperative apnea after regional anesthesia is unclear, multiple studies have shown that there is a significant reduction in apnea in the immediate 0-30 minutes postoperatively (though there may be similar incidence of apnea up to 12 hours postoperatively).

What regional anesthetic technique will provide appropriate surgical anesthesia for this operation?
Options for regional anesthesia are spinal or caudal anesthetic.

Spinal anesthesia is performed with a 25- or 22-gauge needle between vertebral levels L3 and L5 with the patient in lateral or sitting position. A reasonable dose is 0.75 mg/kg of hyperbaric 0.75% bupivacaine.

Caudal anesthesia can be performed with a 22- or 24-gauge angiocath. The dose is 2.5 mg/kg of 0.25% bupivacaine (see Case 5).

With either of these techniques, the patient can breathe spontaneously without requiring endotracheal intubation.

How does neonatal respiratory physiology differ from that of adults?
In neonates, tidal volume is relatively fixed, respiratory muscles fatigue more easily, functional residual capacity (FRC) is smaller, and closing capacity (CC) is larger.

Minute ventilation is given by

$$minute\,ventilation = respiratory\,rate \times tidal\,volume$$

In adults, the thorax expands laterally and anteriorly with inspiration. In neonates, the ribs are horizontal, so the thorax expands inferiorly with inspiration. This causes tidal volume to remain relatively constant, so minute ventilation is primarily dependent upon respiratory rate.

Neonatal muscles contain fewer type I muscle fibers, which are often referred to as slow twitch fibers. Type I muscle fibers contain more mitochondria and myoglobin than type II muscle fibers, and can generate more ATP for longer periods of time. Therefore, type I muscle fibers are more resistant to fatigue. With fewer type I muscle fibers, neonatal respiratory muscles fatigue more easily.

FRC is the amount of volume remaining in the lungs at the end of normal expiration, when the outward force of the chest wall is equal to the inward force of the elastic recoil of the lungs. In neonates, the chest wall is cartilaginous and more compliant compared to adults. This causes easier recoil and lower FRC compared to adults. In the supine position, the large abdomen forces the diaphragm cephalad, further decreasing FRC. Smaller FRC results in faster oxygen desaturation during apnea.

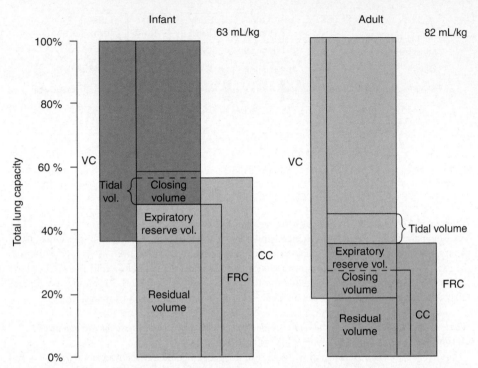

Fig. 8.2 Lung volumes in infants and adults. Notice that in adults tidal volume respiration occurs at lung volumes well above the closing volume. However, in infants, tidal volume respiration occurs at the same volume as closing volume. *CC*, Closing capacity; *FRC*, functional residual capacity; *VC*, vital capacity. (From Marciniak, B. [2019]. Growth and development. In C. J. Coté, J. Lerman, & B. J. Anderson [Eds.], *A Practice of Anesthesia for Infants and Children* [6th ed., Chapter 2, p. 8–24.e3, Fig. 2.7]. Philadelphia, PA: Elsevier.)

Additionally, neonates have higher basal metabolic rates. Neonatal oxygen consumption based on body weight is two to three times higher than that of adults. Increased oxygen consumption further shortens the time to oxygen desaturation during apnea.

CC is the lung volume at which small airways collapse. As a percentage of total lung capacity, neonates have higher CC compared to adults. In adults, normal tidal volume breathing occurs at lung volumes greater than CC. In neonates, normal tidal volume breathing occurs at lung volumes that are the same as CC (Fig. 8.2). Due to the poor elastic properties of infant lungs, their closing volume is greater than their FRC, with terminal airway closure occurring during normal tidal ventilation. This results in air trapping. To overcome this small airway closure during normal respiration, neonates dynamically increase their FRC by breathing at a fast respiratory rate and adducting their vocal cords in expiration to increase expiratory airway resistance.

After a discussion with the patient's mother, you plan for general anesthesia with endotracheal intubation.

What are the options for induction of anesthesia in this patient, and how is each performed?
There are three options for induction of general anesthesia: inhalational (i.e., mask) induction, intravenous (IV) induction, and intramuscular (IM) induction. Inhaled and IV inductions are most commonly used.

To perform a mask induction, begin by having the patient breathe anesthetic gas (usually sevoflurane, sometimes starting with nitrous oxide). Once the patient is fully anesthetized, secure

IV access, then administer a neuromuscular blocking agent (e.g., rocuronium, cisatracurium) and intubate the patient.

An IV induction requires securing IV access in an awake patient. Administer an IV anesthetic agent (usually propofol) followed by a neuromuscular blocking agent, and then intubate the patient.

IM induction is most commonly used in children who will not tolerate a mask induction and IV catheter placement. Ketamine (3–5 mg/kg IM) is the most commonly used IM induction agent, and takes 3–5 minutes for onset of action. Oftentimes, IM glycopyrrolate (10 mcg/kg) is used as an adjunct to reduce secretions during induction.

> You plan for inhalational induction.

How will you intubate the patient?
Direct laryngoscopy or video laryngoscopy may be used. However, it has been shown that video laryngoscopy increases the rate of success of the first attempt, and potentially reduces episodes of oxygen desaturation.

What type of laryngoscope blade will you use?
Straight blade laryngoscope (e.g., Miller) is preferred, as it is easier to pick up the epiglottis during laryngoscopy.

What size endotracheal tube (ETT) should you use for this patient?
This patient weighs 3050 g. Given that proper ETT size can be estimated by

$$ETT\ size = age/4 + 3.0\ or\ 3.5$$

so a size 3.0 or 3.5 ETT is appropriate for our patient.

Table 8.1 shows the appropriate size of ETT based on the patient's weight. Remember to consider that this is a generalization, and each patient's needs may vary.

What is the difference between a cuffed and uncuffed ETT? Which should you use for this patient?
A cuffed ETT has an inflatable balloon near the distal end. An uncuffed ETT does not.

Neonates born at term are generally intubated with a cuffed ETT. Anesthesiologists prefer cuffed ETT as a cuff will be useful to ventilate at higher pressures if needed. Neonatologists generally prefer uncuffed ETT, so most neonates in the neonatal intensive care unit (NICU) will have an uncuffed ETT.

TABLE 8.1 ■ **Appropriate Endotracheal Tube Size Based on Patient Weight.**

weight (g)	Endotracheal Tube Size (internal diameter in mm)
<1000	2.5
1000–2000	3.0
2000–3000	3.5
>3000	3.5–4.0

> Before inflating the cuff on the ETT, you give a few manual breaths, and do not hear an air leak around the ETT.

Inhaled induction and intubation with a size 3.5 Cuffed ETT are uneventful. What is going on?

Once the ETT is in place, there should be an air leak starting at airway pressures around 20 cm H_2O. If there is no leak with airway pressure above 20 cm H_2O, even with the cuff fully deflated, consider downsizing the ETT to avoid trauma to the trachea from prolonged pressure.

There is a risk of pressure injury to the trachea when an inappropriately large ETT is used. Consider downsizing to a size 3.0 uncuffed ETT.

> You exchange the size 3.0 cuffed ett for a size 3.0 Uncuffed ETT.

How deep should the ETT be placed?

The proper depth of insertion in centimeters is given by

$$depth\ of\ insertion\ =\ patient\ weight\ (in\ kg) + 6$$

or

$$depth\ of\ insertion\ =\ internal\ diameter\ (in\ mm) \times 3$$

In this patient, the depth of insertion should be 9–10 cm. Always listen for bilateral breath sounds to confirm proper ETT placement.

What ventilator settings will you use?

Pressure control or volume control ventilation may be used, with the goal of tidal volumes of 4–6 cc/kg of body weight. PEEP can also be added. Fraction of inspired oxygen (FiO_2) should be kept less than 40% to prevent complications such as retrolental fibroplasia.

What is retrolental fibroplasia? What are other possible complications of administration of high concentrations of oxygen?

In utero, the environment is relatively hypoxic compared to room air. Neonates are susceptible to oxidative damage via reactive oxygen species. Therefore, too much supplemental oxygen can cause toxicity in multiple organ systems.

Retrolental fibroplasia is also known as retinopathy of prematurity (ROP). High amounts of supplemental oxygen can cause inhibition of neuronal and retinal vessel growth in the premature infant, then vasoproliferation occurs and can result in retinal detachment. Other complications of high oxygen concentrations include bronchopulmonary dysplasia (BPD), intraventricular hemorrhage (IVH), necrotizing enterocolitis (NEC), and periventricular leukomalacia.

TABLE 8.2 ■ Normal Heart Rate, Blood Pressure, and Cardiac Output for Neonates, Children, and Adults.

	Neonate	Child	Adult
Heart rate (beats/minute)	120–200	80–120	50–90
Systolic blood pressure (mm Hg)	50–90	95–110	90–140
Diastolic blood pressure	25–50	55–70	60–90
Cardiac output (cc/kg/min)	200–250	100–150	80–100

The patient's blood pressure is 68/34 mm Hg, with A mean arterial pressure (Map) of 42 mm Hg.

Is that acceptable?
This blood pressure is appropriate for this patient. The minimum acceptable MAP for neonates is equal to PCA; for example, this neonate at 41 weeks PCA should have a minimum MAP of 41 mm Hg.

Table 8.2 shows normal hemodynamic parameters for neonates, children, and adults.

During the operation, the patient's blood pressure drops to 55/30 mm Hg.

How do you treat hypotension in a neonate under general anesthesia?
In our patient with a goal MAP of at least 41 mm Hg, bolus IV fluid (10 mL/kg) and/or decrease anesthetic agents to improve the MAP.

What is the main determinant of cardiac output in neonates?
Cardiac output is given by

$$cardiac\ output = heart\ rate \times stroke\ volume$$

In neonates, stroke volume is relatively fixed, so cardiac output is dependent on heart rate. Therefore, it is critical to avoid bradycardia.

STEP 2 PEARL
One of the most common causes of bradycardia in pediatric patients is hypoxia.

What IV maintenance fluid should you use? At what rate should you administer maintenance fluid?
Normal saline (NS) 0.9% sodium chloride (NaCl) or lactated Ringer's solution with dextrose should be given to neonates and infants to prevent hypoglycemia. Intraoperatively, 0.45% NaCl solution with 5% dextrose (D5 0.45% NaCl) or 0.9% NaCl with 5% dextrose (D5 NS) are commonly used. Use the 4-2-1 rule to calculate the rate of maintenance fluid administration.

What is the 4-2-1 rule?
To calculate the rate of maintenance fluid
- 4 cc/kg/h for the first 10 kg of body weight
- 2 cc/kg/h for the next 10 kg of body weight
- 1 cc/kg/h for every kg of body weight above that.

For this patient, who weighs roughly 3 kg, maintenance fluid will be
$$3\,kg \times 4\,cc/kg/hr = 12\,cc/hr$$

What are the risk factors for hypoglycemia?
Hypoglycemia may occur in healthy neonates, but it is more common in those with respiratory diseases, severe infection, brain damage, or those who are small for gestational age. Hypoglycemia may develop due to low hepatic glycogen stores and lack of glucose source (e.g., from feeding difficulty). Neonates born to mothers with diabetes mellitus may have islet cell hyperplasia, which increases the risk of hypoglycemia.

The surgeon begins closing the incision, and the resident asks if the patient should receive morphine for postoperative pain control.

Narcotics can contribute to postoperative apnea. A better first-line analgesic is acetaminophen 10–15 mg/kg IV.

The surgery concludes, and extubation is uneventful. In the recovery room, the patient's mother asks when she can take her son home.

TABLE 8.3 ■ Congenital Anomalies and the Anesthetic Implications

Anomaly	Description	Anesthetic considerations
Gastrointestinal anomalies		
Pyloric stenosis	Most common cause of intestinal obstruction in infancy. 2–4 per 1000 live births. More common in males than females (4:1), first born males, Caucasians and those born preterm. Physical exam demonstrates the "olive" sign in the majority of infants; firm mass palpated at lateral edge of rectus abdominis in right upper quadrant. Diagnose with abdominal ultrasound.	• Not a surgical emergency • Resuscitation, optimize electrolytes • Full stomach precautions • Nasogastric suctioning before rapid sequence intubation • Awake extubation
Tracheoesophageal fistula and esophageal atresia (TEF)	A: isolated esophageal atresia B: proximal fistula with distal atresia C: proximal atresia with distal fistula (most common) D: double fistula with intervening atresia E: isolated fistula (H-type) See Fig. 8.3 for anatomy of types of TEF	• Orogastric tube • Mask or IV induction • Spontaneous ventilation for rigid bronchoscopy and isolation of fistula by surgeons • ETT tip beyond fistula • Post repair transport to the intensive care unit intubated and ventilated
Hirschsprung disease	Congenital aganglionic megacolon. Most common cause of lower intestinal obstruction in full-term neonates. May present at birth as bowel obstruction with delayed passage of meconium, irritability, bilious vomiting, failure to thrive, and abdominal distension. Diagnose with full-thickness biopsy. 1:5000 live births. More common in males than females.	• Full stomach precautions • Nasogastric suctioning before rapid sequence intubation • Awake extubation
Necrotizing enterocolitis (NEC)	Most common neonatal medical and surgical emergency. Characterized by varying degrees of mucosal or transmural necrosis of the intestine, most often involving terminal ileum and proximal colon. 1–3:1000 live births. 90% of cases in preterm infants.	• Emergency • Surgery in NICU • Total intravenous anesthesia (TIVA) with fentanyl and rocuronium • Bleeding and coagulation issues • Have blood products available

(continued)

TABLE 8.3 ■ Congenital Anomalies and the Anesthetic Implications—cont'd

Anomaly	Description	Anesthetic considerations
Omphalocele	Defect of the anterior abdominal wall that permits external herniation of the abdominal viscera through the base of the umbilical cord. Defect is >4 cm. **Hernia sac is present** and made of peritoneal membrane and amniotic membrane. More than 50% of cases are associated with other anomalies, often cardiac. More prevalent in males, 30% cases seen in preterm infants. Surgical intervention is not urgent.	• Not an emergency • Consider echocardiogram to evaluate for cardiac anomalies prior to repair
Gastroschisis	Defect of anterior abdominal wall that permits external herniation of abdominal viscera, usually lateral to the umbilical cord. Defect usually <5 cm. **Hernia sac is absent.** Exposed viscera is in direct contact with amniotic fluid. Surgical intervention is urgent to limit evaporative and thermal losses.	• Decompress stomach with oro/nasogastric tube to reduce risk of aspiration, regurgitation, and further bowel distention • Rapid sequence intubation. ETT should allow for peak inspiratory pressures of >20 cm H_2O as primary closure may require higher pressures initially • Watch out for high peak pressures during closure
Diaphragmatic hernia	Defect in diaphragm associated with variable amount of intraabdominal organ extrusion into the thoracic cavity. 1:2500–3000 live births. Other anomalies seen in 50% of cases. Associated with Beckwith-Wiedemann, colomba of the retina, heart abnormalities, atresia of the choanae, retarded growth and mental development, genital hypoplasia in males, ear abnormalities (CHARGE), and trisomy 21 and 18.	• Repair may occur within a few days after birth • Larger defects require intubation immediately after birth • Consider oro/nasogastric tube to decompress the stomach • Consider repair at bedside as patients may be on extracorporeal membrane oxygenation (ECMO)/Oscillator
Neural Tube Defects		
Myelomeningocele	Severe form of spina bifida. Spinal cord and nerves develop outside of the body, which are contained in meninges. Often have loss of function and sensation below the level of the defect if not repaired in a timely manner.	• Careful positioning during induction to prevent compression of the meningocele • Surgery is performed in a prone position • Neural tube defects are associated with elevated serum α-fetoprotein

Cardiac Anomalies		
Type	**Blood Flow**	**Examples**
Left-to-right shunts	Pulmonary-to-systemic flow ratio (Qp/Qs) is > 1 Pulmonary circulation is greater than systemic circulation Concern for volume-overloaded ventricle and development of congestive heart failure (CHF)	• Atrial septal defect (ASD) or ventricular septal defect (VSD) with severe aortic stenosis or low right heart pressures • atrioventricular (AV) canal defect • Patent ductus arteriosus (PDA)
Right-to-left shunts	Pulmonary-to-systemic flow ratio (Qp/Qs) is < 1 Pulmonary circulation is less than systemic circulation Concern for pressure overloaded ventricle, hypoxemia Usually cyanotic	• Tetralogy of Fallot • Pulmonary atresia • VSD • Eisenmenger syndrome

TABLE 8.3 ■ **Congenital Anomalies and the Anesthetic Implications—cont'd**

Mixing Lesions	Mixing of pulmonary and systemic circulation is so great that systemic and pulmonary artery O_2 saturations approach each other. Pulmonary-to-systemic flow ratio Qp/Qs is independent of shunt size, and completely dependent on vascular resistance or outflow obstruction.	• ASD • VSD • PDA • Transposition of the great vessels with VSD • Tricuspid atresia • Anomalous venous return • Univentricular heart
Obstructive lesions	Obstructive lesions range from mild to severe. Severe lesions manifest in the newborn period with a pressure-overloaded, diminutive, or profoundly dysfunctional ventricle proximal to the obstruction. Concern for ventricular dysfunction, pressure-overloaded ventricle, and ductal dependence	• Interrupted aortic arch • Critical aortic stenosis • Critical pulmonic stenosis • Hypoplastic left heart • Coarctation of the aorta • Mitral stenosis

Ductal-dependent lesions	Without patent ductus arteriosus, these patients would not survive after birth	Lesions that PDA provides **systemic** flow (obstructive lesions):
		  • Coarctation of the aorta
		  • Interrupted aortic arch
		  • Hypoplastic left heart
		  • Critical aortic stenosis
		Lesions that PDA provides **pulmonary** flow (R-L lesions):
		  • Pulmonary atresia
		  • Critical pulmonary stenosis
		  • Severe subpulmonic stenosis with VSD
		  • Tricuspid atresia with pulmonic stenosis

ETT, Endotracheal tube; *IV*, intravenous; *NICU*, neonatal intensive care unit.

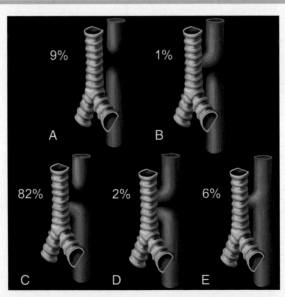

Fig. 8.3   Classification and relative frequency of the types of tracheoesophageal fistulas. (From Merrow, A. C., & Hariharan S. [2018]. Esophageal atresia and tracheoesophageal fistula. In A. C. Merrow & S. Hariharan [Eds.], *Imaging in pediatrics* [pp. 44–45]. Philadelphia, PA: Elsevier.)

What do you tell her?
Neonates and infants are usually monitored for at least 12 hours postoperatively, as the risk for postoperative apnea is highest in this very young population. This patient underwent general anesthesia, rather than regional anesthesia, and therefore, his risk of postoperative apnea is high. He should be monitored in t 67he hospital for at least 12 hours postoperatively.

BEYOND THE PEARLS

- The most common congenital anomalies are heart defects (5–7 per 1000), cleft lip and palate (1.5 per 1000), and neural tube defects (0.3 per 1000).
- Ventricular septal defects (VSDs) are the most common congenital cardiac defect and are often asymptomatic. Many self-resolve over time. Table 8.3 describes congenital anomalies and their anesthetic implications.
- During the fetal period, a right to left shunt is normal through a ductus arteriosus and foramen ovale, both of which close soon after birth with the increase in oxygen tension.

References

Marciniak, B. (2019). Growh and development. In C. J. Coté, J. Lerman, & B. J. Anderson (Eds.), *A practice of anesthesia for infants and children* (6th ed., Chapter 2, pp. 8–24.e3). Philadelphia, PA: Elsevier.

ACOG committee opinion no 579: Definition of term pregnancy. (2013). *Obstetrics and Gynecology, 122*(5), 1139–1140.

McGregor, K. (2017). Principles of anaesthesia for term neonates. *Anaesthesia and Intensive Care Medicine. 18*(2), 75–78.

Alexander, P. (2019). Respiratory physiology for intensivists. In R. M. Ungerleider, J. N. Meliones, K. N. McMillan, D. S. Cooper, & J. P. Jacobs (Eds.), *Critical heart disease in infants and children* (3rd ed., Chapter 14, pp. 134–149.e2). Philadelphia, PA: Elsevier.

Green, G. E. & Ohye, R. G. (2021). Diagnosis and management of tracheal anomalies and tracheal stenosis. In P. W. Flint, H. W. Francis, B. H. Haughey, M. M. Lesperance, V. J. Lund, K. T. Robbins, et al. (Eds.), *Cummings otolaryngology: Head and neck surgery* (7th ed., Chapter 210, pp. 3107–3118.e3, Fig. 210.5). Philadelphia, PA: Elsevier.

Davidson, A. J., Morton, N. S., Arnup, S. J., de Graaff, J. C., Disma, N., Withington, D. E., et al. (2015). Apnea after awake regional and general anesthesia in infants: The general anesthesia compared to spinal anesthesia study—comparing apnea and neurodevelopmental outcomes, a randomized controlled trial. *Anesthesiology, 123*(1), 38–54. https://doi.org/10.1097/ALN.0000000000000709.

Diu, M.W., & Mancuso, T. J. (2018). Pediatric diseases. In R. L. Hines & K. E. Marschall (Eds.), *Mancuso Stoelting's anesthesia and co-existing disease* (7th ed., Chapter 30, pp. 635–670). Philadelphia, PA: Elsevier.

Elsevier Point of Care. (2020). *Ventricular Septal Defect. Clinical Overview.* Philadelphia, PA: Elsevier.

Frumiento, C., Abajian, J. C., & Vane, D. W. (2000). Spinal anesthesia for preterm infants undergoing inguinal hernia repair. *Archives of Surgery, 135*(4), 445–451. https://doi.org/10.1001/archsurg.135.4.445.

Gregory, G. A., & Brett, C. M. (2017). Neonatology for anesthesiologists. In P. J. Davis & F. P. Cladis (Eds.), *Smith's anesthesia for infants and children* (9th ed., Chapter 23, pp. 513–570.e15). Philadelphia, PA: Elsevier.

Hall, J. E., & Hall, M. E. (Eds.). (2021). Fetal and neonatal physiology. *Guyton and Hall textbook of medical physiology* (14th ed., Chapter 84, pp. 1061–1070). Philadelphia, PA: Elsevier.

Kliegman, R. M., & St Geme, J., (2020). Acyanotic congenital heart disease: Left-to-right shunt lesions. In R. M. Kliegman, J. W. St Geme, N. J. Blum, S. S. Shah, R. C. Tasker, & K. M. Wilson (Eds.), *Nelson textbook of pediatrics* (21st ed., pp. 2373–2384.e1.). Philadelphia, PA: Elsevier.

Martin, J. A., Hamilton, B. E., Osterman, M. J., Driscoll, A. K., & Mathews, T. J. (2017). Births: Final data for 2015. *National Vital Statistics Reports, 66*(1), 1.

Marshall, W. J., Lapsley, M., Day, A., & Shipman, K. (2021). Disorders of carbohydrate metabolism. In *Clinical chemistry* (9th ed., Chapter 13, pp. 225–254). Philadelphia, PA: Elsevier.

Motoyama, E. K., & Finder, J. D. (2017). Respiratory physiology. In P. J. Davis & F. P. Cladis (Eds.), *Smith's anesthesia for infants and children* (9th ed., Chapter 3, p. 23–72.e15). Philadelphia, PA: Elsevier.

Gropper, M. A., Miller, R. D., Cohen, N. H., Eriksson, L. I., Fleisher, L. A., Leslie, K., et al. (Eds.). (2020). *Miller's anesthesia* (9th ed., chapter 77). Philadelphia, PA: Elsevier.

Rainaldi, M. A., & Perlman J. M. (2017). Neurologic effects of respiratory support. In J. P. Goldsmith, E. H. Karotkin, M. Keszler & G. K. Suresh (Eds.), *Assisted ventilation of the neonate* (6th ed., Chapter 42, pp. 451–458.e2). Philadelphia, PA: Elsevier.

Stewart, D. L., Barfield, W. D. & Committee on Fetus and Newborn. Updates on an at-risk population: Late-preterm and early-term infants. *Pediatrics, 144*(5), e20192760. https://doi.org/10.1542/peds.2019-2760.

Stork, J. E., & Ohliger, S. (2020). Anesthesia in the neonate. In R. J. Martin, A. A. Fanaroff & M. C. Walsh (Eds.), *Neonatal–perinatal medicine* (11th ed., Chapter 39, pp. 634–653). Philadelphia, PA: Elsevier.

Tipple, T. E., & Ambalavanan, N. (2019). Oxygen toxicity in the neonate: Thinking beyond the balance. *Clinics in Perinatology, 46*(3), 435–447.

Obstetrics

A 26-Year-Old Primigravid Woman at 39 Weeks' and 4 Days' Gestation Presenting With 6 Hours of Cramping Abdominal Pain

Ian Brooks ■ Paul Neil Frank

A 26-year-old primigravid woman at 39 weeks and 4 days gestation presents to labor and delivery triage with 6 hours of cramping abdominal pain and a large gush of clear fluid 1 hour ago. She is otherwise healthy and takes only a daily prenatal vitamin. She denies vaginal bleeding or loss of fetal movement. Her vital signs are blood pressure 107/68 mm Hg, pulse 78/min, respiration rate 18, oxygen saturation 99% on room air, and temperature 36.9°C. Exam shows that her cervix is dilated to 3 cm and is 40% effaced, and the fetus is at −1 station.

What are the stages of labor? What stage of labor is our patient in?
Labor is divided into four stages, described in Table 9.1. Stage one consists of cervical dilation and can be subdivided into latent and active phases. The first stage typically lasts 8–12 hours in nulliparous women and 5–8 hours in multiparous women. Stage two consists of fetal descent, stage three consists of placental delivery, and stage four consists of monitoring for return of uterine tone (see Fig. 9.1).

Our patient is in the latent phase of the first stage of labor.

The patient is complaining of back pain. Is this normal? What causes pain during labor?
Pain during the first stage of labor is caused by lower uterine and cervical dilation. These areas are innervated by visceral afferent nerve fibers. Because visceral pathways cause poorly localized pain, referred pain to other sites including the lower back are common.

Pain during the second stage of labor is caused by cervical dilation as in the first stage and also by distension of the vagina, pelvic floor, and perineum. These areas have somatic innervation via the pudendal nerve. Thus pain during the second stage of labor includes the visceral pain experienced in the first stage, with the addition of well-localized pain in the vagina and perineum. Fig. 9.2 shows the innervation of the uterus, cervix, and vagina as well as the appropriate regional nerve block to treat pain arising from each area.

STEP 1 PEARL

Oxytocin is a hormone produced by the posterior pituitary gland that causes the uterus to contract. During pregnancy, uterine oxytocin receptors are upregulated. Oxytocin stimulates uterine smooth muscle contraction during labor. After birth, oxytocin plays a role in maternal milk release and maternal-infant bonding.

TABLE 9.1 ■ **Endpoints and Characteristics of the Stages of Labor**

Stage	Description
First Stage (Latent Phase)	• Increase in intensity and frequency of uterine contractions • Moderate cervical change
First Stage (Active Phase)	• Acceleration in the rate of cervical change • Ends with full dilation of cervix to 10 cm
Second Stage	• Full cervical dilation to delivery of the fetus • Characterized by fetal descent in the pelvis
Third Stage	• Delivery of the placenta
Fourth Stage	• Reestablishment of uterine tone after placental delivery

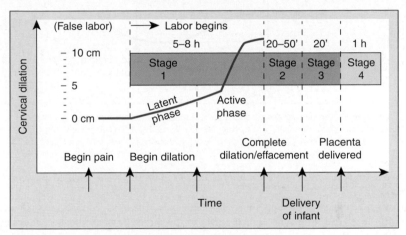

Fig. 9.1 The normal duration of each stage of labor. These vary somewhat based on the parity of the patient. (Walls, R., Hockberger, R., & Gausche-Hill, M. [2017]. *Rosen's emergency medicine: Concepts and clinical practice* [Chapter 181, pp. 2296–2312.e2, Figure 181.1].)

What techniques are available to treat pain during labor?

Systemic opioid administration, inhaled nitrous oxide, and regional and neuraxial anesthesia are all used to provide analgesia in labor.

Systemic opioids are inexpensive and easy to administer, but these agents can cause maternal and fetal respiratory depression, as well as decreased fetal heart rate (FHR) variability. All opioids readily cross the placenta. Side effects tend to be more related to opioid dose than the type of opioid selected. Although judicious administration of short-acting opioids is safe early in labor, this should be avoided closer to delivery.

Inhaled nitrous oxide use is more common in Europe than in the United States. It is typically administered by facemask in a 50% nitrous oxide and 50% oxygen mixture. It has a very quick onset and has not been shown to have any harmful effects on neonates. The most common maternal side effect is nausea and vomiting, with a reported incidence of up to 33%. Like opioid administration, inhaled nitrous oxide is less effective than neuraxial anesthesia. Nonetheless, some studies have shown improved maternal satisfaction with nitrous oxide even in the absence of significantly improved analgesia.

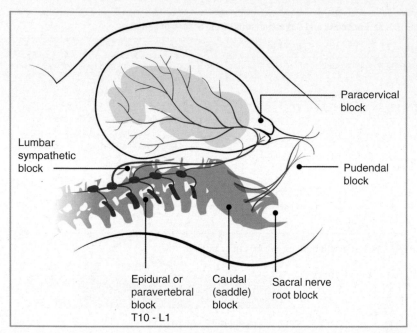

Fig. 9.2   Innervation of the uterus, cervix, and vagina as well as the appropriate regional block for each. (Chestnut, D. H., Wong, C. A., Tsen, L. C., Kee, W. D. N., Beilin, Y., Mhyre, J. M. et al. [Eds.]. [2020]. *Chestnut's obstetric anesthesia* [Chapter 20, pp. 422–440]. Philadelphia, PA: Elsevier. Figure 20.5.)

Would a paracervical nerve block be helpful in this context? What about a pudendal nerve block?

A paracervical block is not the best choice for labor pain. The block consists of local anesthetic injection in the vaginal fornix and vaginal aspect of the cervix. Some of the local anesthetic will diffuse and block the visceral nerves innervating the cervix and uterus. It will provide analgesia during the first stage of labor but will not provide relief from somatic pain during the second stage as the patient progresses. Paracervical blocks are associated with a higher risk of fetal bradycardia and have fallen out of favor for this reason. Paracervical blocks are commonly used for cervical dilation and uterine curettage procedures but are not used for labor analgesia.

Obstetricians may perform pudendal nerve blocks to help with pain from the second stage of labor, episiotomy during delivery, or vaginal laceration repair afterward. This block involves injection of local anesthetic near the pudendal nerve (S2–S4) as it travels near the ischial spines. Pudendal nerve blocks are associated with rapid maternal uptake of local anesthetic.

Epidural anesthesia is a better option for pain control for this patient.

The patient asks how epidural anesthesia differs from spinal anesthesia.

The most common types of neuraxial anesthesia are epidural and spinal anesthesia. Spinal anesthesia is generally administered as a single injection directly into the subarachnoid space, while epidural anesthesia involves placement of a catheter in the epidural space. Analogous to an intravenous (IV) catheter, an epidural catheter allows for ongoing administration of medications, such as local anesthetics and opioids, to provide continuous analgesia. In addition, higher doses of stronger medications may be administered via an epidural catheter to provide adequate surgical anesthesia should a cesarean delivery (C-section) become necessary.

TABLE 9.2 ■ **Comparison of Epidural and Spinal Anesthesia**

	Epidural	Spinal
Anatomic location	Epidural space, between the ligamentum flavum and the dura mater (see Fig. 9.5)	Inside the thecal sac, in solution with cerebrospinal fluid (CSF)
Primary site of action	Spinal nerve roots	Spinal cord
Most common type of needle	Touhy (17- or 18-gauge)	• Blunt tip (more common, lower risk of spinal headache) • Cutting (Quincke)
Spread affected by baricity of solution	No	Yes
Risk of total spinal	No	Yes
Mode of administration	Catheter	Single-shot
Time to block onset	10–20 min	2–8 min

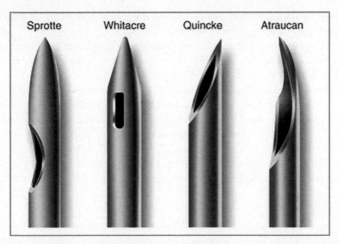

Fig. 9.3 Common types of spinal needles. Pencil-point needles such as Sprotte and Whitacre designs are associated with lower incidence of postdural puncture headache than the cutting Quincke needle. (Chestnut, D. H., Wong, C. A., Tsen, L. C., Kee, W. D. N., Beilin, Y., Mhyre, J. M. et al. [Eds.]. [2020]. *Chestnut's obstetric anesthesia* [Chapter 12, pp. 238–270]. Philadelphia, PA: Elsevier. Figure 12.6.)

Due to its limited duration of action and the need to repeat the entire procedure to repeat a dose of medication, spinal anesthesia is rarely used for labor analgesia but is often used for C-sections.

Table 9.2 outlines key differences between spinal and epidural anesthesia. Figs. 9.3 and 9.4 show needles used for spinal injection and epidural catheter placement, respectively.

What is baricity? How does it affect the spread of spinal anesthesia?
The baricity of a solution is its density relative to cerebrospinal fluid (CSF). A hyperbaric solution, or one that is denser than CSF, will tend to distribute toward dependent areas of the spinal canal (i.e., gravity pulls it down). For example, in a patient sitting upright, a hyperbaric spinal bolus will tend to sink and affect more caudal dermatomal levels. Conversely, a hypobaric solution, or one less dense than CSF, would tend to rise in an upright patient and affect more cephalad dermatomes. Isobaric spinal solutions have the same density as CSF and are not significantly influenced by gravity. Note that the concept of baricity applies only to spinal injections; it does not apply to epidural medications, which are not injected into CSF.

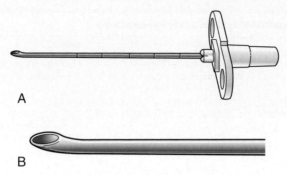

Fig. 9.4   (A) The shape of a Tuohy epidural needle is illustrated. (B) The upturned tip of the needle is used to direct the epidural catheter cephalad on insertion into the epidural space. (Yentis, S., Hirsch, N., & Ip, J. [2018]. *Anaesthesia, intensive care and perioperative medicine A-Z* [Chapter E, pp. 197–224, Figure 64].)

Which dermatomal levels must be covered by epidural anesthesia to provide analgesia during labor? What levels must be covered for a C-section?

During the first stage of labor, pain is primarily related to distension of the lower uterine segment and cervix, which have visceral innervation from spinal levels T10–L1. Thus an epidural must cover T10–L1 to provide analgesia during the first stage of labor.

Pain during the second stage of labor is caused by the same areas as the first stage of labor, as well as by distension of the vaginal side of the cervix, vagina, and perineum, which are innervated by somatic fibers originating from spinal levels S2–S4. Thus, to provide analgesia for the second stage of labor, an epidural must provide coverage for the levels T10–S4.

Although cesarean delivery is most commonly performed with a horizontal (Pfannenstiel) incision around T11–12 dermatomes, visceral pain may be sensed significantly higher than that. Anesthesia for C-section should cover levels as cephalad as the T4–T6 dermatomes.

STEP 1 PEARL

Commonly tested dermatomes include:
T4—nipple level
T10—umbilicus level
L1—inguinal ligament level
L4/L5/S1—medial, top, and lateral aspects of the foot, respectively

---

The patient's husband is nervous. He asks about the potential complications of epidural placement.

Risks of epidural placement include postdural puncture headache, epidural hematoma, epidural abscess, or total spinal anesthesia (in the event of inadvertent intrathecal placement). The causes, presentations, and management of these complications are listed in Table 9.3. Neurological injury is rare.

Some studies of epidural anesthesia have shown a mild increase in the length of the second stage of labor of up to 15 minutes, but there is no association between epidural anesthesia and risk of needing a C-section.

When during labor should an epidural be placed?

There is no designated time or degree of cervical dilation at which an epidural should be placed. American Society of Anesthesiologists (ASA) guidelines state that patient request is an appropriate indication , assuming there are no contraindications (e.g. coagulopathy, overlying infection,

TABLE 9.3 ■ Pathophysiology, Presentation, and Management of Complications of Epidural Anesthesia

Complication	Pathophysiology	Diagnosis/Presentation	Management
Dural puncture ("wet tap")	Touhy needle violates the dura and enters the thecal sac	• Gush of warm fluid through Touhy needle • Positional headache (worse sitting up, better lying down), known as a "spinal headache" or "postdural puncture headache" • photophobia, other neurological symptoms	• IV fluids • Caffeine • Blood patch if persistent symptoms or associated neurological symptoms
Intrathecal catheter placement	Touhy needle violates the dura and enters the thecal sac; this then goes unrecognized and the epidural catheter is threaded into the thecal sac, where epidural (higher) doses of medications are inadvertently given intrathecally	• Aspiration of CSF via catheter • "Total spinal" (severe hypotension, apnea, cardiovascular collapse)	Emergent endotracheal intubation and hemodynamic support until resolution
Spinal hematoma Epidural hematoma	Bleeding within the spinal canal or epidural space that causes hematoma compressing the spinal cord or nerve roots	Persistent or progressive numbness, weakness, or paralysis after discontinuation of epidural	• CT or MRI of spine • Emergent neurosurgical consult for decompression
Epidural or spinal abscess	Infection within epidural or subarachnoid space	• Localized pain → radicular pain → motor/sensory deficits → paraplegia • Fever • Symptoms may present days after placement of neuraxial anesthesia	• CT or MRI of spine • Emergent neurosurgical consult

CSF, Cerebrospinal fluid; *CT*, computed tomography; *IV*, intravenous; *MRI*, magnetic resonance imaging.

hemodynamic instability). Patients should be made aware that changes—including possible dietary restriction, bedrest, and urinary catheter insertion—may be required after an epidural is placed.

The patient agrees to epidural placement.

What are the steps of the procedure?

The patient should be positioned in a way that exposes the lower back and expands the spaces between lumbar vertebrae. Typically, this is done in a sitting position, but lateral positioning may be considered as well. The patient's iliac crests should be palpated as a landmark because they usually correspond to the L4–L5 spinal levels. This helps identify the interspaces between vertebrae. The patient's back should be palpated to determine an appropriate needle entry point, usually midline between the spinous processes of L4–5 or L3–4, although this may

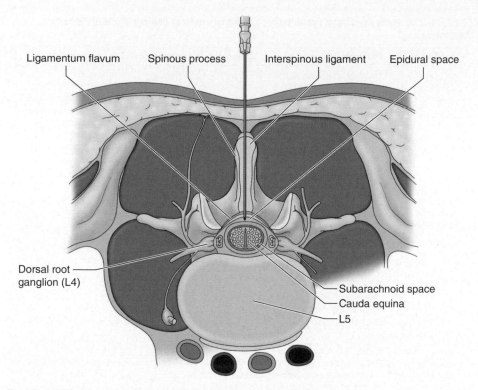

Fig. 9.5   Midline lumbar epidural approach and related anatomy. (Hyder, O., & Rathmell, J. P. *Basics of 2018 Anesthesia* [Chapter 44, pp. 770–787, Figure 44.4]. Redrawn from Rathmell, J. P. [2006]. *Atlas of image-guided intervention in regional anesthesia and pain medicine* [p. 47]. Philadelphia: Lippincott Williams & Wilkins.)

vary in cases of scoliosis or other aberrant anatomy, or when a paramedian epidural approach is attempted.

Next the back is prepped with a sterile cleaning solution, and a sterile drape is applied. Local anesthetic (typically lidocaine) is injected subcutaneously for patient comfort. An epidural needle, often a 17-gauge Tuohy needle, is inserted and advanced. When the needle is felt to have engaged with supraspinous or interspinous ligament, a specialized syringe filled with air and/or saline is attached. As the needle is slowly advanced, the plunger on the syringe is compressed, either in a continuous or intermittent fashion. When the syringe depresses easily, this is known as a "loss of resistance" and can indicate that the tip of the needle is past the ligamentum flavum and in the epidural space. The epidural catheter is then threaded into the epidural space. The epidural needle is removed, and the catheter is aspirated to check for accidental intravascular or intrathecal insertion. If aspiration is negative (i.e., there is no return of clear fluid or blood), the catheter can be secured and a test dose of medicine may be given through it.

Assuming a midline approach, what structures does the needle tip pass through on the way to the epidural space?

The structures passed through are, in order: skin/subcutaneous tissue, supraspinous ligament, interspinous ligament, ligamentum flavum, epidural space. Anatomy related to lumbar epidural placement is shown in Fig. 9.5.

Epidural placement is uneventful.

What is a test dose, and why is it necessary?

A test dose is a small bolus of short-acting local anesthetic mixed with epinephrine given after epidural placement to ensure that the catheter is not in a blood vessel or the subarachnoid space. If the catheter is inadvertently placed intravascularly, the epinephrine may cause tachycardia and the local anesthetic may cause neurological side effects (e.g., perioral numbness or tingling). If the catheter is inadvertently placed intrathecally, profound sensory and motor block will occur. Patients should be asked to report these symptoms when receiving a test dose.

The patient is still awaiting pain relief 5 minutes after the first dose through the epidural.

Could other techniques have been used to provide quicker analgesia?

After bolus of a standard epidural, block onset may take 10–20 minutes. If faster onset is desired, combined spinal-epidural (CSE) or dural puncture epidural (DPE) techniques may be considered instead.

CSE offers the rapid onset of a spinal while facilitating ongoing neuraxial anesthesia via the epidural catheter. To perform a CSE, an epidural needle is placed with its tip in the epidural space, as it is during usual epidural placement. A long spinal needle is then passed through the epidural needle and into the intrathecal space, where a dose of spinal anesthetic is deposited. The spinal needle is withdrawn, and the epidural catheter is threaded through the epidural needle into the epidural space. Studies have not shown an increase in the incidence of postdural puncture headache or C-section with CSE compared with labor epidural alone. CSE technique is demonstrated in comparison to traditional epidural placement in Fig. 9.6.

DPE technique is almost identical to CSE; the key difference is that no intrathecal medication is given after the spinal needle punctures dura mater. Instead, the purpose of the small dural puncture with DPE is to allow some of the medication from the epidural catheter to diffuse intrathecally. Some studies have shown evidence of decreased time to onset of analgesia and better analgesia with DPE when compared to standard labor epidural.

What medicines can you give the patient through her epidural catheter? Should they be short or long acting?

Local anesthetics and opioids are the most common medicines given with epidural catheters. Epidural α_2 agonists have been shown to improve analgesia and reduce local anesthetic requirement when used as an adjunct, but these are generally not recommended in obstetric patients due to the risk of hypotension and bradycardia. Epidural clonidine use in obstetrics is more common in Europe than the United States.

The ideal epidural block maximizes sensory blockade and minimizes motor blockade; it also has a duration to match the duration of the painful stimulus. Thus long-acting medicines are best for labor. Bupivacaine and ropivacaine are excellent choices for labor analgesia. They are long acting and have a favorable sensory-to-motor blockade profile. They may be given as a continuous infusion, patient-controlled boluses (patient-controlled epidural analgesia [PCEA]), or provider-administered boluses.

Lidocaine and chloroprocaine are better choices for analgesia for shorter procedures. Lidocaine may be given with epinephrine, which can increase both block duration and density (i.e., more numbness). Chloroprocaine is rapidly metabolized by plasma esterases, allowing for a higher safe maximum dose compared with other local anesthetics. Because of the higher doses used, it has the fastest onset of any of the local anesthetics and is often used when rapid analgesia is needed for emergency surgery.

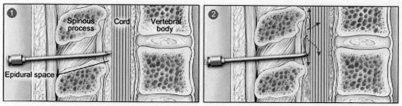

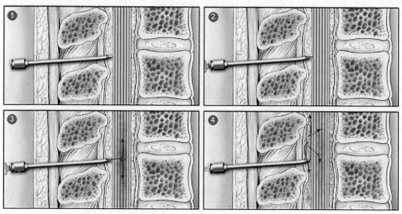

A Epidural Analgesia

B Combined Spinal-Epidural Analgesia

Fig. 9.6   Epidural and combined spinal-epidural (CSE) placement techniques. (A) Epidural catheter place-ment for labor analgesia: (1) The Tuohy epidural needle is advanced through the interspinous ligament and ligamentum flavum into the epidural space. (2) The epidural catheter is threaded through the Tuohy needle and into the epidural space. The catheter is then used to infuse epidural medicines. (B) CSE technique: (1) The Tuohy needle is advanced into the epidural space in the same manner as traditional epidural placement. (2) The spinal needle is passed through the Tuohy needle; dural puncture is confirmed by cerebrospinal fluid return. (3) A bolus of local anesthetic, opioid, or both is given intrathecally through the spinal needle. (4) The spinal needle is removed and an epidural catheter is threaded into the epidural space. Note that the special CSE Tuohy needle design prevents the catheter from passing through the spinal needle opening on the back of the bevel. The catheter is used to infuse medicine during labor. (Lucero, J., & Rollins, M. *Basics of Anesthesia* [Chapter 33, pp. 553–586, Figure 33.5]. From Eltzschig, H. K., Lieberman, E. S., & Camann, W. R. [2003]. Regional anesthesia and analgesia for labor and delivery. *The New England Journal of Medicine. 348*, pp. 319–332.)

Opioids, including fentanyl, morphine, and sufentanil, may be administered in the epidural space as well. When used in conjunction with local anesthetics, they decrease local anesthetic requirements.

The test dose is negative, and you bolus the epidural catheter with ropivacaine and fentanyl. Thirty minutes later, the patient says her pain is nearly gone, but now she feels itchy.

What's going on?
Diffuse pruritus is the most common side effect of epidural opioid administration.

Will an antihistamine such as diphenhydramine help?
No. The mechanism of opioid-induced pruritus is poorly understood but is not histamine medi-ated, so antihistamines are typically not helpful. Instead, systemic opioid antagonists or partial agonists are better choices for this indication.

After another bolus of local anesthetic through the epidural catheter, the patient's blood pressure is now 82/40 mm hg and her pulse is 105/min. She feels nauseated.

What's going on? What can you do?

Both epidural and spinal anesthesia commonly cause hypotension due to sympathetic blockade, known as sympathectomy. The level of sympathectomy is often several dermatomes more cephalad than the level of the sensory block. The sympathectomy causes arterial and venous vasodilation, resulting in decreased systemic vascular resistance and blood return to the heart (i.e., preload).

Our patient is most likely experiencing hypotension due to vasodilation from epidural local anesthetic. She should be treated with IV fluids, phenylephrine, and/or ephedrine. Antiemetics may be considered, but if the primary etiology of her nausea is believed to be related to her hypotension, then her blood pressure should be addressed first. The gravid uterus may also compress the inferior vena cava if the patient is supine. Tilting the patient to her left (i.e., left uterine displacement) will help improve blood pressure.

To minimize this risk of hypotension from neuraxial anesthesia, patients should be given IV fluids shortly before or during initiation of neuraxial anesthesia. Studies have shown conflicting data about the ideal fluid volume, but 0.5–1 L is considered reasonable. Care should be taken to avoid initiating neuraxial anesthesia in hypovolemic patients.

STEP 1 PEARL

Adrenergic receptors of the sympathetic nervous system include α_1 receptors, which cause vasoconstriction; $\beta 1$ receptors, which cause increased heart rate and contractility; and β_2 receptors, which cause vasodilation and bronchodilation. Phenylephrine is a vasopressor that is an α receptor agonist.

What are the other possible effects of neuraxial anesthesia?

Neuraxial anesthesia also has noncardiovascular effects. Sympathectomy in the T6–L1 distribution can cause unopposed gastrointestinal parasympathetic activity resulting in hyperperistalsis and nausea. Atropine is the most effective treatment.

Neuraxial anesthesia can also cause decreased functional residual capacity in the lungs and decreased renal blood flow, but these are rarely clinically significant.

The patient's blood pressure improves with a bolus of fluid. The cardiotocograph is shown in Fig. 9.7.

What is a cardiotocograph? How do you interpret this?

A cardiotocograph is a graph showing both FHR and uterine contractions on the same time axis, allowing for the relationship between the two to be analyzed. FHR is used to monitor fetal well-being and oxygenation. Normal FHR varies between 110 and 160/min. Fetal bradycardia is the initial response to acute fetal hypoxemia. Different timing of episodes of fetal bradycardia relative to uterine contractions (i.e., decelerations) on cardiotocograph correspond with different types of either benign or pathologic situations.

The cardiotocograph in Fig. 9.7 shows the onset of the fetal bradycardia right at the start of uterine contractions and a return to normal FHR at the end of the uterine contractions. This is called an early deceleration. Early deceleration is caused by compression of the fetal head by uterine contraction, which causes a transient vagal response by the fetus. Early decelerations are a normal, nonconcerning finding.

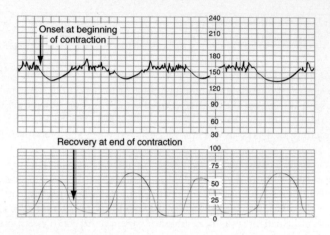

Fig. 9.7 Early deceleration of fetal heart rate resulting from fetal head compression and subsequent fetal vagal output. (Vasquez, V., & Desai, S. [2017]. *Rosen's emergency medicine: Concepts and clinical practice* [Chapter 181, pp. 2296–2312.e2]. Philadelphia, PA: Elsevier. Modified from Fig 181.6. Vasquez V, Desai S. [Modified from Lowdermilk, D. L., Bobak, I. M., & Perry, S. E. [1997]. *Maternity and women's health care* [6th ed.]. St. Louis: Mosby].

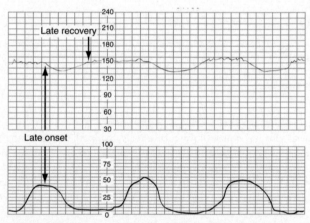

Fig. 9.8 Late decelerations of fetal heart rate resulting from uteroplacental insufficiency. (Vasquez, V., & Desai, S. *Rosen's emergency medicine: Concepts and clinical practice* [Chapter 181, pp. 2296–2312.e2, Fig. 181.6]. [Modified from Lowdermilk, D. L., Bobak, I. M., & Perry, S. E. [1997]. *Maternity and women's health care* [6th ed.]. St. Louis: Mosby].)

Furthermore, in Fig. 9.7, moderate variability in the FHR is observed between the early decelerations. A moderate degree of variability in the baseline FHR is an indicator of fetal well-being because it suggests an intact fetal central nervous system (CNS) and parasympathetic activation of the fetal heart. Decreased FHR variability, which would appear as a flatter tracing, suggests fetal hypoxia, sleep, neurological abnormality, or medication (i.e., opioid) effect.

What if the tracing had looked like the one in Fig. 9.8? Or Fig. 9.9?
The cardiotocograph shown in Fig. 9.8 shows late decelerations. A late deceleration is characterized by a gradual, delayed drop in FHR that does not reach its nadir until after the peak of the uterine contraction; recovery occurs more slowly and only after the contraction has resolved. Late

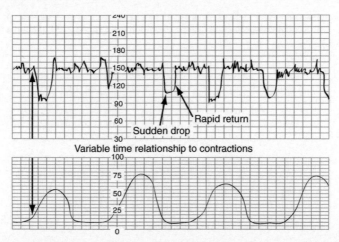

Fig. 9.9   **Variable decelerations of fetal heart rate resulting umbilical cord compression.** (Vasquez, V., & Desai, S. *Rosen's emergency medicine: Concepts and clinical practice* ([Chapter 181, pp. 2296–2312.e2, Fig. 181.6]. Vasquez V, Desai S. [Modified from Lowdermilk, D. L., Bobak, I. M., & Perry, S. E. [1997]. *Maternity and women's health care* [6th ed.]. St. Louis: Mosby].)

TABLE 9.4 ■ **Types of FHR Decelerations and Their Characteristics**

Type of Deceleration	Relationship to Uterine Contraction	Etiology	Association With Fetal Well-being
Early	Coincides with start of contraction	Fetal head compression and vagal response to mild hypoxia	Not concerning for compromised well-being
Variable	Variable, often with abrupt onset and offset	Umbilical cord compression	Usually tolerated if the fetus is healthy and FHR remains >80
Late	Starts 10–30 s after contraction initiation	Uteroplacental insufficiency, fetal hypoxemia	Concerning for fetal distress, especially when seen with decreased FHR variability

FHR, Fetal heart rate.

decelerations indicate insufficient oxygen supply to the fetus, called uteroplacental insufficiency. Late decelerations are a nonreassuring finding.

The cardiotocograph in Fig. 9.9 shows variable decelerations. As the name implies, variable contractions have a variable temporal relationship to uterine contractions. Their shape is characterized by steep FHR descents and often by similarly rapid recoveries. Variable decelerations are caused by periods of umbilical cord compression and are more common when amniotic fluid volume is decreased. Variable decelerations may be well tolerated by a healthy fetus but can be nonreassuring if the bradycardia periods are profound or frequent. The types of FHR decelerations are summarized in Table 9.4.

How does a cardiotocograph guide management? Should any changes be made to our patient's care?
FHR tracings are described as category I, II, or III. Criteria for the three categories are listed in Table 9.5. A category I FHR tracing is reassuring and only indicates the need for intermittent

TABLE 9.5 ■ FHR Tracing Categorization Criteria. Modified from Box 8.2 of Chestnut's Obstetric Anesthesia (2020)

Category I FHR tracing	Must include all:
	• Baseline FHR 110–160/min
	• Moderate FHR variability
	• No late or variable decelerations
	• Presence or absence of early decelerations
Category II FHR tracing	Any tracing not category I or III
Category III FHR tracing	Sinusoidal pattern
	OR
	Absent FHR variability and any of the following:
	• Bradycardia
	• Recurrent late decelerations
	• Recurrent variable decelerations

FHR, Fetal heart rate.

TABLE 9.6 ■ Chorioamnionitis Diagnostic Criteria and Risk Factors

Chorioamnionitis, or Intra-amniotic Infection	
Diagnostic Criteria	Risk Factors
Maternal temperature ≥38°C and any of the following: • Fetal tachycardia • Maternal WBC >15,000 • Purulent fluid from cervical os on exam • Amniotic fluid result with evidence of infection	• History of chorioamnionitis with prior delivery • Low parity • Increased number of vaginal exams • Prolonged labor • Prolonged rupture of membranes • Intrauterine monitors

reevaluation. A category II or III tracing may indicate the need for further evaluation or intervention depending on the clinical context. Interventions may target improving fetal oxygenation, alleviating umbilical cord compression, or reducing the intensity of uterine contractions. Possible interventions include maternal positional changes, IV fluids or vasopressors, tocolytic medicines (to decrease uterine contractions), or amnioinfusion (only if cord compression is suspected). A category III tracing that does not improve may be an indication for urgent delivery.

Our patient's fetus has a category I tracing, meaning FHR is between 110 and 160/min with moderate variability and no variable or late decelerations. Only periodic reevaluation is indicated.

Four hours later, the patient has a temperature of 38.1°C. Laboratory analysis shows a newly elevated maternal white blood cell count of 26,000/µl, and fetal tachycardia is noted.

What is the diagnosis?

These findings are consistent with chorioamnionitis, or intra-amniotic infection. Diagnostic criteria and risk factors for this condition are listed in Table 9.6. Chorioamnionitis has been associated with maternal preterm labor, postpartum hemorrhage, intensive care unit (ICU) admission, and mortality, as well as neonatal pneumonia, meningitis, and mortality. Early antibiotic therapy is indicated. Our patient should be treated with ampicillin and gentamicin. Chorioamnionitis alone is not an indication for C-section, but if she were to require a C-section later, clindamycin or metronidazole should be added to decrease the risk of endometritis.

STEP 2, 3 PEARL

Several lab changes are normal during pregnancy. They include:
- Blood hemoglobin concentration decreases, even though total body hemoglobin amount increases. This is due to expansion of total blood volume. This is known as "physiologic anemia of pregnancy" (see Case 10).
- Thyroxine (T4) levels increase but so do thyroid-binding globulin levels, so free T4 levels remain the same.
- Blood urea nitrogen (BUN) and serum creatinine decrease because the glomerular filtration rate in the kidneys increases.

Should you remove the epidural catheter since the patient has chorioamnionitis?
There is no need to remove the epidural catheter, especially if appropriate antibiotic therapy is started. Studies, albeit small retrospective ones, have not demonstrated increased CNS infection risk with neuraxial anesthesia in the setting of chorioamnionitis. In 2017, the ASA issued a Practice Advisory for the Prevention, Diagnosis, and Management of Infectious Complications Associated with Neuraxial Techniques. It concluded that during systemic infection, neuraxial technique may be considered on a case-by-case basis and that, when neuraxial techniques are administered to patients with suspected or known bacteremia, antibiotics should be considered.

The baby is delivered 36 hours after the start of labor. One minute after birth, the neonate's heart rate is 76/min, respirations are irregular, his body is pink but his limbs are dusky, he is limp, and he does not response to suctioning.

What is his apgar score? How is this information used clinically?
His Apgar score is 3, which indicates the need for immediate resuscitation.

Apgar scoring was developed by Dr. Virginia Apgar, an anesthesiologist, as a quick and relatively objective way to assess newborns. Its primary purpose is to help identify newborns who require resuscitation. It is calculated at 1 and 5 minutes after delivery. The scoring criteria are listed in Table 9.7. A score of three or less suggests the need for immediate resuscitation, whereas a score of 8–10 is normal. The evaluation does not replace the physical exam and is not a reliable predictor of long-term outcomes. Its use is commonplace, although its value remains subject to debate.

TABLE 9.7 ■ **Apgar Score Criteria. Modified from Table 9.1 in Chestnut's Obstetric Anesthesia (2020)**

Apgar Category	2 Points	1 Point	0 Points
Heart rate	>100	<100	Absent
Respiratory status	Crying	Irregular, slow, or gasping respirations	Absent
Color	Pink	Pink body, cyanotic extremities	Cyanotic
Muscle tone	Movement	Some extremity flexion	Limp
Grimace/response to nasal or oral suctioning	Coughing or sneezing	Grimace	Absent

STEP 2, 3 PEARL

Uterine atony is an overdistension, or lack of appropriate contraction, of the uterus after birth. Atony increases risk of postpartum hemorrhage. Prolonged labor ("tired uterus"), extended use of oxytocin, and a large number of previous pregnancies are risk factors for atony. Treatments to help with contraction include oxytocin, manual stimulation (uterine massage), ergonovine, prostaglandin f2α, and misoprostol (see Case 10).

The mother is stable, and an anesthesiology colleague takes over her care while you resuscitate the newborn.

What supportive measures should be taken?

A heart rate less than 100/min is an indication to begin immediate resuscitation of a neonate, regardless of respiratory status. Positive pressure ventilation (PPV) with bag-mask ventilation should be started and continued until the heart rate is greater than 100/min. An algorithm for neonatal resuscitation is shown in Fig. 9.10.

The first breath given should include an end-inspiratory recruitment maneuver in which a pressure of 30 cm H_2O is held for 4–5 seconds to open alveoli. Breaths should then be given at a rate of 40–60/min with a pressure of 20–30 cm H_2O.

If you are the sole anesthesia provider in the room, ensure the mother is stable prior to addressing the neonate.

Should you provide PPV with 100% fraction of inspired oxygen (FiO₂ 1.0)?

No. Room air should be used for PPV because higher fractions of inspired oxygen have been associated with worse outcomes in neonates. Meta-analyses published in 2004 and 2008 aggregated studies that compared neonatal resuscitation with 21% oxygen (room air) and 100% oxygen; pooled data in both analyses showed significant mortality benefit in the groups ventilated with room air. The 2008 meta-analysis also showed a trend towards decreased risk of hypoxic ischemic encephalopathy with use of room air. Furthermore, oxygen toxicity in preterm infants is thought to be a contributing factor to retinopathy of prematurity. Current guidelines recommend minimizing FiO_2 during initial neonatal resuscitation.

An assistant places the pulse oximeter probe on the baby's left hand.

What should you do?

Move the probe to the baby's right hand. It should be applied to the right upper extremity because the right arm receives preductal circulation (i.e., oxygenated blood ejected from the left ventricle into the ascending aorta and aortic arch before it is potentially mixed with deoxygenated blood from the ductus arteriosus). Preductal oxygen saturation is representative of the blood flowing to the brain and heart. Blood flowing to the left upper extremity and both lower extremities may contain a mixture of oxygenated and deoxygenated blood until the ductus arteriosus closes as the baby transitions from fetal to neonatal circulation. The ductus arteriosus is illustrated in Fig. 9.11.

What is the ductus arteriosus? Describe fetal circulation.

Oxygen diffuses from maternal circulation through the placenta. Oxygenated fetal blood travels from the placenta to the fetus via the umbilical vein; deoxygenated blood returns from the fetus to the placenta via the umbilical arteries. Blood moves from the right ventricle to systemic circulation,

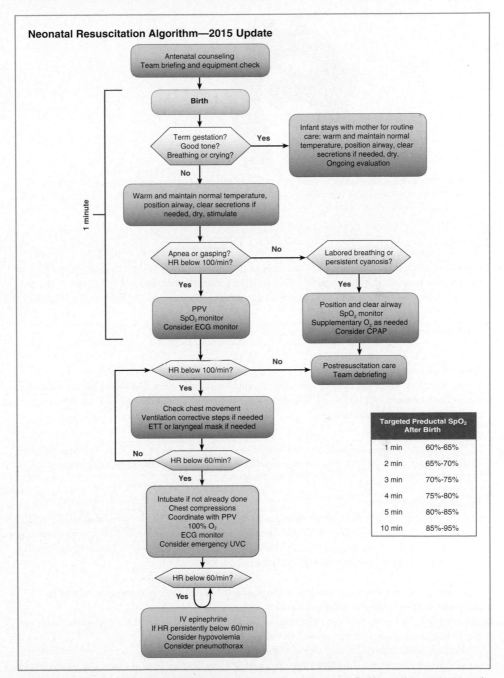

Fig. 9.10　Neonatal resuscitation algorithm. (Aucott, S. W., & Murphy, J. D. Neonatal assessment and resuscitation. *Chestnut's obstetric anesthesia* [Chapter 9, pp. 171–198. Fig. 9.3].)

HR, heart rate; *ETT*, endotracheal tube; *PPV*, positive pressure ventilation; *IV*, intravenous; *CPAP*, continuous positive airway pressure; *ECG* electrocardiogram; *UVC*, umbilical venous catheter.

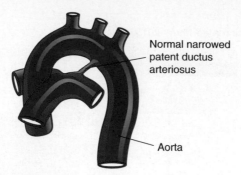

Normal narrowed patent ductus arteriosus

Aorta

Fig. 9.11   The ductus arteriosus. In fetal circulation, blood is shunted from the pulmonary artery to the aorta via the ductus arteriosus. After birth, the duct closes and becomes the ligamentum arteriosum. (Moore, K., Persaud, T., & Torch, M. [2020]. *Before we are born*. [Chapter 14, pp. 175–208.e1, Figure 14.34].)

bypassing the fetal lungs, which are not oxygenated, by two right-to-left shunts: an opening in the septum between the right and left atria called a foramen ovale, and a shunt between the pulmonary artery and aorta called the ductus arteriosus. These structures are illustrated in Fig. 9.12.

Despite ppv, the baby's heart rate drops to 55/min.

What should you do?
If the heart rate decreases to less than 60/min, intubation and chest compressions are indicated. Chest compressions will inhibit PPV, and thus the two need to be staggered in a 3:1 ratio with 90 compressions and 30 breaths/min.

The baby's condition improves, and he is admitted to the neonatal icu. On postpartum day 1, the patient (the mother) complains of new numbness and burning over her right anterolateral thigh.

What's going on?
Our patient's condition, known as meralgia paresthetica, is the result of isolated injury to the lateral femoral cutaneous nerve. It is the most common obstetric neurological injury, caused by compression of the nerve as it courses by the anterior superior iliac spine or beneath the inguinal ligament. Reassure the patient that this will resolve on its own.

What other nerve injuries are common in parturients? Are they more commonly related to labor and delivery or to neuraxial anesthesia?
Other peripheral nerves that can be injured in the peripartum period include the obturator, femoral, sciatic, and peroneal nerves, as well as the lumbosacral trunk.

Forceps used during delivery can compress the obturator nerve against the maternal pelvis, causing nerve injury. An obturator nerve palsy may cause sensory changes over the medial thigh or gait changes due to hip adduction weakness.

Prolonged lithotomy positioning, squatting, or pressure on the lateral aspect of the knee can injure the common peroneal nerve as it courses by the head of the fibula. Common peroneal nerve palsy may present with sensory changes over the anterolateral calf or dorsum of the foot or with foot drop (i.e., inability to dorsiflex the foot).

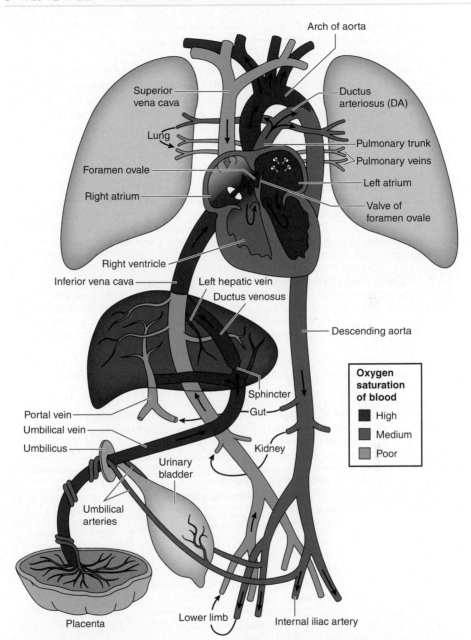

Fig. 9.12 Fetal circulation. Oxygenated blood travels from the placenta through the umbilical vein to the fetus. After returning to the fetal right ventricle, oxygenated blood largely bypasses the nonoxygenated fetal lungs and moves to systemic circulation by two shunts: the foramen ovale (between the right and left atria) and the ductus arteriosus (between the pulmonary artery and aorta). Note that inferior vena cava blood (IVC) is more oxygenated than superior vena cava (SVC) blood. Due to the anatomical relationships of the structures in the right atria, the more oxygenated IVC blood tends to pass through the foramen ovale and supplies the entire aortic arch, whereas the less oxygenated SVC blood tends to pass through the right ventricle and pulmonary artery and ultimately to the ductus arteriosus, which does not supply the aortic arch. (Moore, K. L., Persaud, T. V. N, Torchia, M. G. [2020]. *The Developing Human* [Chapter 13, pp. 263–314, Figure 13.46].)

Prolonged hip flexion, abduction, or external rotation (often seen with a prolonged second stage of labor) increases risk of femoral nerve injury near the inguinal ligament. Femoral nerve palsy may cause weakness of hip flexion.

Although neurological injuries related to neuraxial anesthesia are possible, they are much more commonly due to pregnancy, labor, or delivery. Obstetric neurological injuries tend to affect the peripheral nerves, whereas injuries from neuraxial anesthesia are more likely to affect the CNS. While not the direct cause of injury during labor, epidural anesthesia can prevent a patient from realizing she is positioned in a way that compresses a nerve. Accordingly, patients should be counseled not to remain in hip flexion for prolonged periods during labor.

BEYOND THE PEARLS

- If a patient is on anticoagulation, American Society of Regional Anesthesia and Pain Medicine (ASRA) guidelines should be followed regarding timing of anticoagulant therapy and neuraxial intervention. This will minimize risk of hematoma formation and neurological injury. For instance, if a patient is on daily prophylactic enoxaparin, epidural placement should occur no sooner than 12 hours after the last dose. After epidural removal, daily prophylactic enoxaparin can be restarted no sooner than 4 hours later. ASRA offers a clinical decision-making app with information from its most recent guideline.
- The factors that affect block height in spinal anesthesia are different from those that affect block height in epidural anesthesia. With spinal anesthesia, block height is primarily determined by dose of local anesthetic, baricity of anesthetic solution, patient positioning, and CSF volume. For epidural anesthesia, the volume of anesthetic solution administered plays a greater role.
- A given dose of epidural medication has greater block height spread in pregnant patients than nonpregnant patients. This may be due to engorged epidural veins compressing the epidural space.
- Placental abruption is a full or partial separation of the placenta from the decidua basalis of the uterus. Common clinical findings include vaginal bleeding, uterine tenderness, and a nonreassuring fetal heart tracing, but the absence of any of these does not rule out abruption. Patients should be monitored closely for shock and coagulopathy.
- Opioid antagonists such as naloxone should not be given to neonates. Opioid reversal can cause seizures and worsen hypoxic neurological injury. If opioid effect is suspected after delivery, supportive care should be administered.
- The only veins that carry oxygenated blood are the umbilical vein (in fetal circulation) and the pulmonary veins (in adult circulation).

References

Aucott, S. W., & Murphy, J. (2020). Neonatal assessment and resuscitation. In D. H. Chestnut, C. A. Wong, L. C. Tsen, W. D. N. Kee, Y. Beilin, J. M. Mhyre, et al. (Eds.), *Chestnut's obstetric anesthesia* (Chapter 9, pp. 171–198). Philadelphia, PA: Elsevier.

Banayan, J., Hofer, J., & Scavone, B. (2020). Antepartum and postpartum hemorrhage. In D. H. Chestnut, C. A. Wong, L. C. Tsen, W. D. N. Kee, Y. Beilin, J. M. Mhyre, et al. (Eds.), *Chestnut's obstetric anesthesia* (Chapter 37, pp. 901–936). Philadelphia, PA: Elsevier.

Bauer, M., Albright, C., Segal, S., & Wlody, D. (2020). Infection. In D. H. Chestnut, C. A. Wong, L. C. Tsen, W. D. N. Kee, Y. Beilin, J. M. Mhyre, et al. (Eds.), *Chestnut's obstetric anesthesia* (Chapter 36, pp. 879–900). Philadelphia, PA: Elsevier.

Blair, T., & Pedigo, R. (2018). Embryology. *Crush step 1: The ultimate USMLE step 1 review* (Chapter 4, pp. 77–107). Philadelphia, PA: Elsevier.

Brull, R., Macfarlane, A., & Chan, V. (2020). Spinal, epidural and caudal anesthesia. In M. A. Gropper, R. D. Miller, N. H. Cohen, L. I. Eriksson, L. A. Fleisher, K. Leslie, et al. (Eds.), *Miller's anesthesia* (Chapter 45, 9th ed., pp. 1413–1449). Philadelphia, PA: Elsevier.

Chestnut, D. (2020). Alternative regional analgesic techniques for labor and vaginal delivery. In D. H. Chestnut, C. A. Wong, L. C. Tsen, W. D. N. Kee, Y. Beilin, J. M. Mhyre, et al. (Eds.), *Chestnut's obstetric anesthesia* (Chapter 24, pp. 540–552). Philadelphia, PA: Elsevier.

Choi, J., Germond, L., & Santos, A. Obstetric regional anesthesia. *New York School of Regional Anesthesia.* Accessed 2021. Retrieved from https://www.nysora.com/foundations-of-regional-anesthesia/sub-specialties/obstetric/obstetric-regional-anesthesia/.

Davis, P. G., Tan, A., O'Donnell, C. P. F., & Schulze, A. (2004). Resuscitation of newborn infants with 100% oxygen or air: A systematic review and meta-analysis. *Lancet, 364*(9442), 1329–1333. doi:10.1016/S0140-6736(04)17189-4.

Frölich, M. A. Obstetric anesthesia. In J. F. Butterworth IV, D. C. Mackey, J. D. Wasnick (Eds.). *Morgan & Mikhail's clinical anesthesiology* (6th ed.). New York, NY: McGraw Hill. Accessed July 12, 2021. https://accessmedicine.mhmedical.com/content.aspx?bookid=2444&sectionid=193562808.

Horlocker, T. T., Vandermeulen, E., Kopp, S. L., Gogarten, W., Leffert, L. R., & Benzon, H. T. (2018). Regional anesthesia in the patient receiving antithrombotic or thrombolytic therapy: American Society of Regional Anesthesia and Pain Medicine Evidence-Based Guidelines (fourth edition). *Regional Anesthesia and Pain Medicine, 43*, 263–309. https://doi.org/10.1097/AAP.0000000000000763.

Livingston, E. (2020). Intrapartum fetal assessment and therapy. In D. H. Chestnut, C. A. Wong, L. C. Tsen, W. D. N. Kee, Y. Beilin, J. M. Mhyre, et al. (Eds.), *Chestnut's obstetric anesthesia* (Chapter 8, pp. 155–170). Philadelphia, PA: Elsevier.

O'Connell, T. X. (2018). USMLE step 2 secrets. *Obstetrics* (Chapter 25, pp. 195–214). Philadelphia, PA: Elsevier.

O'Connell, T. X., Blair, T., & Pedigo, R. (2015). Pregnancy, labor, delivery, fetus, and the newborn. *USMLE step 3 secrets* (Chapter 12, pp. 189–214). Philadelphia, PA: Elsevier.

O'Connell, T. X., & Storage, T. R. (2018). Reproductive system. *Crush step 1: The ultimate USMLE step 1 review* (Chapter 16, pp. 580–599). Philadelphia, PA: Elsevier.

Pan, P., & Booth, J. (2020). The pain of childbirth and its effect on the mother and fetus. In D. H. Chestnut, C. A. Wong, L. C. Tsen, W. D. N. Kee, Y. Beilin, J. M. Mhyre, et al. (Eds.), *Chestnut's obstetric anesthesia* (Chapter 20, pp. 441–452). Philadelphia, PA: Elsevier.

Pedigo, R. (2018). Cardiology. *Crush step 1: The ultimate USMLE step 1 review* (Chapter 8, pp. 236–284). Philadelphia, PA: Elsevier.

Practice advisory for the prevention, diagnosis, and management of infectious complications associated with neuraxial techniques: An updated report by the American Society of Anesthesiologists Task Force on Infectious Complications Associated with Neuraxial Techniques and the American Society of Regional Anesthesia and Pain Medicine. (2017). *Anesthesiology, 126*(4), 585–601. https://pubs.asahq.org/anesthesiology/article/126/4/585/19809/Practice-Advisory-for-the-Prevention-Diagnosis-and.

Saugstad, O. D., Ramji, S., Soll, R. F., & Vento, M. (2008). Resuscitation of newborn infants with 21% or 100% oxygen: an updated systematic review and meta-analysis. *Neonatology, 94*(3), 176–182. https://doi.org/10.1159/000143397.

Setty, T., & Fernando, R. (2020). Systemic analgesia: Parenteral and inhalational agents. In D. H. Chestnut, C. A. Wong, L. C. Tsen, W. D. N. Kee, Y. Beilin, J. M. Mhyre, et al. (Eds.), *Chestnut's obstetric anesthesia* (Chapter 22, pp. 453–473). Philadelphia, PA: Elsevier.

Sharpe, E., & Arendt, K. (2020). Anesthesia for obstetrics. In M. A. Gropper, R. D. Miller, N. H. Cohen, L. I. Eriksson, L. A. Fleisher, K. Leslie, et al. (Eds.), *Miller's anesthesia* (Chapter 62, 9th ed., pp. 2006–2041). Philadelphia, PA: Elsevier.

Singh, M. (2018). Neurology. *Crush step 1: The ultimate USMLE step 1 review* (Chapter 13, pp. 457–511). Philadelphia, PA: Elsevier.

Sviggum, H., & Reynolds, F. (2020). Neurological complications of pregnancy and neuraxial anesthesia. In D. H. Chestnut, C. A. Wong, L. C. Tsen, W. D. N. Kee, Y. Beilin, J. M. Mhyre, et al. (Eds.), *Chestnut's obstetric anesthesia* (Chapter 31, pp. 752–776). Philadelphia, PA: Elsevier.

Wong, C. (2020). Epidural and spinal analgesia: Anesthesia for labor. In D. H. Chestnut, C. A. Wong, L. C. Tsen, W. D. N. Kee, Y. Beilin, J. M. Mhyre, et al. (Eds.), *Chestnut's obstetric anesthesia* (Chapter 23, pp. 474–539). Philadelphia, PA: Elsevier.

A 36-Year-Old Primigravida at 36 + 0 Weeks' Gestation Complaining With Severe Abdominal Pain

Paul Neil Frank

A 36-year-old primigravida presents to the labor and delivery unit at 36+0 weeks' gestation complaining of severe abdominal pain. She has a past medical history of lupus and obstructive sleep apnea. She denies vaginal bleeding. Her body mass index (BMI) is 32 kg/m². Vital signs show blood pressure 168/110 mm Hg, pulse 110/min, respirations 22/min, oxygen saturation 100% on room air, and temperature 36.1°C.

What is the differential diagnosis of abdominal pain in this patient?
Table 10.1 shows the common causes of abdominal pain in parturients. Because this patient is in her third trimester, obstetric causes are always high on the differential. However, it is important to consider nonobstetric etiologies as well.

Repeat blood pressure measurement is 162/114 mm Hg. She also complains of a new headache.

What's going on?
These findings are concerning for severe preeclampsia.

What laboratory studies should you order?
Hemoglobin and hematocrit studies may identify hemoconcentration (if elevated hemoglobin and hematocrit) or hemolysis (if low hemoglobin and hematocrit). Serum creatinine level and a 24-hour urine protein study (or urine protein/creatinine ratio) will identify acute kidney injury (AKI). Serum aminotransferase levels will identify lysis of hepatic cells from liver damage.

Platelet count will identify thrombocytopenia (if low platelet count), which may help in diagnosis of Hemolysis, Elevated Liver enzymes, and Low Platelets syndrome ("HELLP syndrome") syndrome. Prothrombin time (PT), international normalized ratio (INR), and partial thromboplastin time (PTT) will also identify coagulopathy and liver dysfunction. All of these coagulation parameters will guide decision-making regarding neuraxial anesthesia.

Finally, a type and crossmatch for at least 2 units of red blood cells should be ordered in case the patient requires a blood transfusion. If thrombocytopenia or other coagulopathy is identified, fresh frozen plasma (FFP) and platelets should be ordered.

What is a type and crossmatch?
This is a laboratory assay to ensure that blood transfused to a patient is an appropriate match. The patient's ABO blood type and rhesus (Rh) status will be confirmed. In a crossmatch, the patient's

TABLE 10.1 ■ **Causes of Acute Abdominal Pain in Pregnant Patients**

Etiology	Pathophysiology
Normal labor	Uterine contractions
Preeclampsia/severe preeclampsia	Vascular hyperreactivity due to abnormal placentation; mechanism incompletely understood
HELLP syndrome	Hemolysis, elevated liver enzymes, low platelets; a more advanced form of preeclampsia
Uterine rupture	Rupture of the uterus into the pelvic or abdominal cavity
Nonobstetric	Traumatic, biliary, pancreatic, intestinal, urologic, musculoskeletal causes

TABLE 10.2 ■ **Expected Cardiovascular Changes in Pregnancy**

Parameter	Change (%)
Plasma volume	↑45–55
Red blood cell volume	↑20–30
Cardiac output	↑40–50
Stroke volume	↑25–30
Heart rate	↑15–25
Systemic vascular resistance	↓20

Because the plasma volume increases more than does the red blood cell volume, dilutional decreases in hemoglobin and hematocrit are expected. Increased heart rate and intravascular volume (i.e., preload), as well as decreased systemic vascular resistance, contribute to increased cardiac output.

plasma is mixed with red blood cells from a proposed donor. If agglutination is observed, the patient has antibodies against the donor red blood cells, and the patient cannot receive red blood cells from that donor. If there is no agglutination, it is likely safe for the patient to receive those red blood cells.

What are the cardiovascular changes expected in a healthy pregnancy?
Table 10.2 shows the expected cardiovascular changes at full term in a healthy pregnancy compared with the nonpregnant state.

STEP 2 PEARL

Signs of preeclampsia are
- systolic blood pressure ≥140 mm Hg and/or diastolic blood pressure ≥90 mm Hg on two measurements at least 4 hours apart measured after 20 weeks' gestation in a patient with previously normal blood pressure
- proteinuria >300 mg in 24 hours

STEP 2 PEARL

Signs and symptoms of severe preeclampsia are
- systolic blood pressure ≥160 mm Hg and/or diastolic blood pressure ≥110 mm Hg
- thrombocytopenia with platelet ≤100,000/µL
- oliguria (urine output less than 500 mL / 24 hours)

- elevated liver enzymes
- persistent epigastric or right upper quadrant pain
- pulmonary edema (may result in dyspnea or hypoxia)
- neurological symptoms (e.g., headache, vision changes)

Lab studies show platelet count of 55,000/μL, aspartate transaminase (ast) 650 IU/L, and alanine transaminase (alt) 574 IU/L.

What is the diagnosis?

This patient meets criteria for severe preeclampsia.

STEP 2, 3 PEARL

Risk factors for preeclampsia include
- Nulliparity
- Multiple gestations
- Personal or family history of preeclampsia
- African American ethnicity
- Chronic hypertension
- Diabetes (pregestational or gestational)
- Thrombophilia
- Systemic lupus erythematosus
- BMI greater than 30 kg/m^2
- Antiphospholipid antibody syndrome
- Maternal age ≥35 years
- Kidney disease
- Assisted reproductive technology
- Obstructive sleep apnea

What is the treatment for severe preeclampsia?

The definitive treatment is delivery of the fetus. In the meantime, this patient requires intravenous magnesium, antihypertensive medication (labetalol and hydralazine are commonly used), and judicious fluid resuscitation.

Why magnesium?

Magnesium is effective at preventing seizures in patients with severe preeclampsia and eclampsia. It also reduces blood pressure.

The fetal heart tones are nonreassuring (see case 9), and the obstetrician calls for an emergency cesarean section.

Assuming the patient does not already have an epidural catheter in place, can you offer this patient neuraxial anesthesia?

There are two primary considerations here.

First is the urgency of the cesarean section. If there is an urgent or emergent need for delivery, as in the case of severe fetal distress or maternal bleeding, the fastest option is general anesthesia. Assuming a typical obstetric airway, rapid sequence intubation can have the patient ready for surgery in less than 2 minutes. Even in expert hands, placement of an epidural catheter or spinal anesthetic, including patient positioning, prep, and drape, can take 5 minutes or more. Surgery is further delayed until an adequate level of anesthesia is achieved, which can take several minutes.

The second concern is the patient's coagulation status. Placement of neuraxial anesthesia carries the risk of epidural or intrathecal bleeding. Expansion of the hematoma within the fixed volume of the spinal canal can compress the spinal cord or nerve roots, causing paralysis. Therefore neuraxial anesthesia is only offered to patients with normal coagulation profiles. Minimum coagulation parameters are platelet count 50,000 to 80,000/µL and INR of 1.4 or less, although there is some disagreement about the exact cutoffs.

Because this patient is thrombocytopenic and requires emergency cesarean delivery, she will require general anesthesia.

The patient has not had anything to eat for 9 hours. Can this operation be done with laryngeal mask airway (LMA)?

No, the gold standard is endotracheal intubation, which will protect the airway from aspiration of gastric contents. LMA sits in the pharynx, overlying the larynx and esophagus. The airway is not protected. Patients in the second half of their pregnancies have an elevated risk of aspiration.

However, if laryngoscopy is unsuccessful, an LMA may be placed to facilitate oxygenation and ventilation as a rescue measure until a definitive airway (i.e., endotracheal tube) can be achieved.

Why do pregnant patients have an elevated risk of aspiration?

Pregnant patients have decreased tone of the lower esophageal sphincter. The anatomic relationship between the diaphragm and the stomach changes as the uterus enlarges, and progesterone causes smooth muscle relaxation. In addition, an enlarged uterus will increase intraabdominal pressure. Finally, although pregnancy itself does not cause delayed gastric emptying, gastric emptying does slow during the late stages of labor. This can be caused by pain, and opioids.

In addition to the increased likelihood of aspiration, pregnant patients are at increased risk of harm from aspiration because the character of the aspirate itself may be more damaging to the lungs. The placenta secretes gastrin, which stimulates secretion of stomach acid and may lower the pH of gastric fluid. Aspiration of fluid with a pH less than 2.5 is more harmful than aspiration of an equivalent amount of fluid with a higher pH.

Any special precautions for the obstetric airway?

Yes. If there is time, obstetric patients undergoing general anesthesia should receive a nonparticulate oral antacid (e.g., Bicitra) and H2 receptor blocker or proton pump inhibitor (PPI) preoperatively. They may also benefit from a promotility agent such as metoclopramide. As with any other patient with a potentially full stomach, rapid sequence intubation (see Case 13) should be performed. Positioning the patient in a slight head up or reverse Trendelenburg position may reduce the risk of aspiration, increase functional residual capacity (FRC), and make laryngoscopy easier.

STEP 1 PEARL

Parietal cells in the stomach secrete acid. This is stimulated by multiple pathways including direct innervation by the vagus nerve (cranial nerve X), release of histamine from enterochromaffin-like (ECL) cells, and release of gastrin from G cells (see Fig. 10.1). H2 blockers work by blocking the binding of histamine to H2 receptors on parietal cells, which prevents activation of the H+/K+-ATPase. PPIs work by directly inhibiting the function of the H+/K+-ATPase on parietal cells. Oral antacids work by neutralizing acid in the lumen of the stomach. Figure 10.1 shows the mechanisms of these acid-blocking agents.

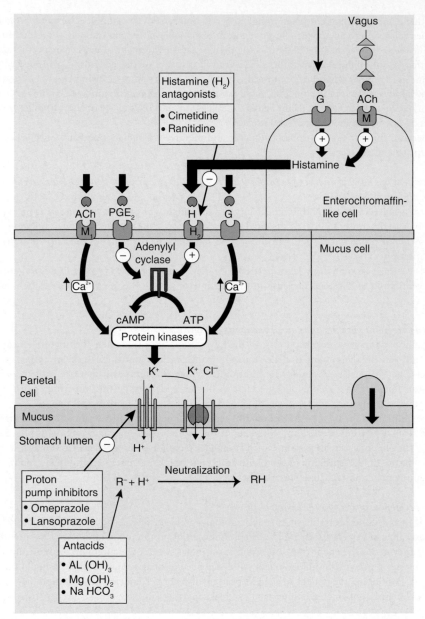

Fig. 10.1 There are multiple mechanisms involving vagal and gastrin stimulation of enterochromaffin-like cells and parietal cells, as well as histamine stimulation of parietal cells, to generate gastric acid. *ACh*, acetylcholine; *PGE2*, prostaglandin E2; *H*, histamine; *cAMP*, cyclic adenosine monophosphate; *ATP*, adenosine triphosphate; *G*, gastrin. (Blair, T. E. [2017]. Gastroenterology. In: T. X. O'Connell, R. A. Pedigo, & T. E. Blair [Eds.], *Crush step 1: The ultimate USMLE step 1 review* [pp. 330–364]. Philadelphia, PA: Elsevier. Fig 10.30.)

Why is airway management more challenging in obstetric patients?

Laryngoscopy and intubation can be more challenging in pregnant patients for several reasons. Pregnancy itself causes soft tissue swelling which can affect the airway. This can be exaggerated in patients with preeclampsia. Additional airway challenges include increased mucosal vascularity (which predisposes to bleeding), weight gain, and increased breast size.

Complicating matters is the fact that obstetric patients become hypoxic with shorter periods of apnea than do nonobstetric patients. This is because of reduced FRC and increased oxygen consumption.

What is FRC, and why is it relevant?
FRC is a measurement of the resting volume of the lungs after a normal exhalation. Normally, this volume is filled with ambient air, which contains an oxygen concentration of 21%. During preoxygenation, this volume of ambient air is replaced with pure oxygen. During the apneic period between induction (i.e., administration of propofol) and mechanical ventilation, the FRC acts like internal scuba tanks, maintaining normal oxygen saturation for up to 8 minutes of apnea in healthy, nonobstetric patients.

In obstetric patients, the large gravid uterus increases intraabdominal pressure, which is then transmitted to the chest cavity, thereby decreasing FRC. In these patients, smaller "scuba tanks" result in less oxygen reserve.

What other respiratory changes occur in pregnancy?
Table 10.3 shows the expected respiratory changes at full term in a healthy pregnancy compared to the nonpregnant state.

You plan to use succinylcholine for neuromuscular blockade.

Because pregnant patients have decreased levels of pseudocholinesterase, should you give a smaller dose of succinylcholine?
Although it is true that pregnant patients have 25% to 30% lower plasma activity of pseudocholinesterase, the duration of action of succinylcholine is unchanged in this population. Therefore the standard dose of 1 mg/kg is appropriate.

How does pregnancy affect minimum alveolar concentration (MAC) of inhaled agents?
Pregnancy decreases MAC by 20% to 30%.

Should the magnesium infusion be continued during surgery?
Yes. In fact, the physiologic stress of delivery may reduce the seizure threshold, making eclamptic seizures more likely.

TABLE 10.3 ■ **Changes of Respiratory Parameters in Pregnancy**

Parameter	Change
Minute ventilation	↑50%
Respiratory rate	↑0%–15%
Tidal volume	40%–50%
Functional residual capacity (FRC)	↓20%
Expiratory reserve volume (ERV)	↓20%–25%
Residual volume (RV)	↓15%–20%
Vital capacity	No change
Inspiratory capacity	↑5%–15%
Oxygen consumption (term, prelabor)	20%–35%
Oxygen consumption (first stage of labor)	↑40% above prelabor
Oxygen consumption (second stage of labor)	↑75% above prelabor

The increase in minute ventilation is mainly due to the increase in tidal volume. The decrease in FRC is due to decreases in both ERV and RV. The decrease in FRC, combined with an increase in oxygen consumption, means pregnant patients will become hypoxic after shorter periods of apnea compared with nonobstetric patients.

How will magnesium therapy affect anesthetic management?

Magnesium augments the effects of nondepolarizing neuromuscular blockers. Therefore smaller doses and longer dosing intervals are appropriate.

Induction and intubation are uneventful. After delivery of a healthy baby girl, the obstetrician complains that the uterus is not contracting.

What can you do to help?

Halogenated anesthetic agents (e.g., sevoflurane, desflurane) cause uterine relaxation. Reduce the concentration of these agents and supplement with nitrous oxide (N_2O), which does not cause uterine relaxation. Alternatively, consider switching to total intravenous anesthesia ("TIVA"). Oxytocin can be given intravenously as a bolus or infusion to augment uterine contraction. Rapid administration of a bolus of oxytocin can cause vasodilation and hypotension.

Despite these changes, the uterus is still boggy. The obstetrician asks you to give intramuscular methylergonovine.

What do you say?

Although methylergonovine improves uterine tone, it can also cause significant vasoconstriction and hypertension. It is therefore contraindicated in patients with preeclampsia. It is also contraindicated in patients with pulmonary hypertension, stroke, or ischemic heart disease.

You could consider giving the patient prostaglandin F2α intramuscularly. Beware that this can cause bronchospasm, and it should therefore be avoided in patients with asthma.

The surgery is completed and the patient is extubated postoperatively. In the postanesthesia care unit (pacu), the patient is flushed and lethargic. She complains of weakness.

What should you do?

This patient is receiving magnesium for severe preeclampsia, and these symptoms are concerning for magnesium toxicity. Stop the magnesium infusion and check a serum magnesium level. Administer calcium to antagonize the effect of the magnesium. Loop diuretics will decrease magnesium levels. In extreme cases, the patient may require reintubation, hemodynamic support, and hemodialysis.

What is the goal serum magnesium level in treating preeclampsia, and at what levels do complications arise?

The therapeutic serum magnesium level for treatment of preeclampsia is approximately 5 to 9 mg/dL. Table 10.4 shows the effects of supratherapeutic magnesium levels.

On the morning after delivery, the patient has a seizure and then becomes unresponsive.

TABLE 10.4 ■ **Patients with Elevated Levels of Magnesium May Develop Respiratory Depression and Eventually Cardiac Arrest**

Magnesium Level (mg/dL)	Symptoms
9–12	Diminished deep tendon reflexes
>12	Respiratory depression
>30	Asystole

What happened?
This patient has likely developed eclampsia. Remember the eclampsia may first manifest *after* delivery of the fetus, as it has in this patient.

What should you do?
Support the patient's ventilation and oxygenation by mask ventilating with 100% fraction inspired oxygen (FiO_2). Closely monitor vital signs, particularly blood pressure and oxygen saturation. Treat hypertension if blood pressure is 160/110 mmHg or greater. If the seizure does not quickly resolve or if the patient is unstable and requires intubation, propofol can also break seizures. Continue magnesium infusion and consider an additional bolus. Eclamptic patients are at risk for cerebral hemorrhage. If the patient remains unresponsive or if there are focal neurologic findings, obtain a computerized tomography (CT) scan of the head to evaluate for intracranial hemorrhage.

BEYOND THE PEARLS

- Always ask the patient about recent use of antiplatelet or anticoagulant use prior to placement of neuraxial anesthesia. The American Society of Regional Anesthesia (ASRA) has published guidelines regarding the minimum waiting time between the last dose of these agents and the safe placement of neuraxial anesthesia.
- Incompetence of the lower esophageal sphincter returns to prepregnancy levels 48 hours after delivery.
- In a healthy pregnancy at term, pulmonary vascular resistance is 35% less than in the nonpregnant state. There is no change in central venous pressure.
- Gestational hypertension and preeclampsia may not be two unique disease processes. Although they can be distinguished by the absence of proteinuria in gestational hypertension, up to 50% of patients with gestational hypertension will develop proteinuria or other end-organ dysfunction. Gestational hypertension with severe blood pressure should be managed the same way as preeclampsia with severe features.
- HELLP syndrome may first present in the postpartum period. Some patients with HELLP syndrome may present without hypertension or proteinuria.
- Magnesium is eliminated by the kidneys. In patients with acute kidney injury (AKI), particularly if oliguric, magnesium can accumulate to toxic levels.
- Eclamptic seizures may be associated with elevated intracranial pressure.
- Forced expiratory volume in 1 second (FEV1) and forced vital capacity (FVC) do not change during pregnancy. Therefore FEV1/FVC does not change during pregnancy.

References

Dyer, R. A., Swanevelder, J. L., & Bateman, B. T. (2020). Hypertensive disorders In D. H. Chestnut, C. A. Wong, L. C. Tsen, W. D. N. Kee, Y. Beilin, J. M. Mhyre, et al. (Eds.), *Chestnut's obstetric anesthesia* (Chapter 35, pp. 840–878). Philadelphia, PA: Elsevier.

Emery, M. (2018). Blood and blood components. In R. M. Walls, R. S. Hockberger, M. Gausche-Hill, K. Bakes, J. M. Baren, T. B. Erickson, et al. (Eds.), *Rosen's emergency medicine: concepts and clinical practice.* (9th ed., Chapter 111, pp. 1455–1462. e2). Philadelphia, PA: Elsevier.

Espinoza, J., Vidaeff, A., Pettker, C. M., & Simhan, H. (2020). Gestational hypertension and preeclampsia. *American College of Obstetricians and Gynecologists Practice Bulletin Number 222. Obstetrics & Gynecology,* 135(6), e237–e260.

Farber, M. K. (2020). Aspiration: risk, prophylaxis, and treatment. In D. H. Chestnut, C. A. Wong, L. C. Tsen, W. D. N. Kee, Y. Beilin, J. M. Mhyre, et al. (Eds.), *Chestnut's obstetric anesthesia* (Chapter 28, pp. 671–691). Philadelphia, PA: Elsevier.

Sharpe, E. E., & Arendt, K. W. (2020). Anesthesia for obstetrics. In M. A. Gropper, R. D. Miller, N. H. Cohen, L. I. Eriksson, L. A. Fleisher, K. Leslie, et al. (Eds.), *Miller's anesthesia* (Chapter 62, pp. 2006–2041.e8). Philadelphia, PA: Elsevier.

A 38-Year-Old Woman, G5P4004, at 37 Weeks and 3 Days of Gestation With Contractions Every 5 Minutes

Reihaneh Forghany ■ Elizabeth Fung

A 38-year-old woman, G5P4004, at 37 weeks and 3 days of gestation presents to the labor and delivery unit with contractions every 5 minutes. Upon chart review, you come across a prenatal ultrasound with concerns of placenta accreta; however, the patient has since been lost to follow-up. She reports having had three cesarean sections in the past and has been having vaginal spotting over the past week. In triage, her vital signs show blood pressure of 125/63 mm Hg, pulse rate of 90/min, respiration rate of 20/min, and oxygen saturation of 98% on room air.

What does G5P4004 mean?

This an abbreviation to reflect a patient's obstetric history. The number after the G refers to the number of pregnancies a patient has had. The numbers after the P reflect, in order, the number of full-term births, pre-term births, abortions (spontaneous or medical/surgical), and the number of living children the patient has had. Our patient has had 5 pregnancies (including the current one), and has 4 living children.

What is placenta accreta and its spectrum?

Placental implantation beyond the endometrial layer of the uterus gives rise to placenta accreta, which is often described as a spectrum, and there are three degrees of severity or invasiveness. Each subsequent category will adhere to a deeper layer in the uterus, as seen in Fig. 11.1.

STEP 1 PEARL

- Placenta accreta: placental villi are attached to the myometrium (rather than the decidua)
- Placenta increta: placental villi penetrate the myometrium
- Placenta percreta: placental villi penetrate through the myometrium and can attach to uterine serosa or other adjacent organs, such as bowel, bladder, ovaries, or other pelvic organs and vessels

---

STEP 1 PEARL

The placenta is the primary site for the exchange of nutrients, blood gases, and other substances between the mother and fetus. Two other important functions of the placenta are to secrete hormones during pregnancy and to act as a barrier to prevent direct contact between fetal and maternal blood.

STEP 1 PEARL

The placental tissue is composed of two different sources, which include fetal and maternal components. The fetal component is composed of tertiary chorionic villi. The fetal layer secretes human chorionic gonadotropin (hCG) to maintain production of progesterone from the corpus luteum during the first trimester of pregnancy. Meanwhile, the maternal layer of placental tissue is composed of decidua basalis, which is derived from the endometrium of the uterus.

What are the risk factors for developing placenta accreta?

Risk factors for developing placenta accreta include history of cesarean delivery and/or other uterine surgeries. The presence of placenta previa in the setting of a previous cesarean section also significantly increases the risk of developing placenta accreta, especially if the placenta is in the anterior position and overlies the previous uterine scar.

In fact, a multicenter, prospective, observational study assessed the risk of developing placenta accreta in the setting of placenta previa and prior cesarean sections. In patients with placenta previa and no prior cesarean section, there was a 3% incidence of placenta accreta. In patients with placenta previa and one prior cesarean section, incidence was 11%. In patients with placenta previa and two prior cesarean sections, incidence increased to 40%. In patients with placenta previa and three or more prior cesarean sections, incidence was more than 60%, as shown in Table 11.1.

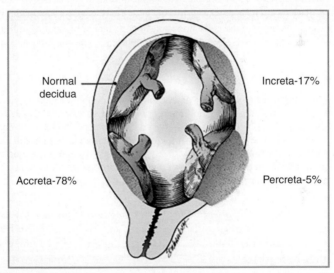

Fig. 11.1 Illustration of the degree of invasiveness of placental villi within the spectrum of placenta accreta, placenta increta, and placenta percreta. The incidence of each type of invasive placentation is also listed. (Banayan, J. M., Hofer, J. E., & Scavone, B. M. [2020]. Antepartum and postpartum hemorrhage. In D. H. Chestnut, C. A. Wong, L. C. Tsen, W. D. N. Kee, Y. Beilin, J. M. Mhyre, et al. (Eds.), *Chestnut's obstetric anesthesia* [6th ed., Chapter 37, pp. 901–936]. Philadelphia, PA: Elsevier. Fig. 37.2.)

TABLE 11.1 ■ **Risk of Developing Placenta Accreta in Patients With Existing Placenta Previa and the Relationship to the Number of Prior Cesarean Deliveries**

Number of Prior Cesarean Deliveries	Percentage of Patients With Placenta Accreta
0	3
1	11
2	40
3	61
4 or more	67

From: Banayan, J. M., Hofer, J. E., & Scavone, B. M. (2020). Antepartum and postpartum hemorrhage. In D. H. Chestnut, C. A. Wong, L. C. Tsen, W. D. N. Kee, Y. Beilin, J. M. Mhyre, et al. (Eds.), *Chestnut's obstetric anesthesia* (6th ed., Chapter 37, pp. 901–936). Philadelphia, PA: Elsevier.

Other risk factors for the development of placenta accreta include Asherman syndrome, submucosal leiomyomata, and maternal age older than 35 years.

How is placenta accreta diagnosed?

The most common screening tool for diagnosis is ultrasonography. In patients who have increased risk of placenta accreta, the sensitivity and specificity of ultrasonography may be reduced. Obtaining magnetic resonance imaging (MRI) may help to confirm the diagnosis in high-risk patients with inconclusive ultrasonographic results, especially if the placenta is situated posteriorly.

If there is no established diagnosis of placenta accreta at the time of delivery, a presenting sign is that the obstetrician can experience difficulty separating the placenta from the uterine wall. At this time, the definite diagnosis can be made by laparotomy.

What are the ultrasound findings for placenta accreta?

In a normal placental attachment, there is a hypoechoic border between the placenta and the bladder, which represents the myometrium and normal retroplacental myometrium vasculature. In the presence of placenta accreta, there is a loss of the normal hypoechoic border, in addition to sonolucent or lacunar spaces within the placenta itself, as portrayed in Fig. 11.2. There is also a loss of the well-delineated bladder wall. Doppler sonography and color flow can show turbulent blood flow in the lacunar spaces within the placenta, as well as increased vascularity at the placenta-uterus interface.

STEP 2 PEARL

Patients with placenta accreta are usually asymptomatic throughout pregnancy and are diagnosed incidentally on routine ultrasound screening in the second trimester. Classic ultrasound findings include placental lacunae, myometrial thinning, and loss of space behind the placenta. The placental lacunae are irregularly shaped spaces in the placental parenchyma filled with maternal blood. They give the placenta a moth-eaten appearance on ultrasound. Attempting to remove the adherent placenta can disrupt these vascular spaces and cause postpartum hemorrhage and hemorrhagic shock.

What is your main concern for this patient with a known diagnosis of placenta accreta?

The main concern here is hemorrhage. Placenta accreta and its spectrum can lead to a tightly adhered placenta that may not be removable without tearing the myometrium, which can result in a life-threatening hemorrhage.

STEP 2, 3 PEARL

Although there are conflicting definitions, the most common definition of postpartum hemorrhage is estimated blood loss (EBL) of greater than 500 mL after vaginal delivery or EBL of greater than 1000 mL after cesarean delivery.

STEP 2 PEARL

The management for placenta accreta spectrum that is diagnosed antenatally is a planned cesarean hysterectomy. There should be coordination between specialized obstetricians, anesthesiologists, and the blood bank. Due to high rates of hemorrhagic shock, disseminated intravascular coagulation, and maternal mortality, uterus-preserving techniques of delivery are generally contraindicated. If the patient is diagnosed at the time of the delivery, they will usually require an emergency hysterectomy.

The patient will undergo cesarean delivery followed by hysterectomy.

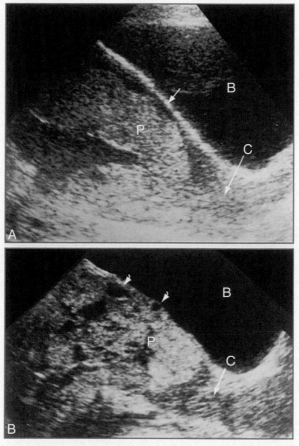

Fig. 11.2 (A) Ultrasound image of a normal placental implantation. The arrow shows a hypoechoic area separating the placental tissue and the bladder. (B) Ultrasound image of placenta accreta with the absence of the hypoechoic area separating the placenta and bladder, no well-delineated bladder wall, and presence of sonolucent areas or lacunar spaces within the placenta. *B*, Bladder, *C*, cervix, *P*, placenta. (From: Hull, A. D., Resnik, R., & Silver, R. M. [2019]. Placenta previa and accreta, vasa previa, subchorionic hemorrhage, and abruptio placentae. In R. Resnik, C. J. Lockwood, T. R. Moore, M. F. Greene, J. A. Copel, & R. M. Silver (Eds.), *Creasy and Resnik's maternal-fetal medicine: Principles and practice* [8th ed., Chapter 46, pp. 786–797.e4]. Philadelphia, PA: Elsevier. Fig. 46.3.)

What is your anesthetic plan for this patient?
Given that this patient is hemodynamically stable and appears to be euvolemic, it is reasonable to proceed with placement of an epidural catheter as the primary anesthetic. However, the neuraxial technique may fail due to a number of reasons: (1) prolonged operative time, (2) the need for more extensive surgical retraction, or (3) the need for a still surgical field with muscle relaxation. It is important to discuss the possibility of intraoperative conversion to general anesthesia with your patient prior to proceeding with neuraxial anesthesia.

You should be prepared for massive hemorrhage with adequate, large-bore intravenous (IV) access, arterial catheter, and availability of blood products. Cell salvage equipment should also be considered. The patient should also be counseled about the likelihood of blood transfusion.

Epidural placement is uneventful, and a healthy baby boy is delivered by cesarean delivery. Shortly thereafter, the obstetrician reports significant bleeding. The patient's blood pressure drops to 70/50 mm Hg with a pulse of 140/min.

What should you do?

In an emergency situation with active hemorrhage, conversion to general anesthesia is required. Secure the patient's airway with rapid-sequence induction and endotracheal intubation (see Case 13). Your induction agent depends on the degree of hemodynamic instability of the patient. Typically, low-dose propofol, ketamine, or etomidate can be used for induction.

In the setting of massive hemorrhage, massive transfusion protocol may need to be activated with aggressive administration of packed red blood cells (RBCs), fresh frozen plasma (FFP), platelets, and fibrinogen. These are often administered in ratios similar to trauma resuscitation to avoid dilutional coagulopathy (see Case 13).

STEP 1 AND 2 PEARL

Postpartum hemorrhage is the most common cause of maternal morbidity and mortality worldwide. The main causes of postpartum hemorrhage are uterine atony, trauma, coagulopathy, retained products of conception, abnormal placental separation, and velamentous cord insertion. Uterine atony is failure of the uterus to adequately contract following delivery of the placenta and makes up approximately 80% of cases of postpartum hemorrhage.

Would tranexamic acid (TXA) be helpful in this situation?

There have been numerous randomized controlled trials concluding that the use of TXA significantly decreased postpartum hemorrhage; however, the studies have not adequately discussed the safety of the use of empiric TXA. There is currently an ongoing trial (the World Maternal Antifibrinolytic [WOMAN] trial), which is an international, randomized, double-blinded placebo-controlled trial with approximately 20,000 enrolled patients. This study is aimed to determine the effect of early administration of TXA on mortality, hysterectomy, and other morbidities in women with clinically diagnosed postpartum hemorrhage.

Profuse bleeding continues despite aggressive treatment of coagulopathy and surgical bleeding.

What else can be done?

If postpartum hemorrhage is not controlled with standard pharmacologic measures, consider uterine artery ligation, uterine compression sutures, intrauterine balloon placement for tamponade, or arterial embolization by interventional radiology if the patient is stable enough for transport.

STEP 1, 2 PEARL

The uterine vessels are contained in the transverse cervical (cardinal) ligament, which connects the cervix to the side wall of the pelvis. The uterine artery arises from the anterior division of the internal iliac artery and serves as the main blood supply to the uterus. The ureter travels underneath the uterine vessels and is therefore at risk of injury during ligation of the uterine vessels.

The bleeding subsides with placement of an intrauterine balloon. The surgery concludes, and the patient is taken to the intensive care unit. On postpartum day 2, she attempts to breastfeed her newborn but has no milk.

What's going on?
The inability to breastfeed after significant hemorrhage is concerning for Sheehan syndrome.

STEP 2, 3 PEARL

During pregnancy, the pituitary gland will double in size while the amount of blood supply the gland stays relatively constant. This makes the pituitary gland prone to infarction and ischemic necrosis from hypovolemic shock, which is a sequela of postpartum hemorrhage. Sheehan syndrome, postpartum necrosis of the pituitary gland, is also known as postpartum hypopituitarism. Although a rare occurrence, Sheehan syndrome can present acutely after pregnancy or may go unnoticed for years before it is diagnosed.

STEP 1 PEARL

The anterior pituitary gland, which is derived from oral ectoderm (Rathke pouch), produces and secretes follicle-stimulating hormone (FSH), luteinizing hormone (LH), adrenocorticotropic hormone (ACTH), growth hormone (GH), thyroid-stimulating hormone (TSH), and prolactin. The posterior pituitary gland is derived from neuroectoderm and secretes vasopressin (antidiuretic hormone [ADH]) and oxytocin. Both ADH and oxytocin are made in the hypothalamus and then transported to the posterior pituitary by carrier proteins called neurophysins.

STEP 2, 3 PEARL

The presenting symptom of Sheehan syndrome is often the mother's inability to breastfeed. This is due to a lack of prolactin, which is secreted by the anterior pituitary gland. Other presenting symptoms depend on loss of specific hormones from the pituitary gland. Patients can experience amenorrhea, hot flashes, and vaginal atrophy due to decreased FSH and LH. Decreased TSH can lead to lethargy, dry skin, bradycardia, and other signs of hypothyroidism. ACTH deficiency may present as weight loss, hypotension, and anorexia. Lack of growth hormone is often asymptomatic in adults but can result in weight gain, loss of lean body mass, and weakness. Treatment entails supplementation of pituitary hormones.

What is the optimal obstetric management of placenta accreta?
Most patients with a known placenta accreta should undergo planned, preterm cesarean delivery and hysterectomy with the placenta left in place. *Any attempt at removing the placenta from the uterus can lead to massive hemorrhage.* In the event that there is only a small focal area of abnormal placental attachment, more conservative treatment options can be used, such as medical management or curettage.

A planned delivery with multidisciplinary collaboration has been shown to be associated with less maternal morbidity, fewer blood transfusions, and fewer intensive care unit admissions when compared with emergency deliveries. The preferred time for planned delivery is often around 34 weeks' gestational age.

What prophylactic interventions may help in the event of postpartum hemorrhage?
Insertion of preoperative internal iliac artery balloon catheters helps to control hemorrhage during a cesarean delivery. However, this is controversial because there are multiple complications that can arise from their placement, including disruption of lower extremity blood flow leading to lower extremity ischemia and even fetal bradycardia, leading to the need for emergency delivery.

In addition, based on a meta-analysis of observational studies, the prophylactic use of resuscitative endovascular balloon occlusion of the aorta (REBOA) has been shown to reduce blood loss during placenta accreta cesarean deliveries.

BEYOND THE PEARLS

- Placenta accreta exists on a spectrum of abnormal placental implantation, involving an adherent placenta that can lead to postpartum hemorrhage if there is an attempt to manually remove the placenta.
- If a patient has placenta previa and a history of Cesarean deliveries in the past, maintain a high clinical suspicion for concurrent placenta accreta. The greater the number of Cesarean deliveries in the past, the higher the incidence of placenta accreta.
- Placenta accreta is most commonly diagnosed with ultrasonography but can also be diagnosed or confirmed with MRI in high-risk patients, particularly if the placenta is located posteriorly.
- The value of TXA in postpartum hemorrhage is currently under investigation in the WOMAN trial. This is an international, randomized, double-blinded placebo-controlled trial assessing the effect of early administration of TXA on mortality, hysterectomy, and other morbidities in women with clinically diagnosed postpartum hemorrhage.
- A patient with a known placenta accreta will typically undergo planned, preterm cesarean delivery around 34 weeks.
- The anesthetic management of postpartum hemorrhage involves general anesthesia with endotracheal intubation, large-bore IV access, arterial line catheter, availability of colloid/crystalloid, and blood products such as RBC/FFP/platelets, and fibrinogen.
- A planned, multidisciplinary approach to managing patients with placenta accreta has been shown to be associated with less maternal morbidity, fewer blood transfusions, and fewer intensive care unit admissions.
- Abnormal placentation is a risk factor for amniotic fluid embolism (AFE). AFE may present with respiratory distress, hypoxia, coagulopathy, and cardiovascular collapse.

References

Banayan, J. M., Hofer, J. E., & Scavone, B. M. (2020). Antepartum and postpartum hemorrhage. In D. H. Chestnut, C. A. Wong, L. C. Tsen, W. D. N. Kee, Y. Beilin, J. M. Mhyre, et al. (Eds.), *Chestnut's obstetric anesthesia* (6th ed., Chapter 37, pp. 901–936). Philadelphia, PA: Elsevier.

Frolich, M., & Bucklin, B. A. (2016). Obstetric emergencies. In C. Baysinger, B. Bucklin & D. Gambling (Eds.), *A practical approach to obstetric anesthesia* (2nd ed., Chapter 16, pp. 307–338). Philadelphia, PA: Elsevier.

Hull, A. D., Resnik, R., & Silver, R. M. (2019). Placenta previa and accreta, vasa previa, subchorionic hemorrhage, and abruptio placentae. In R. Resnik, C. J. Lockwood, T. R. Moore, M. F. Greene, J. A. Copel, & R. M. Silver (Eds.), *Creasy and Resnik's maternal-fetal medicine: Principles and practice* (8th ed., Chapter 46, pp. 786–797.e4). Philadelphia, PA: Elsevier.

Lucero, J. M., & Rollins, M. D. (2018). Obstetrics. In M. C. Pardo & R. D. Miller (Eds.), *Basics of anesthesia* (7th ed., Chapter 33, pp. 553–586). Philadelphia, PA: Elsevier.

Toledo, P. (2020). Embolic disorders. In D. H. Chestnut, C. A. Wong, L. C. Tsen, W. D. N. Kee, Y. Beilin, J. M. Mhyre, et al. (Eds.), *Chestnut's obstetric anesthesia* (6th ed., Chapter 38, pp. 937–955). Philadelphia, PA: Elsevier.

Walton, Z., Snegovskikh, D., & Braveman, F. (2018). Pregnancy-associated diseases. In R. L. Hines & K. E. Marschall (Eds.), *Stoelting's anesthesia and co-existing disease* (7th ed., Chapter 31, pp. 671–693). Philadelphia, PA: Elsevier.

General

A 32-Year-Old Woman Undergoing Laparoscopic Ovarian Cystectomy

Paul Neil Frank

A 32-year-old woman is undergoing laparoscopic ovarian cystectomy. She has smoked 1 pack of cigarettes per day for the last 12 years. The patient says she was nauseous for days when she underwent repair of a tibial fracture after a skiing accident as a teenager. She is otherwise healthy and takes no medications at home. Preoperative vital signs show blood pressure 124/70 mm Hg, pulse 82/min, respirations 10/min, oxygen saturation 100% on room air, and temperature 36.9°C.

What risk factors does this patient have for postoperative nausea and vomiting (PONV)? What protective factors does she have?

Patient characteristics that increase the risk for PONV include:
- female gender
- history of PONV
- age less than 50 years
- nonsmoker status
- history of motion sickness

Surgical factors that increase the risk of PONV include:
- laparoscopy
- orchiopexy
- gynecologic surgery
- ear surgery
- intra-abdominal surgery

Anesthetic factors that increase the risk of PONV include:
- use of nitrous oxide (N_2O)
- use of halogenated inhaled anesthetic gases
- use of opioids
- prolonged duration of anesthesia
- general anesthesia (instead of regional anesthesia)

This young woman with a history of motion sickness undergoing a laparoscopic gynecologic procedure is at an increased risk for PONV. While her use of cigarettes is by no means good for her, it is protective against PONV. The mechanism is unknown.

What prophylactic options are there to prevent PONV?

Table 12.1 shows the classes of drugs that have been shown to reduce the risk of PONV.

In addition to the drugs in Table 12.1, adequate hydration with intravenous fluids has also been shown to reduce the incidence of PONV.

TABLE 12.1 ■ Several Classes of Drugs Can Help Prevent Postoperative Nausea and Vomiting

Drug Class	Examples	Side Effects/Contraindications
Serotonin antagonist	Ondansetron, granisetron	• Can cause serotonin syndrome in patients taking serotonergic medications (e.g., selective serotonin reuptake inhibitor (SSRI), serotonin and norepinephrine reuptake inhibitor (SNRI), monoamine oxidase inhibitor (MAOI), tramadol) • Prolonged QT interval is usually clinically insignificant but can be dangerous in patients with prolonged QT intervals at baseline
Glucocorticoids	Dexamethasone	• Can cause elevated blood sugar in patients with poorly controlled diabetes • Can cause perineal itching and burning on administration in awake patients
Dopamine antagonist	Droperidol, prochlorperazine	• Can worsen movement symptoms in patients with Parkinson disease • Black box warning for droperidol for sudden cardiac death (in high doses for psychiatric patients)
Neurokinin-1 antagonist	Aprepitant	• Inhibits CYP 3A4; co-administration with other inhibitors (e.g., fluoxetine) can cause toxicity
Anticholinergic	Scopolamine	• Can cause blurry vision, dry mouth • Transdermal patch takes several hours to have an effect
α2 adrenergic agonist	dexmedetomidine, clonidine	• Can cause hypotension • Dexmedetomidine can cause sedation
Gabapentinoids	Gabapentin	• Can accumulate in patients with renal failure
Benzodiazepine	Midazolam	• Can accumulate in patients with liver failure
Propofol	Propofol	• Causes sedation, pain on injection

It is important to be cognizant of the potential side effects of these drugs.

STEP 1, 2 PEARL

The QT interval is a measurement on an electrocardiogram (ECG) from the start of the QRS complex to the end of the T wave. This is the duration of time comprising ventricular depolarization and repolarization. Fig. 12.1 shows a cardiac rhythm strip with important intervals labeled. Generally, the QT interval shortens as the heart rate increases. To account for this, a corrected QT interval, QTc, is calculated using Bazett formula:

$$QTc = \frac{QT\ interval}{\sqrt{RR\ interval}}$$

The RR interval is the length of time from one R wave to the next R wave, expressed in seconds. Normal QTc duration is 390–450 milliseconds for males and 390–460 milliseconds for females. Patients with prolonged QTc are at increased risk for ventricular dysrhythmia, particularly torsade de pointes. Fig. 12.2 shows a rhythm strip as the patient develops torsade de pointes.

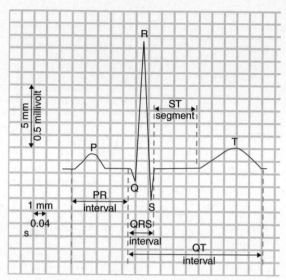

Fig. 12.1 Electrocardiogram showing the most commonly measured intervals, including QT interval. The QT interval is the duration of time from ventricular depolarization (QRS interval) through repolarization (T wave). (Modified from Fig. 48.2 in Ganz, L., & Link, M. S. [2020]. Electrocardiography. In L. Goldman, & A. I. Schafer (Eds.), *Goldman-Cecil medicine* [26th ed., pp. 246–253.e1]. Philadelphia, PA: Elsevier.)

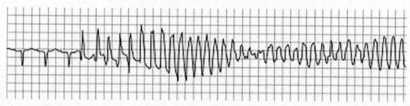

Fig. 12.2 Rhythm strip showing a torsade de pointes. (Haque, M. E., & Sethurman, R. [2018]. Complications in anesthesia. In L. A. Fleisher, & S. H. Rosenbaum (Eds.), *Long QT syndromes and torsades de pointes* [3rd ed., pp. 600–604]. Philadelphia, PA: Elsevier.)

STEP 1 PEARL

Parkinson disease is caused by a loss of dopaminergic neurons from the substantia nigra in the brain due to intracellular accumulation of Lewy bodies, comprised of the protein α-synuclein. Ultimately this leads to reduced activation of the motor cortex.

STEP 1, 2, 3 PEARL

The symptoms of Parkinson disease include bradykinesia, muscle rigidity, and a resting tremor. Difficulty with gait and posture occur late in the disease process. Other symptoms include mood disorders, sleep disturbance, constipation, urinary dysfunction, orthostatic hypotension, and weight loss.

The patient is nervous before surgery.

What can you do?
The best anxiolytic is a reassuring discussion with the anesthesiologist. A small dose of an intravenous benzodiazepine can also be helpful. Be sure to check with the preoperative and operating room nursing staff to make sure all consents and other paperwork have been signed before giving any sedatives.

You will induce general anesthesia with propofol. What is the mechanism of action of propofol?
Propofol works via agonism and potentiation of γ-aminobutyric acid A ($GABA_A$)-induced chloride channels. It also inhibits N-methyl-D-aspartate (NMDA) glutamate receptors.

How is propofol metabolized and eliminated from the body?
Propofol is primarily metabolized by the liver, although some metabolism occurs in the kidneys and lungs as well. Metabolites are not active and are eliminated by the kidneys.

STEP 2, 3 PEARL

Patients receiving high-dose propofol infusions, as well as those with sepsis and severe brain injury, are at risk of propofol infusion syndrome. The signs of propofol infusion syndrome include severe metabolic acidosis, rhabdomyolysis, hyperkalemia, hepatomegaly, lipemia, heart failure, bradycardia, and asystole. Although propofol infusion syndrome was first described in children, it has been observed in adults as well.

After preoxygenation, you induce the patient with propofol. Her eyes close and she becomes apneic. You then administer succinylcholine. The patient starts twitching then stops.

Why is that happening?
Succinylcholine is a depolarizing neuromuscular blocker. It works by activating, or depolarizing, the motor endplate at the neuromuscular junction. The chemical structure of succinylcholine is that of two acetylcholine molecules bound together. This compound binds the ligand-gated ion channels at the neuromuscular junction, which depolarizes muscle fibers, causing them to twitch, or fasciculate. Once the muscle fibers have been depolarized, the fasciculations stop and the patient is paralyzed until the effect wears off, usually within several minutes in healthy patients.

STEP 2 PEARL

Succinylcholine is a triggering agent for malignant hyperthermia. Propofol is not a triggering agent for malignant hyperthermia.

Intubation is uneventful. 5 minutes later, while the patient is being prepped and draped, her blood pressure is 76/44 mm Hg.

What's going on? What should you do?
Induction of general anesthesia with a bolus of propofol can cause hypotension. This is primarily due to systemic vasodilation and a decrease in systemic vascular resistance (SVR). There is also a decrease in cardiac output, likely due to decreased sympathetic stimulation of the heart as well as a decreased venous return to the heart (i.e. preload).

Treat with a bolus of intravenous fluid or a small dose of vasopressor or ephedrine.

The patient's blood pressure returns to baseline, and the operation begins. During insufflation of the abdomen, the patient's heart rate drops from 80/min to 35/min.

What should you do?

Bradycardia is a relatively common response to abdominal insufflation. It is mediated by the vagus nerve (cranial nerve X) stimulating muscarinic receptors on the heart, which slows the heart rate. It is important to keep a close eye on the patient's vital signs during insufflation to watch for this reaction. In extreme circumstances, the patient can become asystolic.

Ask the surgeons to release the insufflation. Treat with an anticholinergic drug like glycopyrrolate or atropine. These drugs competitively inhibit the activation of muscarinic acetylcholine receptors. Atropine is faster-acting and more potent, but also shorter-lasting compared to glycopyrrolate.

STEP 1 PEARL

There are two clinically important types of acetylcholine receptors: nicotinic and muscarinic. Nicotinic receptors are ligand-gated ion channels found at the neuromuscular junction and in autonomic ganglia. Muscarinic receptors are G-protein coupled receptors (GPCRs) that are found throughout the body, including in the brain, heart, and salivary glands. Stimulation of muscarinic receptors on the heart causes bradycardia. Atropine and glycopyrrolate antagonize these receptors, preventing or reversing the bradycardic response.

What are the hemodynamic consequences of abdominal insufflation, or pneumoperitoneum?

Increased intraabdominal pressure compresses the inferior vena cava (IVC), which reduces venous return to the heart, and hence, preload. Pneumoperitoneum also increases SVR and mean arterial pressure (MAP). Cardiac output tends to decrease with abdominal insufflation. Aside from the bradycardic response to insufflation, heart rate can increase with laparoscopy.

What are the ventilatory consequences of pneumoperitoneum?

Abdominal insufflation is achieved with carbon dioxide (CO_2), which readily diffuses into the bloodstream, causing elevated arterial CO_2 tension ($PaCO_2$). Hypercarbia causes decreased SVR, increased pulmonary vascular resistance (PVR), and increased pulmonary artery pressure. Hypercarbia can also increase the risk of cardiac arrhythmia.

Elevated intraabdominal pressure displaces the diaphragm cephalad (i.e., toward the head). This decreases the compliance of the lungs, thereby increasing peak airway pressure (i.e. the maximum amount of pressure generated by the ventilator to inflate the lungs). The cephalad displacement of the diaphragm also causes atelectasis. This can also cause endobronchial intubation, where the distal tip of the endotracheal tube migrates from the trachea into a main bronchus.

STEP 2, 3 PEARL

Pulmonary artery pressures and airway pressures *are not the same thing*. Pulmonary artery pressures refer to the blood pressure within the pulmonary arterial system. Airway pressures refer to the amount of resistance encountered by the ventilator in pushing air into the lungs.

What is hypoxic pulmonary vasoconstriction?

Hypoxic pulmonary vasoconstriction is an reflex to maintain adequate blood oxygenation. The pulmonary vasculature decreases blood flow to areas with low alveolar oxygen levels by vasoconstriction. For example, less blood would flow through a segment of the lung blocked by a mucus plug. This reduces shunting. Inhaled anesthetic gases inhibit this reflex to some degree.

What is shunting? What is dead space?

Ideally, alveolar ventilation and blood flow would be evenly matched, such that all blood flowing through the alveolar capillaries takes up oxygen from the air spaces. In this scenario, there would be no wasted perfusion (i.e., blood that does not receive oxygen) and no wasted ventilation (i.e., oxygen that does not get taken up by the blood). The reality is that ventilation and perfusion are never perfectly matched—there are always areas of the lung that receive more blood than oxygen and vice versa.

In areas of the lung where there is excess blood flow relative to the amount of oxygen to be taken up by the blood, this is known as shunting. This results in deoxygenated blood returning to the left atrium, where it will flow to the systemic circulation. Shunting can be physiologic, as in the natural distribution of perfusion and ventilation throughout the lung, or pathologic, as in lobar pneumonia, atelectasis, or mucus plugging. In all of these cases, there is perfusion, but inadequate ventilation.

In areas of the lung where there is excess ventilation, and hence oxygen, relative to the amount of blood to take it up, this is known as dead space. Dead space can be physiologic, anatomic (i.e., ventilation of the trachea and other conducting airways, where no gas exchange occurs), or pathologic (i.e., pulmonary embolism). In all of these cases, there is ventilation but inadequate perfusion.

STEP 1 PEARL

In patients standing upright, both ventilation and perfusion are greatest at the base of the lung.

You administer glycopyrrolate and the patient's heart rate normalizes. Pneumoperitoneum is achieved. Fifteen minutes after insufflation, the oxygen saturation on the pulse oximeter (SpO_2) begins to drop. SpO_2 after intubation was 99%, and it is now 90%.

What's going on?
Table 12.2 shows the primary causes of hypoxemia during laparoscopy.

What should you do?
Manually ventilate with 100% fraction inspired oxygen (1.0 FiO_2) and assess lung compliance. Auscultate both lung fields. Suction the endotracheal tube. Try recruiting alveoli by holding 30 cm water of inspiratory pressure for 30 seconds. Check the patient's chest and neck for crepitus, as this may be a sign of subcutaneous emphysema. Pass a fiberoptic scope through the endotracheal tube to identify the carina and rule out main stem intubation and mucus plugging. If the saturation continues to drop, ask the surgical team to release pneumoperitoneum or decrease the insufflation pressure. Examine the patient for evidence of tracheal deviation or neck vein engorgement suggestive of tension pneumothorax. If the hypoxemia does not improve order a chest radiograph (CXR) and arterial blood gas.

Breath sounds are normal over the right side and absent over the left side.

Now what?
The presence of unilateral breath sounds is suggestive of endobronchial intubation (i.e., main stem intubation). Pneumothorax is also a possibility Withdraw the endotracheal tube slowly until breath sounds are auscultated over both lung fields. You may also consider passing a fiberoptic scope down the endotracheal tube to identify the carina and confirm correct placement. If you are still unsure, order a CXR.

The oxygen saturation improves and surgery proceeds. At the conclusion of the operation, 2 hours after administration of succinylcholine, the patient does not have any twitches on train of four monitoring. No other neuromuscular blocking agent has been given.

What's going on?
The effect of succinylcholine should last 4–6 minutes. When the patient remains paralyzed for significantly longer than that, first be sure to rule out drug error (i.e., make sure you didn't accidentally give some other neuromuscular blocking agent). Assuming succinylcholine was administered as intended and the patient still has no twitches after 2 hours, the patient may have pseudocholinesterase deficiency.

TABLE 12.2 ■ **The Differential Diagnosis of Hypoxemia During Laparoscopy**

Etiology	Pathophysiology
Endobronchial intubation	• Elevated intraabdominal pressure displaces the diaphragm, lungs, and bronchial tree cephalad, causing the tip of the endotracheal tube to migrate into either the right or the left main bronchus.
Hypoventilation/hypercarbia	• CO_2 used for abdominal insufflation diffuses into the bloodstream. • Elevated intraabdominal pressure is transmitted to the lungs reducing tidal volumes and causing CO_2 retention. • Atelectasis causes shunting.
Pneumothorax/capnothorax	• Loss of negative pressure within the pleural space can cause the collapse of a lung, greatly reducing the tidal volumes it receives from the ventilator. • High airway pressures can cause pneumothorax. • Capnothorax can occur due to diaphragmatic injury or CO_2 spreading to the pleura via subcutaneous tissue or retroperitoneum. • If gas continues to accumulate in the pleural space and the pressure rises, a tension pneumothorax may develop.
Tension pneumothorax	• Accumulation of gas, CO_2 from insufflation in this case, within the pleural space collapses the lung and can shift the mediastinum into the contralateral thorax. • This can cause severe hypotension and must be addressed quickly. Insufflation should be released, and a needle thoracostomy may be necessary.
Bronchospasm	• Bronchospasm increases resistance to flow and decreases tidal volumes delivered. • This can be caused by a drug reaction, asthma, aspiration, or stimulation of the carina by the endotracheal tube.
Pulmonary embolism	• A blood clot becomes lodged in the pulmonary arterial system, increasing pulmonary vascular resistance and dead space ventilation. • This may cause hemodynamic instability or cardiovascular collapse in extreme cases.

Communication with the surgical team is critical as you work through the diagnostic possibilities.

Normally, succinylcholine is metabolized and inactivated by pseudocholinesterase. However, some individuals have one or two genetic alleles that produce a mutant variant of pseudocholinesterase that does not inactivate succinylcholine. This variant is called atypical pseudocholinesterase, and this condition is referred to as pseudocholinesterase deficiency.

How is pseudocholinesterase deficiency diagnosed?

This diagnosis is made by the dibucaine test. Dibucaine is a local anesthetic that inhibits normal pseudocholinesterase much more than it inhibits atypical pseudocholinesterase. A sample of the patient's plasma is mixed with dibucaine. The percentage activity of pseudocholinesterase is then measured.

The dibucaine number is a measure of *the percent of inhibition of activity* of pseudocholinesterase. Since normal pseudocholinesterase is very susceptible to inhibition by dibucaine, the dibucaine number of a patient with two normal (i.e., homozygous typical) alleles for pseudocholinesterase is 80, meaning dibucaine has inhibited 80% of its activity. The dibucaine number for a patient with one normal allele and one atypical allele (i.e., heterozygous) is 50. Meanwhile, the dibucaine number of a patient with two abnormal alleles (i.e., homozygous atypical) is 20.

What can be done for this patient?
The prolonged effect of paralysis is different from delayed emergence. Although this patient may be completely paralyzed, she will be fully awake if the anesthetic wears off. Be sure to continue anesthetic or sedative while she remains paralyzed to avoid awareness, recall, and risk of post-traumatic stress disorder.

If the patient still has no twitches at the end of the operation, begin by ruling out other causes of prolonged paralysis. Make sure succinylcholine, and no other neuromuscular blocking agent, was given. Check electrolytes, specifically calcium, magnesium, and phosphate, and ensure these are normal. Make sure the patient is normothermic. Rule out significant acidosis.

If all other reversible causes have been ruled out, treatment is supportive. The patient should remain intubated and sedated. The paralysis should wear off within 24 hours. A dibucaine test should be sent, however, the result of this test will take days or weeks to return, so while it will be helpful for the patient in the future, it will not help you make decisions intraoperatively.

Once the paralysis has worn off and the patient is awake and extubated, she should be advised to tell future anesthesiologists caring for her that she had a prolonged response to succinylcholine.

BEYOND THE PEARLS

- In addition to abdominal insufflation, the vagal response and subsequent bradycardia or asystole can be caused by pressure on the eyeball (see Case 7), manipulation of the uterus, laryngoscopy, manipulation of the carotid sinus (see Case 32), traction on the dura, and patient anxiety.
- The presence of a nasogastric tube, obesity, and supplemental oxygen are not risk factors for PONV.
- Obese patients have increased levels of pseudocholinesterase and a larger extracellular fluid volume, so they generally require larger doses of succinylcholine. Dose succinylcholine based on total body weight, not ideal body weight.
- Modern practice is to dose succinylcholine just once for intubation, and then use a nondepolarizing neuromuscular blocker to maintain paralysis. Patients who receive multiple doses or an infusion of succinylcholine are at risk for developing a phase II block, where the twitch pattern looks like that of a nondepolarizing neuromuscular blocker.
- Propofol does not inhibit hypoxic pulmonary vasoconstriction (see Case 21).
- After administration of succinylcholine, it is good practice to wait until twitches return prior to administration of another paralytic. This will rule out pseudocholinesterase deficiency as a cause of prolonged paralysis.

References

Berg, S. M., & Braehler, M. R. (2020). The postanesthesia care unit. In M. A. Gropper, R. D. Miller, N. H. Cohen, L. I. Eriksson, L. A. Fleisher, K. Leslie, et al. (Eds.), *Miller's anesthesia* (9th ed., Chapter 80, pp. 2586–2613.e5). Philadelphia, PA: Elsevier.

Gan, T. J., Diemunsch, P., Habib, A. S., Kovac, A., Kranke, P., Meyer, T. A., et al. (2014). Consensus guidelines for the management of postoperative nausea and vomiting. *Anesthesia & Analgesia, 118*(1), 85–113.

Schumacher, M., & Fukuda, K. (2020). Opioids. In M. A. Gropper, R. D. Miller, N. H. Cohen, L. I. Eriksson, L. A. Fleisher, K. Leslie, et al. (Eds.), *Miller's anesthesia* (9th ed., Chapter 24, pp. 680–741.e15). Philadelphia, PA: Elsevier.

Tate, J. (2022). Parkinson disease. In R. D. Kellerman, & D. P. Rakel (Eds.), *Conn's current therapy* (pp. 757–761). Philadelphia, PA: Elsevier.

Vuyk, J., Sitsen, E., & Reekers, M. (2020). Intravenous anesthetics. In M. A. Gropper, R. D. Miller, N. H. Cohen, L. I. Eriksson, L. A. Fleisher, K. Leslie, et al. (Eds.), *Miller's anesthesia* (9th ed., Chapter 23, pp. 638–679.e10). Philadelphia, PA: Elsevier.

A 21-Year-Old Man With a Gunshot Wound Through the Right Lower Quadrant of his Abdomen

Paul Neil Frank ■ David C. Asseff

A 21-year-old man is brought to the operating room for emergency exploratory laparotomy after he was found unresponsive with a gunshot wound through the right lower quadrant of his abdomen. He is unable to provide a history. His blood pressure is 64/37 mm Hg via the blood pressure cuff, and his heart rate is 152/min. His respiratory rate is 6/min and irregular. His oxygen saturation is 84%. His extremities are cool. He has a 20-gauge IV in his left hand.

What are the priorities in treating this patient?

Advanced trauma life support (ATLS) provides a framework for the rapid assessment of trauma patients.

- A—Airway: ensure the patient's airway is patent. Obstruction may be a direct result of trauma, such as facial injury, or it may be the result of a depressed level of consciousness from brain injury or intoxication. If there is airway obstruction or if you believe airway obstruction is imminent, intubate the patient. If conventional methods of intubation are unsuccessful, cricothyrotomy or other surgical airways may be necessary.
- B—Breathing: ensure the patient is adequately ventilating. Inadequate ventilation may be a direct result of trauma, such as a pneumothorax or cervical spine injury (leading to diaphragmatic paralysis), or it may be the result of a depressed level of consciousness. As above, if the patient is not breathing adequately, intubation and possible surgical airway may be necessary. Chest tubes should be placed as necessary to relieve pneumothorax or hemothorax.
- C—Circulation: sites of active hemorrhage should be identified. Tourniquets, pelvic binder, and direct pressure should be applied as necessary. Proceed emergently to the operating room for surgical control of hemorrhage.
- D—Neurologic Disability: assess the patient's global neurologic status by calculating their Glasgow Coma Scale (GCS, see Case 26). Look for focal signs such as asymmetric pupils. If the patient is hemodynamically stable, obtain a computerized tomography (CT) of the head to rule out operative emergencies, such as epidural hematoma or impending herniation.
- E—Exposure: remove all the patient's clothing and conduct a head-to-toe search for visible injuries (e.g., deformed bones, swelling, bruising). Triage any additional injuries.

What is the differential diagnosis of hypotension?

In the case of an unstable trauma patient, the differential is short. We expect the patient to be hypotensive and tachycardic. Hemorrhage is extremely likely—in fact, it should be your working diagnosis until definitively ruled out. It is important to consider other causes of tachycardia and hypotension that may result from trauma. Table 13.1 shows the differential diagnosis and initial management in a hypotensive trauma patient.

TABLE 13.1 ■ **Differential Diagnosis of Hypotension in Trauma**

Etiology	Pathophysiology/Diagnosis	Treatment
Hemorrhagic shock	• Severe acute intravascular volume loss • Diagnosed by clinical observation, imaging, or invasive examination	• Large-bore IV access • Volume resuscitation (ideally with blood) • Stop the bleeding with tourniquets, direct pressure, and surgical repair as necessary
Pericardial tamponade	• Fluid accumulation within the pericardial sac inhibits diastolic filling of the heart • Diagnosed echocardiographically (Fig. 13.1)	• Large-bore IV access • Volume resuscitation • Maintain tachycardia and systemic vascular tone (i.e., afterload) • Avoid positive pressure ventilation if possible • Emergent percutaneous or surgical decompression of tamponade
Tension pneumothorax	• Air leak into the pleural space creates positive pressure that inhibits venous return to the heart, thereby reducing preload and stroke volume • Diagnosed clinically or on chest radiograph (Fig. 13.2)	• Decompressive needle thoracostomy with a large-bore needle
Neurogenic shock	• High spinal cord injury (high thoracic level or above) inhibiting sympathetic efferent signaling causing bradycardia and reduced vascular tone (see Case 24)	• Hemodynamic support including volume resuscitation, vasopressors, and inotropes as necessary

Note that these diagnoses may not be mutually exclusive. For example, the patient may be hemorrhaging and have a tension pneumothorax.

What is the most likely diagnosis?

The patient has sustained penetrating trauma. He is hypotensive and tachycardic. This is hemor-rhagic shock until proven otherwise. *Beware of missed injury, such as additional gunshot wound, or tension pneumothorax.*

STEP 1 PEARL

The body's initial response to shock is mediated by the baroreceptor reflex. Stretch receptors in the walls of the aortic arch and carotid sinuses sense a drop in wall tension as blood pressure falls. They signal the brainstem to upregulate sympathetic tone which increases heart rate, cardiac contractility, and systemic vascular resistance. Blood flow is shunted away from the skin and gastrointestinal tract in order to maintain perfusion to the heart, brain, and kidneys.

What should you do?

Surgery needs to begin quickly. Place basic monitors (e.g., pulse oximeter, blood pressure cuff, and electrocardiogram leads), secure the airway, and begin aggressive resuscitation. Ideally, there are multiple team members present, so these things can be accomplished simultaneously.

After the airway is secured and resuscitation is underway, place additional monitors: arterial line, temperature probe, twitch monitor, indwelling urinary catheter, orogastric tube (assuming there is no concern for skull base injury), and processed electroencephalogram (EEG) monitor.

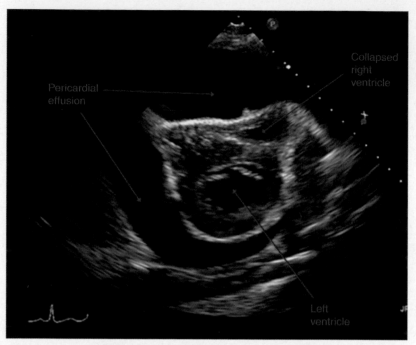

Fig. 13.1   Transthoracic echocardiogram (TTE) showing a large fluid collection surrounding the heart causing collapse of the right ventricle during diastole. (Modified from Holt, B. D., & Oh, J. K. [2020]. Pericardial diseases. In L. Goldman, & A. I. Schafer [Eds.], *Goldman-Cecil medicine* [26th ed., pp. 428–436.e1]. Philadelphia, PA: Elsevier, Fig. 68.4.)

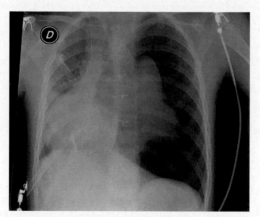

Fig. 13.2   CXR showing a left-sided tension pneumothorax causing rightward shift of the mediastinum and trachea. (Reproduced from Federici, D., Vavassori, A., Mantovani, L., Cattaneo, S., Ciuffreda, M., Seddio, F., et al. (2013). Complete rightward cardiac luxation caused due to left tension pneumothorax. *Annals of Thoracic Surgery, 96*[2], 693–694, Fig. 1.)

How should you induce this patient?

The most commonly used drug for induction in a trauma patient is etomidate, although ketamine may also be used. While the classic teaching is that etomidate and ketamine help maintain blood pressure, it is important to note that these agents can cause hypotension, especially in a patient who is severely hypovolemic. A small dose of benzodiazepine can also be given. Consider using a reduced dose of induction agent or even no induction agent, depending on the stability, or lack thereof, of the patient.

How should you secure the airway?

In this hemorrhaging trauma patient with depressed mental status and hypoxemia undergoing emergent exploratory laparotomy, endotracheal intubation is mandatory. Have suction, a video laryngoscope, and a bougie ready. Preoxygenate with 100% fraction inspired oxygen (1.0 FiO_2) while the induction drugs are administered. Remember that only a small dose of induction agent will be needed. Paralysis for rapid sequence intubation can be accomplished with succinylcholine (1 mg/kg) or rocuronium (1.2 mg/kg).

What are the contraindications to succinylcholine?

Table 13.2 shows other contraindications to succinylcholine. Be sure to quickly check for these contraindications prior to giving succinylcholine to any patient. In the setting of a trauma, you will not have time to obtain a thorough history, so you must rely on your clinical observations (e.g. does the patient have a crush injury?).

What is rapid sequence intubation, and why is it advisable in this scenario?

Rapid sequence intubation entails giving induction drugs followed immediately by paralytic without any mask ventilation. In ordinary (i.e., not rapid sequence) intubations, induction drugs are given, and then the patient is mask ventilated while paralytic is administered and takes effect. In this emergency case, the goal is to secure the airway as quickly as possible. Rapid sequence intubation minimizes the risk of aspiration of gastric contents, especially in a patient with unknown *nil per os* (NPO) status.

If the patient's oxygen levels quickly drop with induction, it may be necessary to provide mask ventilation prior to intubation. Avoid large tidal volumes and high airway pressures.

What is cricoid pressure, and is it a good idea in this scenario?

Cricoid pressure is the application of manual force by an assistant to the patient's cricoid ring during induction and laryngoscopy, usually with the thumb and index finger. The goal is to compress the esophagus to prevent the aspiration of gastric contents. This is often done during rapid sequence intubation. Opinions regarding the efficacy of cricoid pressure are mixed.

After induction, but before intubation the patient starts vomiting.

TABLE 13.2 ■ **Contraindications to Succinylcholine**

Contraindication	Comments
Crush injury	• Succinylcholine in the setting of crush injury can cause severe hyperkalemia.
Personal or family history of malignant hyperthermia	• Succinylcholine can trigger malignant hyperthermia, resulting in rhabdomyolysis, metabolic acidosis, and death.
History of stroke, remote spinal cord injury, or prolonged period of being bed-bound (such as from chronic illness)	• When a neuromuscular group is unused for an extended period of time (as in the thigh muscles of a paraplegic patient), the muscle develops "immature" nicotinic receptors outside of the neuromuscular junction that release much more potassium than do normal nicotinic receptors when stimulated. • The development of these immature receptors takes time, so if a previously healthy patient comes in with a new stroke or spinal cord injury, it is still safe to use succinylcholine.
Burns	• As with stroke patients, burn patients will develop immature ligand-gated ion channels over time. • It is safe to use succinylcholine in the first 24 h after the burn.
Muscular dystrophy	• Succinylcholine can cause rhabdomyolysis in these patients.

What should you do?

If cricoid pressure is being applied, it should be immediately released. The patient should be placed in Trendelenburg position (this prevents gastric contents from passively flowing down the trachea, see Fig. 13.3) and, if the cervical spine has been cleared (i.e., there is no concern for cervical spine injury), turn the patient's head to the side. Suction out the mouth and oropharynx thoroughly. Once the patient has stopped vomiting, proceed with laryngoscopy and intubation. After the endotracheal tube is in proper position and the cuff is inflated, use a soft suction catheter to suction out the airway via the endotracheal tube.

What are the best options for intravenous access?

The goal here is reliable large-bore access. The fastest way of accomplishing this is with one or more large peripheral IV catheters, usually 18-gauge or larger. Remember, a smaller gauge number means a larger caliber IV catheter. For example, an 18-gauge catheter is larger than a 20-gauge catheter, which is larger than a 22-gauge catheter. If no peripheral IV can be established, an intraosseous line or central venous catheter can be placed. These require specialized equipment and expertise.

Regardless of the type of access, it is best to have access above the level of the injury. In this case, there is likely intraabdominal hemorrhage. It is possible that fluids transfused through IV access below the level of the injury, such as the femoral vein, may simply bleed out through the vascular injury and not return to the heart.

Where can intraosseous access be obtained?

Sites for intraosseous access include the proximal or distal tibia, distal femur, proximal humerus, iliac crest, and sternum. The intraosseous catheter infuses into the intramedullary venous plexus within the bone.

What are the contraindications to intraosseous access?

Do not obtain intraosseous access in an extremity that has sustained a fracture or crush injury or in a bone where prior intraosseous placements have been attempted. Do not place intraosseous access near the sites of prior orthopedic procedures or near the site of infection or burns. Patients with brittle bones, such as those with osteogenesis imperfecta, should not undergo intraosseous line placement. Finally, patients with right-to-left intracardiac shunts are at increased risk of fat or bone marrow embolization to the systemic circulation, and intraosseous access should be avoided in this population.

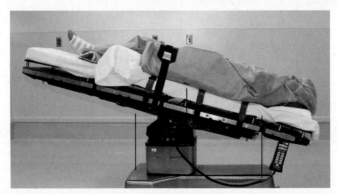

Fig. 13.3 Trendelenburg position, showing the patient supine on the operating table with the head below the level of the feet. ([2020]. Trendelenburg. *AORN Journal, 112*[5], P19–P20.)

Where can central venous access be obtained?
Sites for central venous cannulation include the internal jugular, subclavian, and femoral veins (see Case 31).

Initial labs drawn in the ambulance show a hematocrit of 42%.

Do you still need to transfuse?
Yes, patients bleed whole blood. In other words, patients lose RBCs and plasma in the same ratio that it exists in their bodies. A sample of the patient's blood taken from the floor of the ambulance would also have a hematocrit of 42%. The reason that the hemoglobin and hematocrit levels drop with blood loss is that, over the course of hours to days, interstitial fluid will be mobilized into the intravascular space, and the kidneys will retain free water. This will increase the patient's circulatory volume without increasing RBC content, thereby reducing the concentration of RBCs, resulting in decreased hemoglobin and hematocrit.

What fluids should be used for resuscitation?
Blood! Be sure to activate the massive transfusion protocol as soon as possible—this may be done automatically when the hospital receives the notification of an incoming trauma patient. This will notify the blood bank to release uncrossmatched blood products to facilitate initial resuscitation.

In most civilian hospitals, blood comes as separate products: red blood cells (RBCs), fresh frozen plasma (FFP), platelets, and cryoprecipitate. These products are given in a 1:1:1 (RBC:FFP:platelets) ratio during initial resuscitation until coagulation studies show that the ratio should be changed. This resuscitation schema replaces oxygen-carrying capacity (i.e., RBCs), while also replacing hemostatic agents (i.e., FFP, platelets).

What else can help maintain hemostatic mechanism?
The literature has shown a survival benefit for patients who receive tranexamic acid, an antifibrinolytic agent, during the first hour of resuscitation. Give 1 g over 10 minutes, then another gram over 8 hours. Calcium administration should begin with the first unit of blood. Monitor fibrinogen levels to determine the need for cryoprecipitate.

While the patient is still hemorrhaging, the blood pressure is 143/85 mm Hg. Is that acceptable?
No, high blood pressure can exacerbate bleeding. During initial resuscitation, the goal systolic blood pressure should be 80 to 100 mm Hg. This is known as permissive hypotension.

After 8 RBC, 8 FFP, and 8 platelets have been administered, you notice the cardiac rhythm strip looks unusual, as in Fig. 13.4.

What's going on? What should you do?
Peaked T waves on ECG or rhythm strips are suggestive of hyperkalemia. Banked blood contains relatively high levels of potassium. As multiple units are given, the patient's serum potassium will increase.

Acute hyperkalemia can be treated in multiple ways:
- calcium (this does not reduce potassium levels, but it does stabilize cardiac myocyte membranes) and can increase contractility in the case of citrate toxicity
- insulin and 50% dextrose solution (D50), usually 10 units of insulin intravenously and 12.5 g of D50
- furosemide
- beta-agonists (e.g., albuterol, epinephrine)
- hemodialysis

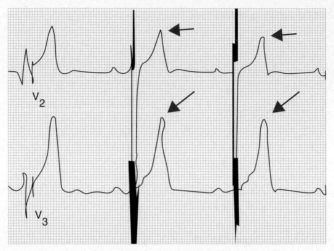

Fig. 13.4   Peaked T waves, denoted by *red arrows*. (Modified from Kopyt, N., & Yee, J. [2021]. Hyperkalemia. In F. F. Ferri [Ed.], *Ferri's clinical advisor* [pp. 723–728.e1]. Philadelphia, PA: Elsevier, Fig. E2.)

STEP 2, 3 PEARL

Massive blood transfusion causes multiple electrolyte abnormalities, not just hyperkalemia. The citrate in stored blood chelates calcium and magnesium in the patient's blood, resulting in hypocalcemia and hypomagnesemia. This can be treated with IV calcium and magnesium.

The patient's temperature is 33.4°C. Should you be concerned?
Yes, hypothermia can be lethal in trauma patients. It is one component of the lethal triad of trauma, along with coagulopathy and metabolic acidosis.

To warm the patient, increase the temperature of the room, apply a convection heating blanket (or warm blankets) to as much body surface area as possible, and administer fluids via a fluid warmer.

What are the mechanisms of heat loss under general anesthesia?
There are four primary mechanisms of heat loss in patients under general anesthesia:
- radiation: heat leaves the body into the surroundings
- convection: cold air saps heat from the body as it circulates in the room
- evaporation: this is most significant with open body cavities such as the thorax or abdomen
- conduction: patient's body loses heat to a cold surface

This trauma patient is also receiving a large volume of blood, which has been stored cold. It is therefore recommended that blood products and other fluids be administered warm via a fluid warmer or rapid transfuser.

The surgeons have control of the bleeding.

How will you know that your resuscitation is adequate?
The underlying cause of hemorrhagic shock is hypovolemia. As the hypovolemia resolves, stroke volume, and hence blood pressure, will increase. As the stretch receptors in the walls of the aortic arch and carotid arteries sense that blood pressure is adequate, the activation of the sympathetic nervous system will be reduced. Heart rate will start to trend down to the normal range. Urine

output should also improve, although this can be a lagging indicator. Laboratory abnormalities such as lactic acidosis will resolve.

At the end of the surgery, the patient received 22 units of RBC, 18 units of FFP, 10 units of platelets, and 4 units of cryoprecipitate. Estimated blood loss is 10 L. The patient's pulse is 112/min, his blood pressure is 106/68 mm Hg, and his oxygen saturation is 94%.

Should you extubate this patient?
No, it is safer for the patient to remain intubated for now. This patient has received many liters of fluid resuscitation to compensate for a massive hemorrhage. There is high risk for airway edema in this case. Additional respiratory risks include pulmonary edema from transfusion-associated lung injury (TRALI) or transfusion-associated circulatory overload (TACO), which can impair oxygenation.

Furthermore, the patient had a depressed mental status when he first arrived, and his current mental status is unknown. It is therefore unclear whether his ventilatory drive and airway protective reflexes are intact. It would be prudent to bring this patient to the intensive care unit (ICU) intubated and sedated. He will require hemodynamic and respiratory monitoring, assessment for missed injuries, management of coagulopathy, assessment of neurologic status, and pain control.

BEYOND THE PEARLS

- Trauma patients have a high incidence of intraoperative recall. With severe hypotension, it may be necessary to turn off the anesthetic agent. A dose of benzodiazepine early in the case can reduce the risk of recall.
- Shock is a strong anesthetic—it takes very little induction agent to induce general anesthesia in a hemorrhaging trauma patient. A full induction dose of propofol, etomidate, or ketamine can exacerbate hypotension and lead to cardiovascular collapse.
- Cricoid pressure may or may not be helpful in preventing passive aspiration (i.e., the reflux of gastric contents up the esophagus and into the airway without retching), but it will not prevent active aspiration (i.e., retching and vomiting). Application of cricoid pressure during active vomiting by the patient can cause esophageal rupture.
- In acute bleeding, hemoglobin and hematocrit will not change quickly enough to indicate the need for additional transfusion. In this setting, it is better to rely on hemodynamics (e.g., heart rate, blood pressure) and clinical observation (e.g., how fast are the suction canisters filling up?) to guide resuscitation.

References

Ball, J. W., Dains, J. E., Flynn, J. A., Solomon, B. S., & Stewart, R. W. (Eds.). (2019). Neurologic system. In *Seidel's guide to physical examination* (Chapter 23, pp. 567–606). Philadelphia, PA: Elsevier. Fig. 23.25.

Fisher, A. D., Washburn, G., Powell, D., Callaway, D. W., Miles, E. A., & Baker, J. (October 2018). Damage control resuscitation in prolonged field care (CPG ID: 73). *Joint Trauma System Clinical Practice Guideline*.

Galvagno, S. M., Steurer, M. P., & Grissom, T. E. (2020). Anesthesia for trauma. In M. A. Gropper, R. D. Miller, N. H. Cohen, L. I. Eriksson, L. A. Fleisher, K. Leslie, et al. (Eds.), *Miller's anesthesia* (9th ed., Chapter 66, pp. 2115–2155.e8). Philadelphia, PA: Elsevier.

Jarris, R. F., & Fowler, G. C. (2020). Intraosseous vascular access. In G. C. Fowler, B. A. Choby, D. Iyengar, T. X. O'Connell, F. G. O'Connor, B. Reddy, et al. (Eds.), *Pfenninger and Fowler's procedures for primary care* (4th ed., Chapter 226, pp. 1510–1514). Philadelphia, PA: Elsevier.

Tobin, J., Barras, W., Bree, S., Williams, N., McFarland, C., Park, C., et al. (April 2021). Anesthesia for trauma patients (CPG ID: 40). *Joint Trauma System Clinical Practice Guideline*.

A 50-Year-Old Man With a History of Morbid Obesity

Bahar Kasimi ■ Elizabeth C. Fung ■ Paul Neil Frank

A 50-year-old man with a history of morbid obesity (body mass index, BMI of 63 kg/m²), diabetes mellitus type 2 (DM2) on insulin, and obstructive sleep apnea (OSA) on nighttime continuous positive airway pressure (CPAP) at home is scheduled to undergo Roux-en-Y gastric bypass surgery for weight loss. He has adequate exercise tolerance and is able to climb three flights of stairs without shortness of breath or chest pain. In the preoperative area, his vital signs are blood pressure 144/82 mm Hg, pulse 94/min, respirations 16/min, oxygen saturation 97% on room air, and temperature 35.8 C.

STEP 1, 2 PEARL

OSA is characterized by intermittent closure of the upper airway during sleep, often due to decreased pharyngeal muscle tone. It is most commonly associated with obesity. Clinical features include loud snoring, restless sleep, daytime sleepiness, and morning headaches. OSA is diagnosed with polysomnography and initial treatment involves weight loss and CPAP.

STEP 1, 2 PEARL

Sequelae of OSA include systemic hypertension, pulmonary hypertension, and depression. Intermittent upper airway obstruction during sleep results in hypoxia and hypercarbia. This leads to activation of the sympathetic nervous system, causing systemic and pulmonary vasoconstriction. Untreated pulmonary hypertension can lead to right ventricular failure. Transient hypoxia will also lead to increased red blood cell production and erythrocytosis.

How is obesity categorized?

According to the Centers for Disease Control (CDC), 39.5% of the US population 20 years old and older was overweight as of 2016. Higher BMI correlates with the higher risk of comorbidities such as diabetes mellitus, hypertension, cardiovascular disease, OSA, restrictive lung disease (see Case 21), and more (Table 14.1). Patients are categorized as overweight or obese based on the following criteria:

- Overweight: BMI 25–29.9 kg/m²
- Class I obesity: BMI 30–34.9
- Class II "severe" obesity: BMI 35–39.9
- Class III "morbid" obesity: BMI 40+

The American Society of Anesthesiologists Physical Status scoring (on a scale of 1 through 6) is used perioperatively to communicate the presence and severity of a patient's comorbidities. This score can be used in conjunction with other information to help estimate the perioperative risk of adverse events for this patient. A patient with BMI greater than 40 kg/m² is categorized at least as an American Society of Anesthesiologists (ASA) 3.

TABLE 14.1 ■ **Health Risks Associated with Elevated Body Mass Index**

Comorbidity	Comments
Type 2 diabetes	• 90% of people with type 2 diabetes have a BMI of >23 kg/m^2
Hypertension	• 5× greater risk of hypertension in patients with obesity
	• 85% of diagnoses of hypertension are associated with a BMI >25 kg/m^2
Coronary artery disease	• Significantly increased risk of coronary artery disease
	• Overweight/obesity plus hypertension is associated with increased risk of ischemic stroke
Respiratory effects (e.g., obstructive sleep apnea)	• Neck circumference of >43 cm in men and >40.5 cm in women is associated with obstructive sleep apnea, daytime somnolence, and development of pulmonary hypertension
Cancer	• 20% of all cancer deaths among nonsmokers are related to obesity (30% of endometrial cancers)
Osteoarthritis	• Frequent association in the elderly with increasing body weight— the risk of disability attributable to osteoarthritis equal to heart disease and greater to any other medical disorder of the elderly
Liver and gall bladder disease	• Overweight and obesity are associated with nonalcoholic fatty liver disease and nonalcoholic steatohepatitis (NASH). 40% of NASH patients are obese; 20% have dyslipidemia
	• 3× risk of gall bladder disease in women with a BMI of >32 kg/m^2; 7× risk if BMI of >45 kg/m^2

Obesity can affect multiple organ systems. *BMI*, Body mass index.

What is a roux-en-Y gastric bypass surgery?

Many individuals look to medicine for help with weight loss when diet and lifestyle changes are unsuccessful. The Food and Drug Administration (FDA) has approved several medications that may help with weight loss, although they do not have the same success rate as surgical intervention. Patients with severe obesity, after attempting all non-surgical methods of weight loss, may be candidates for bariatric surgery.

Roux-en-Y gastric bypass surgery is considered to be the gold standard of bariatric surgery. This procedure involves a complex anatomic rearrangement resulting in both restriction (a smaller stomach) and malabsorption (ingested food bypasses much of the absorptive area of the small intestine), as in Fig. 14.1. This also results in a change in the secretion of gastric hormones and an eventual change in the gut microbiome. The net effect is weight loss. The procedure is often done laparoscopically.

STEP 2 PEARL

Initial attempts to decrease weight are diet and exercise. However, if these conservative measures are not enough, medication or surgery may be indicated. Failure of medication treatment is not necessary in order to consider bariatric surgery, and the two are often used together. Medication, such as orlistat or lorcaserin, can be considered for patients with a BMI ≥30 kg/m^2 or in patients with a BMI 25 to 29.9 kg/m^2 who have associated comorbidities such as diabetes or hypertension. Bariatric surgery is considered in patients with a BMI of 40 kg/m^2 or more. Those with a BMI ≥35 kg/m^2 and weight-related complications may also be candidates for weight loss surgery. The two most common types of bariatric surgeries are sleeve gastrectomy and Roux-en-Y gastric bypass.

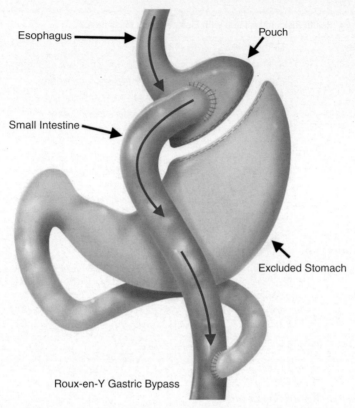

Esophagus

Pouch

Small Intestine

Excluded Stomach

Roux-en-Y Gastric Bypass

Fig. 14.1   Diagram of roux-en-Y anatomy. Ingested food enters a small pouch of stomach and then enters a distal portion of the small intestine. The proximal small intestine and excluded stomach are bypassed. (Gandhi, D., Boregowda, U., Sharma, P., Ahuja, K., Jain, N., Khanna, K., & Gupta, N. [2021]. A review of commonly performed bariatric surgeries: imaging features and its complications. *Clinical Imaging, 72*, 122–135. https://doi.org/10.1016/j.clinimag.2020.11.020. Modified from Fig. 6.)

STEP 2 PEARL

Although Roux-en-Y surgery is a common operation, it can have significant complications. Early complications include anastomotic leak and bowel ischemia. Late complications include anastomotic stricture, dumping syndrome, marginal ulcers, small bowel obstructions, cholelithiasis, and vitamin B12 deficiency.

STEP 1 PEARL

Vitamin B12 absorption starts when stomach acid releases the vitamin from ingested food. Vitamin B12 is then bound by an R binder protein. In the duodenum, this bond is cleaved and vitamin B12 is subsequently bound by the intrinsic factor, which is produced by the parietal cells of the stomach. This complex is then absorbed in the terminal ileum. A Roux-en-Y surgery disrupts this process and can result in a deficiency of B12.

The most common cause of vitamin B12 deficiency is pernicious anemia, which is an auto-immune condition preventing the formation of the vitamin B_{12}-intrinsic factor complex. Other causes of B12 deficiency include low dietary intake of B12, small intestinal bacterial overgrowth, malabsorption, medications such as proton pump inhibitors, and parasitic infections.

STEP 1, 2 PEARL

Clinical manifestations of vitamin B12 deficiency include megaloblastic anemia, cognitive impairment, paresthesia, glossitis, and other neurologic symptoms. Subacute combined degeneration is classically associated with vitamin B12 deficiency due to demyelination of the dorsal columns, corticospinal tracts, and spinocerebellar tracts of the spinal cord. Damage to these areas can result in many of the neurologic symptoms associated with vitamin B12 deficiency such as loss of proprioception and vibration sense (dorsal columns), spastic paresis (corticospinal tracts), and ataxia (spinocerebellar tracts).

What preoperative lab tests/studies will you order for this patient?
If the patient has a history of diabetes mellitus, check their serum glucose level on the morning of surgery. A recent hemoglobin A1c (measure of glycated hemoglobin) should also be noted, as it is a good marker of the patient's blood glucose control over the past few months.

Patients with poorly controlled diabetes are at risk for diabetic nephropathy, which may manifest as elevated creatinine, and in severe forms of chronic kidney disease, electrolyte abnormalities including hyperkalemia. Check serum electrolytes preoperatively.

Chronic hypoxia can stimulate increased erythropoietin secretion, resulting in increased erythrocyte production, which manifests as elevated hemoglobin and hematocrit. Check a complete blood count.

Patients with OSA are at increased risk of right ventricular hypertrophy due to chronic night-time hypoxia and hypercarbia, both of which increase pulmonary vascular resistance and right ventricular afterload. Order an electrocardiogram (ECG). If the patient has any history, signs, or symptoms of heart failure, an echocardiogram should be ordered as well.

STEP 1, 2 PEARL

Diabetic nephropathy is the most common cause of end-stage renal disease in the United States. Diabetes causes glomerular hypertrophy, increased renal plasma flow, and increased filtration fraction. This leads to glomerular hyperfiltration and an elevated glomerular filtration rate. Kimmelstiel-Wilson nodules are classically seen in diabetic nephropathy due to nodular glomerulosclerosis.

STEP 1, 2, 3 PEARL

Early detection of diabetic nephropathy is important for preventing further kidney damage in diabetic patients. The rapid decline in estimated glomerular filtration rate (eGFR) and microalbuminuria (30–300 mg/day) are early signs of diabetic nephropathy. The urine microalbumin/creatinine ratio is one of the most sensitive screening tests for diabetic nephropathy. The most effective intervention for slowing progression is good blood pressure control. Angiotensin-converting enzyme (ACE) inhibitors are the first line due to their protective effect on the kidneys.

In patients who have not formally been diagnosed with OSA, how can you screen for it?
A quick screening for OSA can be done using the STOP BANG score (Table 14.2). A response of
"yes" to 3 or more questions indicates a high risk for OSA; the patient should be notified of their
risks and may benefit from a sleep study.

The patient's ECG is shown in Fig. 14.2.

What does this show?
This ECG shows a right bundle branch block. This is suggestive of right ventricular overload,
which is a known sequela of chronic pulmonary hypertension.

Patients who have OSA, especially if untreated, are at risk of developing right heart strain
and pulmonary hypertension. They can have ECG findings such as right axis deviation, right
bundle branch block, widened QRS, as well as deep S waves in the lateral leads. It is important to maintain normotension, normocarbia, and adequate oxygenation throughout the surgery.

TABLE 14.2 ■ **STOP BANG Score Helps Predict a Patient's Risk for Having Obstructive Sleep Apnea**

STOP BANG	Question
Snoring	Do you snore loudly enough to be heard through closed doors?
Tired	Do you often feel tired, fatigued, or sleepy during the daytime?
Observed	Has anyone observed you stop breathing during sleep?
Pressure	Do you have high blood pressure?
BMI	Body mass index >35 kg/m²?
Age	Age >50 years?
Neck circumference	Neck circumference >40 cm?
Gender	Male?

A response of "yes" to 3 or more questions indicates a high risk of OSA, and less than 3 indicates a low risk.

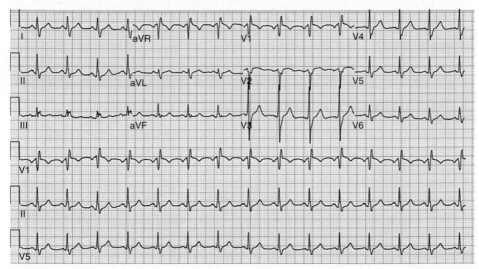

Fig. 14.2 Right bundle branch block on electrocardiogram. Notice the biphasic QRS pattern in the V1
lead. (Mu, Y., & Supino, M. [2019]. Elusive cardiac dysrhythmia in high-risk syncope. *American Journal of
Emergency Medicine, 37*[10], 1992e1–1992e2. Fig. 1.)

Maintaining normocarbia can be particularly challenging during laparoscopic surgery when the peritoneal cavity is insufflated with carbon dioxide (see Case 12). Have hemodynamic medications (e.g., vasopressors, vasodilators) available and maintain blood pressure within 20% of the patient's preoperative baseline.

In the preoperative area on the morning of surgery, the patient's blood sugar is 284 mg/dL.

What should you do?
Ask the patient when he last took insulin and how much he took. While exact cutoffs may vary, by institution studies suggest that a perioperative blood glucose value of 140–180 mg/dL is optimal. Perioperative hyperglycemia is associated with increased morbidity and mortality. In particular, patients with hyperglycemia are at an elevated risk of myocardial infarction, sepsis, surgical site infection, and death. This applies to both diabetic and nondiabetic patients.

What is a normal hemoglobin A1c?
According to the CDC, a normal hemoglobin A1c is less than 5.7%, and a hemoglobin A1c ≥6.5% indicates diabetes. Hemoglobin A1c between 5.7% and 6.5% is considered prediabetes.

STEP 1, 2 PEARL

Hemoglobin A1c reflects the blood glucose over the previous 3 months by measuring glycated hemoglobin. The life span of red blood cells is about 3 months. Therefore, any condition that increases red blood cell turnover can falsely alter this measurement.

How will you determine whether this patient may have a difficult airway?
Airway management is often challenging in obese patients. Bariatric surgery requires general anesthesia with endotracheal intubation due to the level of invasiveness, length of procedure, need for abdominal muscle relaxation, and prevention of aspiration.

Safe airway management starts with a thorough preoperative interview and examination. Ask the patient if they have ever been told that they have a difficult airway or have ever required an awake intubation. Review prior anesthetic records if any are available.

A "difficult airway" may mean the patient is challenging to mask ventilate and/or challenging to intubate. The risk factors for these are listed in Table 14.3.

TABLE 14.3 ■ **Predictors of Difficult Mask Ventilation and Difficult Intubation**

Predictors of Difficult Mask Ventilation	Predictors of Difficult Intubation
• BMI >30 kg/m²	• History of difficult intubation
• Age >55 years	• Long upper incisors
• Presence of a beard	• Limited mandibular protrusion
• Edentulous (lacking teeth)	• Mallampati class 3 or 4
• History of snoring or OSA	• Thyromental distance <6 cm
• Abnormal neck or pharyngeal anatomy	• Sternomental distance <12 cm
• Male gender	• Limited neck mobility
• Large tongue	• Neck circumference >40 cm
• Poor atlanto-occipital extension	
• Mallampati class 3 or 4	

BMI, Body mass index; *OSA*, obstructive sleep apnea.

TABLE 14.4 ■ **American Society of Anesthesiologists Standard Monitors**

Parameter to Be Measured	Method
Blood oxygenation	Pulse oximetry
Inspired gas oxygen content (when anesthesia machine is used)	Oxygen analyzer
Ventilation	End-tidal carbon dioxide or visual observation of chest excursion if end-tidal carbon dioxide cannot be measured due to nature of patient or procedure
Circulation	Continuous electrocardiogram; arterial blood pressure (at least once every 5 min); monitor heart rate via palpation, arterial catheter, or pulse oximetry
Body temperature	Monitor temperature when clinically significant changes in body temperature are anticipated or suspected; site of measurement not specified

What are ASA standard monitors?
ASA guidelines describe minimum physiologic monitoring for patients receiving care from an anesthesiologist or other anesthesia provider. The measured parameters and means of measurement are described in Table 14.4.

Will you want any special monitors beyond the ASA standard monitors?
Given the presence of right ventricular pathology on ECG, place an arterial catheter to allow for continuous hemodynamic monitoring. An arterial line will also allow you to draw labs intraoperatively.

What labs do you want to monitor intraoperatively?
Arterial blood gas (ABG), specifically partial pressure of oxygen (PaO_2) and partial pressure of carbon dioxide ($PaCO_2$) will indicate whether the patient is being adequately oxygenated and ventilated.

Blood glucose level will determine whether the patient's glucose is in the desired range.

Hemoglobin and hematocrit will be useful in the event of bleeding and volume resuscitation.

How will you intubate this patient?
Once the patient is moved to the operating table and standard monitors have been applied, place the anesthesia circuit mask on the patient's face and administer 100% oxygen. Adequate preoxygenation usually requires tidal volume breathing for 3 to 5 minutes or eight deep breaths within 1 minute. The goal here is to fill the lungs, specifically the functional residual capacity (FRC), with as much oxygen as possible. Position with a ramp to improve mask ventilation and intubating conditions, as in Fig. 14.3.

Functional residual capacity is the sum of expiratory reserve volume (ERV, the amount of air that can still be forcibly blown out after a normal exhalation) and residual volume (RV, the leftover volume after a forced exhalation) (see Fig. 14.4). Patients who are obese have a decreased ERV, and in turn, FRC. The lower the FRC, even with adequate preoxygenation, the less time available for endotracheal tube placement before oxygen desaturation. Consider putting the operating room table in reverse Trendelenburg position to maximize FRC.

Consider placing a high-flow nasal cannula (HFNC) on the patient prior to induction. This can facilitate passive oxygenation. With oxygen flows of up to 60 L/min, HFNC will increase the

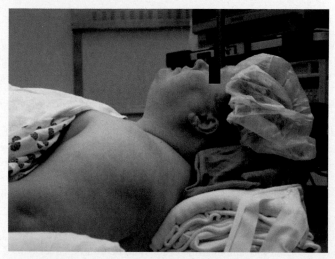

Fig. 14.3 Place folded blankets or pillows under the patient's head and upper back to create a ramp and consider placing the operating room table in the reverse Trendelenburg position. A ramp allows horizontal alignment between the sternal notch space and the external auditory meatus, improving intubating conditions in obese patients. Reverse Trendelenburg positioning improves functional residual capacity by shifting weight off of the chest wall and reducing cephalad displacement of the diaphragm by the obese abdomen. (Collins, J. S., Lemmens, H. J., Brodsky, J. B., Brock-Utne, J. G., & Levitan, R. M. [2004]. Laryngoscopy and morbid obesity: A comparison of the "sniff" and "ramped" positions. *Obesity Surgery, 14*[9], 1171–1175.)

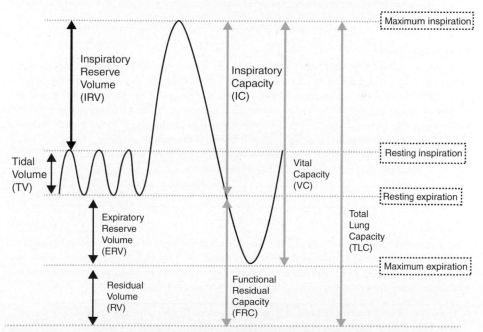

Fig. 14.4 Lung volumes and capacities. Note that FRC is the sum of the ERV (volume remaining in the lungs after a normal exhalation during tidal volume breathing) and RV (volume remaining in the lungs after full forced exhalation). (Lutfi, M. F. [2017]. The physiological basis and clinical significance of lung volume measurements. *Multidisciplinary Respiratory Medicine,12,* Article 3, Figure 1. Retrieved from https://mrmjournal.biomedcentral.com/articles/10.1186/s40248-017-0084-5/figures/1.)

time to oxygen desaturation once the patient becomes apneic after induction. This will be useful if intubation proves difficult.

Always have a backup plan in case intubation with direct laryngoscopy is unsuccessful. Note where your airway equipment is before every case. Have a video laryngoscope and bougie available and consider awake intubation if the suspicion of difficult airway is high.

What is end-tidal carbon dioxide (CO_2)? How can you tell if you are ventilating the patient after induction of anesthesia?

End-tidal CO_2 is a measure of the partial pressure of carbon dioxide that a patient exhales with each breath. It is measured by a sampling line that connects from the Y connector of the breathing circuit to the anesthesia machine, and both the quantitative measurement (i.e., maximum expiratory CO_2 tension) and waveform are displayed. Consistent capnography with each breath, along with other clinical signs (chest rise, refilling of the reservoir bag, breath sounds) suggest adequate ventilation.

How is end-tidal CO_2 measured?

The most common method by which the anesthesia machine measures CO_2 is infrared spectroscopy. Exhaled gas from the sampling line is dehumidified, and then a beam of infrared light is passed through the gas. A photodetector measures the intensity of infrared light that passes through the gas sample. CO_2 absorbs light with a wavelength of 4.26 μm. The greater the concentration of CO_2 present in the exhaled gas, the more infrared light will be absorbed, and the less infrared light that will reach the photodetector. The partial pressure of exhaled CO_2 is determined based on the intensity of transmitted infrared light.

> After induction, the patient becomes apneic and you administer paralytic. You attempt to mask ventilate the patient, but there is no end-tidal CO_2 on the capnogram.

What should you do?

You are not adequately ventilating the patient. Assuming the CO_2 detection equipment is functioning properly, this may be due to a poor seal between the ventilator mask and the patient's face and/or airway obstruction caused by the excess soft tissues of the patient's upper airway.

Use of airway assistive devices may relieve the obstruction. An oropharyngeal airway (OPA), as shown in Fig. 14.5, is a curved hollow plastic device that can be placed in the mouth and helps move the tongue forward to stent open a path between the tongue and the posterior oropharynx, which relieves the obstruction and allows movement of air. A nasopharyngeal airway (NPA) serves a similar purpose but is inserted through the nostril.

> You place an OPA, but there is still a leak between the patient's face and the ventilator mask.

Now what?

Two-handed ventilation can be used. Place your hands at the angle of the mandible bilaterally, and pull the patient's mandible up into the ventilator mask. Use your thumbs to press the mask onto the patient's face (Fig. 14.6). An assistant can administer breaths by squeezing the reservoir bag, or the ventilator can be turned on to automatically administer breaths.

> With two-handed mask ventilation and an OPA in place, there is adequate ventilation and end-tidal CO_2. On video laryngoscopy, you have the view shown in Fig. 14.7.

What do you see? What should you do?

This is a grade III laryngopharyngeal view. The vocal cords are not visible behind the epiglottis. The inability to visualize the vocal cords presents a challenge for the anesthesiologist. If direct laryngoscopy is being attempted, try using a video laryngoscope instead. If this is unsuccessful,

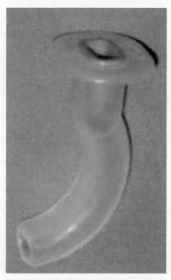

Fig. 14.5 Oropharyngeal airway devices can help improve ventilation by relieving upper airway obstruction caused by the tongue and other soft tissues. Schmölzer, G. M., Agarwal, M., Kamlin, C. O., & Davis, P. G. [2013]. Supraglottic airway devices during neonatal resuscitation: An historical perspective, systematic review and meta-analysis of available clinical trials. *Resuscitation, 84*[6], 722–730. https://doi.org/10.1016/j.resuscitation.2012.11.002. Modified from Fig. 1.)

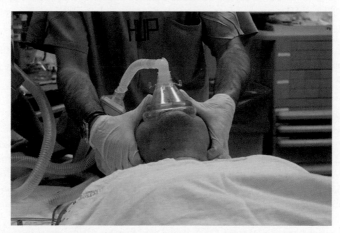

Fig. 14.6 Two-handed mask ventilation. Notice the thumbs are on the mask and the first and second fingers are behind the angle of the mandible. *Mask Ventilation*. Elsevier Procedure Videos. Fig. 11.

consider using a bougie (Fig. 14.8). A bougie is a long, thin, and relatively rigid device that can assst with intubation when the vocal cords cannot be visualized. While maintaining your view with the laryngoscope, advance the bougie into the oropharynx, under the epiglottis, and through the vocal cords even if the cords cannot be visualized. If you feel the bumps of the cartilaginous tracheal rings as the bougie is advanced, the bougie is through the cords into the trachea. Once the bougie is past the vocal cords, the endotracheal tube can be advanced over it and into the trachea, and the bougie subsequently removed. If this is unsuccessful, follow the ASA Difficult Airway Algorithm, shown in Fig. 14.9.

Cormack-Lehane classification describes the view of the vocal cords during laryngoscopy, as seen in Fig. 14.10. Grade I view means the entire glottis is visible, correlating with likely easy

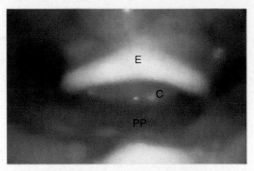

Fig. 14.7   Grade III view on video laryngoscopy. *C*, Corniculate cartilage; *E*, epiglottis; *PP*, posterior pharynx. (Cheng, K. I., Yun, M. K., & Chang, M. C. [2008]. Fiberoptic bronchoscopic view change of laryngopharyngeal tissues by different airway supporting techniques: Comparison of patients with and without open mouth limitation. *Journal of Clinical Anesthesia, 20*[8], 573–579. Modified from Fig. 2.)

Fig. 14.8   The bougie can be used to aid in difficult intubation. (Lauria, A., & Macdonald, J. [2018]. Equipment for airway management. *Anaesthesia and Intensive Care Medicine,* 19(8), 389–396. Modified from Fig. 7.)

intubation. Grade II means part of the glottis is visible. Grade III would only allow visualization of the epiglottis (cannot see the vocal cords), and grade IV indicates that you can only see the soft palate. Grade III and IV views indicate a more challenging endotracheal intubation.

> The patient is successfully intubated with a bougie, and the case proceeds uneventfully. The patient is extubated at the end of surgery and is taken to the postanesthesia care unit (PACU). He was sleepy but breathing comfortably. Thirty minutes later, the nurse calls you because the patient was complaining of pain, and his oxygen saturation is now 84%.

What's going on? What should you do?
Start by administering supplemental oxygen via nasal cannula or facemask. Assess the patient's level of consciousness and respiratory effort. Provide chin tilt and jaw thrust if you suspect an obstruction. Consider sending an ABG to assess oxygenation and ventilation status and a chest radiograph (CXR) to evaluate for lung expansion and to rule out pneumothorax (see Case 12). The differential diagnosis of hypoxia in PACU includes upper airway obstruction (particularly common in obese patients and those with OSA), central hypoventilation, atelectasis, incomplete reversal of neuromuscular blockade, and pneumothorax.

Since this patient has a history of OSA, make sure that his CPAP machine, or one with the same settings, is available in PACU. As the anesthetic continues to wear off, he is still at risk for upper airway obstruction. Consider placing an oral airway prior to extubation in patients with OSA. The patient will remove it when he is awake enough to do so.

Obese patients are at an increased risk of atelectasis, particularly after prolonged laparoscopic surgeries when intraabdominal pressure is increased by peritoneal insufflation. CXR may show the collapse of the lower lung segments. Increasing CPAP (if the patient is using it) or administering intermittent positive pressure ventilation (IPPV) can be helpful in recruiting collapsed alveoli.

It is also possible that the neuromuscular blocking agent used intraoperatively has not been fully reversed and the patient may still be weak. Consider checking twitches on the train of four monitoring, making sure they have received reversal, and if appropriate, give more reversal medication.

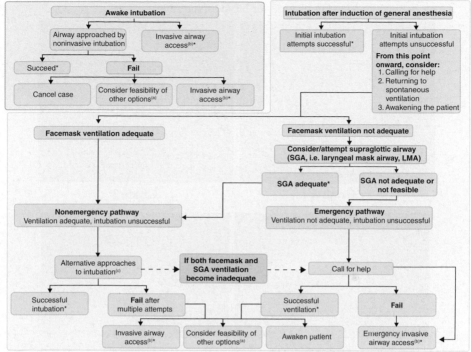

*Confirm ventilation, tracheal intubation, or supraglottic airway (SGA) placement with exhaled CO_2.

a: Consider additional further anesthetizing the airway, or consider using laryngeal mask airway (LMA) or facemask during the operation.

b: Options for invasive ventilation include transtracheal jet ventilation, retrograde intubation, and surgical airway.

c: Alternative approaches include video laryngoscopy, fiberoptic intubation, and intubating LMA.

Fig. 14.9 ASA Difficult Airway Algorithm. If the patient cannot be intubated after induction of general anesthesia, the next steps are based on whether or not the patient can be ventilated with the ventilator mask or supraglottic airway (SGA) (e.g., laryngeal mask airway, LMA). If the patient can be ventilated, this allows time for attempts at other noninvasive intubation techniques. If the patient cannot be ventilated, emergency airway access such as cricothyrotomy may be necessary. (Artime, C. A., & Hagberg, C. A. [2020]. Airway management in the adult. In M. A. Gropper, R. D. Miller, N. H. Cohen, L. I. Eriksson, L. A. Fleisher, K. Leslie, et al. (Eds.), *Miller's anesthesia* [9th ed., Chapter 44, pp. 1373–1412]. Philadelphia, PA: Elsevier. Modified from Fig. 44.1.)

If the patient has severe oxygen desaturation and/or hypercarbia that is not improved with other interventions, the patient may require reintubation.

The patient barely opens his eyes in response to sternal rub. His respiratory rate is 4/minute. His pupils are pinpoint bilaterally. He has four strong twitches on the train of four monitoring.

What's going on? What should you do?
These findings are consistent with opioid overdose.

Administration of naloxone will reverse the respiratory depressant effects of opioids. Naloxone is an opioid antagonist used to reverse the opioid overdose that works at mu (μ), delta (δ), and kappa (κ) receptors. It reverses respiratory depression, pruritus, and sedative effects of opioids, but also reverses the analgesic effect. Side effects of naloxone can include nausea, vomiting, tachycardia, seizures, and pulmonary edema.

One could also consider reintubating the patient and allowing the opioid to be metabolized prior to extubation.

Viewing of Anterior laryngopharyngeal tissue

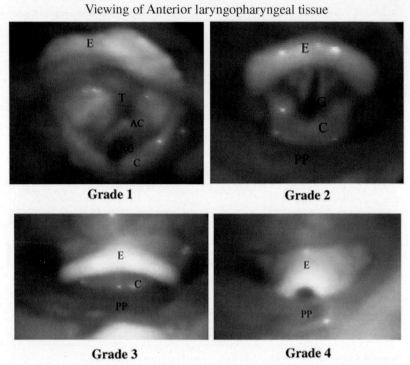

Grade 1   Grade 2

Grade 3   Grade 4

Figure 14.10 Cormack-Lehane classification of laryngoscopic views of the airway. *AC*, Anterior commissure of vocal cords, *C*, corniculate cartilage; *E*, epiglottis; *PP*, posterior pharynx; *RG*, rima glottidis; *T*, tubercle of the epiglottis. Grades I and II usually indicate easier intubation, while grades III and IV usually indicate more challenging intubation. (Cheng, K. I., Yun, M. K., Chang, M. C., Lee, K. W., Huang, S. C., Tang, C. S., et al. [2008]. Fiberoptic bronchoscopic view change of laryngopharyngeal tissues by different airway supporting techniques: Comparison of patients with and without open mouth limitation. *Journal of Clinical Anesthesia*, *20*[8], 573–579. Modified from Fig. 2.)

STEP 1, 2 PEARL

Signs of an acute opioid overdose include respiratory depression which can manifest as decreased respiratory rate and shallow breaths. Waning mental status, miosis, decreased gag reflex, bradycardia, and decreased bowel sounds are also signs of opioid intoxication. Opioid overdose is also known to cause seizures.

STEP 1, 2 PEARL

Opioid withdrawal can occur with dose reduction or cessation after prolonged use of opioids. Withdrawal is often characterized by flu-like symptoms such as fever, nausea, vomiting, rhinorrhea, piloerection, chills, myalgias, and arthralgias. Patients may also experience sweating, dilated pupils, lacrimation, yawning, and diarrhea. Opioid withdrawal is often managed with opioid agonists such as methadone or buprenorphine along with non-opioid adjunctive medication.

The nurse says he gave the patient hydromorphone 4 Mg over the last 30 minutes. You give the patient naloxone 0.4 Mg and he wakes up. His oxygen saturation and respiratory rate normalize.

Can he be discharged from pacu to the ward now?
No, the duration of action of naloxone is much shorter than that of most opioids, such as hydromorphone. Therefore, as naloxone wears off, the patient may become obtunded again. It may be necessary to redose naloxone.

How could this have been prevented?
Obese patients are particularly sensitive to opioids. Use short-acting opioids and minimize the total dose. In order to minimize opioid administration, use a multimodal pain management technique including regional anesthesia and non-opioid analgesics. Regional anesthesia nerve blocks such as a transversus abdominis plane (TAP) block will reduce incisional pain after abdominal surgery. Non-opioid analgesic medication such as dexmedetomidine, acetaminophen, and ketorolac may also be helpful.

How is a TAP block performed?
A TAP block is performed by injection of local anesthetic into the fascial plane between the internal oblique and transversus abdominis muscles, as shown in Fig. 14.11.

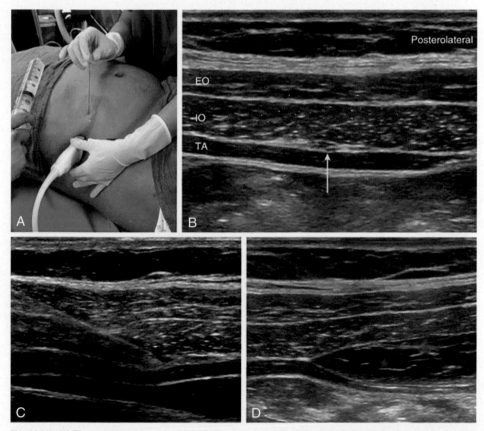

Fig. 14.11 (A) The proper patient positioning, ultrasound probe placement, and needle direction for a TAP block. The patient is supine, and the needle is advanced parallel to the ultrasound beam, known as "in-plane." (B) Normal ultrasonographic anatomy of the abdominal wall, showing external oblique (EO), internal oblique (IO), and transversus abdominis (TA) muscles. The yellow arrow indicates the target location for the block—the fascia between the internal oblique and transversus abdominis muscles, which is the location of parietal nerves. (C) In-plane ultrasonographic view of needle placement. (D) Appropriate spread of local anesthetic identified by the red star. (Johnson, R. L., Kopp, S. L., & Kessler, J. [2020]. Peripheral nerve blocks and ultrasound guidance for regional anesthesia. In M. A. Gropper, R. D. Miller, N. H. Cohen, L. I. Eriksson, L. A. Fleisher, K. Leslie, et al. (Eds.), *Miller's anesthesia* [9th ed., pp. 1450–1479.e3]. Philadelphia, PA: Elsevier. Modified from Fig. 46.25.)

Will a TAP block treat all surgical pain?
No, a TAP block anesthetizes the nerves of the anterior abdominal wall. This will treat most somatic pain arising from the skin, muscle, and parietal peritoneum. However, a TAP block will not treat visceral pain arising from internal structures (e.g., intestine, stomach).

BEYOND THE PEARLS

- Roux-en-Y procedure is the gold standard of bariatric surgery, and involves the complex rearrangement of the gastrointestinal system, leading to malabsorption and changes in hormonal signaling, leading to weight loss.
- Obese patients have multiple complex anesthetic considerations due to metabolic, circulatory, and ventilatory risks. Appropriate preoperative workup is important. If the patient is not medically optimized for an elective case, the case should be rescheduled.
- Mask ventilation conditions can be improved by administering jaw thrust, placing an OPA or NPA, or using the two-hand masking technique while another person administers breaths, or the ventilator is turned on to administer breaths.
- The anesthesiologist must be prepared for difficult airway management, particularly in the obese patient population. Do a thorough preoperative airway examination looking for predictors of difficult airway, use reverse Trendelenburg positioning, ramp the head and shoulders, provide use adequate preoxygenation, and consider passive oxygenation with HFNC.
- Have backup airway equipment available such as a video laryngoscope and a bougie. Be familiar with the ASA Difficult Airway Algorithm.

References

"All about your A1c." *Centers for Disease Control and Prevention.* https://www.cdc.gov/diabetes/managing/managing-blood-sugar/a1c.html#:~:text=A%20normal%20A1C%20level%20is,for%20developing%20type%202%20diabetes. Accessed February 1, 2021.

Baraka, A. S., Taha, S. K., & Auoad, M. T. (1999). Preoxygenation: Comparison of maximal breathing and tidal volume breathing techniques. *Anesthesiology*, *91*, 612. https://doi.org/10.1097/00000542-199909000-00009

Bariatric Surgery Procedures: ASMBS. (n.d.). Retrieved October 10, 2020, from https://asmbs.org/patients/bariatric-surgery-procedures

Brodsky, C., Herzig, S., Tuot, D., Görges, M., Barrett, K., & Barsuk, J. (n.d.). *Weighing in on surgical safety.* Retrieved January 30, 2021, from https://psnet.ahrq.gov/web-mm/weighing-surgical-safety

Chung, F., Subramanyam, R., Liao, P., Sasaki, E., Shapiro, C., & Sun, Y. (2012). High STOP-Bang score indicates a high probability of obstructive sleep apnoea. *British Journal of Anaesthesia*, *108*(5), 768–775. https://doi.org/10.1093/bja/aes022

Collins, J. S., Lemmens, H. J., Brodsky, J. B., Brock-Utne, J. G., & Levitan, R. M. (2004). Laryngoscopy and morbid obesity: A comparison of the "sniff" and "ramped" positions. *Obesity Surgery*, *14*(9), 1171–1175.

Committee on Economics. (2014, October 15). *ASA Physical Status Classification System, American Society of Anesthesiologists.* Retrieved from https://www.asahq.org/standards-and-guidelines/asa-physical-status-classification-system

Committee on Standards and Practice Parameters. (2020, 13 December). *Standards for Basic Anesthetic Monitoring, American Society of Anesthesiologists.* https://www.asahq.org/standards-and-guidelines/standards-for-basic-anesthetic-monitoring. Accessed August 28, 2021.

Ding, S., McKenzie, T., Vernon, A. H., & Coldfine, A. B. (2016). Bariatric surgery. In J. L. Jameson, L. J. De Groot, D. M. de Krester, L. C. Guidice, A. B. Grossman, S. Melmed, et al. (Eds.) *Endocrinology: Adult and pediatric* (7th ed., Chapter 27, pp. 479–490). Philadelphia, PA: Elsevier.

Donald, M. J., & Paterson, B. (2006). End tidal carbon dioxide monitoring in prehospital and retrieval medicine: A review. *Emergency Medicine Journal: EMJ*, *23*(9), 728–730. https://doi.org/10.1136/emj.2006.037184.

Egan, T. D., & Newberry, C. (2018). Opioids. In M. C. Pardo, & R. D. Miller (Eds.), *Basics of anesthesia.* (7th ed., Chapter 9, pp. 123–138). Philadelphia, PA: Elsevier.

FastStats—Overweight Prevalence. (2021, January 11). Retrieved from https://www.cdc.gov/nchs/fastats/obesity-overweight.htm

Goerg, S. M., Agarwal, M., & Kamlin, O. F. (2012). Supraglottic airway devices during neonatal resuscitation: An historical perspective, systematic review and meta-analysis of available clinical trials. *Resuscitation*, *84*(6), 722–730.

Gropper, M. A., & Miller, R. D. (2020). Inhaled Anesthetics: Delivery Systems. In M. A. Gropper, R. D. Miller, N. H. Cohen, L. I. Eriksson, L. A. Fleisher, K. Leslie, et al. (Eds.), *Miller's anesthesia* (9th ed., pp. 572–637). Philadelphia, PA: Elsevier.

Khalil, M., & Rifaie, O. (2004, May 14). *Electrocardiographic changes in obstructive sleep apnoea syndrome*. Retrieved January 30, 2021, from https://www.sciencedirect.com/science/article/pii/S0954611198900270

Lutfi, M. (2017, February 09). *The physiological basis and clinical significance of lung volume measurements*. Retrieved from https://mrmjournal.biomedcentral.com/articles/10.1186/s40248-017-0084-5/figures/1

Malhotra, G. & Eckmann, D. M. (2020). Anesthesia for bariatric surgery. In M. A. Gropper, R. D. Miller, N. H. Cohen, L. I. Eriksson, L. A. Fleisher, K. Leslie, et al. (Eds.), *Miller's anesthesia* (7th ed., Chapter 58, pp. 1911–1928).

McGill, J. (2007, August). Airway management in trauma: An update. *Emergency Medicine Clinics of North America*, *25*(3), 603–622.

Reed, A. P. (2014). The difficult airway. In A. P. Reed & F. S. Yudkowitz (Eds.), *Clinical cases in anesthesia* (Case 43, pp. 204–214). Philadelphia, PA: Elsevier.

Sudhakaran, S., & Surani, S. (2015). Guidelines for perioperative management of the diabetic patient. *Surgery Research and Practice*, *2015*, 1–8. https://doi.org/10.1155/2015/284063

Yentis, S. M., Hirsch, N. P., & Ip, J. K. (Eds.). (2019). Difficult intubation. In *Anaesthesia, intensive care and perioperative medicine A-Z* (6th ed., pp. 299–333). Philadelphia, PA: Elsevier.

A 28-Year-Old Man With a History of Sickle Cell Disease and Cholelithiasis

Alice Seol ■ Elizabeth C. Fung ■ Paul Neil Frank

A 28-year-old man with a history of sickle cell disease and cholelithiasis is undergoing cholecys-tectomy. He takes hydroxyurea and oral morphine daily. He has a history of multiple hospitaliza-tions for acute chest syndrome. Vital signs show blood pressure 122/72 mm Hg, pulse 80/min, respirations 9/min, oxygen saturation 97% on room air, and temperature 37°C.

What is sickle cell disease?

Sickle cell disease (SCD) is caused by a mutation of the gene that codes for the β globin peptide of hemoglobin. This results in a change of the sixth amino acid in the peptide, from valine to glu-tamic acid. The resulting abnormal hemoglobin molecules (HbSS) are composed of two abnormal β subunits and two normal α subunits.

In a hypoxic environment, HbSS molecules form long polymers that bend and distort the shape of the erythrocyte. The accumulation of these sickled cells causes infarcts and tissue destruc-tion that cause many of the symptoms of SCD.

Patients who are homozygous (i.e., have two abnormal alleles) for the disease (HbSS) suffer from the most severe forms of the disease. In contrast, patients who are heterozygous (i.e., have one normal allele and one abnormal allele) for the abnormal gene are said to have sickle cell trait (HbAS). This is not usually clinically significant because hemoglobin molecules with sickle cell trait will sickle when oxygen saturation is less than 20%. Table 15.1 describes the peptide compo-sition of common types of hemoglobin.

What is the structure of hemoglobin?

Hemoglobin is a tetrameric molecule consisting of four peptides. Each peptide subunit contains a heme group, which binds oxygen. In healthy patients, more than 90% of hemoglobin molecules are hemoglobin A (HbA), which consists of two α peptides and two β peptides. In fetuses, at least 75% of hemoglobin molecules are fetal hemoglobin (HbF), which consists of two α peptides and two γ peptides. By 6 months of age, most of the hemoglobin in circulation is HbA.

STEP 1 PEARL

The vast majority of oxygen carried in blood is stored on hemoglobin. Each molecule of hemoglobin can carry four molecules of oxygen (O_2), one on each heme group. As hemoglobin binds one molecule of O_2, its affinity for a second molecule of O_2 increases, and that second molecule of O_2 increases its affinity for a third, and so on. This is called positive cooperativity, and it is for this reason that the hemoglobin-oxygen dissociation curve is sigmoidal (Fig. 15.1).

TABLE 15.1 ■ **Peptide Components of Hemoglobin**

Hemoglobin Type	Subunits	Comments
HbA	Two α subunits, two normal β subunits	Normal adult hemoglobin
HbF	Two α subunits, two γ subunits	Normal fetal hemoglobin
HbSS	Two α subunits, two abnormal β subunits	Homozygous for sickle cell trait—these patients manifest with symptoms of sickle cell disease
HbAS	Two α subunits, one normal β subunit, one abnormal β subunit	Heterozygous for sickle cell trait—these patients are usually asymptomatic

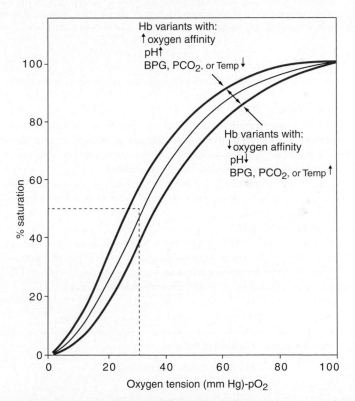

Fig. 15.1 Hemoglobin-oxygen dissociation curve showing the relationship between partial pressure of oxygen (pO_2) and hemoglobin saturation. *BPG*, Bisphosphoglycerate. (Steinberg, M. H., Benz, E. J., Adewoye, A. H., & Ebert, B. L. Pathobiology of the human erythrocyte and its hemoglobins. In R. Hoffman, E. J. Benz, L. E. Silberstein, H. E. Heslop, J. I. Weitz, J. Anastasi, et al. (Eds.), *Hematology: Basic Principles and Practice* (Chapter 33, pp. 447–457). Philadelphia, PA: Elsevier. Modified from Fig. 33.3.)

STEP 1 PEARL

The affinity of hemoglobin for oxygen changes with physiologic and pathologic factors. Increased hemoglobin affinity for oxygen results in higher hemoglobin saturation for a given oxygen tension (pO_2). This results in a shift to the left of the hemoglobin-oxygen dissociation curve. Conversely, decreased hemoglobin affinity for oxygen results in lower hemoglobin saturation for a given pO_2. This results in a shift to the right of the hemoglobin-oxygen dissociation curve. The simplest way to express this left or right shift is the P50, which is the pO_2 corresponding to a hemoglobin saturation of 50%. A lower P50 corresponds to a left shift, and a higher P50 corresponds to a right shift.

STEP 1 PEARL

Physiologic changes that cause left shift of the hemoglobin-oxygen dissociation curve include decreased temperature, elevated pH, and lower carbon dioxide tension (pCO_2). Conversely, increased temperature, lower pH, and increased pCO_2 result in a right shift of the curve. This is beneficial in that working muscle generates heat, acid, and carbon dioxide. All of these factors facilitate release of O_2 by hemoglobin.

What triggers sickling of red blood cells?
Hypoxia, acidosis, hypothermia, and hypovolemia may cause sickling of erythrocytes.

What are the manifestations of SCD?
Recurring episodes of severe pain, often in the extremities, chest, or back, are a common manifestation of this illness. SCD causes chronic organ damage as the abnormal erythrocytes occlude microvasculature in the lungs, kidneys, bones, skin, spleen, and central nervous system. Table 15.2 illustrates the different manifestations of SCD by organ system.

When there is an acute vascular occlusive event in the lungs, it is called acute chest syndrome (ACS). This is the leading cause of death and the second most common complication of SCD.

How is SCD managed chronically?
Hydroxyurea is the mainstay of overall management of SCD. It reduces the incidence of vasoocclusive crises (e.g., pain crises and ACS) and improves the quality of life of patients with SCD. Although the exact mechanism of action is incompletely understood, hydroxyurea induces HbF production. Unlike HbSS, HbF is not affected by the sickle cell gene and does not sickle.

TABLE 15.2 ■ **Manifestations of Sickle Cell Disease**

Organ System	Effects of Sickle Cell Disease
Central nervous system	Ischemic stroke, retinopathy
Musculoskeletal	Osteonecrosis, acute and chronic pain
Genitourinary	Renal insufficiency, priapism
Lymphatic	Splenomegaly, splenic sequestration, abdominal pain, susceptibility to infection by encapsulated organisms
Vascular	Vasculopathy
Hematologic	Chronic hemolytic anemia
Skin	Leg ulcers
Cardiopulmonary	Acute chest syndrome, pulmonary hypertension, right ventricular dysfunction/hypertrophy, cardiac iron overload (from chronic blood transfusions)

STEP 2 PEARL

Treatment with hydroxyurea is indicated in sickle cell patients with frequent pain crises, symptomatic anemia, and/or a history of ACS. Patients who respond well to hydroxyurea with an improvement in symptoms will usually have 10%–30% HbF on gel electrophoresis. Hydroxyurea is a relatively safe drug but does have a dose-limiting side effect of myelosuppression.

Blood transfusions are used in SCD to treat life-threatening complications or prophylactically to decrease the incidence of complications. Transfusion of normal erythrocytes reduces the concentration of HbSS molecules in circulation. Chronic blood transfusions are often used as secondary prevention of stroke, ACS, pain crises, priapism, and pulmonary hypertension.

STEP 1, 2 PEARL

Patients with SCD tend to infarct their spleens over time and are therefore susceptible to certain infections. Children with SCD should receive penicillin prophylaxis. They should also receive immunizations against encapsulated bacterial organisms, such as *Streptococcus pneumoniae, Haemophilus influenzae type B*, and *Neisseria meningitidis*. *S. pneumoniae* (usually nonvaccine serotypes) remains overwhelmingly the most common cause of sepsis in patients with SCD. If sepsis is suspected, treatment with an intravenous (IV) third-generation cephalosporin should be initiated. In addition, yearly influenza vaccinations are recommended.

Describe the structure of the spleen.

The spleen is a lymphoid organ whose anatomy is divided into three major areas: red pulp, white pulp, and a marginal zone that separates them. Some of the blood that enters the spleen is directed into splenic parenchyma, hence the name red pulp. To reenter the vascular system, erythrocytes must squeeze between slits in the endothelium of the venous sinuses. The white pulp is composed entirely of lymphoid tissue; B cells in the white pulp of the spleen are critical in humoral immunity and produce immunoglobulin M (IgM) antibodies capable of opsonizing encapsulated bacteria.

How does SCD affect the spleen?

Sickled red blood cells (RBCs) can cause chronic, long-term insults by obstructing drainage from the spleen, causing scarring and eventual atrophy. In the early stages of SCD, these are small and usually unnoticed. Repeated obstruction of the spleen leads to fibrosis and atrophy, ultimately causing the organ to be nonfunctional, a term called "autosplenectomy."

What is splenic sequestration crisis?

Splenic sequestration crisis is defined as an acute drop in hemoglobin ($>2\,g/dL$) in combination with splenomegaly in a patient with SCD. Sickled erythrocytes become trapped within the red pulp of the spleen and obstruct larger draining veins. As the obstruction continues, the spleen enlarges, causing the abrupt onset of pallor, weakness, abdominal pain, tachycardia, and hypotension. The sluggish blood flow and low oxygen tension within the spleen encourages further sickling, propagating the cycle of sickling and obstruction. If severe, this can lead to hypovolemic shock, cardiovascular collapse, and death. Infection and splenic sequestration crises are the two leading causes of death in the first decade of life in patients with SCD. For these reasons, recurrent splenic sequestration crises is the most common indication for splenectomy in the SCD population.

What studies should be ordered preoperatively for this patient?
Check a complete blood count, including hemoglobin and hematocrit, as well as white blood cell count. Also check a reticulocyte count. Because SCD can cause kidney dysfunction, check an electrolyte panel.

Patients with dyspnea at rest or with poor functional capacity should have an echocardiogram to assess cardiac function.

Preoperative labs show a hemoglobin concentration of 8.3 g/dL.

Should this patient receive a blood transfusion preoperatively?
This is an area of ongoing controversy. Generally, patients with SCD undergoing major surgery and those with significant histories of SCD complications should receive transfusion to achieve a hemoglobin level of 10 g/dL. Some studies have shown HbSS patients who receive preoperative blood transfusion experience fewer episodes of ACS and serious adverse events overall.

Patients who receive chronic blood transfusions are likely to have been exposed to different antigens in their lifetime; therefore the likelihood of alloantibody presence is high. Crossmatching blood for these patients may take more time than usual; anticipation of this delay is critically important when preparing for a case with potential for significant blood loss.

STEP 2 PEARL

Patients who require chronic blood transfusions are at high risk for iron overload due to the iron content of the transfused red blood cells. Therefore chelation therapy should be initiated in these patients to reduced damage to organs such as the liver and kidneys and to improve overall survival.

What is a type and screen? Type and cross?
The "type" determines the ABO class and Rh status of the patient. To determine ABO type, the patient's blood is mixed with serum known to have anti-A and anti-B antibodies. To determine Rh status, the patient's blood is centrifuged to isolate erythrocytes; these are then diluted and mixed with anti-D reagent. The "screen" refers to screening the patient's blood for common non-ABO antibodies that the patient may have developed against donor erythrocytes, such as Kell, Kidd, and Duffy antigens.

Crossmatching takes this one step further by confirming whether a specific unit of donated blood is appropriate for the patient prior to transfusion. To perform the test, the patient's blood (say, B+) is mixed with a compatible donor unit (also B+). If agglutination is detected, this indicates that there are unknown antigens on the patient's erythrocytes that are targeted by donor antibodies. Even though a type and screen were performed, crossmatching has detected that this donor blood is incompatible and should not be given to the patient.

Preoperative labs show a glomerular filtration rate (GFR) of 35 mL/min/1.73 m².

What is the likely etiology?
Many sickle cell patients develop sickle cell nephropathy, which originates from renal vasculopathy. As sickled RBCs create vascular stasis and occlusion, the kidney experiences both infarction and, when the occlusion resolves, ischemia-reperfusion injury. This is sometimes termed the "perfusion paradox" and recurs in the same organ. This causes, inflammation and endothelial dysfunction. Hypoperfusion of the renal medulla can lead to papillary necrosis, hematuria, and interstitial disease. Hypoperfusion of the renal cortex can cause hyperfiltration, hypertrophy, proteinuria, glomerular disease, and ultimately, chronic kidney disease. As the GFR progressively declines through life, end-stage renal disease

may occur. The patient's renal function at the time of surgery should be documented and kept in mind because liberal fluid administration may be detrimental for patients with severe renal disease.

STEP 2 PEARL

Renal papillary necrosis is a common complication in patients with sickle cell disease or sickle cell trait. The renal papillae become necrotic and slough off, which presents as gross hematuria and proteinuria.

Patients with sickle cell trait or sickle cell anemia can also develop hyposthenuria, which is the inability of the kidneys to concentrate urine. This occurs due to the hypoxic and hyperosmolar environment of the renal medulla which results in sickled cells in the vasa recta, impaired free water absorption, and disruption of the countercurrent exchange. Patients will usually experience polyuria and nocturia even with water restriction and will have a low urine specific gravity with normal serum sodium.

What are the anesthetic options for this case?
As this is a laparoscopic abdominal surgery, general anesthesia with an endotracheal tube is indicated. However, additional consideration should be given to pain management for this patient. In addition to nonopioid analgesics, regional anesthesia in the form of truncal peripheral nerve blocks can be used to target the incisional pain.

Regardless of anesthetic technique, it is vitally important to keep the patient warm, well hydrated, and adequately oxygenated and ventilated.

The use of preoperative and postoperative incentive spirometry prevents atelectasis and has been shown to reduce the incidence of ACS. Postoperatively, pain from rib, sternum, or thoracic spine infarction leads to alveolar hypoventilation and is highly correlated to the development of ACS.

What IV access is appropriate?
Two large-bore peripheral IV lines should be placed for this surgery. In patients with SCD, IV access can prove challenging. With repeated attempts at venous access over time, veins become scarred and sclerosed, making access challenging or impossible. Vasculopathy and endothelial dysfunction are common in SCD and can make peripheral IV access difficult. The pathologic processes that result in vasculopathy are complex and often interplay with one another—this includes chronic nitric oxide release and eventual nitric oxide depletion, nitric oxide resistance, and activation of endothelial adhesion molecules and endothelin.

Surgery and postanesthesia care unit course are uneventful. Overnight, 12 hours after surgery, the patient has significant pain in his legs, requiring frequent pain medication. On postoperative day 1, the patient complains of intense chest pain. His breathing becomes rapid and shallow, and he feels short of breath. A stat chest radiograph is shown in Fig. 15.2.

What is going on?
Intense, abrupt chest pain in a postoperative patient with SCD is highly concerning for ACS caused by microvascular occlusion of the lungs. Other possible etiologies include acute coronary syndrome, pulmonary embolism, and pneumothorax.

What is ACS?
ACS is defined by a new pulmonary infiltrate on CXR or computed tomography (CT), in combination with fever, cough, dyspnea, chest pain, or hypoxia. It is a phenomenon of

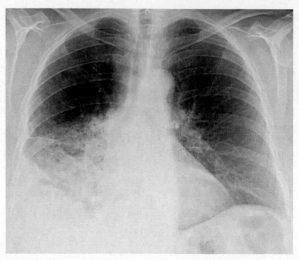

Fig. 15.2 Chest radiograph showing a pulmonary consolidation of the right lower lobe. (Chung, J. H., & Walker, C. M. [2019]. In C. M. Walker, J. H. Chung, S. B. Hobbs, B. P. Little, & C. C. Wu [Eds.], *Muller's imaging of the chest* [2nd ed., pp. 57–70.e1]. Philadelphia, PA: Elsevier. Modified from Fig. 2.2.)

pulmonary sequestration of sickled erythrocytes. Treatment is centered around pain control, maintaining adequate hydration with intravenous fluids, antibiotics, supplemental oxygen, and blood transfusion if needed. Every attempt should be made to achieve adequate analgesia.

STEP 2 PEARL

Patients with sickle cell disease are at risk for developing chronic dyspnea through several mechanisms. They are at higher risk for pulmonary fibrosis, especially in those with recurrent episodes of ACS. Repeated pulmonary infarction will cause parenchymal scarring, and patients can present with exertional dyspnea, crackles, and low diffusing capacity of the lungs for carbon monoxide (DLCO).

Sickle cell patients may also develop pulmonary hypertension. Repeated intravascular hemolysis in sickle cell disease leads to pulmonary vascular remodeling and increased pulmonary vascular resistance. Patients may present with exertional dyspnea and findings of right ventricular failure.

How should you treat this patient?

Careful attention should be given to the patient's volume status, using intravenous fluids to maintain adequate hydration. Although "how much is too much" is unknown, attempts should be made to strike a balance between hypovolemia-induced ACS and hypervolemia-induced pulmonary edema.

ACS is often associated with infection. *Chlamydia pneumoniae* and *Mycoplasma* are the most common pathogens. Therefore, when ACS is suspected, antibiotic therapy with cefuroxime or cefotaxime in combination with a macrolide is indicated.

Provide supplemental oxygen. Beware that oxygen saturation measured with pulse oximetry (SpO$_2$) typically underestimates the patient's arterial oxygen tension because these measurements are based on a normal oxyhemoglobin dissociation curve. Patients with SCD have a right-shifted curve due to the presence of HbSS.

Noninvasive positive pressure has been used to correct hypoxemia and decrease the work of breathing in ACS, but invasive mechanical ventilation may be needed.

Would a blood transfusion be helpful?

Both simple and exchange transfusions have been used in the treatment of ACS. The criteria for when to use which is not clearly defined, but in general, severe cases are treated with exchange transfusion. The goal of transfusion is to increase hemoglobin concentration to 10 g/dL and decrease HbSS concentration to less than 30%. Exchange transfusion is used for severe cases because it allows for large volume and rapid transfusion and avoids elevated blood viscosity that can occur with multiple simple transfusions.

BEYOND THE PEARLS

- Myoglobin stores oxygen in muscles. It has a very similar structure to the globin molecules of the hemoglobin tetramer; however, it exists as a monomer.
- Myoglobin has a higher affinity for oxygen than does hemoglobin.
- Children who have multiple acute chest crises can develop progressive pulmonary fibrosis.
- Pulmonary fat emboli have been observed in many cases of acute chest syndrome (ACS) and is suspected as the cause of many cases of adult ACS. Bone marrow ischemia and resultant necrosis of bone and bone marrow can introduce these inflammatory substances into the bloodstream and cause an inflammatory cascade.
- Use of incentive spirometry in the perioperative period will reduce atelectasis and can reduce the risk of ACS.

References

Oprea, A. D. Hematologic Disorders. In R. L. Hines, & S. B. Jones (Eds.), *Stoelting's Anesthesia and Co-Existing Disease* (8th ed., Chapter 23, pp 465–496). Philadelphia, PA: Elsevier.

Steinberg, M. H., Benz, E. J., Adewoye, A. H., & Ebert, B. L. (2018). Pathobiology of the human erythrocyte and its hemoglobins. In R. Hoffman, E. J. Benz, L. E. Silberstein, H. E. Heslop, J. I. Weitz, J. Anastasi, et al. (Eds.), *Hematology: Basic Principles and Practice* (Vol. *33*, pp. 447–457). Philadelphia, PA: Elsevier.

A 32-Year-Old Male With no Significant Medical History After Being Rescued from a Burning Building

Juliann Cho ■ Paul Neil Frank

A 32-year-old male with no significant medical history is brought to the emergency department by paramedics after being rescued from a burning building. Vital signs are: blood pressure 95/52 mm Hg, pulse 118 bpm, respirations 28/min, and oxygen saturation 98% on 4 L/min via nasal cannula. The physical exam reveals that the patient has sustained 70% total body surface area (TBSA) burns to his face, neck, chest, arms, back, and legs. He is moaning, and his voice is hoarse. Breath sounds are diminished and there is diffuse wheezing heard on auscultation of his lungs. There is soot around his mouth and dark sputum inside his mouth.

How is the percentage of TBSA burned calculated?
TBSA only considers partial and full-thickness burns (i.e., second-, third-, and fourth-degree burns). The "rule of nines" method is commonly used to estimate TBSA in adults (Fig. 16.1). Since children have larger heads in proportion to their bodies compared to adults, TBSA estimation is slightly different.

How are burn injuries classified?
Table 16.1 shows the classification of burn injuries by the depth of the burn and the extent of tissue damage.

What burn classifications will require surgical debridement with skin grafting?
Deep second-degree as well as third- and fourth-degree burns will require surgical treatment. First-degree burns generally do not.

Should you be concerned about the soot around the patient's mouth and dark sputum?
Yes, these findings are highly concerning for inhalational injury. Patients with new burn injuries should always be assessed for inhalational injury. Patients burned in an enclosed space, under the influence of illicit drugs or alcohol, found unconscious, and those with facial burns are at the highest risk for inhalational injury. Physical exam may show singed nose hair, soot in the airway, wheezing, and hoarseness. If there is any concern for airway burn injury, the patient should be intubated immediately.

What are the possible mechanisms of inhalation injury?
Inhalation injury can be caused by direct thermal injury to the upper airway, chemical irritation to the lower airway, and systemic chemical or metabolic injury. Patients may be affected by one or more of these types of inhalation injuries.

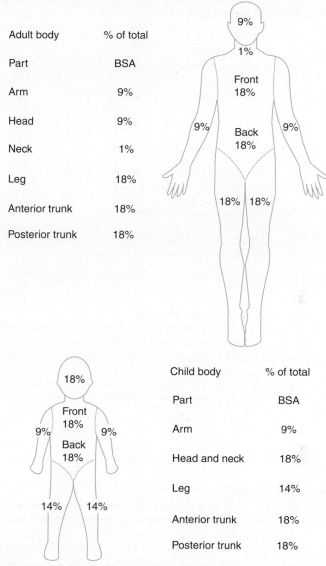

Adult body Part	% of total BSA
Arm	9%
Head	9%
Neck	1%
Leg	18%
Anterior trunk	18%
Posterior trunk	18%

Child body Part	% of total BSA
Arm	9%
Head and neck	18%
Leg	14%
Anterior trunk	18%
Posterior trunk	18%

Fig. 16.1 Rule of nines for adults *(top)* and a child *(bottom)* showing the percentage of body surface area for each part of the body. (Jeschke, M. G., & Herndon, D. N. [2017]. Burns. In C. M. Townsend, R. D. Beauchamp, B. M. Evers, & K. L. Mattox (Eds.), *Sabiston textbook of surgery* [chapter 19, 20th ed., pp. 505–531]. Philadelphia, PA: Elsevier. Modified from Fig. 19.3.)

Direct thermal injury to the upper airway can cause severe swelling of the upper airway and lead to obstruction over the course of hours.

Chemical irritation to the lower airway can cause inflammation, edema, and generation of necrotic debris, ultimately leading to airway plugging and impaired gas exchange. Bronchospasm, atelectasis, and pneumonia may also develop.

Should you wait for chest radiograph (CXR) results to decide whether to intubate the patient?
A CXR is usually normal immediately after burn injury. Do not wait for a CXR prior to securing the airway if you suspect inhalational injury.

TABLE 16.1 ■ **Classification of Burn Injury**

Burn Depth	Description
First degree	• Looks like a sunburn • Only the upper layers of the epidermis are affected • Skin is painful, erythematous, and slightly edematous
Superficial second degree	• Extends into the superficial layer of the dermis • Red in color • Painful blisters may form • Blanches with pressure
Deep second degree	• Extends into the reticular dermis • White or yellow in color • Extremely painful, but sensation may be diminished • Does not blanch with pressure
Third degree	• Dry, leathery, black, or white in color • Painless since nerves are destroyed • Doesn't blanch with pressure
Fourth degree	• Involvement of deeper structures (e.g., muscle, fascia, bone)

You decide to intubate the patient.

Can you use succinylcholine for neuromuscular blockade?
Succinylcholine is safe to use in the first 24 hours after burn injury. Given that the burn happened in the minutes or hours prior to presentation, and assuming the patient has no other contraindication to succinylcholine (see Case 13), it is safe to use succinylcholine to intubate this patient.

The view of the airway is shown in Fig. 16.2. Intubation is uneventful. The oxygen saturation on pulse oximetry is 98%. You draw an arterial blood gas (ABG), and co-oximetry shows an oxygen saturation of 73%.

What's going on?
This is concerning for carbon monoxide (CO) poisoning.

What is carbon monoxide poisoning?
CO is a colorless, odorless gas that is the byproduct of a combustion reaction. Sources of CO poisoning are exhaust fumes, gasoline-powered generators, poorly functioning heating systems, and inhaled smoke. In fact, CO poisoning is one of the most common causes of death in fires. When CO binds with hemoglobin, carboxyhemoglobin (CO-Hb) is formed. CO-Hb has approximately 200 times more affinity for oxygen than does hemoglobin alone. The hemoglobin-oxygen dissociation curve is shifted to the left (see Case 15), which results in impaired oxygen unloading at the cellular level and tissue hypoxia. When fewer oxygen binding sites on hemoglobin are available, the blood oxygen content is reduced.

Additionally, CO binds cytochrome oxidase within mitochondria, thereby impairing the production of adenosine triphosphate (ATP), which is critical for cellular metabolism. CO poisoning can lead to lactic acidosis and other metabolic derangements.

Why isn't CO poisoning reflected in pulse oximetry readings?
CO-Hb and oxyhemoglobin (oxygen bound to hemoglobin) have similar absorption spectra. In other words, they absorb similar frequencies of light. As a result, the color of CO-Hb may appear similar to normal oxygenated hemoglobin and have a light red color. This explains why patients with CO poisoning do not present with cyanosis, but rather a "cherry red" appearance. Given the

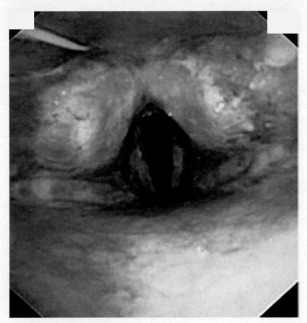

Fig. 16.2   Mucosal edema and erosion of the airway consistent with inhalational injury. (Ikonomidis, C., Lang, F., Radu, A., & Berger, M. M. [2012]. Standardizing the diagnosis of inhalation injury using a descriptive score based on mucosal injury criteria. *Burns*, *38*[4], 513–519. Modified from Fig. 2.)

spuriously elevated value on pulse oximetry, co-oximetry is used instead to determine CO-Hb levels in the setting of CO poisoning.

How does a pulse oximeter work?

A pulse oximeter relies on the fact that oxyhemoglobin and deoxygenated hemoglobin absorb different amounts of light.

A two-sided sensor, most commonly placed on the fingertip, has two components: one side contains light-emitting diodes, and the other side contains a photodetector. The diodes emit light at two wavelengths: 660 nm (red) and 940 nm (infrared). Blood and tissue absorb some of the emitted light, and the rest is transmitted to the photodetector. The amount of light absorbed by capillary and venous blood, and by tissue, remains constant over time. The amount of light absorbed by arterial blood, however, is cyclical, as each beat of the heart transiently increases the amount of blood in the arterioles between the light-emitting diodes and the photodetector (Fig. 16.3). It is this cyclical change in light absorbance that is attributable to arterial blood. The ratio of the cyclical absorbance of light of a 660-nm wavelength to the constant absorbance of light of a 660-nm wavelength is given by

$$S_{660} = \frac{cyclical\ absorbance_{660}}{constant\ absorbance_{660}}$$

The ratio of the cyclical absorbance of light of a 940-nm wavelength to the constant absorbance of light of a 940-nm wavelength is given by

$$S_{940} = \frac{cyclical\ absorbance_{940}}{constant\ absorbance_{940}}$$

The ratio R, given by

$$R = \frac{S_{660}}{S_{940}}$$

correlates to an oxygen saturation (SpO_2) based a calibration curve assumed to be constant across the human species. This curve is shown in Fig. 16.4.

CO-Hb interferes with this measurement because it absorbs light in a manner similar to that of oxyhemoglobin. Significant hypotension and anemia can cause falsely low pulse oximetry readings. Methemoglobin also interferes with pulse oximetry—pulse oximetry tends to read 85% in the presence of methemoglobinemia.

STEP 1 PEARL

Oxyhemoglobin absorbs more infrared light (940 nm wavelength), while deoxyhemoglobin absorbs more red light (660 nm wavelength).

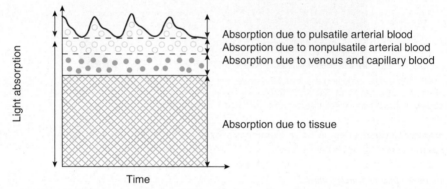

Fig. 16.3 Absorbance of light by tissue and non-pulsatile blood is constant, whereas absorption of light by pulsatile blood is cyclical. (Baker, S. J. [2021]. Pulse oximetry. In J. Ehrenwerth, J. B. Eisenkraft, & J. M. Berry (Eds.), *Anesthesia equipment* [3rd ed., pp. 253–270]. Philadelphia, PA: Elsevier. Modified from Fig. 11.5.)

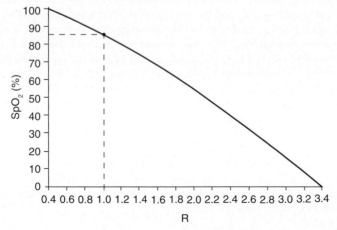

Fig. 16.4 Calibration curve relating the ratio of cyclical absorbances (R) to an SpO_2 measurement. (Baker, S. J. [2021]. Pulse oximetry. In J. Ehrenwerth, J. B. Eisenkraft, & J. M. Berry (Eds.), *Anesthesia equipment* [3rd ed., pp. 253–270]. Philadelphia, PA: Elsevier. Modified from Fig. 11.6.)

STEP 2 PEARL

Dark-colored nail polish (e.g., blue, green, purple) can create falsely low pulse oximetry readings when the sensor is placed on the patient's fingertip.

How should you manage CO poisoning in this patient?
The main treatment for CO poisoning is the administration of 100% oxygen. This allows for faster displacement of CO from hemoglobin. When the patient is breathing room air (21% oxygen), the elimination half-life of CO is 4 hours. When the patient is breathing 100% oxygen, the elimination half-life of CO is shortened to 74 minutes.

What about hyperbaric oxygen therapy?
Hyperbaric oxygen is typically reserved for patients with neurologic impairment, pregnancy, cardiac abnormalities, or a CO-Hb level greater than 25%–50%. This usually requires transferring the patient to a specialized burn center.

> Bedside transthoracic echocardiogram (TTE) shows moderately decreased left ventricular systolic function. The patient's wife says he has no history of cardiac disease and is an avid runner.

What's going on?
Impaired systolic and diastolic cardiac function may be noted in the first 24–36 hours after significant burn injury.

How should much intravenous fluid will you give this patient?
Fluid resuscitation is key to correct hypovolemia and optimize organ perfusion during this critical period to avoid burn shock and other complications. Burn injuries have a high rate of fluid and protein loss, especially during the first 12 hours. This is primarily due to the generalized increase in capillary permeability leading to loss of fluid and proteins into the interstitial tissue.

The goal of fluid resuscitation is to maintain a urine output of 0.5 mL/kg/h, which is a good indication of adequate renal perfusion. The most common formula used to guide resuscitation is the *Parkland Formula*. This involves giving a total of 4 mL/kg/% TBSA of intravenous fluid (crystalloid, such as lactated Ringer's solution, can be used) over 24 hours. The first half of this volume is given in the first 8 hours. The remaining volume is administered over the next 16 hours.

Some institutions may use the more conservative *modified Brooke formula*. This suggests the administration of 2 mL/kg/% TBSA of lactated Ringer's solution.

It is important to remember that these formulas for fluid resuscitation are merely guidelines, and the patient's hemodynamic and physiologic status should be frequently reassessed, with fluid administration adjusted accordingly.

How much fluid would our 80-kg patient who sustained a 70% TBSA burn require using the parkland formula or the modified brooke formula?
Using the Parkland Formula, our patient would require an approximate total of 22.4 L within the first 24 hours after the injury. Given that half of this amount needs to be given within the first 8 hours, our patient would require 11.2 L of fluids during the first 8 hours.

$$Fluid\ requirement = TBSA\ burned\ (\%) \times weight\ (kg) \times 4\,mL$$

$$= 70\% \times 80\,kg \times 4\,mL = 22,400\,mL\ or\ 22.4\,L$$

Using the modified Brooke formula, our patient would require 11.2 L of lactated Ringer's solution.

$$\text{Fluid requirement} = \text{TBSA burned (\%)} \times \text{weight (kg)} \times 2\,\text{mL}$$

$$= 70\% \times 80\,\text{kg} \times 2\,\text{mL} = 11,200\,\text{mL or } 11.2\,\text{L}$$

> In the intensive care unit (ICU), you notice that the patient's pulse is 130/min and blood pressure is 95/68 mm Hg. ABG shows pH 7.12, $PaCO_2$ 42 mm Hg, PaO2 87 mm Hg, and bicarbonate 12 mEq/L. The lactate level is 13 mmol/L.

What's going on?

This is concerning for cyanide toxicity. Cyanide binds the cytochrome oxidase of mitochondria, thereby inhibiting cellular respiration. Cyanide toxicity is rare, but when present is rapidly fatal. High clinical suspicion is required for diagnosis. Cyanide exposure may occur after incomplete combustion of carbon- and nitrogen-containing compounds. Common symptoms include loss of consciousness, anion gap metabolic acidosis (see Case 30), cardiopulmonary failure, and neurologic symptoms (e.g., anxiety, headache, seizures, coma). Patients may initially present with bradycardia and hypertension progressing to hypotension with reflex tachycardia before asystole.

Patients with inhalation injury and CO poisoning are frequently found to have concomitant cyanide toxicity.

How should you treat this patient?

Ensure that the patient is ventilated with 100% FiO_2. Pharmacologic options include sodium thiosulfate, hydroxocobalamin, and induction of methemoglobinemia with sodium nitrite. Beware that induction of methemoglobinemia can be harmful in the presence of CO poisoning because oxygen carrying capacity of hemoglobin is further reduced.

Should you wait to check blood cyanide levels prior to starting treatment?

No. Laboratory assays may be slow to show results and should not delay acute management.

> Several hours later, the patient's right arm is pale and cool. The arm feels very firm.

What's going on?

These findings are consistent with compartment syndrome of the right arm. Compartment syndrome is caused by an increase in pressure within a fascial compartment that exceeds the vascular perfusion pressure (i.e., arterial blood pressure) of that compartment. This ultimately leads to decreased blood flow and tissue ischemia. In particular, burn injuries can result in compartment syndrome from accumulation of interstitial fluid or by extrinsic compression due to the burned tissue acting as a tourniquet. As a result, high pressures are generated in a closed fascial space. Compartment syndrome is most commonly seen in patients who received high-voltage electrical burns or those with circumferential third-degree burns. When deeper layers of the skin are affected, edema and severe tissue restriction are more likely.

STEP 1, 2, 3 PEARL

Compartment syndrome is characterized by the 6 Ps: pain, pallor, paresthesia (tingling or unusual sensations), paralysis, pulselessness, and poikilothermia (uncontrolled temperature regulation usually presenting as decreased temperature).

STEP 2, 3 PEARL

The most appropriate treatment for compartment syndrome is immediate fasciotomy or escharotomy to decompress the tissue compartments.

The burn surgeon says he will perform an escharotomy.

What is that?
An escharotomy is a surgical procedure that relieves pressure in areas such as the neck, torso, or limbs affected by significant swelling from thickened skin after a burn injury. Specifically, it is used to treat circumferential, full-thickness (third-degree) burns. Such burns can cause a tourniquet effect, leading to reduced circulation, tissue edema, and limited muscle movement. Circumferential burns to the chest or abdomen can lead to shallow respiratory effort from restricted chest and abdominal wall movement. Circumferential burns in the extremities can lead to distal ischemia and tissue necrosis if left untreated. Thus, escharotomy may be done prophylactically or shortly after a severe burn injury. An incision is made deep enough to release pressure by reaching the subcutaneous fat and into the underlying healthy skin. Unlike a fasciotomy, escharotomy incisions do not break through the deep fascial layer.

The patient is extubated on post-burn day 3. On post-burn day 4, he is scheduled to undergo debridement and skin grafting. You plan for endotracheal intubation.

What concerns do you have regarding airway management in this patient?
This patient sustained an airway injury and received aggressive fluid resuscitation. Both of these factors may contribute to upper airway swelling and a narrowed glottic opening. Burns to the face may be covered in dressings or topical agents, and a nasogastric tube may be in place. These factors may complicate mask ventilation. In patients with remote burn injuries, scar formation will limit neck and jaw range of motion as well as mouth opening. Interstitial edema and opioids can delay gastric emptying, predisposing the patient to aspiration.

Once the endotracheal tube is secured, adhesive tape will not be effective over burned skin. A circumferential tube tie will be more effective.

You want to induce anesthesia with propofol.

How will his burn affect your dosing?
In patients with burn injuries beyond the first 24–48 hours of injury, the clearance and volume of propofol distribution are increased compared to a patient without burns. Therefore, this patient may require a larger dose of propofol compared to a patient with no burns.

What neuromuscular blocking agents are safe?
Beginning 24 hours after injury, burn patients are more sensitive to succinylcholine. Succinylcholine should be avoided as it may result in hyperkalemia. Burned, damaged tissue generates upregulation of extra-junctional acetylcholine receptors. These receptors stay open longer when stimulated and can cause potentially fatal hyperkalemia when succinylcholine is given.

On the other hand, burn patients are less sensitive to nondepolarizing muscle relaxant agents such as rocuronium. Thus, they may require significantly increased doses to achieve and maintain paralysis compared to healthy patients.

Induction and intubation are uneventful. The surgeon plans to excise burns from the patient's neck, arms, and chest—about 28% TBSA.

How much blood loss should you expect?
Burn excision causes significant bleeding. It has been estimated that a patient may lose 3.5%–5% of their blood volume for every 1% TBSA burn excised. Therefore, in this patient, you would expect him to lose at least his total blood volume during surgery. Application of tourniquets and epinephrine-soaked gauze can reduce bleeding. *Be prepared with multiple reliable points of vascular access and copious blood products in the operating room. Blood should be administered via a fluid warmer.*

Why is the operating room kept so warm?
Burn injury inhibits the patient's ability to retain body heat. Anesthesia causes vasodilation, which also contributes to heat loss. Burn patients do not tolerate hypothermia, as this can significantly increase oxygen consumption.

Therefore, every effort must be taken to prevent hypothermia. In addition to increased ambient temperature, thermal mattresses, forced-air warming blankets, and wrapping the head and extremities in insulating materials can help maintain normothermia.

The patient remains intubated postoperatively.

How can you treat his pain?
Intravenous narcotics are a mainstay of pain management in severe burns. Intravenous ketamine is also frequently used. In addition to its analgesic affects, ketamine may also prevent central pain sensitization. Acetaminophen and gabapentin are helpful adjuncts.

What about ketorolac?
Nonsteroidal anti-inflammatory drugs (NSAIDs) such as ketorolac can interfere with normal kidney function, cause gastrointestinal ulceration, and increase bleeding risk by inhibiting platelet function. Therefore, NSAIDs are generally avoided in patients with severe burns.

What are some special features of electrical burns?
Overall care for electrical burns is similar to thermal burns. However, the extent of injury can be misleading on presentation. The outer layer of skin may appear normal. However, areas of devitalized tissue may be present. Thus, the extent of superficial injury or lack thereof may result in the underestimation of initial fluid resuscitation requirements. Myoglobinuria is a common sign. As a result, urine output must be kept high to avoid renal damage. Neurological complications, such as peripheral neuropathies or spinal cord deficits, are common.

BEYOND THE PEARLS

- Three main factors are associated with increased mortality in burn patients: advanced age, size of burn injury, and presence of inhalational injury.
- Burn depth can be better determined with the use of laser Doppler imaging.
- CO-Hb levels above 50% are generally considered lethal.
- A normal response to muscle relaxants may be reestablished after the patient has completely healed from burn injury, which may take several years.
- During intubation of a burn patient, be sure to examine the larynx and document any pathologic findings.
- Fetal hemoglobin has similar absorbance of light and therefore does not interfere with pulse oximetry.
- Intravenous dyes such as indigo carmine and indocyanine green can cause transient decreases in pulse oximetry readings.

References

Baker, S. J. (2021). Pulse oximetry. In J. Ehrenwerth, J. B. Eisenkraft, & J. M. Berry (Eds.), *Anesthesia equipment* (3rd ed., pp. 253–270). Philadelphia, PA: Elsevier.

Besner, G. E. (2011). Burns. In: P. Mattei (Ed.), *Fundamentals of pediatric surgery*. New York, NY: Springer.

Bittner, E. A., Jeevendra, M. A. J., & Sjöberg, F. (2020). Acute and anesthetic care of the burn-injured patient. In M. A. Gropper, R. D. Miller, N. H. Cohen, L. I. Eriksson, L. A. Fleisher, K. Leslie, et al. (Eds.), *Miller's anesthesia* (9th ed., Chapter 87, pp. 2476–2773.e6). Philadelphia, PA: Elsevier.

Breen, P. H. (2018). Cyanide poisoning. In L. A. Fleisher, M F. Roizen, & J. D. Roizen (Eds.), *Essence of anesthesia practice* (4th ed., p. 122). Philadelphia, PA: Elsevier.

Mehta, M., & Tudor, G. J. (2020). *StatPearls [Internet]*. Treasure Island, FL: StatPearls Publishing. Parkland Formula.

Pruitt, B. A., Dowling, J. A., & Moncrief, J. A. (1968). Escharotomy in early burn care. *Archives of Surgery, 96*(4), 502–507.

Regan, A., & Hotwagner, D. T. (2020). *StatPearls [Internet]*. Treasure Island, FL: StatPearls Publishing. Burn Fluid Management.

Wong, L., & Spence, R. J. (2000). Escharotomy and fasciotomy of the burned upper extremity. *Hand Clinics, 16*(2), 165–174, vii.

A 60-Year-Old Man With Cirrhosis due to Chronic Hepatitis B Infection

Tom Hughes ■ Mike Priem ■ Paul Neil Frank

A 60-year-old man with cirrhosis due to chronic hepatitis B infection is undergoing liver resection for hepatocellular carcinoma. In the preoperative area, his vital signs are blood pressure 100/57 mm Hg, pulse 94/min, respirations 16/min, oxygen saturation 95% on room air, and temperature 35.6°C.

What is the anatomy and blood supply of the liver?

The liver is the body's largest solid organ, comprising 2% of total body mass. Key structures of the hepatobiliary system include:

- gallbladder and the cystic duct
- common hepatic duct
- common bile duct
- second portion of the duodenum

At rest, the liver receives 25% of total cardiac output and accounts for 20% of oxygen consumption. The liver has a dual blood supply: 25% from the hepatic artery and 75% from the deoxygenated low-pressure portal vein that drains the intestines, spleen, and gallbladder.

Although the portal vein contributes a larger portion of the blood flow, the oxygen content of portal venous blood is much less than that of hepatic arterial blood. Therefore, the portal vein and the hepatic artery each contribute about 50% of the hepatic oxygen supply. When portal blood flow is compromised, the hepatic artery can increase flow by as much as 100% to maintain oxygen delivery. The spongy nature of the liver combined with the contractile potential of the stellate cells allows the liver to either store or augment systemic blood volume as necessary.

STEP 1 PEARL

The smallest functional unit of the liver is the acinus. Each acinus has a portal tract (containing branches of the hepatic artery, portal vein, and bile duct) at the center and a central vein (a tributary to the hepatic vein) peripherally. Blood flows from the portal tracts (specifically the branches of the portal vein and hepatic artery) through hepatic sinusoids to the central vein (Fig. 17.1).

STEP 1 PEARL

Hepatic sinusoids are lined with sinusoidal epithelial cells separated by fenestrations to allow passage of some macromolecules (e.g., plasma proteins, pharmaceutical molecules) into the space of Disse while keeping erythrocytes and other large structures within the sinusoids.

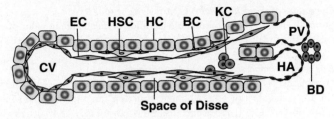

Space of Disse

Fig. 17.1 A hepatic sinusoid lined with epithelial cells (EC). Blood flows from the terminal branches of the portal vein (PV) and hepatic artery (HA) through the sinusoid to the central vein (CV). Kupffer cells (KC) are specialized immune cells found within the sinusoids. Macromolecules pass through fenestrations between the EC to enter the space of Disse, which is bound by EC and hepatocytes (HC). The space of Disse also contains hepatic stellate cells (HSC). Hepatocytes secrete bile into bile canaliculi (BC). (Njoku, D. B., Chitilian, H. V., & Kronish, K. [2020]. Hepatic physiology, pathophysiology, and anesthetic considerations. In M. A. Gropper, R. D. Miller, N. H. Cohen, L. I. Eriksson, L. A. Fleisher, K. Leslie, et al. (Eds.), *Miller's Anesthesia*, [Vol. 16, 9th ed., pp. 420–443.e8]. Philadelphia: Elsevier. Modified from Fig. 16.3B.)

STEP 1 PEARL

Hepatic stellate cells are found within the space of Disse. In the event of liver injury, these cells are activated by inflammatory mediators differentiated into myofibroblasts, which take part in inflammation and fibrosis within the liver.

STEP 1 PEARL

Kupffer cells are macrophages found within the sinusoids of the liver.

What are the essential functions of the liver?

The liver is a complex organ with multiple critical functions.

- Bile synthesis and regulation: Hepatocytes produce roughly 500 mL of bile daily. Bile is composed of bilirubin, cholesterol, and bile salts. Bile facilitates lipid emulsification and the absorption and secretion of toxins and lipophilic drugs.
- Protein synthesis: Includes all of the plasma proteins (except gamma globulins produced by plasma cells), vitamin K-dependent (II, VI, IX, X, protein C, protein S) and independent clotting factors, albumin, angiotensinogen, and fibrinogen. These factors can be measured as an indicator of hepatic synthetic function.
- Protein breakdown and synthesis: Amino acid transamination and deamination to form ketoacids, which are used to synthesize new essential amino acids and the formation of urea from ammonia.
- Hemoglobin metabolism: Process iron generated from the splenic breakdown of senescent red blood cells (erythrocytes) in the form of unconjugated (indirect) bilirubin to either recycle iron for other uses or conjugate bilirubin with glucuronic acid to form water-soluble (direct) bilirubin for excretion in the bile.
- Immune host defense: Direct exposure of ingested toxins to the hepatocyte, Kupffer, and dendritic cells cleanses portal venous blood before it enters systemic circulation (the first-pass effect).
- Nutrient storage: The precursor of glucose (glycogen) and fat-soluble vitamins.
- Drug metabolism and excretion:
  - Phase 1 reactions (cytochrome P450, CYP, superfamily) depend on liver blood flow and alter existing chemical groups via hydrolysis, oxidation, or reduction, making compounds more hydrophilic.
  - Phase 2 reactions involve conjugation reactions, enhancing the secretion of lipid-soluble drugs.

What signs and symptoms are associated with hepatic dysfunction?
Signs and symptoms of liver dysfunction include jaundice, rash, change in color of urine or stool, fatigue, abdominal pain, pruritus, easy bruising, scleral icterus, ascites, and asterixis.

What preoperative studies should you order for this patient?
Alanine aminotransferase (ALT) and gamma glutamyltransferase (GGT) are made almost exclusively in the liver and do not assess hepatic function but rather hepatocellular damage. Profound elevations of ALT, GGT, and aspartate aminotransferase (AST) usually indicate acute hepatitis or other causes of acute hepatocellular damage and are usually a contraindication to elective surgery. Hepatitis serologies document the presence, progression, or resolution of viral infection. Elevations in alkaline phosphatase (ALP) and 5′-nucleotidase indicate biliary tract disease.

Elevated unconjugated bilirubin is consistent with hemolysis or impaired hepatocellular function. Elevated conjugated bilirubin suggests biliary obstruction. Increased levels of both unconjugated and conjugated bilirubin suggest hepatocellular disease.

Prothrombin time and international normalized ratio (INR) tests the synthetic function of the liver, specifically the production of clotting factors. INR greater than 1.5 is common in cirrhotic patients. A low level of fibrinogen in association with low platelets ($<50,000 \times 10^3/\mu$L) may be the best predictor of perioperative hemorrhage. Measuring the serum albumin level is useful to help categorize risk, although albumin has a relatively long half-life of 20 days.

Cirrhotic patients undergoing major surgery should be screened preoperatively with resting echocardiography to document pulmonary artery pressure and ventricular function.

STEP 1, 2 PEARL

Alpha-fetoprotein is used to screen for hepatocellular cancer. CA-19-9 screens for cholangiocarcinoma.

The results of the patient's hepatitis serologic testing are:
- hepatitis B surface antigen (HBsAg): positive
- antibody to hepatitis B surface antigen (anti-HBs): negative
- IgG antibody to hepatitis B core antigen (anti-HBc IgG): positive
- IgM antibody to hepatitis B core antigen (anti-HBc IgM): negative

What does this mean?
This pattern on serologic testing is consistent with chronic hepatitis B infection. Common patterns and the significance of each are listed in Table 17.1.

TABLE 17.1 ■ Interpretation of Serologic Testing for Hepatitis B

	HBsAg	anti-HBs	anti-HBc IgG	anti-HBc IgM
Immune due to recovery from prior infection	–	+	+	–
Immune due to vaccination	–	+	–	–
Acute infection	+	–	+	+
Chronic infection	+	–	+	–
Susceptible to infection	–	–	–	–

What are the common causes of chronic liver disease?
Common causes of liver disease include hepatitis B and C, alcohol abuse, and non-alcoholic fatty liver disease.

What is cirrhosis and portal hypertension?
Cirrhosis involves gross and microscopic scarring and fibrous bridging with functional decline. Tissue scarring and humoral factors lead to hepatic resistance to inflow from the low-pressure portal vein circuit, resulting in portal hypertension and its complications.

STEP 1 PEARL

Resistance to hepatic venous outflow (Budd-Chiari) is seen less often but can result in hepatic congestion and portal hypertension as well.

Cirrhosis and portal hypertension may result in significant sequelae including:
- Hemostatic: Abnormal procoagulants and abnormal fibrinolysis often balance, hence these patients usually are not coagulopathic unless the platelet count is less than $50,000 \times 10^3/\mu L$. Splenic sequestration of platelets in the engorged red pulp accounts for the majority of the coagulation defect, which is partially offset by an increase in the von Willebrand factor.
- Cardiac: Increased cardiac output with decreased mean blood pressure and effective circulating volume. Overall, total blood volume is increased due to pooling in the portal venous circulation. Cardiomyopathy may be present in up to 50% of patients. These patients are usually comfortable at rest but exhibit a blunted cardiovascular response to exercise and stress. They are typically refractory to ordinary doses of vasopressors.
- Renal: Baseline renal perfusion is compromised in these patients due to endogenous vasoconstrictors. An acute illness or stress can provoke acute renal failure (known as hepatorenal syndrome) with shunting of blood away from the kidneys due to splanchnic vasodilation.
- Pulmonary: Hepatopulmonary syndrome is characterized by abnormal arterial oxygenation from intrapulmonary shunts in the setting of liver disease and/or portal hypertension. Roughly 25% of patients with severe chronic liver disease will manifest pulmonary involvement.
- Ascites: Ascites can cause abdominal distention and increased intraabdominal pressure, which impairs respiratory function and predisposes the patient to aspiration during intubation. The presence or degree of ascites is measured in the Child-Turcotte-Pugh (CTP) classification and may persist in compensated cirrhosis.
- Spontaneous bacterial peritonitis (SBP): Intraabdominal infection associated with cirrhosis, portal hypertension, and ascites. Bacteria that cause SBP are *Escherichia coli*, *Klebsiella pneumoniae*, and *Streptococcus pneumoniae*.
- Hepatic encephalopathy: Altered or depressed mental status up to and including coma.
- Enlarging or bleeding esophageal and gastric varices. Varices decompress the portal vein, and rupture may cause catastrophic bleeding. Primary prophylaxis includes either a beta-blocker or endoscopic banding.

Preoperative labs show total bilirubin 2.4 mg/dL, Albumin 3 g/dL, and Inr 1.6. Based on preoperative imaging, the patient has moderate ascites. He is fully alert and oriented.

What is his child turcotte pugh class?
The *CTP Classification for Severity of Liver Disease* assigns points (1–3) based on the criteria in Table 17.2. Based on our patient's laboratory studies, mental status, and quantity of ascites, he has

TABLE 17.2 ■ Child-Turcotte-Pugh Score Is Based on the Presence and Severity of Encephalopathy and Ascites, as Well as Derangements in bilirubin, albumin, and international normalized ratio

	Encephalopathy	Ascites	Bilirubin	Albumin	INR
1 point	None	None	<2 mg/dL	>3.5 g/dL	<1.7
2 points	Altered mood/confusion, somnolence	Slight	2–3 mg/dL	2.8–3.5 g/dL	1.7–2.3
3 points	Markedly confused, stuporous, comatose	Moderate	>3 mg/dL	<2.8 g/dL	>2.3

INR, International normalized ratio.

TABLE 17.3 ■ CTP Classification and Operative Mortality

Points	CTP Class	Perioperative Mortality (%)
5–6	A	2–10
7–9	B	12–31
10–15	C	12–82

9 points, which corresponds to class B (Table 17.3). A higher CTP score correlates to an increased risk of mortality. This patient (Childs B) has a significant likelihood of mortality after a major open intraabdominal procedure.

Does this patient have acute hepatic failure?
No. Acute hepatic failure is called fulminant hepatic failure. This is a critical illness typically requiring intensive care unit (ICU) admission. It is defined as the appearance of encephalopathy together with coagulopathy (usually an INR >1.5) in a patient with no history of liver disease for the 25 weeks prior to the acute illness.

Etiologies include drug-induced (50% of cases, 80% of which are acetaminophen related), autoimmune, viral, Wilson disease, and hypoxemic injury. Forty-five percent of patients spontaneously recover, 25% receive liver transplants, and 30% die, usually due to cerebral edema. Acute hepatic failure is a contraindication to all but the most emergent surgery.

What can be done to reduce the risk of perioperative mortality in this patient?
Less invasive approaches such as laparoscopy may reduce risk. Metabolic factors can contribute to encephalopathy, some of which may be modified by anesthetic management. Hypoxia, hypovolemia, alkalemia, hypoglycemia, hypokalemia, and hyponatremia can all precipitate encephalopathy and should be avoided.

Hypotension, high airway pressures, and sympathetic stimulation should also be avoided to the extent possible. These patients are often less responsive to endogenous and exogenous vasopressors. The action of opioids is prolonged, and these patients often have an enhanced response to sedatives.

The patient is anxious in the preoperative area.

Should you give him midazolam?
The elimination of midazolam is impaired in patients with liver dysfunction. This may lead to prolonged sedation. It is best not to give midazolam to this patient.

Is it Safe to Use Propofol for This Case?

Yes. Intravenous anesthetics such as propofol, thiopental, etomidate, and methohexital are not harmful to the liver. However, patients with cirrhosis may be more sensitive to the hypnotic effects of these drugs.

Is it safe to use sevoflurane?

Yes. The currently used volatile anesthetics (e.g., isoflurane, sevoflurane, and desflurane) are not associated with hepatotoxicity. Sevoflurane and isoflurane result in very little reduction of hepatic blood flow at 1 minimum alveolar concentration (MAC). However, maintenance of circulatory volume and renal perfusion is essential.

The patient has moderate ascites. How will that affect your induction and intubation strategy?

Patients with ascites are at an increased risk of pulmonary aspiration of gastric contents and should undergo rapid sequence intubation (see Case 13). Ascites causes cephalad pressure on the diaphragm, which reduces functional residual capacity (FRC). Therefore, patients with ascites will tolerate shorter periods of apnea prior to developing hypoxia.

Can you intubate using succinylcholine?

Yes, succinylcholine is safe to use in liver disease. Patients with liver disease have decreased levels of pseudocholinesterase, the enzyme responsible for succinylcholine metabolism. Therefore, succinylcholine may have a prolonged duration of action.

Induction and intubation are uneventful. The effect of succinylcholine wears off, and the patient starts breathing on his own. The surgeon asks that the patient be fully relaxed.

What neuromuscular blocking agent should you give?

Cisatracurium is a good choice for neuromuscular blockade in this patient, as its duration of effect will be unchanged in this patient compared to a patient without liver disease. As with all nondepolarizing neuromuscular blocking agents, cisatracurium is a competitive antagonist at nicotinic acetylcholine receptors. Cisatracurium is unique in the mechanism of its metabolism—it undergoes spontaneous degradation into inactive metabolites. This process does not depend on an enzyme, and the rate of metabolism depends only on temperature and pH. This is known as Hofmann elimination. Since the liver is responsible for the metabolism of many pharmacologic agents, the duration of effect of other nondepolarizing neuromuscular blocking agents (which undergo enzymatic metabolism) may be prolonged in patients with liver disease. However, the duration of effect of cisatracurium will be unchanged in patients with liver disease.

The surgeon asks you to minimize fluid administration during the resection and to keep the central venous pressure (CVP) low.

Why?

Maintaining a low CVP (<5 mm Hg) may help reduce blood loss. Lower CVP reduces the pressure in the inferior vena cava and hence the hepatic vein. Venous congestion can contribute to venous bleeding in the liver. Be aware that low CVP does increase the risk of air entrainment, leading to venous air embolism (see Case 23).

What else can be done to reduce blood loss and the need for blood transfusion?

Acute normovolemic hemodilution (ANH) may also be helpful. Before significant bleeding, or ideally before incision, the anesthesiologist sequesters whole blood from the patient via an arterial or intravenous catheter. The blood is stored in a blood bag with citrate for anticoagulation. That volume is then replaced by crystalloid (3 mL crystalloid for 1 mL blood removed) or colloid (1 mL colloid for 1 mL blood removed). This blood is then returned to the patient at the end of the operation. The advantage here is that every mL of intravascular volume lost intraoperatively contains a lower number of erythrocytes, clotting factors, and platelets.

In order to be a candidate for ANH, the patient must have an adequate starting hemoglobin level (usually ≥12 g/dL). Always consider comorbidities, such as cardiac, pulmonary, and renal disease, when deciding whether to use ANH.

There is significant bleeding during the hepatic resection, and the surgeon says she will perform the pringle maneuver.

What's the pringle maneuver? What hemodynamic changes would you expect?

The Pringle maneuver entails occluding the hepatoduodenal ligament, which contains the portal vein, hepatic artery, and common bile duct (Fig. 17.2). This occludes the blood supply to the liver and allows time for localization and repair of bleeding. The Pringle maneuver causes increases in mean arterial pressure and systemic vascular resistance, as well as decreases in cardiac output and left ventricular preload.

The operation is complete. The neuromuscular blockade has been maintained with cisatracurium. As the dressings are being applied to the incisions, the patient has two out of four twitches on train of four monitoring.

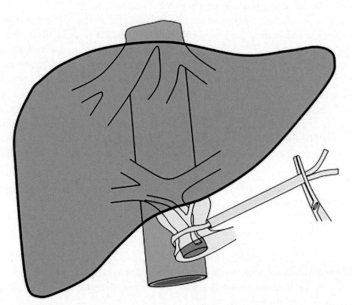

Fig. 17.2 Occlusion of the hepatic pedicle, which blocks blood flow from the hepatic artery and the portal vein. (Cauchy, F., Scatton, O., Belghiti, J., & Soubrane, O. [2017]. In W. R. Jarnagin, P. J. Allen, W. C. Chapman, M. I. D'Angelica, R. P. DeMatteo, R. K. G. Do, et al. [Eds.], *Blumgart's Surgery of the Liver, Biliary Tract, and Pancreas* [Vol. *106*, pp. 1612–1622.e2]. Philadelphia: Elsevier. Fig. 106.2.)

Can you reverse neuromuscular blockade with sugammadex?
No, sugammadex is only effective at reversing the effects of neuromuscular blocking agents of the aminosteroid type (i.e., rocuronium, vecuronium). *Sugammadex is not effective in reversing the neuromuscular blocking effects of cisatracurium.*

How can you reverse the neuromuscular blockade in this patient?
The neuromuscular blockade can be reversed by administering an acetylcholinesterase inhibitor (e.g., neostigmine). Acetylcholinesterase inhibitors prevent the breakdown of acetylcholine at the neuromuscular junction. This allows for more acetylcholine to bind and activate nicotinic receptors at the neuromuscular junction, thereby reversing the effect of the neuromuscular blockade.

Shortly after the administration of neostigmine, the heart rate drops from 82/min to 43/min.

What's going on?
Acetylcholinesterase inhibitors increase the activity of acetylcholine at all cholinergic receptors in the body, including nicotinic receptors and muscarinic receptors. Muscarinic receptors are responsible for, among other things, the negative chronotropic effect (i.e., slowing of the heart rate) by the vagus nerve on the heart. When an acetylcholinesterase inhibitor is given, this potentiates the stimulation of muscarinic receptors on the heart, thereby causing bradycardia.

What should you do?
Glycopyrrolate is an antagonist of muscarinic cholinergic receptors. This will block the effect of the excess acetylcholine at these receptors. It will not have an effect on nicotinic cholinergic receptors at the neuromuscular junction.

If neuromuscular blockade will be reversed with neostigmine, glycopyrrolate should be given at the same time to prevent bradycardia.

The patient's heart rate normalizes and he is taken to the ICU. Over the next several hours, the patient's urine output decreases to 15 mL/h.

What should be done?
Liver disease can cause progressive renal dysfunction. Vasoconstrictors (e.g., norepinephrine or vasopressin) may be beneficial in these patients.

When should albumin be given?
Albumin may be helpful in preventing or treating renal dysfunction in patients with liver disease. Common indications for albumin administration include:
- Hepatorenal syndrome, where oncotic pressure is beneficial in conjunction with splanchnic vasoconstrictors
- After large volume (4–5 L) paracentesis
- In the presence of SBP to prevent renal impairment

BEYOND THE PEARLS

- Since the liver performs so many functions, no single group of tests or assessments exists to determine the overall health of the liver.
- Hypoalbuminemia can be caused by factors other than impaired hepatic synthetic function, such as renal losses, expansion of plasma volume (i.e., dilution), and catabolism.

- Cirrhotic patients undergoing cardiac surgery do very poorly. A Childs A score estimates 20% mortality at 1 year, a Childs B score 55% mortality, and Childs C score 84% mortality at 1 year compared with a 2% yearly mortality of noncirrhotic patients. Elective high-risk abdominal and cardiac procedures for patients in the Childs C category should be deferred until after improvement of liver function or liver transplantation.
- If the patient has a history of esophageal varices, they are likely taking a beta-blocker for primary prophylaxis against variceal bleeding. This increases the risk of perioperative hypotension.
- Warfarin is a commonly used oral anticoagulant. It works by inhibiting carboxylation of vitamin K-dependent clotting factors, thereby preventing the activation of the clotting factors.
- When portal venous blood flow increases, hepatic arterial blood flow decreases, and when portal venous blood flow decreases, hepatic arterial blood flow increases. This is known as the hepatic arterial buffer response, and it maintains hepatic blood flow relatively constant. Portal venous blood flow does not change in response to hepatic arterial blood flow.
- The Model for End-Stage Liver Disease (MELD) is a scoring system used in the allocation of liver transplants. It is usually calculated based on patients' values for bilirubin, creatinine, and INR. A MELD Score of >21 documents severe liver disease and a high perioperative mortality of up to 70% for major surgery.

References

Carrion, A. F., & Martin, P. (2021). Cirrhosis. In R. D. Kellerman, & D. P. Rakel (Eds.), *Conn's current therapy* (pp. 190–200). Philadelphia: Elsevier.

Gold Standard, Inc. Cisatracurium. Drug monograph. Published February 27, 2021. www.clinicalkey.com. (Accessed May 5, 2021).

Dudley, M., Miller, R. D., & Turnbull, J. H. (2020). Patient blood management: Transfusion therapy. In M. A. Gropper, R. D. Miller, N. H. Cohen, L. I. Eriksson, L. A. Fleisher, K. Leslie, et al. (Eds.), *Miller's anesthesia* (Vol. 49, 9th ed., pp. 1546–1578.e5). Philadelphia: Elsevier.

Fischer, M., Arslan-Carlon, V., & Melendez, J. (2017). Intraoperative and immediate postoperative management. *Blumgart's surgery of the liver, biliary tract, and pancreas, 24*, 423–436.e3.

Gold Standard, Inc. Glycopyrrolate. Drug monograph. Published February 22, 2021. www.clinicalkey.com. (Accessed May 5, 2021).

Gold Standard, Inc. Neostigmine. Drug monograph. Published February 22, 2021. www.clinicalkey.com. (Accessed May 5, 2021).

Njoku, D. B., Chitilian, H. V., & Kronish, K. (2020). Hepatic physiology, pathophysiology, and anesthetic considerations. In M. A. Gropper, R. D. Miller, N. H. Cohen, L. I. Eriksson, L. A. Fleisher, K. Leslie, et al. (Eds.), *Miller's anesthesia* (Vol. 16, 9th ed., pp. 420–443.e8). Philadelphia: Elsevier.

Cardiothoracic

A 45-Year-Old Female With Worsening Dyspnea on Exertion

Nicole Shirakawa Wei ■ Paul Neil Frank

A 45-year-old female with worsening dyspnea on exertion was found to have severe mitral regurgitation and is scheduled for mitral valve repair. Transthoracic echocardiogram (TTE) showed severe mitral regurgitation with normal biventricular function and no other valvular abnormalities. She has no other significant medical history and takes no medications at home. On the morning of surgery, her vital signs show blood pressure 112/70 mm Hg, pulse 74/min, respirations 11/min, oxygen saturation 100% on room air, and temperature 36°C.

Describe the anatomy of the mitral valve
The mitral valve consists of two leaflets (anterior and posterior, each divided into scallops 1, 2, and 3), as well as the annulus, papillary muscles (classically there are two: anterolateral and posteromedial), and chordae tendinae (primary, secondary, and tertiary). This anatomy is shown in Fig. 18.1.

What are papillary muscles?
Papillary muscles are bands of muscle in the left ventricle (LV). Thin fibrous structures called chordae tendinae attach the leaflets of the mitral valve to the papillary muscles. Just like other myocardial muscle, papillary muscles contract during systole. Normally, this contraction tenses the chordae tendinae, which pull the mitral valve closed during systole.

In the preoperative area, you discuss the risks and benefits of your anesthetic plan, including TEE.

What are the risks of TEE?
TEE has a very low complication rate. The most common complications of TEE include odynophagia, dental injury, malposition of the endotracheal tube (i.e., accidental extubation), and upper esophageal bleeding, although the risks of any of these complications is 0.1% or less. The most feared complications of TEE are perforation of the hypopharynx, esophagus, or stomach, although the risk of perforation has been quoted at 0.02% or less.

An important risk of TEE is operator distraction. While performing TEE, it is critical to continue to monitor the patient's vital signs.

What are the contraindications to TEE?
Absolute contraindications to TEE include esophageal stricture, diverticulum, or tumor; recent esophageal suture lines; or known esophageal perforation. Relative contraindications include symptomatic hiatal hernia, esophagitis, coagulopathy, esophageal varices, and unexplained upper gastrointestinal bleeding.

You place an arterial line with the patient awake, and you are now ready to induce the patient.

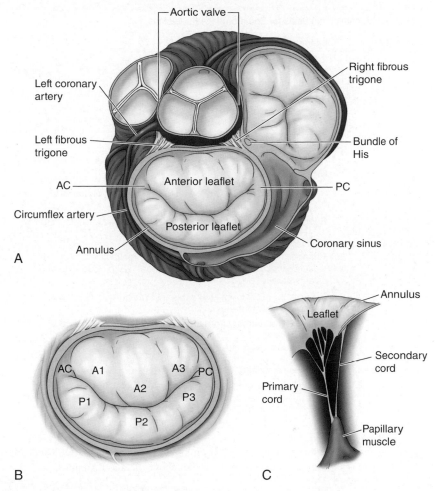

Fig. 18.1 Anatomy of the mitral valve. (A) Mitral valve shown in relationship to other cardiac structures. (B) *En face*, or surgeon's view of the mitral valve. Scallops A1, A2, and A3 of the anterior leaflet labeled, as well as scallops P1, P2, and P3 of the posterior leaflet labeled. The anterior and posterior leaflets join at the anterior commissure (*AC*) and posterior commissure (*PC*). (C) Both leaflets are attached to chordae tendinae from both papillary muscles. (Modified from Sidebotham, D., Legget, M. E., & Sutton, T. (2011). The mitral valve. *Practical Perioperative Transesophageal Echocardiography*, 135–162. Fig. 9.1.)

What are your hemodynamic goals for this patient?

In severe mitral regurgitation, blood in the LV can flow forward across the aortic valve into the aortic root or backward across the mitral valve into the left atrium. The goal is to maximize forward flow and minimize regurgitant (i.e., backward) flow. This can be accomplished by reducing afterload (i.e., systemic vascular resistance) and maintaining a normal or elevated heart rate.

For every valvular pathology, hemodynamics must be carefully monitored and treated to optimize cardiac output and blood pressure. Table 18.1 lists hemodynamic goals for common valvular pathologies. These goals apply for both cardiac and noncardiac surgery.

Induction and intubation are uneventful. You place the TEE probe, and you see the image shown in Fig. 18.2.

TABLE 18.1 ■ Hemodynamic Goals for Common Valvular Lesions

Valvular Pathology	Explanation of Hemodynamic Goals

Aortic stenosis	• Left ventricle (LV) hypertrophy is common
	  • ↓LV compliance → atrial contraction is important for LV filling → **maintain sinus rhythm and euvolemia**
	  • More myocardium to perfuse → high heart rate (HR) will worsen oxygen supply/demand relationship by reducing diastolic perfusion time and increasing myocardial oxygen demand → **avoid tachycardia**
	  • Perfusion of LV reliant on diastolic blood pressure → **maintain or increase afterload**
	• Fixed stroke volume, so bradycardia can cause hypotension → **avoid severe bradycardia**

Aortic regurgitation	• Regurgitant flow occurs during diastole → **maintain higher HR** to limit diastolic time for regurgitant flow • **Reduce afterload** and **maintain contractility** to augment forward flow

Mitral stenosis	• High resistance to flow across mitral valve
	  • **Maintain sinus rhythm** to maintain atrial contraction
	  • Tachycardia will limit diastolic filling time → ↓LV preload → **avoid tachycardia**
	• Fluid accumulation in left atrium (LA) and into pulmonary circulation can cause pulmonary hypertension
	  • **Avoid hypercarbia and hypoxia**, which can worsen pulmonary hypertension
	  • **Avoid fluid overload**

Mitral regurgitation	• **Decrease afterload** to augment forward flow • Regurgitant flow occurs during systole → **maintain higher HR** to limit systolic time for regurgitant flow and diastolic time for overfilling LV

What structures are visible?

Fig. 18.2 shows the midesophageal long axis view on TEE. The posterior mitral leaflet (the P2 scallop in this view) is shown with the body of the leaflet above the mitral annulus.

Is the image shown in Fig. 18.2 taken during systole or diastole? How can you tell?

This image was taken during systole. Notice the aortic valve is open and the mitral valve is closed but prolapsing. Both of these findings suggest that the ventricle is ejecting, which occurs during systole.

You turn on color doppler imaging, and you see the image in Fig. 18.3.

How do you interpret this?

There is a large regurgitant jet (the blue, yellow, and red region) across the mitral valve, consistent with severe mitral regurgitation. The mechanism of the regurgitation helps to determine the direction of the jet, and vice versa. In this case, the cause of the regurgitation is prolapse of the posterior leaflet. When the regurgitation is due to a prolapsing leaflet, the regurgitant jet is directed away from the prolapsing leaflet. In this case, the regurgitant jet is directed anteriorly, and that is consistent with prolapse of the posterior leaflet.

After induction of anesthesia, the rhythm strip shows the pattern in Fig. 18.4. This is a change from preoperatively.

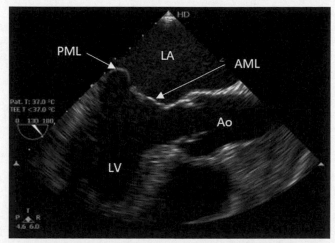

Fig. 18.2 Midesophageal long-axis view on transesophageal echocardiogram *(TEE)* showing prolapse of the P2 scallop of the posterior mitral leaflet (PML). *AML*, Anterior mitral leaflet; *Ao*, aorta; *LA*, left atrium, *LV*, left ventricle. (Modified from Sidebotham, D., Legget, M. E., & & Sutton, T. The mitral valve. *Practical perioperative transesophageal echocardiography*, 135–162. Fig. 9.16.)

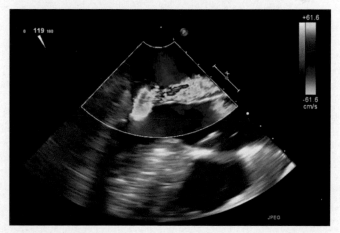

Fig. 18.3 Midesophageal long-axis view on transesophageal echocardiogram *(TEE)* with color flow Doppler showing a large regurgitant jet across the mitral valve during systole. As expected with prolapse of the posterior mitral leaflet, the jet is directed anteriorly, toward the aortic valve (right side of the image). (Modified from Wiener, P. C., Friend, E. J., & Bhargav, R. [2020]. Color doppler splay: A clue to the presence of significant mitral regurgitation. *Journal of the American Society of Echocardiography, 33*(10), 1212–1219.e1. Captured from Supplemental Video 8.)

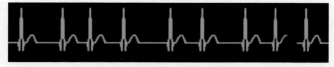

Fig. 18.4 Rhythm strip showing irregularly spaced narrow QRS complexes without P waves consistent with atrial fibrillation. (MedSimLearning.com. Accessed June 20, 2021.)

What is going on?

The rhythm strip shows irregularly spaced QRS complexes without P waves. This is consistent with atrial fibrillation. Atrial fibrillation is due to random and uncoordinated atrial activity. Unlike sinus rhythm, where the ventricle is activated at regular intervals, atrial fibrillation causes ventricular activation at random intervals.

STEP 1, 2, 3 PEARLS

Treatment goals for acute symptomatic atrial fibrillation include slowing the ventricular rate with β-blockers, calcium channel blockers, or digoxin in addition to cardioversion with amiodarone, procainamide, or synchronized electrical cardioversion.

Why do patients with mitral regurgitation tend to develop atrial fibrillation?

Chronic mitral regurgitation leads to increased left atrial volume. Over time, the stretching of the wall of the left atrium can cause arrhythmias such as atrial fibrillation.

The surgeon has performed sternotomy and asks for full-dose heparin to be given in anticipation of going on cardiopulmonary bypass (CPB).

What is the mechanism of action of heparin? What is the typical dose of heparin for CPB?

Heparin binds to and augments the activity of antithrombin III, which inactivates thrombin and clotting factors IX and X. This ultimately inhibits the conversion of fibrinogen to fibrin, thereby inhibiting clot formation. The typical dose of heparin is usually 300–400 units/kg.

Can heparin cause a low platelet count?

Heparin is associated with thrombocytopenia via two mechanisms.

The first mechanism is not immune mediated and results in a decrease in platelet count during the first 2 days of heparin administration. Platelet count typically normalizes without having to discontinue heparin.

The second mechanism is less common and is often referred to as heparin-induced thrombocytopenia (HIT). HIT is an immune-mediated phenomenon wherein antibodies are formed against heparin-platelet factor 4 complexes, resulting in a 50% decrease in platelet count 5–10 days after heparin is initiated. Diagnosis of HIT is typically achieved with a functional assay.

STEP 2, 3 PEARL

Patients with HIT are at elevated risk for intravascular thrombosis, which can lead to stroke, myocardial infarction, or ischemic injury to other organs. Patients with suspected HIT should not receive heparin or low-molecular-weight heparin (LMWH).

Three minutes after heparin has been administered, you run an activated clotting time (ACT) assay on a sample of the patient's blood.

What is ACT?

ACT is a point-of-care (i.e., done in the operating room, not in the laboratory) assay that measures clot formation via the intrinsic and common pathways. It is used as a measure of anticoagulation after heparinization.

The ACT is 180 seconds. Is this adequate to initiate CPB?

No, the ACT should be at least 400 seconds (some institutions have higher ACT requirements) prior to going on bypass due to the risk of clot formation in the bypass circuit with inadequate anticoagulation. Normal baseline ACT (in the absence of heparin) is typically 90–120 seconds.

Why did the ACT only increase by a small amount despite a full dose of heparin?
Heparin resistance is defined as inadequate increase in ACT despite an adequate dose of heparin (and adequate heparin concentration—a separate assay). Some causes of heparin resistance include

- Venous thromboembolism/pulmonary embolism
- Congenital antithrombin III deficiency
- Cirrhosis of the liver
- Nephrotic syndrome
- Disseminated intravascular coagulopathy
- Recent administration of heparin (i.e., heparin infusion preoperatively)

What will you do to achieve adequate anticoagulation prior to going on bypass?
Start by giving an additional dose of heparin. If this is ineffective, the patient likely requires antithrombin III supplementation. Transfusion of fresh frozen plasma (FFP), which contains antithrombin III, or recombinant antithrombin III may be effective.

> You give an additional dose of heparin and 2 units of FFP, and the patient's ACT is now 600 seconds.

What are the next steps prior to initiation of CPB?
After heparin is administered, the next steps involve placement of the arterial and venous cannulas by the surgeon. Typically, the arterial cannula is placed first. The arterial cannula is usually placed in the ascending aorta. The venous cannula(s) will be placed in the superior vena cava, inferior vena cava, and/or right atrium.

What are your hemodynamic goals during arterial cannulation? Why is hemodynamic stability important during this time? What are common complications associated with aortic cannulation?
During aortic cannulation, it is important to maintain a systolic blood pressure less than 110 mm Hg. The risk of aortic dissection increases significantly with blood pressure greater than this. Other potential complications include cannula malposition (e.g., into the head and neck vessels), hemorrhage, and embolism from plaque disruption.

> Placement of arterial and venous cannulas is uneventful, and CPB is initiated.

Describe the basic components of the CPB circuit.
Once arterial and venous cannulas are placed and an adequate ACT is achieved, drainage of blood through the venous cannula collects blood in a reservoir at the CPB machine. This blood is then transported through a heat exchanger, oxygenator membrane, and a filter. Carbon dioxide is removed. Anesthesia gas can be administered through the CPB machine. The blood is also pressurized to arterial pressure (the flow is not pulsatile, so only a mean arterial pressure will be measured) before being returned to the patient through the arterial cannula. Additional components of the CPB circuit include the pump sucker which allows for suctioned blood from the surgical field to return to the venous reservoir, vents to decompress the heart, and cannulas to deliver cardioplegia (see Fig. 18.5).

When can you turn off the ventilator?
Once the flow through the CPB circuit has reached the desired level, usually corresponding to a cardiac index of approximately 2.5 L/min/m^2, the perfusionist will announce that the CPB circuit is running at full flow. It is safe to discontinue ventilation at this time (remember, oxygen is added and CO_2 is removed via the CPB machine). Delivery of inhalational anesthetic via the vaporizer on the anesthesia machine is also discontinued at this time. Volatile anesthetics are administered through the CPB circuit.

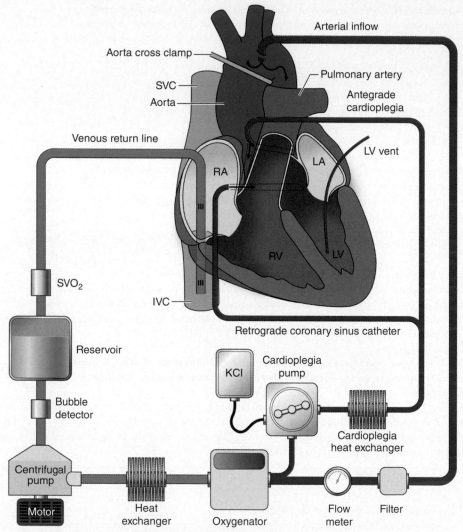

Fig. 18.5 Cardiopulmonary bypass (CPB) circuit. Blood is trained into the venous reservoir. It is then pressurized, heated or cooled, and oxygenated, and CO_2 is removed, prior to returning to the patient. Anesthesia gas may also be added. The aortic cross clamp is placed between the antegrade cardioplegia cannula and the arterial cannula. *SVC*, superior vena cava; *IVC*, inferior vena cav; *RA*, right atrium; *RV*, right ventricle; *LA*, left atrium; *LV*, left ventricle; *SVO2*, mixed venous oxygen; *KCl*, potassium chloride. (Basics of Anesthesia Fig. 25.3.)

What is cardiac index? How does it relate to cardiac output?

Cardiac output is the flow generated by the heart in a given amount of time. This is usually expressed in liters per minute (L/min). Patients of different sizes require different cardiac outputs. To account for this, cardiac index is cardiac output divided by body surface area (there are many formulas to estimate body surface area). A normal cardiac index is 2.2–2.5 L/min/m².

The surgeon repairs the mitral valve and asks if we can start weaning from CPB.

What are the major criteria that must be satisfied prior to weaning CPB?
There are multiple factors that should be evaluated prior to weaning CPB:
- Patient's core temperature is normal (36°C–37°C)
- Electrolytes are within normal range
- Hemoglobin greater than 8 g/dL
- Heart rhythm, rate, and blood pressure are stable and within the desired ranges (with or without infusions of vasoactive or inotropic medications or external pacing)
- Cardiac function is acceptable (again, with or without inotropic medications or mechanical support devices)
- The results of surgical interventions are acceptable (i.e., the mitral regurgitation has resolved)
- There is no air in the heart

Prior to coming off CPB, resume ventilation and ensure that gas exchange is adequate. Lastly, make sure that the patient is adequately anesthetized to avoid intraoperative awareness and recall during this period.

What should you look for on TEE following mitral valve repair?
It is important to assess the repair prior to weaning CPB. Look for regurgitation, stenosis, or left ventricular outflow obstruction due to systolic anterior motion (SAM) of the anterior leaflet of the mitral valve. Residual trace or mild regurgitation is common after valve repair; however, if the regurgitation is moderate or severe, it may be necessary to arrest the heart again (i.e., give more cardioplegia) and modify the repair. It is also important to assess the ventricular function by both visual inspection and with the TEE.

It is good practice to do a full TEE examination to confirm that no other structures were inadvertently damaged.

> The postrepair TEE shows only trace mitral regurgitation. The perfusionist gradually decreases the flow on the CPB circuit, and the patient successfully separates from CPB. Shortly after cessation of CPB, the blood pressure drops to 54/30 mm Hg.

What is going on?
The differential diagnosis of hypotension in the post-CPB period is listed in Table 18.2.

The TEE is shown in Fig. 18.6. How should you treat the patient's hypotension based on these findings?
This image is a transgastric midpapillary short-axis view of the LV in end-diastole and end-systole. The left ventricular volume appears to be reduced in both images, suggesting that the patient is hypovolemic. Treat with volume. This is usually done by the perfusionist, who can rapidly administer volume through the arterial cannula.

> The blood pressure improves after bolus of 500 mL of blood from the CPB reservoir. Left ventricular systolic function appears moderately depressed. You begin an infusion of epinephrine to improve contractility.

Why can ventricular function worsen following mitral valve repairs or replacement?
Patients may develop worsened left ventricular function following mitral repair or replacement due to an increase in the effective afterload against which the ventricle must eject. In severe mitral regurgitation, the ventricle can eject blood forward across the aortic valve into the high-pressure aortic root, or backward across the mitral valve into the low-pressure left atrium. After mitral valve repair or replacement, the ventricle can only eject forward into the high-pressure aortic root. This can cause a reduction in ejection fraction.

TABLE 18.2 ■ Etiologies and Management of Post–Cardiopulmonary Bypass Hypotension

Etiology	Comments
Surgical complication	This can be residual disease (e.g., residual severe mitral regurgitation), injury to other structure (e.g., inadvertent suture ligation of a coronary artery causing ischemia), or graft failure (e.g., suture failure). This usually requires a return to cardiopulmonary bypass (CPB) for repair.
Hypovolemia	Underfilled ventricles on transesophageal echocardiogram (TEE). Treat with volume administration. Communicate with the surgeon as to whether there is significant surgical bleeding.
Vasoplegia	Hyperdynamic, underfilled left ventricle (LV). May have high cardiac output. Treat with vasopressors and volume.
Coronary air embolism	Regional wall motion abnormalities on TEE and ST segment changes on rhythm strip. Treat by augmenting afterload with vasopressors. Nitroglycerin is a coronary vasodilator and may be helpful. In extreme cases, this may cause ventricular failure and necessitate return to CPB.
Global heart failure	Dilated, hypokinetic, or akinetic right ventricle and/or LV. Treat with inotropes. May need to reinitiate CPB.
Left ventricular outflow tract obstruction	After mitral valve repair, most commonly occurs when the anterior leaflet of the mitral valve gets "sucked" into the left ventricular outflow tract during systole, causing mitral regurgitation and decreased stroke volume. Treat with volume, vasopressors, and negative chronotropes (e.g., β-blockers).
Arrhythmia	Ventricular arrhythmias such as ventricular tachycardia and ventricular fibrillation can occur after CPB. These will require defibrillation, which can be performed by the surgeon using internal paddles placed directly on the heart. Especially in elderly patients or those with a thick, noncompliant ventricle, atrial fibrillation can cause hypotension. This requires synchronized cardioversion. Lidocaine, magnesium, and amiodarone may be helpful in preventing or treating arrhythmias. Make sure the patient is adequately rewarmed prior to weaning CPB.

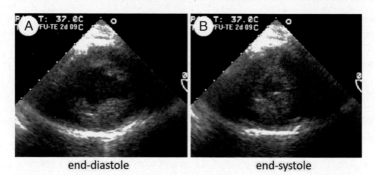

end-diastole   end-systole

Fig. 18.6   Transgastric midpapillary short-axis views of the left ventricle (LV) in end-diastole (A) and end-systole (B) with small LV cross-sectional areas indicative of severe hypovolemia. (Modified from Barclay, D. K., Royster, R. L., & Butterworth, J. [2007]. Rapid recovery of left-ventricular function after intraoperative conversion of atrial fibrillation. *Journal of Cardiothoracic and Vascular Anesthesia, 21*(1), 160–162. Modified from Fig. 2.)

STEP 1 PEARL

Epinephrine and norepinephrine are endogenous catecholamines and direct sympathetic agonists. They bind G protein–coupled receptors (GPCRs). Four GPCRs are most clinically relevant: α_1, α_2, β_1, and β_2. Epinephrine is an agonist of α_1, α_2, β_1, and β_2 that causes vasoconstriction (via α_1 agonism), increased heart rate and contractility (via β_1 agonism), and bronchodilation and increased blood flow to skeletal muscle (via β_2 agonism). Norepinephrine acts primarily on α_1 receptors and is a potent vasoconstrictor. Norepinephrine has some β_1 agonism, but this is less than its α_1 effect.

The patient's hemodynamics stabilize with the epinephrine infusion. You begin to administer prot-amine to reverse the heparin and announce that protamine administration has started. Shortly after, the blood pressure drops significantly.

What is going on?

This is consistent with a protamine reaction. There are several types of protamine reactions that can occur:

- Systemic hypotension due to histamine release and vasodilation.
- Anaphylactoid or anaphylactic reactions. The risk is increased in patients with previous exposure to protamine or neutral protamine Hagedorn (NPH) insulin. Patients with fish allergies are also at increased risk.
- Pulmonary hypertension possibly leading to right ventricular failure and cardiovascular collapse.

Protamine reactions are more likely to occur if large amounts of protamine are infused rapidly; thus a slower administration over 5–10 minutes is ideal. Mild hypotension is usually responsive to vasoconstrictors and judicious fluid administration, but severe refractory hypotension may require return to CPB. *If you have to emergently reinitiate CPB any time after protamine administration, you must give heparin.*

The blood pressure improves with a bolus of norepinephrine. You announce that half of the total protamine dose has been given.

Why is it important to communicate protamine administration with the perfusionist and surgeon?

Once protamine administration has started, it is important for the perfusionist and surgeon to be aware of how much has been given. Depending on the institution, the perfusionist may turn off the pump suckers either as soon as protamine administration begins or when half the dose has been given. The reason for this is to avoid collecting protamine in the CPB circuit, which could precipitate catastrophic clotting in the circuit should you have to reinitiate CPB.

The surgeons also coordinate removal of cannulas with protamine administration, usually starting with removing the venous cannula(s). The arterial cannula is removed after either half or all of the protamine is given.

It has been 15 minutes since protamine was given, and the surgeon states that the patient is very "Oozy." The ACT of a blood sample drawn after protamine was administered (i.e., Postprotamine ACT) was near the patient's baseline.

Why might the patient be coagulopathic? What should you do?

Patients tend to develop coagulopathy following CPB for a few reasons. The interaction of blood with the bypass circuit activates and damages platelets, activates the coagulation cascade, and causes hyperfibrinolysis. In addition, cooling during CPB causes coagulopathy because clotting factors are not as effective at lower temperatures. Longer bypass runs are associated with increased risk of coagulopathy and greater likelihood of transfusion of blood products.

Check coagulation studies such as prothrombin time/international normalized ratio (PT/INR), partial thromboplastin time (PTT), platelet count, and fibrinogen. Viscoelastic testing (i.e., thromboelastogram [TEG]) may also be beneficial at this time because these tests provide infor-mation on both the coagulation cascade and fibrinolytic system (see Case 20).

Coagulation studies show that the INR is 2.3. You transfuse two units of FFP, and the coagulopa-thy improves. As the surgeons pull the sternum closed, the blood pressure begins to decrease again.

What is going on?

Chest closure can cause hypotension. Closure of the sternum may compress the heart and great vessels, which can reduce venous return and hence preload. In patients who have undergone coronary artery bypass grafting, ischemia due to kinking of bypass graft and subsequent myocardial dysfunction can occur during chest closure. Always check the rhythm strip for ST changes in this context. TEE is useful to assess for causes of hypotension such as hypovolemia, ventricular dysfunction, new regional wall motion abnormalities, or pericardial tamponade.

Depending on the findings on TEE, treat with fluid administration, vasopressors, or inotropes or ask the surgeons to reopen the chest to relieve the compression.

BEYOND THE PEARLS

- The tricuspid valve is supported by papillary muscles in the right ventricle.
- Primary chordae tendinae are attached from the papillary muscle to the free end of the mitral valve leaflet. Secondary chordae tendinae are attached from the papillary muscle to the body of the leaflet. Tertiary chordae tendinae attach from the free wall of the LV to the base of the leaflet.
- Due to lack of coordinated atrial contraction, patients with atrial fibrillation are at risk for blood stasis which may result in clot formation and embolization. If clot forms in the left atrium, patients may suffer from an embolic stroke and usually require anticoagulation.
- Chronic atrial fibrillation is typically managed with pharmacologic agents for rate control and anticoagulation. Check for thrombus in the heart with a TEE prior to cardioversion of a patient with chronic atrial fibrillation.
- Patients with preexisting pulmonary hypertension, chronic mitral valve disease, or tricuspid regurgitation may develop right ventricular dysfunction after cardiac surgery.
- Patients with a history of vasectomy may also be at increased risk of anaphylactoid protamine reaction.

References

Feinman, J. W., Savino, J. S., & Weiss, S. J. (2017). Decision making and perioperative transesophageal echo-cardiography. In J. A. Kaplan, G. J. T. Augoustides, G. R. Manecke, T. Maus & D. L. Reich (Eds.), *Kaplan's cardiac anesthesia* (Vol. 16, 7th ed., pp. 635–662). Philadelphia, PA: Elsevier.

Kahn, R. A., Maus, T., Salgo, I., Weiner, M. M., & Sherman, S. K. (2017). Basic intraoperative transesophageal echocardiography. In J. A. Kaplan, G. J. T. Augoustides, G. R. Manecke, T. Maus & D. L. Reich (Eds.), *Kaplan's cardiac anesthesia* (Vol. 14, 7th ed., pp. 427–504). Philadelphia, PA: Elsevier.

Panigrahi, A. K., & Liu, L. L. (2020). Patient blood management: Coagulation. In M. A. Gropper, R. D. Miller, N. H. Cohen, L. I. Eriksson, L. A. Fleisher, K. Leslie, et al. (Eds.), *Miller's anesthesia* (Vol. 50, 9th ed., pp. 1579–1602.e7). Philadelphia, PA: Elsevier.

Paul, A., & Das, S. (2017). Valvular heart disease and anaesthesia. *Indian Journal of Anaesthesia, 61*(9), 721–727.

Sarwar, M. F., Searles, B. E., Stone, M. E., & Shore-Lesserson, L. (2020). Anesthesia for cardiac surgical procedures. In M. A. Gropper, R. D. Miller, N. H. Cohen, L. I. Eriksson, L. A. Fleisher, K. Leslie, et al. (Eds.), *Miller's anesthesia* (Vol. 54, 9th ed., pp. 1717–1814). Philadelphia, PA: Elsevier.

Shore-Lesserson, L., Enriquez, L. J., & Weitzel, N. (2017). Coagulation monitoring. In J. A. Kaplan, G. J. T. Augoustides, G. R. Manecke, T. Maus & D. L. Reich (Eds.), *Kaplan's cardiac anesthesia* (Vol. 19, 7th ed., pp. 698–727). Philadelphia, PA: Elsevier.

Wallace, A. (2018). Cardiovascular Disease. In M. C. Pardo & R. D. Miller (Eds.), *Basics of Anesthesia* (Vol. 25, pp. 415–449). Philadelphia, PA: Elsevier.

A 71-Year-Old Male With Exertional Angina

Tyler Gouvea ■ Paul Neil Frank

A 71-year-old male with exertional angina presents for coronary artery bypass grafting (CABG). Coronary artery catheterization shows high-grade stenosis of the left anterior descending artery (LAD), left circumflex artery (LCx), and right coronary artery (RCA). He had a myocardial infarction (MI) 10 years ago, and a drug-eluting stent (DES) was placed in his LAD at that time. He takes aspirin, metoprolol, and atorvastatin daily. In the preoperative area his vital signs are blood pressure 153/80 mm Hg, pulse 72/min, respirations 10/min, oxygenation 99% on room air, and temperature 35.9°C.

STEP 1 PEARL

Atorvastatin is an inhibitor of hydroxymethylglutaryl–coenzyme A (HMG CoA) reductase. This enzyme catalyzes the rate-limiting step in the conversion of HMG-CoA to mevalonate in the production of cholesterol.

What are the major arteries of the heart?

The arteries of the heart are known as the coronary arteries. The right and left main coronary arteries arise from the aorta at the level of the sinus of Valsalva, just above the aortic valve. The RCA courses circumferentially between the right atrium and right ventricle (RV) toward the posterior aspect of the heart. In the majority of patients, it gives rise to the posterior descending artery (PDA) on the posterior surface of the heart. This is known as right-dominant circulation. The left main coronary artery divides into the LAD and LCx. The LAD courses inferiorly along the anterior surface of the heart toward the cardiac apex, while the LCx courses circumferentially between the left atrium and left ventricle (LV) toward the posterior aspect of the heart. In the minority of patients, the PDA arises from the LCx instead of the RCA. This is known as left-dominant circulation. Normal right-dominant coronary anatomy is shown in Fig. 19.1.

What echocardiographic changes would you expect in the territory of the heart where the MI occurred 10 years ago?

The affected myocardium may not contract inward as much as healthy myocardium (i.e., hypokinesis) or at all (i.e., akinesis) during systole. It may also move outward (i.e., dyskinesis) during systole. Infarcted territory may be thinner than healthy myocardium and may not thicken during systolic contraction. Thrombus may form over the infarcted territory.

What are the possible complications of MI?

Complications from MI vary depending on the time since the MI as well as the location and extent of the MI. Within the first 2 days of MI, the most common serious complication is arrhythmia (e.g., ventricular tachycardia or ventricular fibrillation). Involvement of the conduction system can also lead to bradycardia or complete heart block.

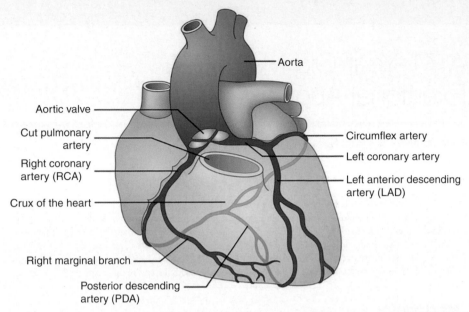

Fig. 19.1 Normal coronary anatomy showing the left main (LM) coronary artery giving rise to the left anterior descending (LAD) artery and left circumflex artery (LCx) and the RCA giving rise to the PDA. *SVC*, superior vena cava; *RA*, right atrium, *IVC*, inferior vena cava; *RV*, right ventricle; *LA*, left atrium; *LV*, left venricle; *SvO₂*, mixed venous oxygen saturation. (Pedigo, R. A., [2017]. Cardiology. In T. X. O'Connell, R. A. Pedigo, & T. E. Blair (Eds.), *Crush step 1: The ultimate USMLE step 1 review* [pp. 605–636]. Philadelphia, PA: Elsevier. Modified from Fig. 8.3.)

After several days, mechanical complications (e.g., compromise of the physical integrity of cardiac structures) can arise. These include free wall rupture, ventricular septal defect, and papillary muscle rupture. These complications can cause acute heart failure or pericardial tamponade.

Several weeks after MI, there is a risk of aneurysmal dilation of the infarcted territory.

What is the mechanism of action of aspirin? Why is this patient taking it?

Aspirin is an irreversible inhibitor of the cyclooxygenase (COX) enzymes. One of the effects of aspirin is inhibition of platelet function. This reduces the risk of in-stent thrombosis in patients who have coronary stents.

STEP 1 PEARL

Ordinarily, phospholipases generate arachidonic acid from phospholipids of the cell membrane. Cyclooxygenase (COX) enzymes convert arachidonic acid to prostacyclins and thromboxane A2. Thromboxane A2 enhances platelet aggregation. Therefore inhibition of COX enzymes by aspirin inhibits platelet aggregation.

Should the patient take his metoprolol on the morning of surgery?

Yes. He should take his usual dose of β-blocker on the morning of surgery.

What are the determinants of myocardial oxygen supply?

Myocardial oxygen supply is determined by the oxygen content of arterial blood (CaO_2) and by coronary blood flow.

CaO_2 is determined primarily by hemoglobin concentration (Hb) and hemoglobin saturation (SaO_2). Arterial oxygen tension (PaO_2) also makes a small contribution. CaO_2 is given by

$$CaO_2 = 1.34 \times Hb \times SaO_2 + 0.003 \times PaO_2$$

Coronary blood flow is determined by coronary perfusion pressure and coronary vascular resistance.

How is coronary perfusion pressure calculated?

For any flow to occur, there must be a pressure gradient, and blood will flow from high pressure to low pressure. In the case of coronary blood flow, blood flows from the aortic root through the coronary arteries. The pressure within each chamber of the heart is transmitted to the walls of the chamber and to the nearby coronary arteries.

During systolic ejection, the pressure inside the LV is equal to or greater than the pressure in the aortic root (this is because LV contraction *is* the source of systolic blood pressure). This LV intracavitary systolic pressure is transmitted to the associated coronary arteries. During systole, the aortic root pressure and the coronary artery pressure are equal, and there is no pressure gradient to drive blood flow. *Therefore LV coronary blood flow does not occur during systole and occurs only during diastole.*

The perfusion pressure for the LV is determined by diastolic pressures: aortic diastolic blood pressure (AoDBP) and LV end diastolic pressure (LVEDP). LV perfusion pressure is given by

$$LV\ perfusion\ pressure = AoDBP - LVEDP$$

Unlike the LV, the RV is perfused during systole and diastole. This is because the pressure within the RV is lower than aortic root pressure (except in cases of extreme pulmonary hypertension) during both systole and diastole.

What are the determinants of myocardial oxygen demand?

Myocardial oxygen demand is determined by heart rate, wall stress, and contractility.

What determines wall stress?

Wall stress increases with intracavitary pressure and with distention of the ventricle, and wall stress decreases as wall thickness increases. These relationships are articulated by the Law of Laplace

$$wall\ stress = \frac{(intracavitary\ pressure) \times (chamber\ radius)}{2 \times wall\ thickness}$$

Intracavitary pressure increases with afterload—the ventricle has to squeeze harder to overcome higher afterload. Chamber radius increases with preload—the more volume in the ventricle, the larger the radius of the ventricle will be. Therefore, to minimize myocardial oxygen demand, decrease heart rate, preload, afterload, and contractility.

The caveat here is that afterload also contributes to oxygen supply by augmenting coronary perfusion pressure during diastole. Maintenance or even increase in afterload will also prevent baroreceptor-mediated tachycardia. This may be helpful in optimizing the oxygen supply-demand relationship.

What special anesthesia setup is required for a cardiac case?

In addition to American Society of Anesthesiologists (ASA) standard monitors (see Case 14):
- 5-lead electrocardiogram (ECG)
- transesophageal echocardiogram (TEE) machine and probe

- temperature probe (e.g., bladder, nasopharyngeal)
- cerebral oximeters
- invasive monitoring lines
  - arterial catheter
  - central venous catheter (CVC)
  - pulmonary artery catheter (PAC)
- hemodynamic medications
  - inotrope (e.g., epinephrine, dobutamine)
  - vasopressor (e.g., norepinephrine, vasopressin)
  - vasodilators (e.g., clevidipine, nitroglycerin)
  - anticholinergic (e.g., atropine)
  - antiarrhythmic (e.g., amiodarone)
- heparin
- antifibrinolytic (e.g., aminocaproic acid)
- transcutaneous pacing/defibrillation pads
- blood products
- temporary external pacemaker box

How is a 5-lead ECG helpful?

A 5-lead ECG is useful to monitor for arrhythmias and ischemia. Typically lead II will be used to evaluate for the presence or absence of P waves, useful in identifying atrial fibrillation. Meanwhile, lead V_5 will be used to identify changes in QRS wave and ST segment morphology indicative of ischemia. The use of lead V_5 increases detection to greater than 80% of ischemic events.

When should the arterial catheter be placed?

Induction of anesthesia and laryngoscopy for intubation can cause significant hemodynamic changes—hypotension with induction, and hypertension and tachycardia with laryngoscopy. In patients with significant cardiovascular disease, invasive blood pressure monitoring via an arterial catheter during this time allows the anesthesiologist to quickly identify and treat hemodynamic changes. Therefore an arterial line should be placed *prior* to induction of anesthesia. Depending on the patient, it may be safe to give a small dose of benzodiazepine or other sedative prior to placement of the arterial line. It is good practice to infiltrate the area with local anesthetic prior to placing an invasive line in an awake patient.

What are the contraindications and risks of arterial line placement?

Contraindications include infection or burn at the planned insertion site, intravascular stent, or synthetic vascular material, vascular insufficiency, and lack of collateral circulation. In CABG, the patient's superficial leg veins are most commonly used as bypass graft. However, the radial artery may be harvested as a bypass graft. This is usually taken from the patient's nondominant hand. It is important to speak with the surgeon prior to placing an arterial line to confirm whether or not they plan on harvesting radial artery.

Complications of arterial line placement include thrombosis, distal ischemia, infection, bleeding, and arterial dissection.

What are the common sites for arterial catheter placement?

Common sites for arterial line placement include:

- radial (most common)
- ulnar
- brachial
- axillary

- femoral
- dorsalis pedis
- aortic root (placed intraoperatively by surgeon)

How do you place a radial arterial line?
The steps for radial artery catheterization are:

1. Position the patient's wrist in extension and secure the hand with tape to the arm board (Fig. 19.2A).
2. Sterilize the volar surface of the wrist using alcohol or other prep solution.
3. Apply a sterile drape or surround the area with sterile towels.
4. Use palpation or ultrasound to identify the radial artery. It is usually found between the radial tuberosity and the flexor tendons.
5. If the patient is awake, infiltrate the area with local anesthetic.
6. Insert the needle and catheter into the skin at an angle of 30 degrees or less aimed proximally along the long axis of the artery (see Fig. 19.2B). Once there is blood return in the catheter, there are two options. Either (1) hold the needle still and thread the guidewire and then catheter into the artery or (2) continue advancing the needle and catheter until the tip of the needle is through the back wall of the artery and blood return in the catheter stops (this is known as the through-and-through technique).

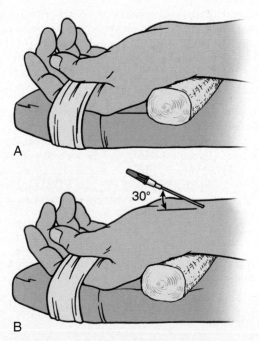

Fig. 19.2   (A) Proper arm and wrist positioning for radial arterial catheterization. The hand is supinated and the wrist is extended. (B) The needle and catheter are inserted into the skin at an angle of no more than 30 degrees. (Fowler, G. C., & Landen, D. A. [2020]. Arterial puncture and percutaneous arterial line placement. In G. C. Fowler, B. A. Choby, D. Iyengar, T. X. O'Connell, F. G. O'connor, B. Reddy, et al. (Eds.), *Pfenninger and Fowler's procedures for primary care* [4th ed., Chapter 225, pp. 1499–1509]. Philadelphia, PA: Elsevier. Fig. 225.10.)

7. If you chose option (1), remove the needle and attach the transducer tubing to the end of the catheter. Secure the catheter with suture or tape, then apply a sterile dressing.

8. If you chose option (2), hold the catheter still and remove the needle. Slowly withdraw the catheter until pulsatile blood returns. Advance a guidewire through the catheter and into the artery. Advance the catheter over the guidewire. Remove the guidewire and attach the transducer tubing to the end of the catheter. Secure the catheter with suture or tape, then apply a sterile dressing.

What are the hemodynamic goals for induction and intubation for this patient?

This patient has coronary artery disease. It is critical to maintain adequate myocardial oxygen supply and minimize myocardial oxygen demand. Avoid tachycardia during laryngoscopy and intubation. It is also important to maintain afterload.

Opioid (e.g., fentanyl) administered several minutes before induction will blunt the tachycardic response to laryngoscopy. Slow administration of hypnotic (e.g., propofol, etomidate), while closely monitoring the arterial pressure, will allow for a smooth and safe induction. Mask ventilation with anesthesia gas (e.g., sevoflurane) will deepen the anesthetic and further blunt the response to laryngoscopy while maintaining relatively stable hemodynamics. Short-acting β-blocker (e.g., esmolol) and vasopressor (e.g., phenylephrine) should be readily available.

In patients with reduced cardiac output, as in the case of poor ventricular function, intravenous anesthetics will take effect more slowly. Be patient when administering intravenous anesthetics to avoid overdose and hypotension. Conversely, inhaled anesthetic agents take effect more quickly in patients with reduced cardiac output.

Once the patient becomes apneic, mask ventilate to avoid hypercapnia and hypoxia. Hypoxia and hypercapnia will reduce myocardial oxygen supply and increase pulmonary vascular resistance, which is problematic in patients with poor right ventricular function.

> Induction and intubation are uneventful. The TEE probe is inserted, and the anterior wall of the LV is hypokinetic.

What coronary artery supplies this territory?

This is in the distribution of the LAD.

The LAD supplies the anterior two-thirds of the interventricular septum, the anterior left ventricular wall from the base through the apex, and the anterolateral papillary muscle (sometimes called the anterior papillary muscle). The LCx supplies the lateral left ventricular wall and the anterolateral papillary muscle. The RCA (including the PDA) supplies the RV, the inferior third of the interventricular septum, and the posteromedial papillary muscle (sometimes called the posterior papillary muscle). This is illustrated in Fig. 19.3.

STEP 1 PEARL

Papillary muscles arise from the left ventricular wall and contract during systole to hold the leaflets of the mitral valve shut (see Case 18).

> After sternotomy and harvesting of bypass grafts, the surgeon asks for heparin to be administered, and you give heparin 300 U/kg.

What will you need to do next?

Three to 5 minutes after administration of heparin, an activated clotting time (ACT) is measured to ensure adequate anticoagulation for cardiopulmonary bypass.

What ACT is adequate for cardiopulmonary bypass?

This varies somewhat by institution, but the threshold is usually an ACT of at least 400 seconds.

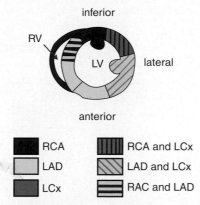

Fig. 19.3 Perfusion territory of each coronary artery. Diagram of the heart corresponding to the transgastric midpapillary short axis view on transesophageal echocardiogram (TEE). Notice inferior is at the top of the image and anterior is at the bottom of the image. *LAD*, Left anterior descending artery; *LCx*, left circumflex artery; *LV*, left ventricle; *RCA*, right coronary artery; *RV*, right ventricle. (Krajewski, M. L., & Mahmood, F. [2020]. Perioperative echocardiography. In M. A. Gropper, R. D. Miller, N. H. Cohen, L. I. Eriksson, L. A. Fleisher, K. Leslie, et al. (Eds.), *Miller's anesthesia* [9th ed., Chapter 37, pp. 1194–1230.e9]. Philadelphia, PA: Elsevier. Modified from Fig. 37.13.)

What is cardiopulmonary bypass?
Cardiopulmonary bypass is an extracorporeal (outside the body) circuit that allows for continued flow of blood through the body even in the absence of cardiac and pulmonary function. There are a wide variety of circuits and cannulation strategies, depending on the institution, the patient, and the operation. Fig. 19.4 shows a typical cardiopulmonary bypass setup for a CABG. The main elements are:
- Venous blood is drained from the superior vena cava, right atrium, and/or inferior vena cava via the venous cannula(s) and enters a reservoir, essentially a collecting bucket for blood.
- Blood from the reservoir is heated or cooled, oxygenated, and pressurized. Carbon dioxide is removed. Anesthesia gas can be added.
- Blood then returns to the patient via an arterial inflow cannula in the ascending aorta.
- Cardioplegia is administered intermittently into the aortic root or coronary arteries (antegrade) or into the coronary sinus (retrograde). This is usually a high-potassium solution that maintains diastolic cardiac arrest.
- An LV vent drains blood from the LV and returns it to the cardiopulmonary bypass circuit to prevent LV distention, which increases myocardial oxygen demand.

What steps should be taken by the anesthesiologist prior to initiation of cardiopulmonary bypass?
Consider redosing neuromuscular blocker and amnestic agents (e.g., midazolam). Confirm with the perfusionist that they have sufficient volatile anesthetic in their vaporizer to ensure adequate depth of anesthesia. Make sure nitrous oxide (N_2O) is turned off to prevent expansion of any air bubbles (see Case 23).

If a PAC has been placed, withdraw it into the main pulmonary artery. This is necessary because decompression of the RV with cardiopulmonary bypass results in distal migration of the tip of the PAC. Withdrawing the PAC reduces the risk of pulmonary artery rupture that can occur with distal placement of the PAC tip.

Take note of baseline cerebral oximetry, urine output, and body temperature.

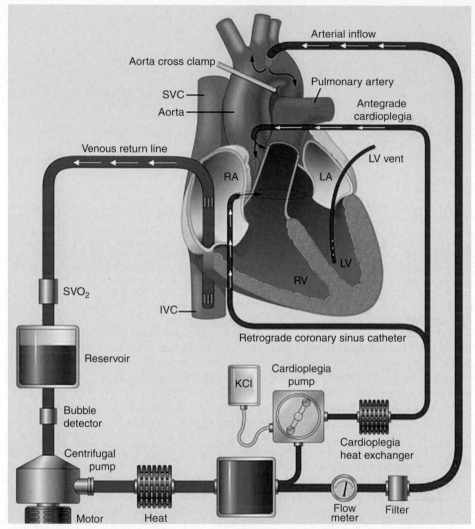

Fig. 19.4   Cardiopulmonary bypass circuit. Blood is drained from the patient via the venous return cannula positioned in the right atrium, superior vena cava, and/or inferior vena cava. From there it flows into the bypass machine, which includes a venous reservoir to sequester blood outside the patient's body, a centrifugal pump to pressurize blood, a heat exchanger to warm the blood, and an oxygenator to oxygenate the blood. Blood then returns to the patient via the arterial inflow cannula located in the ascending aorta or aortic arch. The cardioplegia pump delivers a concentrated solution of potassium, usually potassium chloride (KCl), to arrest the heart. (Wallace, A. [2018]. Cardiovascular disease. In M. C. Pardo & R. D. Miller (Eds.), *Basics of anesthesia* [pp. 415–449]. Philadelphia, PA: Elsevier.)

Which cannula is usually placed first?
The arterial inflow cannula, usually in the ascending aorta, is placed first.

What are your hemodynamic goals during aortic cannulation?
Maintain the systolic blood pressure less than 110 mm Hg or mean arterial pressure less than 70 mm Hg. The risk of aortic dissection with cannulation increases significantly with higher blood pressure.

Aortic cannulation is uneventful. During placement of the venous cannula in the right atrium, the blood pressure suddenly drops to 65/40 mm Hg.

What is going on?

Placement of the venous cannula sometimes requires the surgeon to compress the heart and great vessels to gain adequate exposure. This can precipitate a sudden drop in blood pressure. It is important to communicate with the surgeon and watch the surgical field closely during this time.

The surgeon releases pressure on the heart, and the blood pressure normalizes. The venous cannula is placed. The ACT is 460 seconds. What happens next?

The perfusionist will start the cardiopulmonary bypass pump, and blood will start flowing through the circuit.

What changes will you notice on patient monitor?

The arterial line waveform will become less pulsatile and almost flat. *This is because blood flow in the cardiopulmonary bypass circuit is nonpulsatile.* End-tidal carbon dioxide ($EtCO_2$) levels on the ventilator will decrease. Remember, the CO_2 that contributes to $EtCO_2$ comes from pulmonary blood flow. In cardiopulmonary bypass, there is no flow through the pulmonary circulation.

The surgeon places a cross clamp on the ascending aorta and asks for cardioplegia to be delivered via the cardioplegia cannula. What is cardioplegia? Why is it necessary?

Cardioplegia causes cessation of mechanical and electrical cardiac activity to produce a still surgical field.

Cardioplegia protects the myocardium from ischemic injury by arresting the heart in diastole, thereby reducing the heart's metabolic demand. *Remember, the heart is not perfused with oxygenated blood during CPB once the aortic cross-clamp is applied, so it is critical to reduce the myocardial oxygen demand as much as possible to minimize ischemic injury.*

Most cardioplegia solutions contain a high concentration of potassium, which depolarizes myocardial cells and stops electrical activity. This reduces the heart's oxygen consumption by approximately 90%.

How else is myocardial oxygen demand reduced?

As discussed earlier, wall distention increased oxygen demand. The left ventricular vent ensures that the LV is maximally decompressed (i.e., empty). In addition, the patient is cooled during bypass, which further reduces myocardial oxygen demand.

What are antegrade and retrograde cardioplegia?

Antegrade and retrograde refer to the site of administration and direction of the flow of cardioplegia solution relative to normal coronary blood flow. Antegrade cardioplegia is given into the aortic root (or directly into the opening of the coronary arteries in the aortic root, known as the coronary ostia). It travels in the same direction as normal coronary blood flow. Retrograde cardioplegia is given into the coronary sinus. It travels in the opposite direction as usual coronary blood flow.

STEP 1 PEARL

The normal course of blood flow to the heart is through the aortic valve into the aortic root, through the coronary ostia into the coronary arteries, ultimately into coronary veins and the coronary sinus, and into the right atrium.

A full dose of antegrade cardioplegia is administered. There is still electrical activity on rhythm strip. What is going on?
If it seems like the cardioplegia is not working, there are a few possible explanations. Confirm with the surgeon and perfusionist that cardioplegia solution is actually flowing and that the cardioplegia tubing is not clamped. Assuming cardioplegia solution is flowing, there are several patient factors that can complicate administration of antegrade cardioplegia.

If the patient has coronary artery disease, the same blockages in the coronary arteries that limit the flow of blood may limit the flow of cardioplegia, preventing it from reaching myocardium distal to the blockages. This can be overcome by administration of retrograde cardioplegia.

In the case of aortic regurgitation, cardioplegia given into the aortic root will flow back across the aortic valve into the chamber of the LV, and not into the coronary arteries. This can be overcome by administration of cardioplegia directly into the coronary ostia (still considered antegrade) or into the coronary sinus (i.e., retrograde).

After a few minutes of cardiopulmonary bypass, you notice the patient's face is newly plethoric. What is going on?
This is suggestive of a malpositioned venous cannula that is obstructing venous drainage from the superior vena cava. Ask the surgeon to reposition the cannula.

The surgeon repositions the venous cannula, and the patient's plethora resolves. What should you do during cardiopulmonary bypass?
Closely monitor the cerebral oximeters to ensure there is no drop in cerebral oxygenation. Watch the rhythm strip on the patient monitor to ensure there is no electrical activity, and check the TEE to ensure there is no cardiac motion. Either electrical activity or cardiac motion would suggest inadequate cardiac arrest and the need to redose cardioplegia. Check an arterial blood gas, usually every 30 to 60 minutes, and treat hyperglycemia and anemia as necessary. Monitor urine output. Occasionally, it may be necessary to start a vasopressor or vasodilator to maintain blood pressure in the desirable range during cardiopulmonary bypass. Coordinate this with the perfusionist.

In addition, the anesthesiologist must prepare for separation from cardiopulmonary bypass.

What should the anesthesiologist do to prepare for separation from cardiopulmonary bypass?
Prior to weaning cardiopulmonary bypass, the anesthesiologist should:
- Ensure any necessary blood products are in the room and checked.
- Prepare anticipated inotropes, vasopressors, and other hemodynamic drips.
- Prepare emergency bolus drugs.
- Check the temporary pacemaker box to ensure it has adequate battery and is functioning appropriately.
- Have a plan for protamine administration. Because premature administration of protamine can cause catastrophic clotting of the cardiopulmonary bypass circuit and patient death, institutions have developed different safety mechanisms to prevent accidental protamine administration. Some institutions store protamine outside the operating room and it is only brought into the room when it is safe to give protamine. Other institutions have protamine in a locked box by the anesthesia cart. Know where protamine is and how to get it.

After completing the bypass grafts, the surgeon removes the aortic cross-clamp. Now what?
Ideally the heart will quickly resume beating. Start hemodynamic drips as necessary. Check the patient monitor to ensure the patient is in a perfusing rhythm (ideally sinus rhythm) and not ventricular tachycardia or ventricular fibrillation. Check for widened QRS complexes and ST segment elevations or depressions.

As the heart resumes beating, the arterial pressure waveform will become more pulsatile. In coordination with the surgeon, give several large breaths via the ventilator circuit to recruit the patient's lungs and resume ventilation. Do a thorough TEE exam to rule out new abnormalities (i.e., make sure the surgeon did not inadvertently damage something).

Weaning of cardiopulmonary bypass and administration of protamine are uneventful. LV function is mildly reduced, and you start an infusion of dobutamine. The incision is closed, and you are preparing to transport the patient to the intensive care unit. He is intubated and sedated on an infusion of dexmedetomidine. During transport, his blood pressure begins to drop. What will you do?

Check the rhythm strip and other vital signs for other abnormalities that could contribute to hypotension (e.g., arrhythmia or hypoxia). A bolus of a vasoconstrictor or inotrope may be necessary. Hemodynamic infusions should then be checked to ensure that they are infusing properly.

When a patient will be transported from the operating room intubated and sedated, start the intravenous sedative that will be used for transport and make sure the anesthetic gas has been eliminated (check the expiratory concentration of anesthetic gas) prior to transport. This will allow you a chance to adjust the dose of sedative as necessary in the relative safety of the operating room prior to transport.

Postoperative transport can be a dangerous time for cardiac surgical patients, and preparation is essential. Since most patients remain intubated, have airway equipment available during transport should you have to reintubate after accidental extubation. Patients may also develop rapid hemodynamic changes; monitor vital signs continuously on a portable transport monitor and have emergency medications ready. Since many of these patients are on vasoactive infusions, make sure that the infusion pumps are working and have enough battery life and that the infusion lines are patent.

BEYOND THE PEARLS

- The anterolateral papillary muscle is supplied by both the LAD and LCx, so it is less susceptible to ischemic dysfunction compared with the posteromedial papillary muscle, which is supplied only by the RCA.
- Patients generally receive dual-antiplatelet therapy (DAPT) after placement of coronary stents. DAPT usually consists of low-dose aspirin and a $P2Y_{12}$ adenosine diphosphate (ADP) receptor inhibitor. It is important to know what kind of coronary stent a patient has received, as this will determine the minimum duration of DAPT before stopping the $P2Y_{12}$ ADP receptor inhibitor.
- Platelets lack nuclei, so they cannot produce COX enzymes. Since aspirin irreversibly inhibits COX enzymes, this inhibition lasts for the lifetime of the platelet, which is 5 to 9 days.
- In cardiac cases, heparin is an emergency medication. In the event of unexpected bleeding or heart failure, it may become necessary to initiate cardiopulmonary bypass emergently (i.e., crashing onto bypass). In this scenario, the first thing to do is to give full-dose heparin.
- Right ventricular dysfunction may occur following cardiopulmonary bypass. Given the anterior location of the RV within the chest, there is a risk for air emboli down the RCA, which can result in right ventricular dysfunction. The RV may not be as well protected during cardiopulmonary bypass due to inadequate cooling or inadequate administration of cardioplegia.

References

Atorvastatin Drug Monograph. Accessed January 12, 2021.

Grocott, H. P., & Stafford-Smith, M. (2017). Cardiopulmonary bypass management and organ protection. In J. A. Kaplan, G. J. T. Augoustides, G. R. Manecke, T. Maus, D. L. Reich (Eds.), *Kaplan's cardiac anesthesia* (Vol. *31*, 7th ed., pp. 1111–1161). Philadelphia, PA: Elsevier.

Mauri, L., & Bhatt, D. L. (2019). Percutaneous coronary intervention. In D. P. Zipes, P. Libby, R. O. Bonow, D. L. Mann, G. F. Tomaselli, E. Braunwald (Eds.), *Braunwald's heart disease: A textbook of cardiovascular medicine* (Vol. 62, 11th ed., pp. 1271–1294). Philadelphia, PA: Elsevier.

Shore-Lesserson, L., Enriquez, L. J., & Weitzel, N. (2017). Coagulation monitoring. In J. A. Kaplan, G. J. T. Augoustides, G. R. Manecke, T. Maus, D. L. Reich (Eds.), *Kaplan's cardiac anesthesia* (Vol. 19, 7th ed., pp. 698–727). Philadelphia, PA: Elsevier.

A 69-Year-Old Man Presenting With Stabbing Substernal Chest Pain Radiating to the Back

Gene Kurosawa ■ David Li

A 69-year-old man presents to the emergency department with stabbing substernal chest pain radiating to the back. Past medical history includes poorly controlled hypertension and a 40-pack-year smoking history. Vital signs show blood pressure 198/92 mm Hg, pulse rate 134/min, respiration rate 29/min, and oxygen saturation is 98% on room air. Physical exam reveals a man in acute distress, diaphoretic and clutching his chest in pain. A loud holodiastolic murmur is heard upon auscultation of the chest. Computed tomography angiogram (CTA) shown in Fig. 20.1 reveals an aortic dissection, and cardiothoracic surgery is emergently consulted.

What is the anatomy of the thoracic aorta?

The thoracic aorta consists of the aortic root, ascending aorta, aortic arch, and the descending thoracic aorta (Fig. 20.2). The aortic arch gives rise to several large branches that perfuse the head and upper extremities: the brachiocephalic artery, the left common carotid artery, and the left subclavian artery. The brachiocephalic artery take-off is the boundary between the ascending aorta and the aortic arch. The left subclavian artery take-off is the boundary between the aortic arch and the descending aorta.

STEP 1 PEARL

The aortic wall is comprised of three layers, from innermost to outermost: endothelium-lined intima, a thick tunica media, and the tunica adventitia (see Fig. 20.3). The endothelium-lined tunica intima interfaces directly with circulating blood. The outermost layer contains blood vessels known as vaso vasorum that provide perfusion to the outer half of the aortic wall. A dissection involves disruption of the intimal layer with subsequent exposure of the media to circulating blood.

What is the pathophysiology of an aortic dissection?

An aortic dissection results from a disruption or tear in the tunica intima, subsequently exposing the media to pulsatile arterial blood. This can remain localized to the intimal tear site or it can extend proximally, distally, or both. As pulsatile blood fills the space within the tunica media, a false lumen is created. The true lumen is the normal lumen of the blood vessel. The false lumen is the space between the dissection flap and the remaining layers of the wall of the aorta. The true and false lumens are divided by the dissection flap, and it may be challenging to identify the true and false lumens. Which end-organs are injured depends on the location and extent of the dissection and which branch vessels are involved.

How is aortic dissection diagnosed?

Most patients will present with an abrupt onset of severe chest pain that has a tearing or stabbing quality. Physical exam findings can include a pulse deficit when palpating a radial pulse (i.e., absent

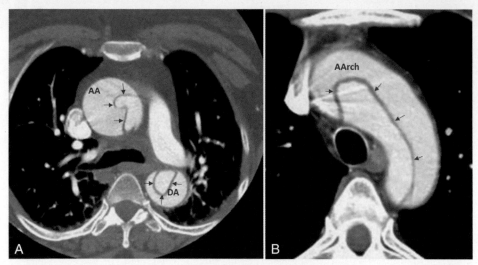

Fig. 20.1 (A) Axial computed tomography angiogram (CTA) showing a dissection flap *(red arrows)* in the ascending *(AA)* and descending *(DA)* aorta. (B) Axial image of CTA showing a dissection flap *(red arrows)* in the aortic arch *(AArch)*. This is a Stanford type A aortic dissection and a surgical emergency. (Modified from Afshar, N. [2013]. Aortic dissection. In J. G. Adams, E. D. Barton, J. L. Collings, P. M. C. DeBlieux, M. A. Gisondi, & E. S. Nadel [Eds.], *Emergency Medicine* [Vol. 65, 2nd ed., pp. 561–570.e1]. Philadelphia, PA: Elsevier. Fig. 65.6.)

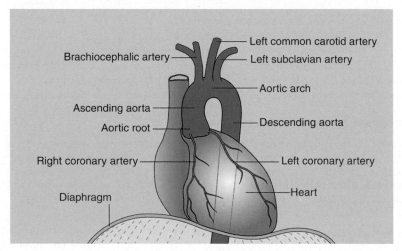

Fig. 20.2 Anatomy of the thoracic aorta. The first branches off of the aorta are the coronary arteries. The aortic arch gives rise to the brachiocephalic, left common carotid, and left subclavian arteries. The takeoff of the left subclavian artery demarcates the end of the aortic arch and the beginning of the descending aorta. (Modified from Ryding, A. [2013]. The aorta. In A. Ryding & J. Newton [Eds.], *Essential Echocardiography* [Vol. 19, 2nd ed., pp. 200–208]. Philadelphia, PA: Elsevier. Fig. 19.1.)

or very weak pulse on one side), a systolic blood pressure difference ≥20 mm Hg between the two arms, new neurological deficits, and a new holodiastolic murmur consistent with aortic regurgitation. Definitive diagnosis is made via CTA, magnetic resonance imaging (MRI), transesophageal echocardiography (TEE), or angiography. Choice of imaging is dependent on immediate availability and patient factors. CTA is most commonly the first imaging modality due to its wide availability.

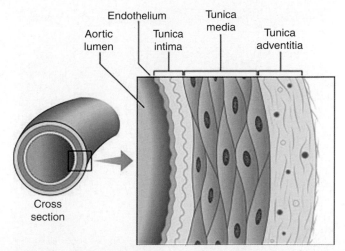

Fig. 20.3 Layers of the aortic wall. The wall of the aorta consists of endothelium, which is exposed to blood in the lumen of the vessel, tunica intima, tunica media, and tunica adventitia (the outermost layer). In aortic dissection, the tunica media is exposed to pressurized blood from the lumen of the aorta. (Reproduced from Lipsitz, M., Soucy, Z. [2020]. Abdominal aorta. In J. P. McGahan, M. A. Schick, & L. D. Mills [Eds.], *Fundamentals of Emergency Ultrasound*. Philadelphia, PA: Elsevier. Fig. 20.13.)

How are aortic dissections classified?

Two schemes exist in grading aortic dissections: DeBakey and Stanford (Fig. 20.4).

DeBakey classifies the dissection into three types: type I and type II, involving the ascending aorta; and type III, involving only the descending aorta.

The Stanford scheme classifies aortic dissections into two types: type A or type B. Type A dissections involve the ascending aorta and/or aortic arch. Type B dissections involve the descending aorta only.

Based on the CTA shown in Fig. 20.1, the dissection involves the ascending and descending aorta. Therefore, this patient has a DeBakey type I, or Stanford type A, dissection. This is a surgical emergency. Surgery aims to repair or replace areas of the diseased aorta and its main branches. Aortic valve replacement and/or coronary artery bypass grafting (CABG) may also be necessary if the aortic valve and/or coronary arteries are affected by the dissection.

What are the possible sequelae of type A aortic dissections?

The sequelae of an aortic dissection depend on the extent of the dissection. Involvement of the aortic root can result in pericardial tamponade, aortic valve regurgitation, and coronary artery disruption, causing myocardial ischemia. Involvement of the major branches of the aortic arch can cause stroke or limb ischemia. Involvement of the descending aorta can cause ischemia and infarction of the spinal cord, kidneys, intestines, and other viscera. Rupture of the dissection can cause massive internal hemorrhage.

The operating room is being prepared.

In the meantime, how will you manage this patient's hemodynamics?

The goals of hemodynamic management in aortic dissections are to minimize the stress on the aortic wall. This can be accomplished by reducing heart rate, the force of ventricular contraction (dP/dt), and blood pressure. Continuous infusion of a beta blocking agent, such as esmolol, should

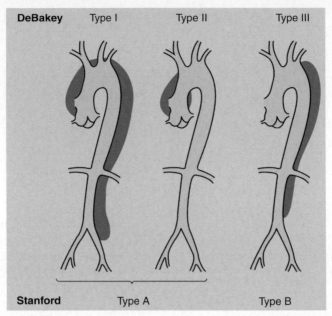

Fig. 20.4　Classification of aortic dissections. Stanford type A dissections involve the ascending aorta, either as part of a more extensive dissection (DeBakey type I), or in isolation (DeBakey type II). Stanford type B dissections (distal, or DeBakey type III) arise distal to the takeoff of the head and neck vessels (i.e., distal to the aortic arch). (Modified from Baig, K., Mahmood, K., Chukwuemeka, A. [2015]. Surgery of the thoracic aorta. *Surgery, 33*(2), 73–77. Fig. 1.)

be started to reduce heart rate to about 60/min and reduce systolic blood pressure to a systolic goal of 100 to 120 mm Hg. Analgesics should be given as pain contributes to the sympathetic response, causing worsening tachycardia and hypertension.

Can you give hydralazine first for blood pressure control?

Hydralazine and other vasodilating drugs should not be used as first-line agents for blood pressure control in aortic dissections, as vasodilation may decrease blood pressure and cause a reflexive increase in heart rate and dP/dt.

Start beta-blockers first to avoid reflex tachycardia. Additional antihypertensive agents (e.g., calcium channel blockers) can be added to manage blood pressure after beta blockade has been initiated.

STEP 2, 3 PEARL

For acute aortic dissections, initiate beta-blockade first prior to starting other antihypertensive agents to avoid reflex tachycardia.

What intraoperative monitors do you want for this case?

In addition to the American Society of Anesthesiologists (ASA) standard monitors, invasive arterial blood pressure monitoring is essential. If the patient is stable, an arterial catheter should be placed prior to induction. The choice of where to place the arterial catheter is dependent on patient factors, institutional practices, and surgical approach, including strategy for cannulation for cardiopulmonary bypass. In many institutions, two arterial catheters are placed—one in the right arm and one in the left arm or in either leg. Arterial catheters are most commonly placed in the radial arteries, although more central arterial pressure monitoring via the brachial, axillary, or femoral arteries may be helpful.

Central venous catheter placement allows for additional hemodynamic monitoring as well as fluid resuscitation and central administration of vasoactive and inotropic infusions. Patients undergoing repair of aortic dissection are prone to significant bleeding in both the pre - and post-cardiopulmonary bypass period. Therefore, large-bore intravenous access is required. This is often accomplished via central venous catheter placement. If there is cardiac dysfunction, a pulmonary artery catheter may also be placed.

TEE will be critical in guiding this operation. TEE will aid in evaluation of the aortic valve, diagnosis of pericardial effusion, assessment of cardiac function and wall motion, identification of the true and false lumens of the aorta, confirming proper placement of cannulas, and evaluating the success of the aortic repair.

An indwelling Foley catheter with temperature measurement capability, as well as a naso-pharyngeal temperature probe, should also be placed. It is common practice to place cerebral oximeters, such as near-infrared spectroscopy (NIRS), to monitor regional oxygen saturation of the frontal cortex as well. Depending on the extent of the aortic dissection, neurophysiologic monitoring of the spinal cord may also be used (see Case 25).

How will you induce general anesthesia for this patient?

When planning an induction of anesthesia for any patient with cardiovascular disease, it is crucial to begin with hemodynamic goals. As discussed above, the goals for an aortic dissection are to minimize dP/dt and avoid hypertension and tachycardia in order to reduce the stress on an already compromised aortic wall, thereby minimizing the risk of rupture. Laryngoscopy is particularly stimulating, so careful attention must be paid to the patient's hemodynamics immediately prior to laryngoscopy and intubation.

There are multiple ways to safely induce general anesthesia in this patient. A combination of intravenous benzodiazepines and opioids, with a judicious amount of propofol or etomidate, may be used. Mask ventilation with volatile anesthetic such as sevoflurane prior to laryngoscopy can further deepen the anesthetic and reduce the risk of a tachycardic response to laryngoscopy. Regardless of which agent or agents are used, the key is to go slowly and pay close attention to the heart rate and blood pressure. Rescue drugs such as esmolol and phenylephrine should be readily available to treat tachycardia and hypotension, respectively.

Induction and intubation are uneventful. The surgeon says he will plan for deep hypothermic circulatory arrest (DHCA).

What is DHCA, and how is it different from cardiopulmonary bypass (CPB)?

In CPB, the entire body except the heart and lungs is perfused with oxygenated, non-pulsatile blood from the CPB circuit (see Case 18). Blood is drained from one or more venous cannulas (usually in the right atrium or the superior and inferior vena cavae) and carried through the bypass tubing to the CPB machine, where carbon dioxide is removed, oxygen is added, the blood is heated and pressurized, and returned to the patient through an arterial cannula (usually in the ascending aorta). This results in a bloodless surgical field and a still heart, allowing the surgeon to operate on the heart and surrounding structures safely. CPB facilitates most cardiac operations, including CABG, valve repair or replacement, and even heart transplantation.

However, when the operation involves the aortic arch, as in the repair of a type A aortic dissec-tion, CPB alone is inadequate to facilitate a bloodless field, as blood from the CPB pump ordinar-ily flows through the aortic arch. In this case, DHCA is required. In DHCA, none of the body is perfused with blood. To achieve DHCA, CPB is first initiated, and then the patient is cooled to as low as 14 degrees Celsius. The CPB pump is then stopped, and the aortic cross-clamp is removed, thereby facilitating a bloodless field for repair of the ascending aorta and aortic arch.

Why does the patient need to be so cold in DHCA?

Since the tissues of the body will not receive oxygenated blood during circulatory arrest, hypothermia decreases the oxygen demand of all organs and protects them from ischemic injury. Hypothermia decreases the metabolic rate and oxygen consumption of all the tissues of the body, including the heart and brain.

The surgeon will cannulate for antegrade cerebral perfusion (ACP) via the right axillary artery and left carotid artery. What does that mean? What is the other option for cerebral perfusion during DHCA?

Remember, in DHCA, none of the tissues in the body receive oxygenated blood. The brain is particularly sensitive to ischemia, even with profound hypothermia. To protect the brain and to allow for a longer duration of circulatory arrest, the brain may be selectively perfused with oxygenated blood (i.e., the brain is the only organ receiving oxygenated blood) during DHCA. This can be accomplished in several ways.

In ACP, the brain is selectively perfused via the carotid artery or arteries via cannulation of a branch or branches of the aortic arch, such as the axillary, subclavian, or carotid artery (see Fig. 20.5). In this case, blood flows up the carotid artery to the brain in the usual direction of blood flow, hence the term *antegrade*.

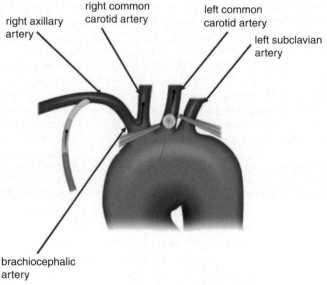

Fig. 20.5 Cannulation for antegrade cerebral perfusion (ACP). An arterial cannula in the right axillary artery delivers oxygenated blood through the axillary artery to the right subclavian and ultimately the brachiocephalic artery. The take-off of the brachiocephalic artery into the aortic arch is clamped, so blood from the arterial cannula flows up the right carotid artery to the brain. Another arterial cannula is placed directly in the left carotid artery to deliver oxygenated blood up the left carotid artery to the brain. Some surgeons prefer to only cannulate the right axillary artery and rely on an intact circle of Willis (see Case 32) to perfuse the contralateral brain. (Modified from Angleitner, P., Stelzmueller, M., Mahr, S. [2020]. Bilateral or unilateral antegrade cerebral perfusion during surgery for acute type A dissection. *Journal of Thoracic and Cardiovascular Surgery, 159*[6], 2159–2167.e2. Fig. 1.)

Alternatively, the brain may be selectively perfused in a retrograde fashion. In this case, blood flows up the superior vena cava to the internal jugular vein to the brain, the reverse of the usual direction of blood flow. This is known as *retrograde* cerebral perfusion (RCP).

> CPB is initiated, then DHCA. After the repair, CPB is reinitiated, and the patient is rewarmed. The patient is weaned from CPB, and protamine is administered. The surgeon says that there is diffuse bleeding in the surgical field.

What factors contribute to coagulopathy after CPB with DHCA?

CPB is known to contribute to coagulopathy by adversely affecting all elements of the coagulation cascade:

- Platelet destruction is caused by exposure to blood-air and blood-tissue interfaces. Dilution and splenic sequestration also contribute to thrombocytopenia. CPB also results in partial activation of platelets, causing a qualitative platelet deficiency.
- CPB causes dilution of clotting factors. Clotting factors are denatured by exposure to the blood-air interface.
- Increased concentration of plasminogen activator during CPB increases fibrinolysis.
- Hypothermia itself is detrimental to the coagulation cascade in many ways. Hypothermia induces splanchnic sequestration of platelets, slows the formation of fibrin, and accelerates fibrinolysis.

> You order a thromboelastogram (TEG). The tracing is shown in Fig. 20.6. The clot lysis index at 30 minutes (LY30) is well above the normal range.

What's going on?

These findings are consistent with hyperfibrinolysis as a result of the CPB with DHCA for aortic repair.

TEG is a viscoelastic assay that can guide treatment of coagulopathy in the perioperative period. The contour as well as the amplitude of the tracing provide information about the patient's coagulation status. Fig. 20.7 shows the measurements taken from a TEG reading as well as the expected changes in these measurements in hyper- and hypocoagulable states. Fig. 20.8 shows the changes in the contour of TEG tracings expected in common hyper- and hypocoagulable states. TEG allows for targeted treatment of coagulopathy.

What should you do?

The mainstay of treatment of fibrinolysis is the administration of an antifibrinolytic agent such as aminocaproic acid or tranexamic acid (see Case 33). Supplement with other blood products as necessary.

How does TEG work?

In TEG, whole blood is placed in a cup that rotates around a stationary pin. As a clot forms, resistance to rotation increases, which is displayed graphically as a larger amplitude of the tracing.

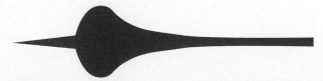

Fig. 20.6 Thromboelastogram (TEG) tracing in your patient with diffuse bleeding after repair of aortic dissection. This is concerning for hyperfibrinolysis. (Modified from Shore-Lesserson, L., Enriquez, L. J., Weitzel, N. [2017]. Coagulation monitoring. In J. A. Kaplan, G. J. T. Augoustides, G. R. Manecke, T. Maus, & D. L. Reich [Eds.], *Kaplan's Cardiac Anesthesia* [Vol. 19, 7th ed., pp. 698–727]. Philadelphia, PA: Elsevier. Fig. 19.18.)

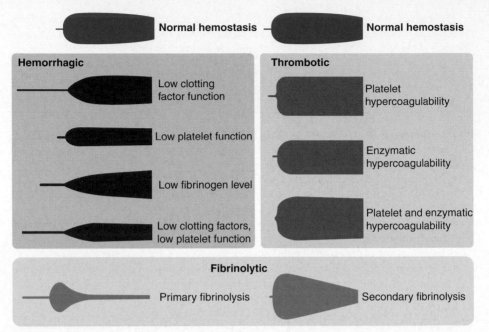

Fig. 20.7   Measurements from a thromboelastogram (TEG) tracing. Changes in the contour of the tracing and in each of the measurements can help identify specific deficiencies within the patient's coagulation status. (Reproduced from Shore-Lesserson, L., Enriquez, L. J., Weitzel, N. [2017]. Coagulation monitoring. In J. A. Kaplan, G. J. T. Augoustides, G. R. Manecke, T. Maus, & D. L. Reich [Eds.], *Kaplan's Cardiac Anesthesia* [Vol. 19, 7th ed., pp. 698–727]. Philadelphia, PA: Elsevier. Fig. 19.18.)

BEYOND THE PEARLS

- Stanford type A dissections are surgical emergencies that require immediate intervention.
- Risks of neurological deficits, cardiogenic shock, and limb ischemia are all possible depending on location and extent of the aortic dissection.
- Deep hypothermic circulatory arrest is necessary for repairs involving the aortic arch. Neuroprotection strategies exist to protect the brain from ischemic and thromboembolic insults.
- Procedures on the aorta often involve large blood volume shifts requiring significant resuscitation. Large-bore intravenous access, central venous access, and multiple arterial lines is often necessary.
- Rotational thromboelastometry (ROTEM) is another viscoelastic assay, somewhat similar to TEG. In ROTEM, whole blood is placed in a cup, but the pin rotates, and the cup is stationary.

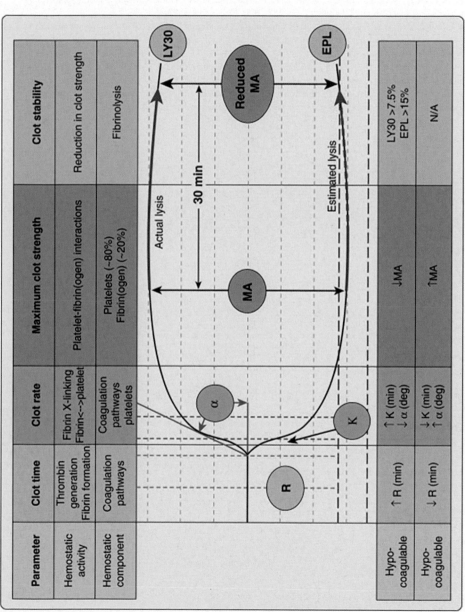

Fig. 20.8 Changes in the contour of a thromboelastogram (TEG) tracing are characteristic of particular coagulation defects. *MA,* maximum amplitude; *EPL,* estimated percentage of lysis. (Reproduced from Shore-Lesserson, L., Enriquez, L. J., Weitzel, N. [2017]. Coagulation monitoring. In J. A. Kaplan, G. J. T. Augoustides, G. R. Manecke, T. Maus, & D. L. Reich [Eds.], *Kaplan's Cardiac Anesthesia* [Vol. 19, 7th ed., pp. 698–727]. Philadelphia, PA: Elsevier. Fig. 19.18.)

References

Augoustides, J. G., Patel, P., Ghadimi, K., Choi, J., Yue, Y., & Silvay, G. (2013). Current conduct of deep hypothermic circulatory arrest in China. *HSR Proc Intensive Care Cardiovasc Anesth*, 5(1), 25–32.

Grecu, L., & Chawla, N. (2018). In R. L. Hines & K. E. Marschall (Eds.), *Vascular disease, Stoelting's anesthesia and co-existing disease* (7th ed., Chapter 12, pp. 237–263). Philadelphia, PA: Elsevier.

Gutsche, J. T., Feinman, J., Silvay, G., Patel, P. , P., Ghadimi, K., Landoni, G., et al. (2014). Practice variations in the conduct of hypothermic circulatory arrest for adult aortic arch repair: Focus on an emerging European paradigm. *Heart Lung Vessel*, 6(1), 43–51.

Kaplan's Cardiac Anesthesia. (2017). In J. A. Kaplan, G. J. T. Augoustides, G. R. Manecke, T. Maus, & D. L. Reich (Eds.), *Cardiac and noncardiac surgery* (7th ed). Philadelphia, PA: Elsevier.

Stein, L. H., & Elefteriades, J. A. (2010). Protecting the brain during aortic surgery: an enduring debate with unanswered questions. *The Journal of Cardiothoracic and Vascular Anesthesia*, 24(2), 316–321.

A 73-Year-Old Male With Past Medical History of Chronic Obstructive Pulmonary Disease and Squamous Cell Carcinoma of the Right Lung

David Li

A 73-year-old male with past medical history of chronic obstructive pulmonary disease (COPD) and squamous cell carcinoma of the right lung is scheduled for video-assisted right upper lobectomy. He has a 50 pack-year smoking history. He has endorsed a persistent cough and shortness of breath upon exertion for the past 6 months. His vital signs during his most recent office visit are blood pressure 155/100 mm Hg, pulse 88/min, respiration rate 12/min, and temperature 36.6°C.

Describe the anatomy of the lungs.

The thorax is a cone-shaped structure with a small apex superiorly and a large inferior portion with the diaphragm attached. The wall of the thorax consists of the bony ribcage along with various muscle groups that surround the vital organs within the chest. Each lung is contained within one hemothorax on either side of the mediastinum.

STEP 1 PEARL

The lung is surrounded by a serous membrane called the pleura: the visceral (adjacent to lung parenchyma) and parietal (adjacent to the deep surface of the wall of the thorax) pleura. The visceral and parietal pleura oppose each other, creating a potential space called the pleural cavity, as in Figs. 21.1 and 21.2.

The left lung consists of the upper lobe, lower lobe, and lingula. The right lung consists of the upper, middle, and lower lobes. The functional structure of the respiratory tract can be divided into three categories:

- Conducting airways facilitate gas transport during inhalation and exhalation, but not gas exchange. Conducting airways start at the pharynx and end at the bronchioles.
- Transitional airways are smaller airway conduits that allow for gas movement and limited gas exchange.
- Respiratory airways are the smallest airways and are primarily responsible for gas exchange. Respiratory bronchioles and alveoli are in this category.

What two vascular systems are found in the lungs?

The lungs contain two major circulatory systems: the pulmonary and bronchial vascular systems. The pulmonary vascular system is responsible for delivering venous blood from the right ventricle

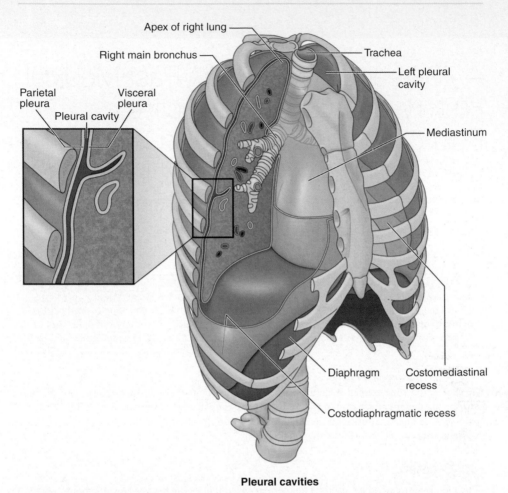

Pleural cavities

Fig. 21.1 Three-dimensional diagram of the thorax showing the visceral pleura against the lung and the parietal pleura against the deep surface of the chest wall. The potential space between the two layers is known as the pleural cavity. (Reproduced from Drake, R. L., Vogl, A. W., & Mitchell, A. W. M. [2021]. Thorax. In *Gray's atlas of anatomy* [3rd ed., pp. 61–132]. Philadelphia, PA: Elsevier.)

to the pulmonary capillary beds for gas exchange, then oxygenated blood is returned to the left atrium via the pulmonary veins. There are usually four pulmonary veins: left upper and lower pulmonary veins and right upper and lower pulmonary veins. The bronchial arterial system, is part of the systemic circulation and supplies oxygenated blood to the conductive airways and walls of the pulmonary vessels.

STEP 2, 3 PEARL

The connections between the bronchial and pulmonary venous systems result in a shunt of 2%–5% of total cardiac output and represents normal physiologic shunt.

Pulmonary function tests (PFTs) 1 week prior to surgery show forced expiratory volume in 1 second/forced vital capacity (FEV_1/FVC) of 0.5 and FEV_1 80% of predicted.

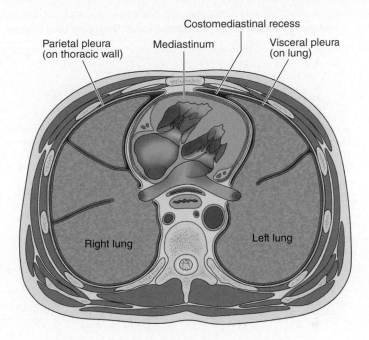

Fig. 21.2   Axial diagram of the thorax, again showing visceral pleura against the lung and parietal pleura against the deep surface of the chest wall. Notice that the visceral and parietal pleura are contiguous with one another. (Reproduced from Drake R. L., Vogl, A. W., & Mitchell, A. W. M. [2021]. Thorax. In *Gray's atlas of anatomy* [3rd ed., pp. 61–132]. Philadelphia, PA: Elsevier.)

What does that mean? What are PFTs?

FEV_1 is the volume of air exhaled in the first second of forceful expiration after maximal inhalation. FVC is the total volume exhaled after maximal inhalation. This patient has a decreased FEV_1 and a decreased ratio of FEV_1/FVC. These findings are consistent with obstructive lung disease.

PFTs are a series of standardized measurements used to quantify aspects of a patient's respiratory physiology. PFTs can assess a patient's airflow status via various lung volume measurements; they can also quantify the capacity of the lungs for gas exchange via measurement of diffusing capacity for inspired carbon monoxide (DLCO). These values are reported as a percentage of a predicted normal value based on a patient's age and height. PFTs are helpful in diagnosis of respiratory disease. Moreover, preoperative PFTs can be valuable in assessing a patient's potential risk for postoperative pulmonary complications.

STEP 1, 2, 3 PEARL

Forced expiratory volume in one second/forced vital capacity (FEV_1/FVC) ratio is helpful in distinguishing between obstructive (e.g., asthma and chronic obstructive pulmonary disease [COPD]) and restrictive (e.g., interstitial lung disease and pulmonary fibrosis) lung diseases, as in Table 21.1.

Which measurement of PFT is most predictive of postoperative respiratory complications?

Predicted postoperative forced expiratory volume in one second (ppoFEV1) is the most predictive of postoperative pulmonary complications: ppoFEV1 greater than 40% represents a relatively

TABLE 21.1 ■ Pulmonary Function Tests in Obstructive Versus Restrictive Lung Disease

PFT Measurements	Obstructive Lung Disease	Restrictive Lung Disease
FEV$_1$	↓↓↓	↓
FVC	↓	↓↓
FEV$_1$/FVC	↓↓↓ (≤80%)	Normal (>80%)

In obstructive lung disease, the decrease in forced expiratory volume in one second (FEV$_1$) is more profound than the decrease in forced vital capacity (FVC). Therefore, the ratio FEV$_1$/FVC decreases significantly. In restrictive lung disease, both FEV$_1$ and FVC are decreased, so the ratio FEV$_1$/FVC is relatively normal.

low risk, whereas ppoFEV1 less than 40% represents a high risk for postoperative pulmonary complications.

It is estimated that right upper lobectomy will remove 15% of the patient's functional lung volume. What is his ppoFEV$_1$?

ppoFEV1 is determined by the amount of functional lung tissue that will remain after lung resection. It is given by

$$ppoFEV1\% = preoperative\ FEV1\% \times \frac{100 - \%\ functional\ lung\ tissue\ removed}{100}$$

for this patient, with preoperative FEV$_1$ 80% of predicted undergoing resection of 15% of functional lung volume.

$$ppoFEV1\% = 80 \times \frac{100 - 15}{100}$$

$$ppoFEV1\% = 80 \times \left(85/100\right)$$

$$ppoFEV1\% = 68\%$$

Describe the different physiologic lung volumes and capacities.

There are several important physiologic lung volumes during normal or forceful respiratory cycles, some of which are obtainable via PFT, as in Fig. 21.3. The tidal volume (V_T) is the volume of air exchanged during each normal breath. The residual volume (RV), on the other hand, is the volume of air that remains in the lungs after maximal exhalation (see Table 21.2 for the rest of the lung volumes).

Lung capacities are composed of two or more lung volumes. For instance, the functional residual capacity (FRC) is the lung volume at the end of normal exhalation, which can be thought of as the sum of RV and expiratory reserve volume (ERV).

The patient's flow-volume loop is shown in Fig. 21.4.

How do you interpret this?

This flow-volume loop, with a concave upward expiratory component, is consistent with obstructive pulmonary disease, as in COPD.

A flow-volume loop (F-V loop) is a graphical representation of a PFT (Figs. 21.4 and 21.5). An F-V loop can be utilized clinically to distinguish between obstructive and restrictive lung

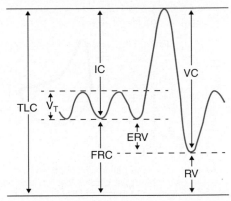

Fig. 21.3 Tracing showing relationships between key physiologic measurements. Total lung capacity *(TLC)*, as the name implies, is the maximum volume of the lungs. Tidal volume (V$_T$) is the volume of a normal breath. Functional residual capacity *(FRC)* is the volume in the lungs after normal exhalation. Inspiratory capacity *(IC)* is the maximum volume that can be inhaled starting after a normal exhalation. Expiratory reserve volume *(ERV)* is the maximum additional volume that can be exhaled starting at the end of a normal exhalation. Residual volume *(RV)* is the volume in the lungs that cannot be exhaled (remember, the lungs remain "sucked" open negative pressure in the pleural space). Vital capacity *(VC)* is the maximum volume that can be inhaled and exhaled, effectively the difference between TLC and RV. (Reproduced from Putnam, J. B. Lung, [2016]. chest wall, pleura, and mediastinum. In C. M. Townsend, R. D. Beauchamp, B. M. Evers, & K. L. Mattox [Eds.], *Sabiston textbook of surgery* [Vol. 57, 20th ed., pp. 1572–1618]. Philadelphia, PA: Elsevier. Fig. 57–6.)

TABLE 21.2 ■ **Lung Volumes and Capacities**

Measurement	Definition	Average Adult Values (mL)
Lung volumes		
Tidal volume (V$_T$)	Volume of a normal breath	500
Inspiratory reserve volume (IRV)	Maximal additional volume that can be inspired beyond V$_T$	3000
Expiratory reserve volume (ERV)	Maximal volume that can be expired below V$_T$	1100
Residual volume (RV)	Volume remaining after maximal exhalation	1200
Lung capacities		
Vital capacity (VC)	Maximum volume of gas that can be exhaled following maximal inspiration	4600
Functional residual capacity (FRC)	The lung volume at the end of normal exhalation, when the inward elastic recoil of the lung approximates the outward elastic recoil of the chest; RV + ERV	2300
Closing capacity (CC)	The volume at which small airways begin to collapse	≈2300 at age 40 years
Total lung capacity (TLC)	The entire lung volume; RV + ERV + V$_T$ + IRV	5000–6000

disease, and identify the location of airway obstruction. The lung volumes are plotted on the *x*-axis and the flow rates on the *y*-axis. An F-V loop starts at FRC, with inspiration represented by the portion of the F-V loop below the *x*-axis, while exhalation is represented by the portion above the *x*-axis. Note that the *x*-axis is numbered in reverse (0 is to the right side of the graph instead of the left).

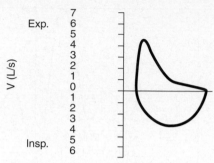

Fig. 21.4 Flow-volume loop showing an obstructive pattern. (Modified From North, I. [2018]. Pulmonary function testing for pathologists. In K. O. Leslie & M. R. Wick [Eds.], *Practical pulmonary pathology: A diagnostic approach* [pp. 15–20]. Philadelphia, PA: Elsevier. Modified from Fig. 2.3.)

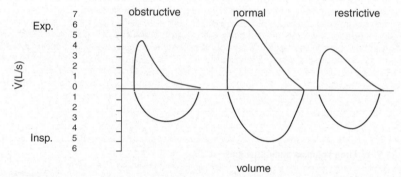

Fig. 21.5 Flow-volume loops. The flow-volume loop from the patient with obstructive disease shows a "scoop" out of the expiratory flow pattern compared to the loop from the patient with normal lungs. Both obstructive and restrictive lung disease have decreased maximal expiratory flow compared to normal lungs. (Modified From North, I. [2018]. Pulmonary function testing for pathologists. In *Practical pulmonary pathology: A diagnostic approach* [pp. 15–20]. Fig. 2.3.)

STEP 2, 3 PEARL

An F-V loop can be utilized clinically to distinguish between obstructive and restrictive lung disease. Patients with obstructive disease have larger lung volumes resulting in F-V loops that are shifted to the left. In comparison, patients with restrictive lung disease have decreased vital capacity, resulting in narrower F-V loops.

What is COPD?

COPD is a spectrum of chronic inflammatory lung disease that includes emphysema and chronic bronchitis. It is typically caused by long-term exposure to lung irritants, such as cigarette smoke and toxic fumes. It ultimately results in airflow obstruction from the lungs, with symptoms including cough, mucus production, shortness of breath, and wheezing.

STEP 2 PEARL

Patients with chronic bronchitis have a chronic cough and frequent sputum production.

How should this patient be optimized prior to elective surgery?
There are a few elements that clinicians should focus on preoperatively: atelectasis, wheezing, mucus secretions, and respiratory tract infections.

Atelectasis may predispose patients to impaired oxygen exchange intraoperatively. It may also increase the risk of pulmonary infection postoperatively. Working with patients to improve their pulmonary hygiene and utilizing incentive spirometry prior to surgery may decrease the degree of atelectasis.

There are various bronchodilators that are available to prevent or treat wheezing, including sympathomimetic agents (e.g., inhaled selective β2–agonists), parasympatholytic agents (i.e., inhaled anticholinergics), and others (see Table 21.3).

Options to reduce respiratory secretions prior to surgery include the use of a humidified inhaler, acetylcysteine, coughing, deep breathing, and incentive spirometry.

If the patient currently smokes, they should be advised to stop.

How can smoking affect this patient?
Smoking and the components of tobacco smoke affect multiple organ systems, as described in Table 21.4.

Surgery is only 1 week away.

Is there still a benefit if the patient stops smoking now?
Yes. The longer a patient can abstain from smoking before surgery, the greater the perioperative benefit. As little as 12–24 hours of smoking cessation is enough to improve oxygen delivery to tissues by reducing CO levels. Mucociliary function improves within 2–3 days of smoking cessation, and sputum production decreases to normal levels within 2 weeks of cessation. Additionally, 3–8 weeks of smoking cessation preoperatively can improve wound healing and decrease respiratory complications.

TABLE 21.3 ■ **Treatment Options for Chronic Obstructive Pulmonary Disease**

Class	Examples	Mechanism of Actions
β-Adrenergic agonists	Albuterol Metaproterenol Terbutaline	Increases adenylate cyclase, increasing cyclic adenosine monophosphate (cAMP) and Ca^{2+}, resulting in decreased smooth muscle tone and bronchodilation.
Methylxanthine	Aminophylline Theophylline	Phosphodiesterase inhibition increases cAMP; potentiates catecholamines resulting in central respiratory stimulation.
Anticholinergics	Atropine Ipratropium	Inhibits acetylcholine at postganglionic receptors, decreasing cyclic guanosine monophosphate (cGMP), resulting in airway smooth muscle relaxation.
Antileukotriene	Montelukast Zileuton	Leukotriene antagonist, inhibits leukotriene production, antiinflammatory.
Membrane stabilizer	Cromolyn sodium	A membrane stabilizer that can prevent mast cell degranulation if given prophylactically.
Corticosteroids	Methylprednisolone Dexamethasone Prednisone	Antiinflammatory, membrane stabilization, and inhibits histamine release.

TABLE 21.4 ■ Smoking Affects Most Organ Systems of the Body

Organ System	Effects
Cardiovascular	• nicotine → ↑sympathetic tone → ↑blood pressure, ↑heart rate (HR), ↑systemic vascular resistance (SVR), ↑contractility • ↑myocardial oxygen demand, ↓myocardial oxygen supply • carbon monoxide (CO) → ↓mitochondrial enzymes in cardiac muscle → ↓contractility • CO → ↑arrhythmia risk
Respiratory	• ↓oxygen delivery to tissues • carboxyhemoglobin → left-shift of hemoglobin-oxygen dissociation curve (see Case 15) • chronic tissue hypoxia → ↑hemoglobin (Hb) • ↑mucus viscosity, ↓ciliary function → ↓clearance of respiratory secretions • ↓small airway diameter → ↑closing capacity →chronic obstructive pulmonary disease (COPD) • ↑pulmonary proteolytic enzyme function → ↓pulmonary elastic recoil → emphysema • ↓surfactant • ↑airway reactivity
Hematologic	• ↑Hb, ↑fibrinogen, leukocytosis, ↑platelets (and ↑platelet activation) → ↑blood viscosity, ↑risk of arterial thromboembolism
Gastrointestinal	• ↓lower esophageal sphincter (LES) tone, however this effect only lasts 8 min, so no increased risk of pulmonary aspiration
Renal	• ↑antidiuretic hormone (ADH) → hyponatremia
Immune	• ↓immune response → ↑risk of infection, neoplasm

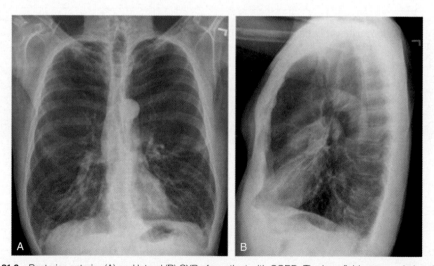

Fig. 21.6   Posterior-anterior (A) and lateral (B) CXR of a patient with COPD. The lung fields appear darker than do those of healthy patients normal patients because there is more air and less lung tissue. The diaphragm is flatter and more caudal, so more ribs are visible. (Reproduced from Washko, G. R. [2012]. The role and potential of imaging in COPD. *Medical Clinics of North America, 96*[4], 729–743. Fig. 1.)

A patient's smoking history heavily impacts their perioperative course. Smoking increases the risk of postoperative complications, including respiratory failure, prolonged intubation, pneumonia, laryngospasm, bronchospasm, and increased need for intensive care unit admission and respiratory therapy services.

The patient's chest radiograph (CXR) is shown in Fig. 21.6.

How do you interpret this?

This patient's CXR shows hyperinflated lungs and a flattened, caudally displaced diaphragm. These findings are expected in patients with COPD.

On the morning of surgery, the patient is wheezing. He says the wheezing is much worse than his usual chronic wheezing. He is also coughing more than usual.

What should you do?

This is concerning for COPD exacerbation. If the patient is actively wheezing at the time of elective surgery and this wheezing is more than what they experience chronically, surgery should be postponed.

Patients with current or recent respiratory tract infection should have their elective surgeries postponed due to increased risks of perioperative respiratory complications, such as bronchospasm, hypoxemia, and prolonged postoperative intubation. Preoperative respiratory tract infections should be treated aggressively prior to proceeding with elective surgery. However, the optimal wait time between recent infection and elective surgery has yet to be clearly defined.

Surgery is postponed. On the morning of the rescheduled surgery, the patient says he is back to his baseline respiratory function.

How will you ventilate this patient during surgery?

Video-assisted thoracic surgery (VATS) requires single lung ventilation (SLV). Other indications for SLV include:
- massive pulmonary/alveolar hemorrhage (to protect the unaffected lung)
- severe pulmonary infection (also to protect the unaffected lung)
- bronchopleural fistula
- bronchial disruption/trauma
- unilateral lung lavage
- repair of thoracic aortic aneurysm
- esophageal surgery

What are contraindications to SLV?

SLV is contraindicated if the patient cannot tolerate SLV, as in severe hypoxia or hemodynamic instability. Patients intubated and dependent on two-lung mechanical ventilation likely will not tolerate SLV.

How will you achieve SLV?

A double-lumen endotracheal tube (DLT) is the most common method to achieve SLV. As its name implies, a DLT is an endotracheal tube that has two lumens of unequal length molded together (see Fig. 21.7). The basic utility of a DLT is to isolate and selectively ventilate one of the two lungs. A DLT consists of a tracheal lumen and a bronchial lumen. A DLT has two inflatable

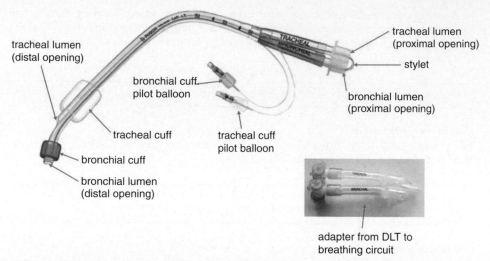

Fig. 21.7 Double-lumen endotracheal tube (DLT). A tubing clamp can be applied to either the tracheal or bronchial arm of the adapter from the DLT to the breathing circuit to direct all flow from the ventilator down the unclamped lumen to the corresponding lung. (Modified from Foley, K. A., & Slinger, P. [2014]. Fiberoptic bronchoscopic positioning of double-lumen tubes. *Anaesthesia and Intensive Care Medicine, 15*[11], 505–508. Modified from Fig. 2.)

TABLE 21.5 ■ Advantages and Disadvantages of Three Main Methods of Lung Isolation

Techniques	Advantages	Disadvantages
DLT	• Quick to place • Easy and more reliable lung isolation • Less repositioning needed • Allows access to both lungs (bronchoscopy or suctioning)	• Difficult to select the proper size • Can be challenging to place during direct laryngoscopy • May result in tracheobronchial injuries due to larger diameter • Not ideal for postoperative ventilation, requiring endotracheal tube (ETT) exchange postoperatively
SLT with BB	• Easy to add to regular single-lumen ETT • Selective lobar isolation • Best device for patient with difficult airway • No need for ETT exchange if postoperative ventilation is required	• Can be cumbersome to place • Unreliable lung isolation • Frequent need for repositioning • Very narrow channel for suctioning
SLT with main stem placement	• Simpler and faster technique • No special equipment necessary • Useful in small children	• SLV may be challenging depending on ETT placement • Cannot suction operative lung • Can result in bronchial injury

BB, Bronchial blocker; *DLT,* double-lumen tube; *SLT,* single-lumen endotracheal tube.

cuffs to facilitate lung isolation: one in the trachea and one in the bronchus. The two lumens are also color-coded: clear for tracheal and blue for bronchial. Modern DLTs have low-pressure, high-volume cuffs to reduce the likelihood of airway trauma. DLTs are available as both a left- and right-sided tube. The "sidedness" refers to the side of the bronchial lumen. Typical sizes of DLTs range from 28 French (F, the smallest), 35 F, 37 F and 39 F, to 41 F (the largest).

What are other options for SLV?

The three techniques for SLV are DLT, single-lumen endotracheal tube (SLT) with a bronchial blocker (BB), and main-stem (i.e. endobronchial) intubation with an SLT. The technique chosen depends on the clinical situation (see Table 21.5).

How is a DLT placed?

After induction of anesthesia and administration of muscle relaxant, laryngoscopy can be performed with a standard laryngoscope or with a video laryngoscope. Once an optimal view of the vocal cord is obtained, the DLT is passed with the distal end cured anteriorly to facilitate its passage through the vocal cords. Once the tip of the DLT is at the vocal cords, the stylet is removed by an assistant. The DLT is then advanced into the airway and rotated into proper position (i.e., the bronchial cuff on the left side for left-sided DLT). The goal is to position the DLT such that the distal opening of the tracheal lumen is above the carina, and the distal opening of the bronchial lumen opening is in the correct bronchus (i.e., in the left bronchus when using a left-sided DLT).

You intubate the patient with the DLT.

How can you confirm that it is properly positioned?

Standard practice is to confirm proper DLT placement by fiberoptic bronchoscopy. If a fiberoptic scope is not available, proper placement can be confirmed by auscultation.

How can proper placement of a left-sided DLT be confirmed via fiberoptic examination?

Fig. 21.8 shows proper placement of a left-sided DLT, with the tracheal lumen above the carina and the bronchial lumen in the left main bronchus. After the DLT is placed, advance the fiberoptic scope down the tracheal lumen. Identify the carina and the bronchial component of the DLT entering the left main bronchus. A sliver of the blue endobronchial balloon should be visible. Advance the scope down the right main bronchus and anteflex (turn the tip of the scope upward) to visualize the takeoff of the right upper lobe, which is classically identified by the presence of three lumens (trifurcation). Placement of the fiberoptic scope down the bronchial lumen will visualize the bifurcation of the left bronchus into the left upper and left lower lobes.

How can proper placement of a left-sided DLT be confirmed via auscultation?

First, with both cuffs inflated and both lumens unclamped, auscultate both lungs to confirm equal bilateral lung sounds. Next, clamp the tracheal lumen of the adapter with a tubing clamp, and verify that breath sounds can be heard over the left but not the right chest. Next, unclamp the tracheal lumen and clamp the bronchial lumen, then verify that breath sounds can be heard over the right, but not the left chest.

You confirm proper position of the DLT.

Why is a left-sided DLT preferred over a right-sided DLT?

Although right-sided DLTs are available for clinical use, left-sided DLTs are much more frequently used due to their ease of placement and adjustment. Unless clinically necessary (e.g., left pneumonectomy for proximal bronchial tumor), a left-sided DLT is preferred.

The right main bronchus is wider and shorter, and the right upper lobe takes off from the right bronchus within 2 cm of the carina. Because of this anatomic difference, it is often more difficult to position a right-sided DLT correctly, often resulting in inability to ventilate the right upper lobe and worsening ventilation/perfusion mismatching during SLV.

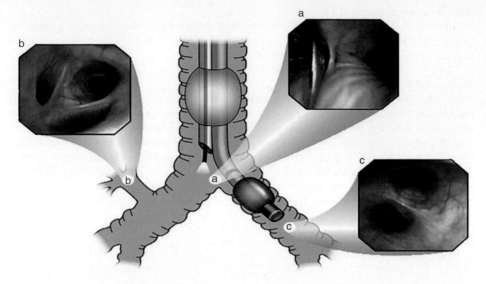

Fig. 21.8   Proper placement of a left-sided DLT. (a) Placement of the fiberoptic scope down the tracheal lumen will identify the carina and the bronchial lumen heading down the left mainstem bronchus. (b) Advancement of the fiberoptic scope farther down the tracheal lumen and into the right main bronchus, along with anteflexing the fiberoptic scope, will allow visualization of the takeoff of the right upper lobe with its trifurcation into the apical, anterior, and posterior segments. This trifurcation is unique to the right upper lobe but is not always present. (c) Placement of the fiberoptic scope down the bronchial lumen will show the bifurcation of the left main bronchus into the left upper and left lower bronchi. (Modified from Foley, K. A., & Slinger, P. [2014]. Fiberoptic bronchoscopic positioning of double-lumen tubes. *Anaesthesia and Intensive Care Medicine, 15*[11], 505–508. Modified from Fig. 4.)

STEP 2, 3 PEARL

The right main bronchus is wider and shorter than the left, and it diverges away from the trachea at a more vertical angle compared to the left main bronchus. Therefore, aspirates such as foreign bodies are more likely to enter the right lung.

You initiate SLV, ventilating only the left lung, and position the patient with their left side down.

How should you manage ventilation during SLV?

Goals during SLV are to maintain adequate ventilation, prevent hypoxemia, and avoid barotrauma. While there is no universal consensus on the lower limit of acceptable oxygen saturation (SpO_2), most clinicians will try to maintain a patient's SpO_2 during SLV $\geq 90\%$. Of course, this can be adjusted as needed based on clinical judgments and a patient's comorbidities.

One critical yet often overlooked factor that can cause intraoperative hypoxemia is incorrect DLT positioning. Confirm proper DLT placement, ideally with a fiberoptic bronchoscope, immediately after intubation and again after any major patient repositioning (such as when the patient is placed in the lateral position). Two-lung ventilation should be continued for as long as possible until SLV is required. On initiation of SLV, start with a fraction of inspired oxygen (FiO_2) of 1.0, and titrate down it as tolerated. Apply 4–6 cm H_2O of positive end-expiratory pressure (PEEP) to help prevent atelectasis in the dependent (i.e., the lung closer to the operating table—generally the operative lung is up, away from the operating table) ventilated lung, thus minimizing ventilation/perfusion mismatching.

To avoid barotrauma, maintain tidal volumes no more than 5–6 cc/kg of ideal body weight. Increasing the respiratory rate to maintain or slightly increase the minute ventilation compared to two-lung ventilation can help maintain appropriate gas exchange during SLV. Pressure-controlled ventilation may be utilized to prevent lung injury during SLV by lowering the peak airway pressures and avoiding sudden airway pressure change caused by surgical manipulation. Avoid long inspiratory-to-expiratory time (I:E) ratios in order to prevent breath stacking, also known as "auto-PEEP," and lung injury.

Over the next 30 minutes, the oxygen saturation decreases from 95%– 84%.

What's going on?

The most significant physiologic change during SLV is mismatching of ventilation (V) and perfusion (Q, blood flow through the lungs). The initiation of SLV stops all ventilation to the nonventilated lung. Blood flow to the nonventilated lung, however, continues. Therefore, all of the blood flowing through the nonventilated lung reaches the pulmonary veins, and ultimately the systemic circulation, without being oxygenated by the lungs. This creates a significant shunt fraction of approximately 50% (i.e., 50% of the total blood flow to the lungs reaches the systemic circulation without taking up oxygen from the lungs).

Fortunately, there are a few mechanisms to reduce the shunt fraction to approximately 25%. Some of these mechanisms include: lateral positioning of the patient leads to an increase in perfusion to the ventilated, dependent lung (gravity pulls blood toward the dependent lung); surgical manipulation of the atelectatic lung reduces blood flow to the nonventilated lung; and hypoxic pulmonary vasoconstriction (HPV) results in diversion of blood flow from the nonventilated regions of the lungs to the ventilated regions of the lungs.

What should you do?

If hypoxemia occurs during SLV, a systemic approach should be applied to troubleshoot the cause in order to improve oxygenation (Table 21.6). Hypoxemia during SLV should prompt immediate fiberoptic bronchoscopic examination, confirming the DLT or BB is properly placed. Suction the ventilated lung. Increase the FiO_2 if it is not already 1.0. Give recruitment breaths to the ventilated lung. Increase PEEP to the dependent lung (beware that excessive PEEP to the ventilated lung may worsen shunt), and apply continuous positive airway pressure (CPAP) to the nondependent, nonventilated lung.

If none of these maneuvers increase oxygen saturation to satisfactory levels, advise the surgeon that you need to resume two-lung ventilation to improve oxygenation. In extreme cases, or when resumption of two-lung ventilation is not possible, the surgeon can clamp the pulmonary artery to the nonventilated lung. This will eliminate perfusion to the nonventilated lung, thereby eliminating the shunt.

What is HPV?

One of the main physiologic adaptations to counter hypoxemia during single-lung ventilation is HPV of the vascular supply to the nondependent, nonventilated lung.

HPV is a physiological phenomenon in which pulmonary arterioles constrict in a region of hypoxia, redirecting blood flow to areas of lung with better oxygenation. In SLV, the effect is to direct more blood flow toward the ventilated lung. As a result of HPV, V/Q mismatch from SLV is decreased, reducing the degree of hypoxemia during SLV.

TABLE 21.6 ■ Troubleshooting Hypoxemia During Single Lung Ventilation

Actions	Consequences
Increase the FiO_2 to 1.0	Will usually increase SpO_2 and allow time for further troubleshooting
Optimize tidal volumes and minute ventilation	To match that of the patient's metabolic demand
Check DLT or BB placement with a fiberoptic bronchoscope	To confirm proper lung portion remains isolated
Suction airway	For removal of secretions, bleeding, and/or mucus plugs
Optimize the patient's hemodynamics	Improving the patient's cardiac output thus improving gas exchange and delivery
Recruit the dependent lung and apply 5–10 cm H_2O of PEEP	To prevent further atelectasis and worsening of shunt
Apply 5–10 cm H_2O of CPAP to the nondependent lung	To allow for passive oxygenation of the nondependent lung thus reducing shunt (although this may be disruptive to the surgeon, especially in VATS)
Returning to two-lung ventilation	Usually as a last resort maneuver, but is needed especially when a patient is becoming hypoxemic
Clamp the pulmonary artery to the nondependent lung	To completely eliminate the shunting of blood to the nondependent lung. This is only done in extreme cases when it is not possible to return to two-lung ventilation.

BB, Bronchial blocker; *CPAP,* continuous positive airway pressure; *DLT,* double-lumen tube; *PEEP,* positive end-expiratory pressure; *VATS,* video-assisted thoracic surgery.

Will volatile anesthesia gas impact HPV? What about other medications?
All volatile anesthetic agents can inhibit HPV in a dose-dependent fashion. However, modern inhaled anesthetics used at doses less than one minimal alveolar concentration (MAC) have clinically insignificant impact on HPV. Some of the main inhibitors of HPV are intravenous (IV) vasodilators, such as nitroglycerin and nitroprusside. Common IV anesthetics, such as propofol and fentanyl, do not have any effect on HPV.

Surgery is uneventful. The patient is extubated and taken to the recovery room. He complains of significant pain at the surgical incision sites and also at his shoulder.

Why is he having shoulder pain?
Visceral pain arising from diaphragmatic irritation can be referred to the shoulder. This is one of the most common and difficult-to-treat pain conditions in thoracic surgical patients.

How can you manage postoperative pain?
Postoperative pain control is essential to recovery after thoracic surgery. A patient may experience anywhere from mild to severe pain after thoracic surgery depending on the surgical approach (e.g., minimally invasive versus open thoracotomy), comorbidities (e.g., baseline chronic pain conditions), and pain tolerance.

Options for postoperative analgesia include:
- Opioids: Most commonly used postoperatively, although they may not provide adequate analgesia alone. Their side-effect profiles, such as respiratory depression and constipation, may impair a patient's recovery.
- Nonsteroidal antiinflammatory drugs (NSAIDs): may be used as an adjunct to reduce opiate consumption postoperatively. They are also good options for addressing shoulder pain.

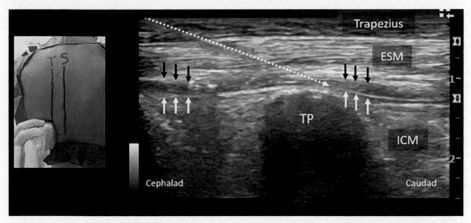

Fig. 21.9 Left: Longitudinal ultrasound probe orientation along the transverse processes (T), lateral to the spinous processes (S), for erector spinae block. Right: Corresponding parasagittal ultrasonographic view showing in-plane needle placement for injection of local anesthetic deep to the erector spinae muscle *(ESM)* and superficial to the transverse process *(TP)* and intercostal muscle *(ICM)*. (Modified from Forero, M., Rajarathinam, M., Adhikary, S., & Chin, K. J. [2017]. Erector spinae plane (ESP) block in the management of post thoracotomy pain syndrome: A case series. *Scandinavian Journal of Pain, 17*, 325–329. Modified From Fig. 1.)

However, they may contribute to gastrointestinal bleeding, decreased platelet function, decreased renal function, and increased bronchial reactivity.
- Acetaminophen: a weak cyclooxygenase inhibitor that may also be considered an analgesic adjunct.
- Other options: low-dose IV ketamine and IV dexmedetomidine may be used to provide additional pain relief and reduce opiate requirements.

What regional anesthetic options may be helpful to this patient?
These regional anesthetics are helpful for reducing opioid consumption and improving patients' recoveries, particularly after more invasive procedures (e.g., thoracotomy):
- Intercostal nerve block: usually performed under direct visualization by the surgeon intraoperatively but can also be performed pre- or postoperatively by an anesthesiologist. Local anesthetic, such as 2–3 mL of 0.5% ropivacaine injection per nerve, can provide 6–24 hours of pain relief. Of note, this usually does not cover shoulder (diaphragmatic) pain.
- Neuraxial and paravertebral analgesia: thoracic epidural or thoracic paravertebral blocks are important regional analgesic options for thoracic surgical patients. Both of these techniques have been shown to provide adequate analgesia postoperatively. However, patients can experience profound hypotension postoperatively due to the resulting inhibition of sympathetic tone (see Case 9).
- Erector spinae plane nerve block: a relatively newer regional anesthesia technique that has been shown to provide good analgesic coverage for the thoracic region (T2–T9 sensory level). Using a 10-cm 18-gauge Tuohy needle, 20 mL of 0.25% ropivacaine local anesthetic is injected to the myofascial plane between the erector spinae muscle and the T5 transverse process followed by placement of a thin catheter for continuous local anesthetic infusion postoperatively (see Fig. 21.9).

What postoperative pulmonary regimen should this patient follow?
It is critical that thoracic surgical patients maintain adequate ventilation and oxygenation postoperatively. Supplemental oxygen delivery can be titrated to the patient's oxygen level (pulse oximeter

and arterial oxygen tension) via devices ranging from nasal cannula to high-flow face-mask. If a patient remains intubated postoperatively, they should be extubated as soon as possible to prevent long-term respiratory complications.

Postoperative pulmonary hygiene should include inhaled β-agonists as needed for control of COPD, acetylcysteine, coughing exercises, chest percussion, deep breathing exercises, ambulation, and incentive spirometry.

On postoperative day 1, the patient complains of tingling at the medial aspect of his right forearm extending to the medial hand and his fourth and fifth fingers.

What's going on?
This is consistent with a stretch injury to the brachial plexus, which is a known risk of lateral positioning for thoracic surgery (Fig. 21.10). Advise the patient that this is likely transient and should improve with time.

What are other potential complications of thoracic surgery exist?
Postoperative complications after thoracic surgery include atelectasis, pneumothorax, respiratory failure, arrhythmias, right heart failure, wound infection, and neuropathies (see Table 21.7).

BEYOND THE PEARLS

- Prior to thoracic surgery, a thorough preoperative evaluation is critical to ensure positive surgical outcome. Cardiopulmonary function testing and respiratory optimization treatments should be considered based on patient's comorbidities and the invasiveness of the surgery to be performed.
- 12–24 hours of smoking cessation is enough to decrease carboxyhemoglobin levels in the blood and shift the oxyhemoglobin dissociation curve rightward, thus increasing oxygen delivery to tissues.
- VATS is one of the absolute indications for single-lung ventilation (SLV), which is required to create enough space in the thorax to facilitate minimally invasive surgery.
- DLT is the most commonly utilized tool for SLV in an adult during thoracic surgery. A stepwise approach should be taken for both placement and troubleshooting of the DLT.
- Hypoxemia may occur during SLV and is usually secondary to shunting—not dead space. Increasing FiO_2 may only improve hypoxemia slightly to provide a small window of opportunity for further troubleshooting.
- Although there is a stepwise approach to dealing with hypoxemia during SLV, one should immediately return to two-lung ventilation if a patient's oxygenation drops precipitously below the acceptable threshold in order to prevent hypoxic end-organ damage.
- Adequate analgesia is critical for a patient's speedy recovery post-thoracic surgery. A multimodal analgesia approach is recommended, which usually includes the utilization of opioids in conjunction with other adjuncts, such as NSAIDs and acetaminophen. Regional anesthesia should also be considered to provide adequate analgesia.
- Most complications after thoracic surgery are respiratory (20%) or cardiovascular (10%) in nature.

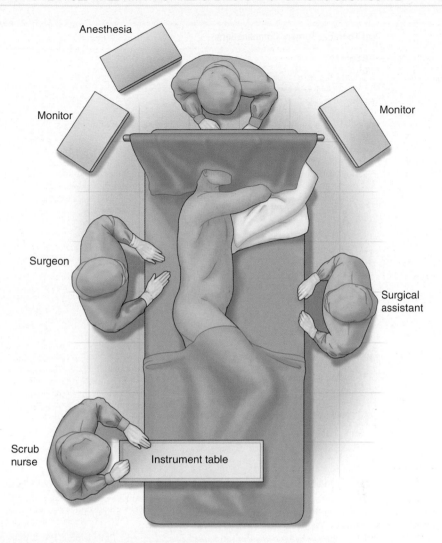

Fig. 29.10   For VATS, the patient is generally placed in the lateral position, with the operative lung up (i.e., non-dependent) and the ventilated lung down (i.e., dependent). The shoulders flexed. It is important to minimize this flexion to reduce the risk of brachial plexus injury. (Reproduced from Lackner, R. P. [2013]. Thoracoscopic lung resections. In C. T. Frantzides & M. A. Carlson [Eds.], *Video atlas of advanced minimally invasive surgery* [Chapter 2, pp. 11–30. Philadelphia, PA: Elsevier]. Fig. 2–1.)

TABLE 21.7 ■ Post Thoracic Surgery Complications

Complication	Etiology	Management
Atelectasis	Common, due to prolonged SLV and poor postoperative pulmonary hygiene	Improve pulmonary hygiene via coughing, mobilization, and incentive spirometry; bronchodilators; improve analgesia.
Pneumothorax	Due to recent invasive thoracic surgery	Apply suction to chest tubes; close follow-up via repeat physical exam and chest radiograph.
Respiratory failure	As a result of poor preoperative pulmonary function, major pulmonary resection, or multifactorial. Defined as PaO_2 <60 mm Hg, $PaCO_2$ >45 mm Hg, or >24 h of postoperative mechanical ventilation.	Thorough preoperative workup and patient optimization; adequate postoperative analgesia, early extubation, early ambulation, and chest physiotherapy.
Arrhythmias	Thought to be linked to postoperative right heart dysfunction. Patient with cardiopulmonary risk factors, such as chronic obstructive pulmonary disease (COPD), are at higher risk.	Antiarrhythmic agents (e.g., diltiazem); correct the underlying problem such as right heart failure and COPD exacerbation.
Right heart failure	There is some degree of right heart dysfunction post pulmonary resections, likely due to the removal of vascular bed during pulmonary resections.	Close monitoring in intensive care unit (ICU); judicious fluid management; inotropic support as needed.
Neuropathies	Secondary to lateral positioning, with the brachial plexus being the most vulnerable (i.e., via stretch injury) (see Case 25).	Proper positioning and padding of the arms during lateral positioning (see Fig. 21.10); frequent intraoperative position checks; conservative treatment and close observation.

References

Barash, P. G. (Ed.), (2013). *Clinical anesthesia* (7th ed.). Philadelphia, PA: Lippincott Williams & Wilkins.
Duke, J. C. (Ed.), (2016). *Duke's anesthesia secrets* (5th ed.). Philadelphia, PA: Elsevier, Saunders.
Hartigan, P. (2014). Anesthesia for video-assisted thoracoscopic surgery (VATS) for pulmonary resection. In T. W. Post (Ed.), *UpToDate*. Waltham, MA: UpToDate Inc. *UpToDate*.
Jaffe, R. A. (Ed.), (2014). *Anesthesiologist's manual of surgical procedures* (5th ed.). Philadelphia, PA: Lippincott Williams & Wilkins.
Miller, R. D. (Ed.), (2015). *Miller's anesthesia* (8th ed.). Philadelphia, PA: Elsevier, Saunders.
Reilly, J. (2020). Chronic obstructive pulmonary disease. In L. Goldman & A. I. Schafer (Eds.), *Goldman-Cecil Medicine* (26th ed., Chapter 82, pp. 535–544.e2). Philadelphia, PA: Elsevier.
Rodrigo, C. (2020). The effects of cigarette smoking on anesthesia. *Anesthesia Progress*. 2000 Winter; *47*(4): 143–150.
Yao, F. F. (Ed.), (2016). *Yao & Artusio's anesthesiology: Problem-oriented patient management* (8th ed). Philadelphia: Lippincott Williams & Wilkins.

A 30-Year-Old Woman Scheduled for Sternotomy for Resection of an Anterior Mediastinal Mass

Harsha Koneru ■ Paul Neil Frank

A 30-year-old woman is scheduled for sternotomy for resection of an anterior mediastinal mass. She initially presented to her primary care physician with complaints of worsening diplopia, ptosis, dysphagia, dysarthria, and new onset of facial swelling. She was diagnosed with myasthenia gravis and prescribed pyridostigmine 90 mg/day. Computerized tomography (CT) of her chest revealed a large mediastinal mass (see Fig. 22.1A). Vital signs show blood pressure 115/74 mm Hg, pulse 88/min, respirations 9/min, oxygen saturation 96% on room air, and temperature 36.6°C.

Describe the anatomy of the mediastinum.
The mediastinum is divided into the superior and inferior mediastinum. The inferior mediastinum is divided into the anterior, middle, and posterior mediastinal compartments as shown in the chest radiograph (CXR) in Fig. 22.2 and diagrams in Fig. 22.3.

What is myasthenia gravis?
Myasthenia gravis is an autoimmune disease wherein antibodies are generated against the post-synaptic nicotinic acetylcholine receptors at the neuromuscular junction. These antibodies prevent acetylcholine from binding and activating the acetylcholine receptor on the motor end plate, preventing depolarization of the muscle. This results in muscle weakness. Typically, ocular, bulbar, respiratory, and proximal skeletal muscles are most affected. Weakness of these muscles can compromise speech, swallowing, and chewing.

How is myasthenia gravis treated?
The goal in treating myasthenia gravis is to improve transmission at the neuromuscular junction to alleviate symptoms. Unfortunately, medical management is not curative. Instead, the medications administered will help mitigate the symptoms. This is achieved by using acetylcholinesterase inhibitors such as pyridostigmine. Medical therapy also includes immunosuppression with corticosteroids. Patients who do not respond to corticosteroids may receive other immunosuppressants. Patients with severe disease may require plasmapheresis or intravenous immunoglobulin (IVIG).

STEP 1 PEARL

Acetylcholinesterase breaks down acetylcholine released into the neuromuscular junction, which limits the duration of action of acetylcholine in stimulating nicotinic receptors. Pyridostigmine inhibits acetylcholinesterase in the neuromuscular junction, thereby preventing the breakdown of acetylcholine. This increases the amount of acetylcholine available to stimulate nicotinic receptors.

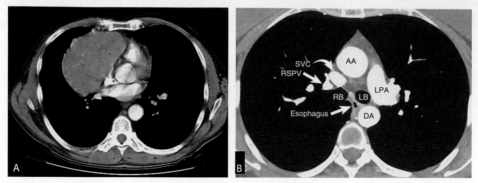

Fig. 22.1 (A) Axial computed tomography (CT) image showing a large mediastinal mass. (B) Axial CT image showing normal anatomy for comparison. *AA*, Ascending aorta; *DA*, descending aorta; *LB*, left bronchus; *LPA*, left pulmonary artery; *RB*, right bronchus; *RSPV*, right superior pulmonary vein; *SVC*, superior vena cava. (Kim, J. Y., & Hofstetter, W. L. [2010]. Tumors of the mediastinum and chest wall. *Surgical Clinics of North America, 90*[5], 1019–1040; Bueno, J., Walker, C. M., Chung, J. H. [2010]. Normal chest radiography and computerized tomography. *Muller's Imaging of the Chest, 1*, 1–56.e2 Modified from Fig. 1.68.)

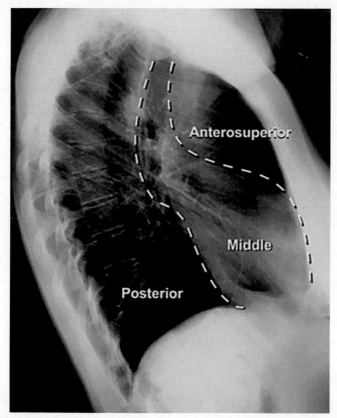

Fig. 22.2 Lateral chest radiograph of normal mediastinum with anterosuperior, middle, and posterior compartments outlined. (Sugarbaker, D. J., et al. [2022]. Chapter 58: Lung, chest wall, pleura and mediastinum. In M. Courtney (Ed.), *Sabiston textbook of surgery*. Townsend: Elsevier, 2021. Fig. 58.38.)

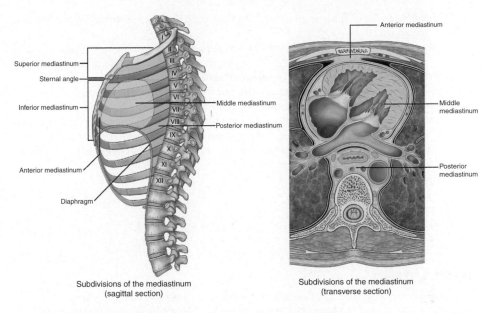

Fig. 22.3 Sagittal and transverse diagrams of the mediastinum. (Drake, R. L., Vogl, A. W., & Mitchell, A. W. M. [2021]. Thorax. *Gray's Atlas of Anatomy, 3*, 61–132.)

STEP 1 PEARL

Glucocorticoids diffuse across the cell membrane and bind to the receptors in the cytoplasm and then enter the nucleus to alter the transcription of certain genes. Chronic use of steroids can cause mood disturbances, abdominal striae, acne, hirsutism, neuropathy, hypertension, osteoporosis, diabetes mellitus, adrenal cortex suppression, immunosuppression, and growth retardation.

In patients with myasthenia gravis found to have a thymoma, thymectomy may be indicated.

What is the primary function of the thymus?
The thymus is a lymphatic gland that is located in the anterosuperior mediastinum. Its primary function is to facilitate maturation and selection of naive T cells from immature T cell precursors that migrated from the bone marrow.

The patient says she has had significant swelling of her face, chest, and arms recently.

What is going on?
These findings are concerning for compression of the superior vena cava (SVC) by the mass. Compression or obstruction of the SVC leads to distention of the veins of the face, neck, and arms, as well as mucosal swelling that can cause dyspnea and congestion. This is known as SVC syndrome.

You notice a large distended vein on the patient's forearm.

Is a good location for an intravenous (IV) catheter?
No. In the setting of SVC compression, medications and fluids administered through an IV line in the arm will have a prolonged and unpredictable return to the central circulation. The same holds

true for medications and fluids administered through central venous catheters in the internal jugular or subclavian veins.

Patients with SVC syndrome should have IV access placed in the groin, legs, or feet.

What are the other possible symptoms of a mediastinal mass?

Symptoms of thymomas may arise from mass effect or from systemic effects.

Mass effects can be caused by direct invasion or compression of nearby structures such as major blood vessels, airways, or nerves. Approximately one third of patients who develop a mediastinal mass may have chest pain, dyspnea, or cough. Symptomatology correlates to the size and location of the mass. Smaller masses are more likely to be asymptomatic, whereas larger masses are more likely to cause

- Cough and hoarseness
- Dyspnea
- Dysphagia
- Horner syndrome
- SVC syndrome

STEP 1, 2, 3 PEARL

Horner syndrome is caused by a loss of sympathetic tone to the one half of the face. Symptoms include miosis, ptosis, anhidrosis, and enophthalmos. In the case of an anterior mediastinal mass, loss of sympathetic tone is caused by tumor invasion or compression of the sympathetic nerves to the face (see Case 1).

What additional preoperative work-up is necessary given the patient's history of mediastinal mass and myasthenia gravis?

Preoperative pulmonary function tests (PFTs) can identify potential airway obstruction caused by the mass. Airway obstruction is classified based on the location the mass and whether it varies during the respiratory cycle: extrathoracic variable obstruction, intrathoracic variable obstruction, and fixed obstruction. Each type of pathology has a characteristic flow-volume loop (see Case 21). *Note, the term "obstruction" in this context refers to large airway obstruction and is different than small airway obstructive pulmonary disease as in chronic obstructive pulmonary disease.*

As demonstrated in Fig. 22.4, extrathoracic masses tend to cause flattening of the inspiratory part of the flow-volume loop during negative pressure inspiration, indicating decreased maximal inspiratory airflow. Intrathoracic masses tend to cause flattening of the expiratory part of the flow-volume loop during expiration, indicating decreased maximal expiratory airflow. Fixed lesions will result in flattening of both the inspiratory and expiratory parts of the flow-volume loop, indicating decreased maximal inspiratory and expiratory airflow.

PFTs will also provide a baseline measure of the strength of respiratory muscles, which may be compromised in patients with myasthenia gravis.

Preoperative evaluation should include a CT scan of the chest for evaluation of the extent of tumor invasion of major airways or cardiovascular structures. Echocardiogram is indicated if there is major cardiac or vascular involvement.

Assessment of baseline strength and symptoms of myasthenia gravis, as well as the patient's history of exacerbations and medications, is also important.

During the preoperative interview you ask the patient whether she can breathe comfortably lying flat and whether she ever becomes lightheaded or faint while lying flat.

Why?
Dyspnea while lying supine is an indication of significant airway obstruction. Lightheadedness or a sensation of impending syncope is concerning for compression of major vessels.

You tell the patient that there is a risk that she will remain intubated at the end of surgery.

What are the classic risk factors for postoperative mechanical ventilation?
A predictive scoring system of controversial efficacy is used to estimate the risk for requiring postoperative mechanical ventilation in patients with myasthenia gravis. This includes the following criteria:
- Duration of disease for longer than 6 years
- Chronic comorbid pulmonary disease
- Pyridostigmine dose >750 mg/day
- Vital capacity <2.9 L.

The patient's flow-volume loop looks like loop C in Fig. 22.4.

Why is it important to distinguish intrathoracic and extrathoracic airway obstruction?
Airway management and emergency rescue procedures are different depending on the location of the obstruction, as shown in Table 22.1.

Although intubation may be "easy" in intrathoracic airway obstruction, ventilation may be extremely challenging if the distal end of the endotracheal tube is past the vocal cords but not past the obstruction. This may necessitate rescue ventilation with a rigid bronchoscope.

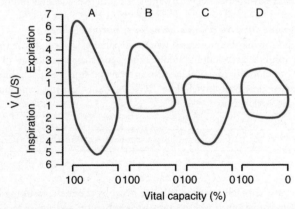

Fig. 22.4 Flow-volume loops showing (A) normal tracing, (B) variable extrathoracic airway obstruction, (C) variable intrathoracic airway obstruction, and (D) fixed upper airway obstruction. (Kraft M. "Approach to the Patient with Respiratory Disease." Goldman-Cecil Medicine. Modified from Fig. 77.1.)

TABLE 22.1 ■ Comparison of Intrathoracic and Extrathoracic Airway Obstruction

	Extrathoracic Obstruction	Intrathoracic Obstruction
mask ventilation	difficult (↑risk of gastric insufflation)	easy
intubation	difficult	easy
rescue procedure	cricothyrotomy or tracheotomy	rigid bronchoscopy

The patient says she becomes short of breath after lying flat for 30 seconds. She sleeps on three pillows at night.

How will you induce anesthesia in this patient?

Since she cannot tolerate lying flat, it is likely that the mass is compressing her airway. Inducing this patient with a hypnotic and then a muscle relaxant (i.e., propofol then rocuronium) will result in loss of spontaneous respiration and muscle tone, which could result in total compression of the airway. Therefore, the safest approach is awake fiberoptic intubation (see Case 24). Keeping the patient spontaneously breathing during intubation will allow for more troubleshooting should you encounter difficulty. Another possibility is an inhaled induction with anesthesia gas to maintain spontaneous respiration with titration of an IV hypnotic, classically ketamine.

It is critical that the distal end of the endotracheal tube be placed distal to the airway obstruction while the patient maintains muscle tone in the upper airway and spontaneous negative pressure ventilation. Be sure that there is a rigid bronchoscope and personnel familiar with using it in the room.

In scenarios in which there is a high risk for total compression of the airway and inability to ventilate, venovenous extracorporeal membrane oxygenation (VV ECMO) may need to be initiated prior to induction of anesthesia. VV ECMO requires systemic heparinization and involvement of a cardiac surgeon, cardiac anesthesiologist, and perfusionist.

Awake intubation is successful, and general anesthesia is induced with propofol and rocuronium.

How does myasthenia gravis affect the patient's sensitivity to neuromuscular blockers?

Patients with myasthenia gravis have increased sensitivity to nondepolarizing neuromuscular blockers and decreased sensitivity to depolarizing agents such as succinylcholine.

How does pyridostigmine affect the pharmacokinetics of succinylcholine?

Effects of succinylcholine may be prolonged when the patient has been taking pyridostigmine

Pyridostigmine inhibits acetylcholinesterase and causes an abundance of acetylcholine at the neuromuscular junction. Pyridostigmine also inhibits plasma pseudocholinesterase, which is responsible for breaking down succinylcholine. Both these mechanisms contribute to the prolongation of action of succinylcholine.

Shortly after induction, the patient's blood pressure decreases from 105/70 to 45/28 mm Hg.

What is going on?

This may be caused by compression of the SVC or heart by the mass, resulting in decreased preload and hypotension. Initiation of positive pressure ventilation and supine positioning may also contribute to hypotension. Ventilate with the lowest possible airway pressure, and aggressively treat with volume replacement and vasopressors.

You maintain neuromuscular blockade with rocuronium. At the end of surgery, you reverse the neuromuscular blockade with sugammadex. Just after extubation, the patient cannot lift her head off the pillow.

What is going on?

The potential causes of weakness after extubation in this patient are

1. Incomplete reversal of neuromuscular blockade: Neuromuscular blockade should be fully reversed prior to extubation. Even with four strong twitches on train of four stimulation, there may be residual neuromuscular blockade. These patients should receive additional reversal agent.
2. Myasthenic crisis: Severe respiratory or bulbar muscle weakness may necessitate reintubation or delayed extubation. Causes of myasthenic crisis include stress of surgery, residual anesthetics, or missed doses of normally administered myasthenia gravis medications. Consult a neurologist for possible plasma exchange or additional immunotherapy.
3. Cholinergic crisis: Increased cholinergic receptor activation caused by overdose of acetylcholinesterase inhibitor. Clinical manifestations include weakness, salivation, lacrimation, urination, diarrhea, gastrointestinal distress, and emesis. In these patients, atropine or glycopyrrolate may be required. This will help counteract the muscarinic effects of excessive cholinergic stimulation.

How does the use of sugammadex help clarify what is happening?
Sugammadex is a modified cyclodextrin molecule that encapsulates and inactivates unbound rocuronium and vecuronium circulating in the plasma. This complex is eliminated in the urine. Sugammadex can be used instead of acetylcholinesterase inhibitors (e.g., neostigmine) for reversal of neuromuscular blockade.

Because acetylcholinesterase inhibitors were not used to reverse neuromuscular blockade, cholinergic crisis is much less likely.

You administer an additional dose of sugammadex, and the patient's strength improves to baseline.

How does myasthenia gravis differ from Lambert-Eaton myasthenic syndrome?
Myasthenia gravis is an autoimmune disorder in which antibodies are generated against postsynaptic nicotinic acetylcholine receptors at the neuromuscular junction. Lambert-Eaton syndrome, also known as myasthenic syndrome, is commonly associated with antibodies against presynaptic voltage-gated calcium channels at the neuromuscular junction. These antibodies hinder the release of acetylcholine from vesicles in the presynaptic nerve terminal in response to an action potential. Patients develop proximal muscle weakness (legs more than arms) and reduced or absent deep tendon reflexes. These patients do not respond to acetylcholinesterase inhibitors. Lambert-Eaton syndrome is most commonly associated with small cell lung cancer. Unlike patients with myasthenia gravis, patients with Lambert-Eaton syndrome may show transient improvement in strength with exercise.

BEYOND THE PEARLS

- Patients with thymomas have 20%–25% incidence of myasthenia gravis. Myasthenia gravis is the most common paraneoplastic syndrome associated with thymoma. Other systemic diseases include red cell aplasia and hypogammaglobulinemia.
- Many drugs can worsen the symptoms of myasthenia gravis. Common culprits include calcium channel blockers, magnesium, aminoglycosides, clindamycin, gabapentin, carbamazepine, and phenytoin.
- Thymomas that are less than 3 cm in size are frequently benign, while thymomas that are greater than 5 cm are often malignant.
- Thymoma is a one of the most common neoplasms of the anterior mediastinum, followed by lymphomas. Thymomas may occur from childhood or adulthood, but the peak incidence is in the third through fifth decades of life.
- Whenever possible, it is advisable to avoid neuromuscular blocking agents in patients with myasthenia gravis. If a procedure can be done with sedation or with regional anesthesia, these options should be given strong consideration.

References

Ashworth, A. (2021). Anaesthesia for surgery of the trachea and main bronchi. *Anaesthesia & Intensive Care Medicine, 22*(3), 156–162.

Campo, E. Jaffe, E. S., & Harris, N. L. (2017). Normal lymphoid organs and tissues. In E. S. Jaffe, D. A. Arber, E. Campo, N. L. Harris, & L. Quintanilla-Martinez (Eds.), *Hematopathology* (2nd ed., pp. 131–152). Philadelphia, PA: Elsevier.

Charlesworth, M., Daroff, R. B., Jankovic, J., Mazziotta, J. C., & Pomeroy, S. L. (2017). Disorders of neuromuscular transmission. In R. B. Daroff, J. Jankovic, J. C. Mazziotta, & S. L. Pomeroy (Eds.), *Bradley's Neurology in Clinical Practice* (pp. 1896–1914). Philadelphia, PA: Elsevier.

Dhallu, M. S., et al. (2017). Perioperative management of neurological conditions. *Health Services Insights, 10* 1178632917711942. https://doi.org/10.1177/1178632917711942.

Gropper, M. A., Miller, R. D., & Cohen, N. H. (2020). Anesthesia for thoracic surgery. In M. A. Gropper, R. D. Miller, N. H. Cohen, L. I. Eriksson, L. A. Fleisher, K. Leslie, et al. (Eds.), *Miller's anesthesia* (9th ed., pp. 1648–1716). Philadelphia, PA: Elsevier.

Townsend, C. M., Sabiston, D. C., Beauchamp, R. D., et al. (2017). Lung, chest wall, pleura, and mediastinum. In *Sabiston textbook of surgery: The biological basis of modern surgical practice*, 1572–1618.

Neurology

A 50-Year-Old Man Scheduled for Resection of a Pineal Gland Tumor

Paul Neil Frank

> A 50-year-old man is scheduled for resection of a pineal gland tumor. He is otherwise healthy. He runs 2 miles 3 days per week. He does not smoke or drink alcohol. In the preoperative area his pulse is 80/min, blood pressure 112/65 mm Hg, respiratory rate 10/min, oxygen saturation 100% on room air, and temperature 36.8°C.

The surgeon wants to do the operation with the patient in the sitting position. What are the hemodynamic implications of the sitting position?

As the name implies, the sitting position keeps the patient's torso fairly vertical (see Fig. 23.1). Preload, stroke volume, cardiac output, mean arterial blood pressure (MAP), and central venous pressure (CVP) will all decrease in the sitting position compared with the supine position. Systemic vascular resistance (SVR) and heart rate (HR) increase to compensate for the drop in MAP.

Sitting position also carries an increased risk of venous air embolism (VAE).

What is a VAE?

Injury to a vein creates an open communication between the intravascular space and the ambient atmosphere. Because the surgical field is above the level of the heart (as in the sitting position), venous pressure may be less than atmospheric pressure. Air can therefore be entrained into the vein through this opening in the vein. When the air is carried to the heart, it creates an air lock (essentially a large bubble) in the right ventricle, significantly reducing the ventricular volume available to fill with and eject blood.

How is MAP calculated?

Given a single reading of systolic and diastolic blood pressure, MAP is calculated by

$$MAP = 1/3 \times systolic\ blood\ pressure + 2/3 \times diastolic\ blood\ pressure$$

This formula assumes that one-third of the cardiac cycle is systole, and two-thirds of the cardiac cycle is diastole.

If blood pressure is measured from an invasive arterial catheter, blood pressure is measured many times per second, and the average of these measurements is used to calculate an average pressure, or MAP.

What is cerebral perfusion pressure (CPP)?

CPP is a measure of the pressure of the blood flow through the brain. If intracranial pressure (ICP) is greater than central venous pressure (CVP), then CPP is given by

$$CPP = MAP - ICP$$

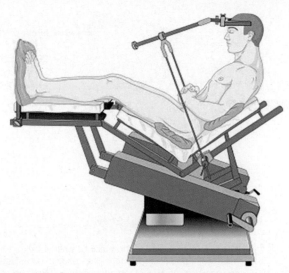

Fig. 23.1 The operating room table, combined with a head holder an appropriate padding of all pressure points, can facilitate maintenance of the sitting position during the operation. Make sure there are at least two finger's breadth between the patient's mandible and sternum once the patient is in the sitting position, to prevent excessive neck flexion. (Modified from Lemkuil, B. P., Drummond, J. C., Patel, P. M., & Lam, A. [2020]. Anesthesia for neurologic surgery and neurointerventions. In M. A. Gropper, R. D. Miller, N. H. Cohen, L. I. Eriksson, L. A. Fleischer, K. Leslie, et al. (Eds.), *Miller's anesthesia* [9th ed., Chapter 66, pp. 1868–1910.e9]. Philadelphia, PA: Elsevier. Modified from Fig. 57.8.)

If CVP is greater than ICP, then CPP is given by

$$CPP = MAP-CVP$$

In otherwise healthy patients in the supine position, ICP is 8–15 mm Hg. CPP should be maintained at 60 mm Hg or greater. In patients with known cerebrovascular disease, hypertension, or cervical myelopathy, higher CPPs may be necessary.

STEP 1 PEARL

ICP is determined by the volume of the things inside the cranium that take up space: brain tissue (including cells and extracellular fluid), blood, and cerebrospinal fluid. As the volume of any of these increases, ICP will increase.

After placing the patient in the sitting position, the arterial line in the patient's left radial artery reads 120/60 mm Hg, with a MAP of 80 mm Hg.

Is that MAP high enough?

No. CPP is based on MAP at the level of the circle of Willis, corresponding to the external auditory meatus—effectively the patient's ear. In patients who are horizontal (either supine or prone), MAP measured at the wrist is the same as MAP at the circle of Willis.

However, this is not the case when the patient is vertical. Blood pressure decreases by 0.75 mm Hg for every centimeter increase in height. Assuming the circle of Willis is 20 cm above the arterial line in the patient's wrist, the MAP at the circle of Willis is

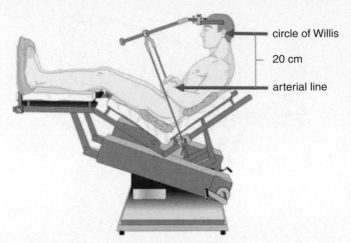

Fig. 23.2 In the sitting position, the radial arterial line at the patient's wrist is well below the circle of Willis. Therefore the blood pressure measured at the level of the arterial line needs to be reduced by 0.75 mm Hg for every centimeter in vertical distance between the level of the arterial line and the level of the circle of Willis to determine what mean arterial blood pressure the brain is receiving. (Modified from Lemkuil, B. P., Drummond, J. C., Patel, P. M., & Lam, A. Anesthesia for neurologic surgery and neurointerventions. In *Miller's anesthesia* [Chapter 57]. 1868-1910.e9 Modified from Fig. 57.8.)

$$MAP_{brain} = MAP_{art\ line} - \Delta_{height} \times 0.75$$
$$MAP_{brain} = 80\ mm\ Hg - \left(20\ cm \times 0.75\ mm\ Hg/cm\right)$$
$$MAP_{brain} = 65\ mm\ Hg$$

Therefore the brain is only receiving a MAP of 65 mm Hg. Fig. 23.2 shows a graphical representation of this change in MAP. In this case, assuming a normal ICP, CPP is given by

$$CPP = MAP - ICP$$
$$CPP = 65\ mm\ Hg - 12\ mm\ Hg$$
$$CPP = 53\ mm\ Hg$$

As discussed above, the CPP should be maintained at 60 mm Hg or greater in otherwise healthy patients.

If the MAP at the circle of Willis increases from 70–80 mm Hg, will cerebral blood flow change?
Assuming the patient is otherwise healthy, cerebral blood flow should remain relatively constant. The arteries of the brain dilate or constrict to maintain constant blood flow to the brain over a wide range of MAP, from 70–150 mm Hg. With MAP less than 70 mm Hg, cerebral vessels are maximally dilated, and blood flow drops with MAP. With MAP greater than 150 mm Hg, cerebral vessels are maximally constricted, and blood flow increases with MAP. This phenomenon is called cerebral autoregulation or myogenic regulation (see Fig. 23.3).

It is important to note that the minimum and maximum MAP, as well as the amount of cerebral blood flow maintained by this mechanism, vary considerably among individuals, as well as with other physiologic factors and disease states. For example, in patients with chronic hypertension, this curve may be shifted to the right, such that cerebral blood flow is constant from MAP of 80–180 mm Hg.

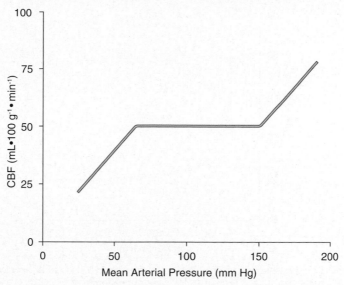

Fig. 23.3 Cerebral autoregulation allows for relatively constant cerebral blood flow over a wide range of mean arterial blood pressure. (Modified from Patel, P. M., Drummond, J. C., & Lemkuil, B. P. Cerebral physiology and the effects of anesthetic drugs. In *Miller's anesthesia* [Chapter 11]. 295–332.e8 Modified from Fig. 11.3.)

What other factors affect cerebral blood flow?
- Cerebral metabolic rate (CMR): Cerebral blood flow increases or decreases with CMR. This relationship is known as neurovascular coupling. The mechanism is complex and incompletely understood, but it is believed that by-products of excitatory neuronal activity, such as glutamate and adenosine, as well as signaling via glial cells, stimulate local vasodilation.
- Temperature: CMR decreases by 7% for every degree Celsius decrease in temperature less than 37°C. Significantly less cerebral blood flow is required at lower temperatures as CMR decreases.
- Arterial carbon dioxide tension ($PaCO_2$): Cerebral blood flow varies directly with $PaCO_2$ within physiologic levels of $PaCO_2$. Cerebral blood flow increases by 1–2 mL/100 g cerebral tissue/min with every increase in $PaCO_2$ by 1 mm Hg. This is why hyperventilation acutely decreases ICP (see Case 26).
- Arterial oxygen tension (PaO_2): Cerebral blood flow remains relatively constant from PaO_2 levels from 60–300 mm Hg. At PaO_2 levels less than 60 mm Hg, cerebral blood flow increases significantly (see Fig. 23.4).
- Other factors such as cardiac output, blood viscosity (affected mainly by hematocrit), and neural control cerebral vascular tone also play a role in regulation of cerebral blood flow.

How do anesthetic agents affect cerebral blood flow?
Except for ketamine and nitrous oxide (N_2O), anesthetic drugs reduce CMR. Inhaled anesthesia gases also alter the relationship between CMR and cerebral blood flow. At doses greater than 1 mean alveolar concentration (MAC), inhaled anesthesia agents cause cerebral vasodilation, resulting in more cerebral blood flow than would ordinarily occur for a given CMR. Cerebral autoregulation is also abolished at higher doses of inhaled anesthesia gas, such that cerebral blood flow is proportional to MAP. Table 23.1 summarizes the effect of common anesthetic agent on CMR and cerebral blood flow.

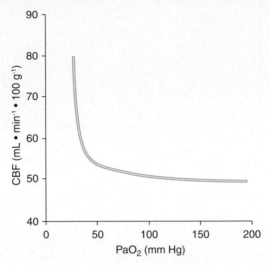

Fig. 23.4   At arterial oxygen tension less than 60 mm Hg, cerebral blood flow increases significantly. (Modified from Patel, P. M., Drummond, J. C., & Lemkuil, B. P. Cerebral physiology and the effects of anesthetic drugs. In *Miller's anesthesia* [Chapter 11]. 295–332.e8 Modified from Fig. 11.7.)

TABLE 23.1 ■ **Changes in Cerebral Metabolic Rate and Cerebral Blood Flow in Response to Anesthetic Agents**

Agent	Change in CMR	Change in Cerebral Blood Flow
N_2O	↑	↑
Halogenated gases (e.g., sevoflurane, desflurane)	↓	↑
Intravenous anesthetics except ketamine (e.g., propofol, barbiturates)	↓	↓
Ketamine	↑	↑

CMR, Cerebral metabolic rate.

What monitors are indicated for this operation?

In addition to American Society of Anesthesiologists (ASA) standard monitors (e.g., pulse oximeter, cardiac rhythm strip, blood pressure cuff, and capnography), the following monitors should be placed:

- arterial line
- indwelling urinary catheter
- temperature monitor
- twitch monitor

Consideration should also be given to a central venous catheter, which will allow for infusions of fluids and vasoactive medications. A specialized multiorifice central venous catheter with the tip at the junction between the superior vena cava and right atrium may allow for aspiration of entrained air in the event of VAE.

Any special monitors to detect VAE?

In any operation where the surgical field is above the level of the heart, maintain a high level of vigilance for VAE. Table 23.2 lists methods of detecting VAE. Methods that are more sensitive are more likely to detect small air emboli.

> You place a transesophageal echocardiogram (TEE) probe. During your exam, you see the image shown in Fig. 23.5.

What is that?

This midesophageal bicaval view on TEE shows a patent foramen ovale (PFO), resulting from incomplete closure of the fossa ovalis, which is a relic of fetal circulation (see Case 9). A PFO allows for communication between the right atrium and the left atrium. Entrained air from VAE will first appear in the right atrium. Although flow through a PFO is usually from the left atrium to the right atrium, changing physiologic conditions can reverse this shunt, allowing blood flow from the right atrium to the left atrium. Air bubbles may enter the systemic circulation. This can lead to stroke, myocardial infarction, or tissue infarction elsewhere in the body and is known as paradoxical air embolism (PAE).

> During the operation, the patient's blood pressure suddenly drops to 40/22 mm Hg, and his HR increases to 150 bpm. End-Tidal carbon dioxide ($EtCO_2$) drops to 18 mm Hg. TEE shows the image in Fig. 23.6.

What happened?

Severe hypotension, tachycardia, and severely decreased $EtCO_2$ in the setting of a surgical field above the level of the heart is consistent with VAE.

TABLE 23.2 ■ **Methods of Detecting Venous air Embolism Listed in Order of Decreasing Sensitivity**

Method	Comments
Transesophageal echocardiography (TEE)	• Most sensitive • Expensive, invasive • Requires expertise • Watch for small bright white dots ("fireflies") in right atrium and right ventricle • Can identify patent foramen ovale (PFO) and other intracardiac shunts
Precordial Doppler	• Placed on the chest on the right or left sternal border, 2nd–4th intercostal space • Listen for high-pitched swishing different from normal blood flow
End-tidal CO_2 ($EtCO_2$)	• Most reliable if patient is intubated and mechanically ventilated • Watch for drop in $EtCO_2$ with decreased cardiac output
Pulmonary artery (PA) catheter	• Invasive, risks of PA rupture • Lumen is too narrow to retrieve entrained air • Watch for increased PA pressure, decreased pulmonary capillary wedge pressure (PCWP)
Electrocardiogram (ECG)/ cardiac rhythm strip	• Watch for ST changes, signs of right ventricle (RV) strain, tachycardia, arrhythmia • Late sign of VAE

VAE, Venous air embolism.

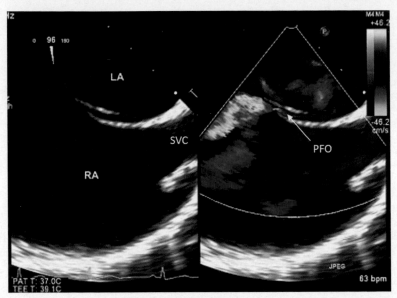

Fig. 23.5   Transesophageal echocardiogram midesophageal bicaval view without *(left)* and with *(right)* color flow Doppler showing a patent foramen ovale *(PFO)* with flow from the left atrium *(LA)* to the right atrium *(RA)*. With changing physiologic conditions, flow across the PFO may be reversed such that blood flows from the RA to the LA. This can carry air bubbles to the systemic circulation and cause paradoxical air embolism. (Modified from DiTullio, M. R. [2010]. Patent foramen ovale: Echocardiographic detection and clinical relevance in stroke. *Journal of the American Society of Echocardiography. 23*[2], 144–155.)

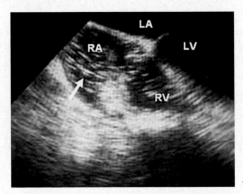

Fig. 23.6   Transesophageal echocardiogram midesophageal four-chamber view showing air bubbles *(white arrow)* within the right atrium *(RA)* and right ventricle *(RV)*. *LA*, Left atrium, *LV*, left ventricle. (Modified from Prabhakar, H., & Bithal, P. K. Venous air embolism. *Complications in Neuroanesthesia. 43*, 435–442. Fig. 1.)

What should you do?

Notify the surgical team and call for help. The surgery team should flood the surgical field with saline or otherwise occlude sources of venous bleeding. Position the patient in Trendelenburg and tilted toward the left (i.e., left lateral decubitus). This will move the air bubble toward the apex of the right ventricle, away from the right ventricular outflow tract. Ventilate with 100% oxygen. Turn off all anesthetic agents. If a central venous catheter is in place, aspirate from it to remove as much intravenous air as possible. If necessary, support cardiac output with epinephrine and begin chest compressions.

The patient had been receiving propofol and N_2O for maintenance of anesthesia prior to the VAE. Why is N_2O problematic here?

N_2O is highly diffusible and can easily diffuse into air-filled spaces within the body, such as the bowel, pleural space (as in a pneumothorax), and even air bubbles in the blood. As N_2O enters an air-filled space, that space will expand. In the case of a bubble from VAE, that air bubble will grow as N_2O diffuses into it, thereby worsening hemodynamic instability. It is particularly important to stop administration of N_2O if VAE is suspected.

Vital signs normalize, and the operation resumes. Eight hours later, at the end of surgery, the patient is neurologically intact and moves all extremities. After extubation, you notice the patient is stridorous.

What is going on?

Upper airway swelling is a known complication of prolonged neck flexion, as in the sitting position for a long neurosurgical case. Patients may develop swelling of the base of the tongue, pharynx, and soft palate.

Another possibility here is incomplete reversal of neuromuscular blockade. Patients with residual neuromuscular blockade after extubation may show signs of respiratory distress. Ensure the patient has four strong twitches on train of four monitoring and does not show fade during 5 seconds of tetanic stimulation (5 seconds of constant muscle contraction in response to constant stimulation from the twitch monitor).

The patient has four strong twitches on train of four monitoring and sustained tetanus. The patient is demonstrating mildly increased work of breathing, but he is maintaining an oxygen saturation of 97%.

What should you do?

In the setting of postextubation stridor, the most important question is whether or not the patient requires immediate reintubation. If the patient has significantly increased work of breathing (e.g., sternal retractions, accessory muscle use) or appears to be "tiring out" or if oxygen saturation drops, the patient should be reintubated immediately.

If respiratory failure is not imminent, several options may temporize the airway edema, potentially eliminating the need for reintubation. Position the patient with the head of the bed elevated at 45–90 degrees, and administer 100% oxygen via nonrebreather facemask to optimize respiratory mechanics and oxygenation. Administer nebulized racemic epinephrine to temporarily reduce airway edema and reverse any concurrent bronchoconstriction. Finally, if the patient maintains adequate oxygenation, heliox may decrease the work of breathing. Heliox is a mixture of 70% helium and 30% oxygen. Dexamethasone 4–8 mg intravenously every 8–12 hours may also help to reduce swelling, but the benefit will take hours to manifest.

How does heliox reduce the work of breathing?

The flow of a gas or liquid through a container (i.e., airway) may be described as laminar or turbulent. In laminar flow, molecules move efficiently in the same direction in an organized fashion. Flow is highest in the middle of the container and lowest near the edges. Conversely, turbulent flow is chaotic. Molecules move in different directions in a disorganized fashion (see Fig. 23.7). Turbulent flow is less efficient. This corresponds to increased work of breathing.

Laminar flow rate is inversely related to the viscosity of the gas. Therefore gases with lower viscosities have higher flow rates than do gases with higher viscosities for the same driving pressure when flow is laminar.

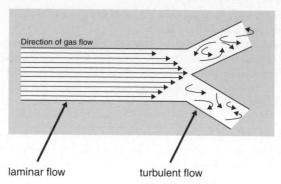

Direction of gas flow

laminar flow   turbulent flow

Fig. 23.7 In laminar flow, all molecules move in the same direction, with ones in the middle of the lumen moving at the highest velocity. In turbulent flow, molecules move in different directions. (Modified from West, T., & Photiou, A. [2018]. Measurement of gas volume and gas flow. *Anesthesia and Intensive Care Medicine. 19*[4], 183–188. Fig. 2.)

Turbulent flow rate is inversely related to the density of the gas. Therefore gases with lower densities have higher flow rates than do gases with higher densities for the same driving pressure when flow is turbulent.

All else being equal, gases with lower densities also are more likely to flow in a laminar, rather than turbulent, fashion. The density of pure oxygen is 1.429 g/L, and the density of helium is 0.178 g/L. This lower density of helium contributes to the low density of heliox. Heliox decreases the work of breathing in two ways:

- The lower density of heliox facilitates laminar, instead of turbulent, flow.
- When flow is turbulent, heliox increases the rate of flow.

After 15 minutes of observation, the patient's oxygen saturation starts to drop, and he appears to be tiring out. He will need to be reintubated. He received rocuronium throughout the surgery for neuromuscular blockade, and he received sugammadex for reversal of the blockade just prior to extubation.

What options for neuromuscular blocking agents are there for reintubation?
Sugammadex is a reversal agent specific for rocuronium and vecuronium. It works by chelating these molecules in the plasma, thereby removing them from the neuromuscular junction. The current recommendation for a patient who needs to be reintubated within 24 hours of receiving sugammadex is to avoid the use of rocuronium and vecuronium. Therefore this patient may receive succinylcholine or cisatracurium (neither of which is chelated by sugammadex) for reintubation. Studies have also shown that high-dose rocuronium (1.2 mg/kg) may still be used for reintubation, albeit with slightly delayed onset of action, within 24 hours of administration of sugammadex.

BEYOND THE PEARLS

- Prolonged neck flexion can result in compression of the ventral spinal cord and may be a cause of quadriplegia postoperatively.
- There are two components to CMR: maintenance of cellular integrity and electrophysiologic function.
- Once enough anesthetic drug has been given to suppress activity on electroencephalogram (EEG), no further reduction in CMR is achieved with higher doses of anesthetic drug. In

contrast, once the temperature has been decreased enough to suppress activity on EEG, CMR can be further reduced by even lower temperature.

- In treating a VAE, it may be helpful to aspirate from a central venous catheter to remove air from the intravascular space. However, if a central venous catheter is not in place, it is generally not recommended to place one specifically to aspirate entrained air in managing VAE.
- In patients with stridor and partial upper airway obstruction, the diminution of stridor may be because the patient is hypoventilating from fatigue of the respiratory muscles. Monitor these patients closely.
- In checking for complete reversal of neuromuscular blockade, four sustained twitches on train of four monitoring and 5 seconds of sustained tetanus do not guarantee complete reversal. No qualitative test has been shown to adequately indicate whether neuromuscular blockade has been fully reversed.
- Many patients scheduled for sitting craniotomy will undergo preoperative echocardiogram to identify a PFO or other intracardiac shunt and may undergo repair prior to craniotomy to reduce the risk of paradoxical air embolism.

References

Lemkuil, B.P., Drummond, J.C., Patel, P.M., & Lam, A. (2020). Anesthesia for neurologic surgery and neurointerventions. In M. A. Gropper, R. D. Miller, N. H. Cohen, L. I. Eriksson, L. A. Fleisher, K. Leslie, et al. (Eds.), *Miller's anesthesia* (9th ed., Chapter 66, pp. 1868–1910.e9). Philadelphia, PA: Elsevier.

Patel, A. (2020). Anesthesia for otolaryngologic and head-neck surgery. In M. A. Gropper, R. D. Miller, N. H. Cohen, L. I. Eriksson, L. A. Fleisher, K. Leslie, et al. (Eds.), *Miller's anesthesia* 9th ed., Chapter 66, pp. 2210–2235.e4). Philadelphia, PA: Elsevier.

Patel, P.M., Drummond, J.C., & Lemkuil, B.P. (2020). Cerebral physiology and the effects of anesthetic drugs. In M. A. Gropper, R. D. Miller, N. H. Cohen, L. I. Eriksson, L. A. Fleisher, K. Leslie, et al. (Eds.), *Miller's anesthesia* (9th ed., Chapter 66, pp. 294–332.e8). Philadelphia, PA: Elsevier.

West, T., & Photiou, A. (2018). Measurement of gas volume and gas flow. *Anesthesia and Intensive Care Medicine, 19*(4), 183–188.

A 34-Year-Old Woman Hit by a Car About to Undergo Emergency Cervical Decompression and Fusion

Paul Neil Frank

A 34-year-old woman who was hit by a car while riding her motorcycle earlier this evening is about to undergo emergency cervical decompression and fusion. She was wearing a helmet and did not lose consciousness. She is fully alert and oriented, although she has no sensation below her mid-chest and cannot move her arms or legs. An Aspen collar is in place. She appears flushed. There is no evidence of active bleeding on imaging. A computerized tomography (CT) scan of her cervical spine shows a fracture of the C6 vertebra. Her vital signs are: pulse 40/min; blood pressure 62/40 mm Hg; respirations 16/min; oxygen saturation 97% on room air; and temperature 33.8°C.

What is the differential diagnosis of hypotension in this patient?

In the setting of trauma, there must always be a high suspicion for hemorrhagic shock (see Case 13). Neurogenic shock should also be high on the differential, especially given the patient's poor neurologic exam. Cardiogenic shock, sepsis, anaphylaxis, and pulmonary embolism are lower on the differential diagnosis.

In this case, since there is no active hemorrhage, and since her neurologic exam presents severe findings, the most likely diagnosis is neurogenic shock.

What is neurogenic shock?

Neurogenic shock is a state of hemodynamic instability (i.e., hypotension) caused by disruption of sympathetic tone to the heart and peripheral vasculature. This is characterized by bradycardia, reduction of systemic vascular resistance (SVR), and hypothermia.

STEP 1 PEARL

Neurons of the sympathetic nervous system travel from the brainstem through the spinal cord and exit at vertebral levels T1 to L2–3. These neurons contribute to the sympathetic chain ganglia on either side of the vertebral column or course to more distal autonomic plexuses, such as the celiac plexus. Preganglionic neurons generally form synapses with postganglionic neurons in the sympathetic chain.

STEP 1 PEARL

Preganglionic neurons release acetylcholine, which stimulates nicotinic receptors on postganglionic neurons. Postganglionic neurons primarily release norepinephrine, which binds adrenergic receptors on the target organ.

What level of spinal cord injury will cause neurogenic shock?
The sympathetic innervation to the heart arises from T1 to T4. Spinal cord injuries at or above T4 can cause neurogenic shock from loss of sympathetic tone to peripheral vasculature and to the heart.

What about respiratory function?
The primary muscle of respiration is the diaphragm. Motor innervation of the diaphragm arises from C3 to C5. Patients with spinal cord injuries at or above C5 will frequently require ventilatory support. Patients with spinal cord injuries below this level may still require ventilatory support, as motor innervation to accessory muscles of respiration may still be lost.

Why is the patient flushed?
Loss of sympathetic tone to the vasculature of the skin results in vasodilation.

What are your priorities when managing this patient?
Hypothermia and hypotension should be addressed immediately. A heating blanket should be applied.

Even in the absence of bleeding, patients with neurogenic shock appear hypovolemic because of significant venodilation, resulting in pooling of blood in the peripheral vasculature. Ordinarily, most of this blood would return to the heart and contribute to preload. To compensate for this loss of preload, this patient should receive warmed crystalloid, or blood products if indicated.

Vasopressors and inotropes (which generally have chronotropic effects) will be required as well. Dopamine or epinephrine is appropriate in this context. These drugs will increase heart rate, contractility, and SVR. Norepinephrine will augment SVR. By increasing SVR, venoconstriction will reduce venous capacitance, thereby driving more intravascular volume back to the heart and increasing preload.

Why not just keep giving fluids instead of giving vasopressors?
As with every type of shock, it is important to treat the underlying cause or causes in order to restore normal hemodynamics. The underlying causes of neurogenic shock are bradycardia, vasodilation, and relative hypovolemia (as stated before, from pooling of blood in the venous system). Overly aggressive fluid resuscitation does not address bradycardia and vasodilation. Additionally, this can lead to spinal cord and pulmonary edema, as well as congestive heart failure.

STEP 1 PEARL

The Frank-Starling law describes the relationship between preload and stroke volume. The underlying principle is that, *up to a certain point*, increased stretch of cardiac sarcomeres (caused by distention from filling of the ventricle) results in increased stroke volume (Fig. 24.1). It is important to note that the curve does not increase indefinitely, and at a certain point, additional stretch of sarcomeres results in decreased force of systolic contraction. This is why judicious fluid resuscitation is important.

Could phenylephrine be used for this patient?
Phenylephrine is not the best choice for initial treatment of this patient. It is a pure α agonist. As such, it will bind α1 receptors on vascular smooth muscle and increase SVR. It has no direct β agonism effect, and the increase in SVR may exacerbate bradycardia via the baroreceptor reflex (see Case 33). Remember, the afferent limb of the baroreceptor reflex, cranial nerves IX and X, is still intact, as is the parasympathetic efferent limb, via cranial nerve X.

What are your hemodynamic goals for this patient?
After spinal cord injury, the mean arterial pressure (MAP) should be maintained at 85 mm Hg for up to 7 days after the injury.

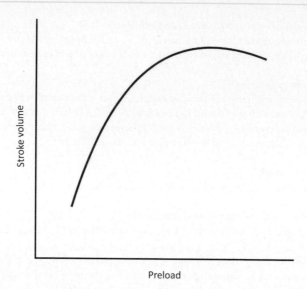

Fig. 24.1   Increased preload causes increased sarcomere length, which results in increased stroke volume. However, on the right side of the curve, corresponding to high preload and long sarcomere length, the force of systolic contraction decreases with additional preload. (Modified from Marks, A. R. [2020]. Cardiac and circulatory function. In L. Goldman & A. I. Schafer [Eds.], *Goldman-Cecil medicine* [26th ed., Chapter 47, pp. 241–245]. Philadelphia, PA: Elsevier. Modified from Fig. 47.3.)

After fluid resuscitation and the initiation of a dopamine infusion, the patient's vital signs are blood pressure 130/75 and pulse 83/min.

How will you intubate this patient?

Assuming the patient is cooperative and has stable hemodynamics and respiratory status, the safest approach is an awake fiberoptic intubation. This approach avoids movement of the cervical spine and allows for a neurological assessment immediately after tube placement to confirm that there are no new neurologic deficits.

What are the contraindications to an awake fiberoptic intubation?

Patients who are uncooperative (e.g., intoxicated, combative), hemodynamically unstable, or who demonstrate actual or impending respiratory failure (e.g., hypoxia, significant airway bleeding) are not candidates for awake fiberoptic intubation.

How do you perform an awake fiberoptic intubation?

Make sure to discuss your plan with the patient before proceeding. Explain why you need to do an awake fiberoptic intubation and tell them what to expect.

The key to an awake fiberoptic intubation is to anesthetize the airway. Adequate anesthesia of the airway requires an understanding of the sensory innervation of each part of the airway (Figs. 24.2 and 24.3).

- The anterior two-thirds of the tongue are innervated by the lingual nerve, a branch of the mandibular (V3) distribution of cranial nerve V (trigeminal nerve).
- The posterior third of the tongue, the soft palate, the oropharynx, and anterior epiglottis are innervated by the glossopharyngeal nerve (cranial nerve IX).

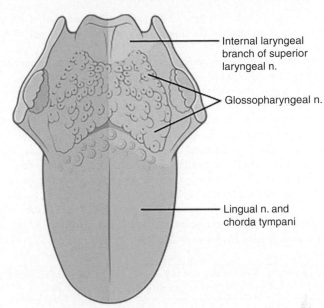

Internal laryngeal
branch of superior
laryngeal n.

Glossopharyngeal n.

Lingual n. and
chorda tympani

Fig. 24.2   Sensory innervation of the tongue. Territories are only labeled unilaterally. Chorda tympani supplies taste sensation. (Reproduced from Klinger, K., & Infosino. A. Airway management. [2018] In M. C. Pardo & R. D. Miller (Eds.), *Basics of anesthesia* [7th ed., Chapter 16, pp. 239–272]. Philadelphia, PA: Elsevier. Fig. 16.3.)

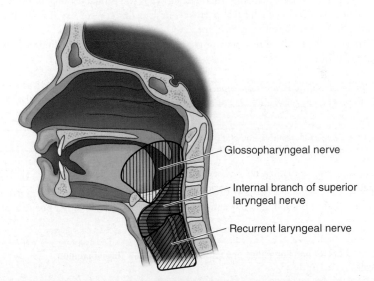

Glossopharyngeal nerve

Internal branch of superior
laryngeal nerve

Recurrent laryngeal nerve

Fig. 24.3   Sensory innervation of the upper airway, sagittal section. (Reproduced from Cabrera, J. L., Auerbach, J. S., Merelman, A. H., & Levitan, R. M. [2020]. The high-risk airway. *Emergency Medicine Clinics of North America, 38*(2), 401–417, Fig. 7. (From Open Access. aimeairway.ca/book#/. Accessed 9.4.2022. Kovacs, G., & Law, A. [2018]. *Airway management in emergencies: The infinity edition*.)

- The posterior epiglottis, base of tongue, and mucosa above the level of the vocal folds are supplied by the internal branch of the superior laryngeal nerve, a branch of the vagus nerve (cranial nerve X).
- The mucosa at and below the vocal folds is innervated by the recurrent laryngeal nerve, another branch of the vagus nerve.

There are multiple ways to anesthetize the airway, including spraying local anesthetic directly onto the mucosa, inhalation of aerosolized local anesthetic, and targeted nerve blocks. These techniques are beyond the scope of this text. It is important to adequately anesthetize all sensory territories of the upper airway in order to facilitate a smooth awake fiberoptic intubation.

An endotracheal tube should be threaded over the fiberoptic scope. A small amount of lubricant may be applied to the scope just distal to the endotracheal tube to allow it to slide into position easily. Once the airway has been anesthetized, pass the fiberoptic scope into the patient's mouth, beyond the posterior tongue, under the epiglottis, and through the vocal cords. Advance the scope until the carina is visualized. An assistant will then thread the ET tube off the fiberoptic scope and inflate the cuff. Withdraw the scope and attach the ventilator circuit. Once end tidal CO_2 is confirmed, induce anesthesia and secure the tube.

Awake fiberoptic intubation is successful, and you induce general anesthesia. During surgery, the anesthesia machine sounds an alarm that the oxygen pipeline pressure is low.

What should you do?

Modern anesthesia machines have redundant sources of fresh gas: oxygen (O_2), air, and nitrous oxide (N_2O). Ordinarily, each of these gases is stored in a large central supply and travels in pipes throughout the hospital to each operating room. Tubes from the wall connect from these pipes directly to the anesthesia machine. This wall supply is the primary source of fresh gas. If this source is depleted or disconnected, backup tanks—or E cylinders—of oxygen, air, and N_2O are attached to the back of the anesthesia machine.

If an alarm sounds that the wall supply of fresh gas is low, open the E cylinders in the back of the anesthesia machine.

Which E cylinder is which? What is the capacity of each cylinder?

Table 24.1 shows the capacity and color of each E cylinder.

You check the oxygen E cylinder, and the pressure gauge is reading 1000 PSI.

How much oxygen is in the tank?

Since oxygen in the E cylinder exists entirely as a gas, the pressure is directly proportional to the volume in the cylinder. If a full tank has a pressure of 2000 psi, a tank with a pressure of half that

TABLE 24.1 ■ Colors and Capacities of each E Cylinder for the Three Common Medical Gases

Fresh Gas	Full Volume (L)	Pressure at Full Volume (pounds per square inch, psi)	Color
O_2	625	2000	Green
air	625	1800	Yellow
N_2O	1590	750	Blue

Note that each cylinder is specific to each gas, and that colors may not be the same in all countries.

amount, or 1000 psi, will contain 312.5 L of gas. The same math works for E cylinders containing air, *but not for E cylinders containing N_2O.*

The N_2O E cylinder shows a pressure of 750 psi. Does that mean the tank has 1590 L of gas in it?

Not necessarily. Unlike oxygen and air, which are both stored entirely as gas, N_2O exists as both a liquid and a gas in E cylinders. Starting with a full tank, as N_2O is removed from the tank, the pressure will remain constant at 750 psi until about three quarters of the tank has been emptied. As gas is removed, liquid N_2O evaporates to replace the gaseous N_2O. Once three quarters of the N_2O has been removed, there will be no more liquid N_2O remaining in the cylinder. At this point, the pressure will start to drop (Fig. 24.4). To determine the amount of N_2O in a blue E cylinder with a pressure reading of 750 psi, the cylinder must be weighed.

The operation concludes. The patient will remain intubated and will be taken to the intensive care unit (ICU). During transport, the patient's oxygen saturation drops from 99% to 85%.

What should you do?

Transport is a dangerous time. There is a risk of complications with equipment, such as accidental extubation, breathing circuit disconnection, oxygen supply depletion, accidental removal of invasive lines, and disconnection of intravenous (IV) tubing. There are also the risks of hemodynamic and ventilatory changes. Meanwhile, the anesthesiologist does not have access to the equipment, drugs, and support staff normally present in an operating room to manage an emergency in transport.

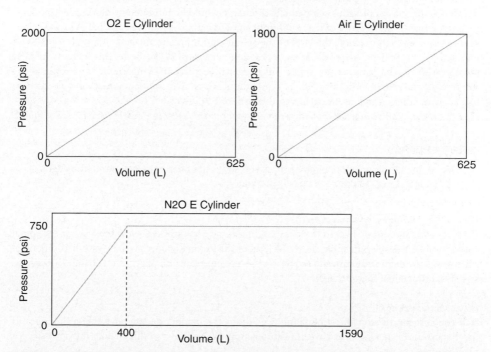

Fig. 24.4 Volume versus pressure for the three common medical gas E cylinders. Notice that there is a linear relationship between volume and pressure for oxygen and air E cylinders, but not for nitrous oxide E cylinders. The pressure of nitrous oxide inside the cylinder stays constant until the volume of gas inside the cylinder is less than 400 L. Courtesy of Paul Frank MD (UC Davis Medical Center, Sacramento, CA).

Check the pulse oximeter tracing to ensure that a normal pulsatile waveform is present; poor contact between the pulse oximeter probe and the patient can create spuriously low readings. Check the transport monitor to ensure a coninuous tracing of end-tidal carbon dioxide ($EtCO_2$). If there is no $EtCO_2$, that is concerning for a breathing circuit disconnect or accidental extubation. Check the oxygen tank to ensure it is not empty. Ideally, this should be done before leaving the operating room. Check the vital signs to ensure that blood pressure is adequate, as significant hypotension or loss of cardiac output can cause a drop in pulse oximeter reading.

If the patient was on high levels of positive end-expiratory pressure (PEEP) in the operating room, it is good practice to maintain that PEEP on transport, whether ventilation is accomplished with the transport ventilator or by hand ventilation with an ambu bag and a PEEP valve. Consider giving a few large recruitment breaths to treat atelectasis, being mindful of the blood pressure, which can drop with elevated intrathoracic pressure.

The patient's oxygen saturation improves to 99% with a few recruitment breaths. You drop her off in the ICU. She has an uneventful hospital course and is discharged to a rehabilitation facility with some motor function of her arms after 2 weeks in the hospital.

Five years later, the patient returns for cystoscopy. Vital signs show blood pressure 133/70 mm Hg, pulse 60/min, respirations 18/min, oxygen saturation 98% on room air, and temperature 36.6°C. You start a propofol infusion and keep the patient breathing spontaneously. After the cystoscope is placed, the blood pressure increases to 205/120 mm Hg and the pulse decreases to 42/min.

What's going on?

This is consistent with autonomic hyperreflexia, which can occur in patients with a remote history of spinal cord injury. Noxious stimulation (i.e., bladder distention) below the level of the spinal cord injury triggers a sympathetic discharge from the corresponding spinal levels. In patients without spinal cord injury, this sympathetic discharge would be inhibited by descending modulatory signaling. In the absence of that inhibitory signaling, the sympathetic discharge causes widespread vasoconstriction below the level of the spinal cord injury. In the case of a high spinal cord injury, as in our patient, there will be vasoconstriction of most of the body. This increase in SVR increases MAP. The baroreceptor reflex will trigger a decrease in sympathetic tone (only above the level of the spinal cord injury, where sympathetic nerve fibers remain intact) and an increase in parasympathetic tone, resulting in vasodilation and bradycardia. *Vasodilation occurs only above the level of the lesion because the inhibitory signal is not carried below the level of the spinal cord injury.*

STEP 1 PEARL

Parasympathetic innervation to the heart, which slows the heart rate, courses in the vagus nerve, so this is not disrupted by spinal cord injury.

What other findings would you expect?

Patients with autonomic hyperreflexia responding to noxious stimuli below the level of the spinal cord lesion may develop flushing above the level of the lesion (again, caused by vasodilation), nasal stuffiness (vasodilation again), and sequelae of severe hypertension (e.g., vision changes, dizziness, seizures, intracranial hemorrhage).

What should you do?

Ask the surgeon to stop the stimulation (i.e., drain the bladder and remove the cystoscope). If the hypertension persists, treat with a short-acting IV arterial vasodilator like nitroprusside or nicardipine.

How could this have been prevented?
General or spinal anesthesia are both effective in reducing the risk of autonomic hyperreflexia.

What is the mechanism of action of nitroprusside?
Nitroprusside is a fast-acting vasodilator. It is administered intravenously. Nitroprusside reacts with sulfhydryl groups on red blood cells and albumin to release nitric oxide (NO)—which stimulates vascular smooth muscle relaxation via the cyclic guanosine monophosphate (cGMP) pathway—as well as cyanide (CN).

Isn't cyanide a poison?
Yes, however the risk of the toxic effects of nitroprusside occurs with prolonged infusions at high doses. A short duration of use is considered safe.

Nitroprusside reacts with hemoglobin to form methemoglobin. CN generally follows one of three metabolic pathways:
- Reaction with methemoglobin to form cyanmethemoglobin
- Reaction with thiosulfate to form thiocyanate
- Binding to mitochondrial cytochrome enzymes, inhibiting cellular utilization of oxygen (see Case 16).

BEYOND THE PEARLS

- Although neurogenic shock and spinal shock are related, they are different entities. As discussed above, neurogenic shock is a hemodynamic state characterized by bradycardia and hypotension. This is usually associated with high spinal cord injury. Meanwhile, spinal shock is a constellation of findings on physical exam also found in the acute period after spinal cord injury.
- Spinal shock is characterized by a loss of reflexes, flaccid paralysis, and sensory dysfunction below the level of the spinal cord injury.
- The rate-limiting step in the synthesis of dopamine, norepinephrine, and epinephrine from the amino acid tyrosine is the conversion of tyrosine to dihydroxyphenylalanine (DOPA) by tyrosine hydroxylase.
- The supply of gas in the E cylinders is limited. The time until depletion of the cylinder is based on the amount of gas in the E cylinder and the fresh gas flow rate.
- Symptoms of cyanide toxicity include abdominal pain, nausea, vomiting, dizziness, acidosis, tachyphylaxis, coma, and death.

References

Gold Standard, Inc. Nitroprusside. Drug monograph. Published February 17, 2021. www.clinicalkey.com. Accessed 8.4.2021.

Pasternak, J.J., & Lanier, W.L. (2018). Spinal cord disorders. In R. L. Hines & K. E. Marschall (Eds.), *Stoelting's anesthesia and co-existing disease* (7th ed., Chapter 14, pp. 305–314). Philadelphia, PA: Elsevier.

Stein, E.J., & Glick, D.B. (2018). Autonomic nervous system. In M. C. Pardo & R. D. Miller (Eds.), *Basics of anesthesia* (7th ed., Chapter 6, pp. 70–82). Philadelphia, PA: Elsevier.

Wang, S., Singh, J.M., & Fehlings, M.G. (2017). Medical management of spinal cord injury. In H. R. Winn (Ed.), *Youmans and Winn neurological surgery* (7th ed., Chapter 303, pp. 2493–2504.e3). Philadelphia, PA: Elsevier.

Williams, K.D. (2021). Fractures, dislocations, and fracture-dislocations of the spine. In F. M. Azar & J. H. Beaty (Eds.), *Campbell's operative orthopaedics* (14th ed., Chapter 31, pp. 1756–1823.e15). Philadelphia, PA: Elsevier.

A 54-Year-Old Man With a History of Chronic Back Pain and Five Prior Spine Operations

Aaron Yim ■ Michael J. Jung ■ Paul Neil Frank

A 54-year-old man with a history of chronic back pain and five prior spine operations is scheduled for a thoracolumbar posterior fusion revision and reinstrumentation from vertebral levels T5 to L3. He takes oxycodone 30 mg three times per day and OxyContin 40 mg twice daily. He also has a permanent pacemaker. Vital signs show blood pressure 140/72 mm Hg, pulse 60/min, respirations 10/min, oxygen saturation 99% on room air, and temperature 37.7°C.

The patient takes oxycodone and oxycontin for his chronic back pain. What else would you like you know regarding his pain management regimen?

Confirm what medications he takes for pain, what doses he takes, when his last dose of each medication was, and what his baseline pain level is. It is also important to note if he has had any nonpharmacologic treatments for pain (e.g., steroid injections, spinal cord stimulator).

Look for signs of opioid misuse, including a history of "lost" prescriptions requiring replacement, history of withdrawal symptoms, or use of illicit drugs. This may include review of the patient's prescriptions in the state's prescription drug monitoring program.

Should this patient receive an opioid-free analgesic regimen perioperatively to reduce the burden of opiate use?

Although it would behoove this patient to decrease his opioid consumption, the perioperative period is not a good time to begin weaning from opioids. Postoperatively, he will have his baseline pain plus significant new surgical pain. The patient can continue his oral opioid medications on the day of surgery. If he cannot take oral medications postoperatively, the oral opioids can be replaced by equivalent intravenous opioids.

For patients with high baseline opioid requirements, methadone, a long-acting opioid, may be helpful. In addition, nonopioid analgesics should be used whenever possible. Nonopioid analgesic options include acetaminophen, cyclooxygenase (COX) inhibitors, gabapentinoids, ketamine, α2 receptor antagonists, magnesium, and intravenous local anesthetics.

Another reason to avoid an opioid-free anesthetic is the risk of opioid withdrawal syndrome. Symptoms of opioid withdrawal include hypertension, tachycardia, altered mental status, and seizures.

STEP 1 PEARL

There are four identified opioid receptors: mu, kappa, delta, and sigma. All are G protein–coupled receptors which cause hyperpolarization of cell membranes and inhibition of the release of excitatory neurotransmitters. They are located in the central nervous system and peripherally.

What is the mechanism of action of ketamine?

Ketamine is a noncompetitive antagonist of the N-methyl-D-aspartate (NMDA) receptor. It causes a dissociative state, sedation, analgesia, and amnesia. In the perioperative setting, it may be beneficial as an adjunctive analgesic due to its reduction in opioid-induced hyperalgesia and "wind-up" phenomenon which can worsen pain. Side effects include nausea, vomiting, hallucinations, and emergence delirium.

What is the mechanism of action of methadone?

Methadone is a long-acting opioid. In fact, it has the longest half-life of any opioid used clinically. It is prepared as a racemic mixture of both L and D isomers. Like ketamine, the D isomer is also an NMDA receptor antagonist. Side effects include decreased respiratory rate, decreased apneic threshold, chest wall rigidity, and slowing of gastrointestinal motility, leading to nausea, vomiting, and constipation. It can also cause prolongation of the QT interval on electrocardiogram (ECG) (see Case 12).

What would you like to know about this patient's pacemaker?

There are several key pieces of information that will help to determine appropriate perioperative management of the patient's pacemaker.

- Why was the pacemaker placed (e.g., complete heart block, tachy-brady syndrome)? *This will tell you the patient's underlying rhythm and underlying cardiac disease.*
- Are they dependent on the pacemaker (i.e., what happens if the pacemaker stops)? *This will help determine whether or not the pacemaker needs to be reprogrammed or have a magnet applied during surgery.*
- What brand is the pacemaker (e.g., Medtronic, Boston Scientific)? *Each brand of pacemaker has a unique reprogramming device and other characteristics. In addition, each brand has its own device representatives who can assist you in understanding the function and reprogramming options of the pacemaker.*
- How many leads are present, and where are they located? *A lead is basically a long thin electrical wire running from the pacemaker box to the heart. Patients can have 1, 2, or even 3 leads. Leads are generally described as atrial or ventricular.*
- When was the pacemaker last interrogated? *Ensure appropriate pacemaker and lead function. An interrogation report will list recent arrhythmias and remaining battery life.*
- In what mode is the pacemaker (e.g. AAI, VVI, DDD)? … *What chamber(s) is/are paced, what chamber(s) is/are sensed, and what is the response?*
- Is it just a pacemaker, or is it an implantable cardioverter defibrillator (ICD)? *All ICDs are pacemakers, but not all pacemakers are ICDs.*

The patient says that his pacemaker was placed 2 years ago for complete heart block after several bouts of syncope. It is not an ICD. His records show that he is pacemaker dependent with an underlying ventricular rate of 30/minute. He has a lead in the right atrium and a lead in the right ventricle. The pacemaker was last interrogated 4 months ago. The battery has 7 years of life left, all leads are functioning appropriately, and the pacemaker is in DDD mode.

What does DDD mean?

There is a standardized way to describe how a pacemaker functions. This code is known as the North American Society of Pacing and Electrophysiology/British Pacing and Electrophysiology Group Code (NBG code). Each letter of the code represents the setting for a particular variable (see Table 25.1).

A cardiac chamber can be sensed or paced by a pacemaker only if a lead is present in that chamber. For example, in a patient with only an atrial lead, the ventricle cannot be paced or sensed.

TABLE 25.1 ■ Standard Cardiac Pacing Modes

What Chamber Is Paced?		What Chamber Is Sensed?		What Is the Response to Sensed Beats?	
A	Atrium	A	Atrium	O	None (no change in pacemaker activity in response to sensed beats)
V	Ventricle	V	Ventricle		
D	Dual (atrium and ventricle)	D	Dual (atrium and ventricle)	I	Inhibited (pacemaker output inhibited in response to sensed beats)
O	None	O	None	T	Triggered (pacemaker output triggered in response to sensed beats)
				D	Dual (pacemaker output inhibited in one lead and triggered in another— only for dual-chamber pacing)

The order is always the same—the first letter describes what chamber(s) is/are paced, the second letter describes what chamber(s) is/are sensed, and the third letter describes the response to sensed beats.

To facilitate dual-chamber pacing (i.e., atrium and ventricle), there must be an atrial lead and a ventricular lead.

Our patient's pacemaker is in DDD mode, also known as dual-chamber pacing. His pacemaker is *pacing* both the atrium and the ventricle (the first D). His pacemaker is *sensing* both the atrium and the ventricle (the second D). The pacemaker can pace the atrium, the ventricle, both, or neither in response to sensed beats (the third D). Possible scenarios for this mode of pacing, DDD, are:

- There is a native atrial beat (i.e., the atrium depolarizes spontaneously). The atrial lead is inhibited (i.e., it does not deliver an electrical impulse). There is no native ventricular beat during a specified amount of time (the preprogrammed atrioventricular (AV) interval), so the ventricular lead paces (i.e., delivers an electrical impulse to depolarize) the ventricle.
- There is no native atrial beat, so the atrial lead paces the atrium. A native ventricular beat is sensed shortly thereafter, so the ventricular lead is inhibited.
- There is no native atrial beat, so the atrial lead paces the atrium. There is no native ventricular beat, so the ventricular lead paces the ventricle.
- There is a native atrial beat, so the atrial lead is inhibited. There is a native ventricular beat, so the ventricular lead is inhibited.

One of these scenarios will occur with every beat of the heart, based on the patient's native heart rate or the desired heart rate programmed into the pacemaker.

The patient's ECG is shown in Fig. 25.1.

How would you describe this? Is this expected?
This ECG shows dual-chamber pacing at 71 beats/min. Given that the patient has a native heart rate of 30 beats/min, it would be expected that all, or nearly all, beats would be generated by the pacemaker. In this ECG, the pacemaker is pacing the atrium and the ventricle.

The patient's pacemaker was interrogated 4 months ago. Is this adequate?
Yes, a pacemaker should have been interrogated within the 12 months prior to surgery. An ICD should be interrogated within 6 months of surgery. If there is no change in clinical status, it is not necessary to interrogate a pacemaker prior to surgery.

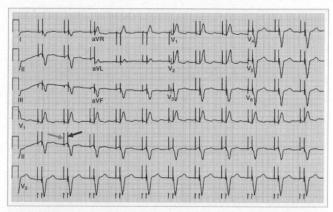

Fig. 25.1 Electrocardiogram (ECG) showing atrial and ventricular (i.e., dual chamber) pacing at 71 beats/min. Notice each systole is associated with two pacing spikes: first an atrial pacing spike *(green arrow)* followed by a P wave and then a ventricular pacing spike *(red arrow)* followed by a wide QRS complex. The QRS complex in wide in the setting of ventricular pacing. (Olshansky, B., Chung, M. K., Pogwizd, S., & Goldschlager, N. [2017]. Cardiac pacing and pacemaker rhythms. *Arrhythmia Essentials, 7*, 278–298. Fig. 7.3.)

STEP 2 PEARL

An ICD is implanted in patients for primary or secondary prevention of cardiac arrest. Primary prevention includes patients who have not had any episodes of ventricular arrhythmias but who are at risk for future events, whereas secondary prevention includes patients who have had prior ventricular arrhythmias. ICDs are able to sense abnormal electrical activity and deliver electrical therapies to terminate ventricular tachycardia or deliver a shock (defibrillation).

How will you manage this patient's pacemaker during surgery?
Pacemakers and ICDs can mistake electrocautery for cardiac activity, a phenomenon known as electromagnetic interference (EMI). Monopolar electrocautery is more problematic than bipolar electrocautery because there is wider spread of the electrical current.

EMI can result in inappropriate pacing, inappropriate inhibition of pacing, or even inappropriate defibrillation (if the patient has an ICD). In this patient, the surgery will be on the thoracic spine, close to the pacemaker. In DDD mode, if the pacemaker mistakes the electrocautery for cardiac activity, the pacemaker output will be inhibited (i.e., the pacemaker "thinks" that the heart is beating on its own and does not need to be paced). With a native ventricular rate of 30/min, the patient may become hypotensive.

To prevent this, the pacemaker should be changed to DOO mode. This is known as asynchronous mode because the pacemaker does not synchronize with native cardiac beats—it paces the atrium and the ventricle (the first D), but it does not sense any chamber (the first O), and the pacemaker behavior does not change in response to sensed beats (the second O).

How does monopolar electrocautery work?
Electrical currents can only flow in a closed loop. With monopolar electrocautery, the current travels from the generator to the electrocautery pencil, through the patient's body to the return pad (usually on the patient's thigh), and then back to the generator.

How can you change the pacemaker to DOO mode?
There are two options: application of a magnet on the patient's chest over the pacemaker (see Fig. 25.2) or reprogramming the pacemaker.

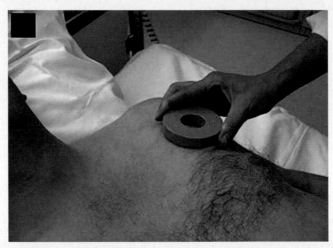

Fig. 25.2 Proper placement of a magnet on the patient's chest over the pacemaker box. (Heidbüchel, H. [2007]. Implantable cardioverter defibrillator therapy in athletes. *Cardiology Clinics, 25*[3], 476–482. Modified from Fig. 7.)

While application of a magnet to the pacemaker usually converts it to an asynchronous mode and increases the pacing rate, this may not always the case. It is good practice to contact the device representative to confirm that application of a magnet over the pacemaker will convert it to asynchronous mode.

If a magnet is not available or if it is not feasible to place a magnet (it may not be feasible if the patient will be in the prone position), the device may be reprogrammed to DOO mode with a specialized device that is unique to each brand of pacemaker. Depending on institution, this can be done by a cardiologist or the device company representative.

Whether a magnet is applied or the device is reprogrammed, it is good practice to apply basic monitors and defibrillation pads prior to initiation of asynchronous pacing.

Why not leave the pacemaker in asynchronous (DOO) mode all the time, even when the patient is not having surgery?

Asynchronous pacing carries the risk of a pacing impulse being delivered when the ventricle is partially depolarized (i.e., between the QRS complex and the T wave) from a native cardiac beat. This can lead to ventricular arrhythmias, including ventricular tachycardia and ventricular fibrillation.

Does this patient's pacemaker need to be placed in an asynchronous mode for all future surgeries?

Not necessarily. The pacemaker should be reprogrammed to asynchronous mode when the patient is undergoing surgery with monopolar electrocautery near the pacemaker (usually above the umbilicus or diaphragm). The risk of EMI is especially high if the surgical field is within 6 inches (15 cm) of the device. If this patient were to undergo a procedure below the umbilicus, the risk of EMI is low and it is not necessary to change the pacing mode.

For example, surgery on the neck using monopolar electrocautery requires the electrical current to flow past the pacemaker on its way to the return pad (on the patient's thigh). The risk of EMI is elevated. By comparison, surgery on the patient's hip using monopolar electrocautery does not require the electrical current to flow close to the pacemaker, so the risk of EMI is low (see Fig. 25.3).

Anytime a patient is pacemaker dependent, even if they are having an operation below the umbilicus, it is good practice to have a magnet in the room in case of unexpected EMI.

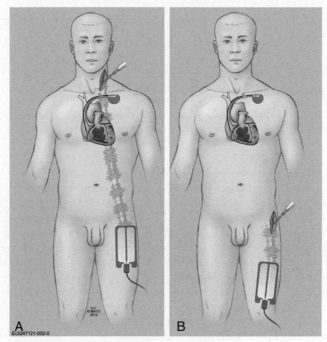

Fig. 25.3 The electrical current in monopolar electrocautery must always flow from the electrocautery pencil to the return pad. (A) When the current passes by the pacemaker, the risk for electromagnetic interference (EMI) is high. (B) When the current does not pass by the pacemaker, the risk for EMI is low. (Mulpuru, S., Madhavan, M., & McLeod, C. J. [2017]. Cardiac pacemakers: Function, troubleshooting, and management. *JACC, 69*[2], 189–210. Fig. 16.)

The surgeon requests intraoperative monitoring of somatosensory evoked potentials (SSEPs) and motor evoked potentials (MEPs) for this procedure.

What are SSEPs and MEPs, and why are they used?

Neuromonitoring, or neurophysiologic monitoring, allows for frequent intraoperative assessment of the integrity of the spinal cord and its associated nerves. If the spinal cord or a peripheral nerve is compressed, stretched, or otherwise injured by surgical manipulation, a change in signal conduction will be noted, and the surgeon may be able relieve the stretch, compression, or other stress to the neural tissue.

SSEPs and MEPs are two commonly used types of intraoperative neuromonitoring. SSEPs assess conduction of a stimulus from a peripheral nerve to the spinal cord and ultimately to the sensory cortex. MEPs assess conduction of a stimulus from the motor cortex to the spinal cord, to a peripheral nerve, and sometimes to a muscle.

STEP 1 PEARL

Sensation of pressure, vibration, and proprioception travels through the dorsal column medial lemniscus pathway of the spinal cord. Peripheral nerves (i.e., first-order neurons) enter the spinal cord and ascend ipsilaterally. These neurons synapse in the medulla with second-order neurons (nucleus cuneatus for sensory information from C2 to T6, nucleus gracilis for information from T7 and below). Second-order neurons decussate (cross the midline) and synapse in the thalamus with third-order neurons. Third-order neurons carry information to the sensory cortex.

STEP 1 PEARL

Voluntary movement is mediated by the lateral corticospinal tract. First-order neurons in the motor cortex descend ipsilaterally through the internal capsule, decussate in the medulla, and descend contralaterally, before synapsing with second-order neurons in the anterior horn of the spinal cord. Second order neurons synapse with muscles at the neuromuscular junction.

How will the use of intraoperative neuromonitoring affect your anesthetic plan?
When SSEPs are monitored, it is recommended to use less than 1 minimum alveolar concentration (MAC)—sometimes less than 0.5 MAC—of volatile anesthetic gas and to supplement with intravenous anesthetics. Halogenated anesthetic gas (e.g., sevoflurane, desflurane) decrease the quality of the signal obtained in SSEP monitoring (i.e., increased latency, decreased amplitude), particularly in patients who are neurologically compromised. Intravenous agents (e.g., propofol) have significantly less effect on signal quality than do an equipotent dose of anesthetic gas.

When MEPs are monitored, neuromuscular blockade can interfere with detection of signal transduction to the muscle. While it is possible to maintain a constant amount of muscle relaxation (with twitch strength approximately 30% of baseline), many anesthesiologists prefer to avoid neuromuscular blockade entirely. Inhaled anesthetic gases tend to depress MEP signals. Total intravenous anesthesia (TIVA) is therefore recommended. If MEPs are monitored and muscle relaxant is not used, place a bite block in the patient's mouth to protect from tongue biting.

It is important to maintain stable levels of anesthetic throughout the operation, to avoid causing a change in neuromonitoring signals that could be confused for neurologic compromise.

What about intraoperative opioids?
Opioids cause small decreases in amplitude and increases in latency of SSEP signals, but this is usually not clinically significant.

Other than surgical manipulation and some anesthetic agents, can anything else affect SSEP and MEP monitoring?
Yes. Hypotension, hypothermia, hyperthermia, hypoxia, and anemia (hematocrit less than 15%) can all reduce the quality of neuromonitoring signals.

In the operating room, you induce and intubate the patient while he is lying on the gurney. He will need to be placed in the prone position.

What are the special considerations for this position?
Secure the endotracheal tube well with tape to prevent accidental extubation while prone or while transitioning the patient between the supine and prone positions.

Be sure the weight of the patient's head is distributed over the bony areas of the face and not on the soft tissue or eyes. Special headrests are available to distribute weight of the head over the forehead, cheekbones, and chin. Once the patient is positioned, it is critical to confirm that the eyes and nose are not compressed. This can be confirmed visually with some headrests with built-in mirrors or by palpation of the face. The neck should be maintained in the neutral position.

The patient's arms should be either tucked at their sides in the neutral position or extended above the head in slight flexion. Abduction of the shoulder greater than 90 degrees increases the risk of brachial plexus injury. The patient's legs should be padded and gently flexed at the knees

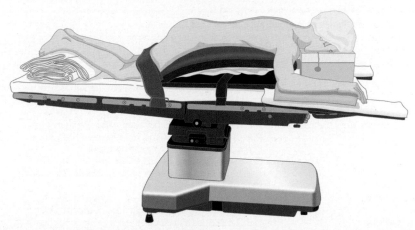

Fig. 25.4 Patient in prone position on a Wilson frame. The face is supported by a specialized soft pillow. The arms are abducted less than 90 degrees. The thorax and pelvis are supported by a Wilson frame. The hips and knees are slightly flexed. All pressure points are padded. (Breyer, K. E. W., & Roth, S. [2020]. Patient positioning and associated risks. In M. A. Gropper, N. H. Cohen, L. I. Eriksson, et al. [Eds.], *Miller's anesthesia* [pp. 1079–1112]. Philadelphia, PA: Elsevier. Fig 34.15.)

and hips. The breasts should be offloaded and positioned medially to the thorax supports. The genitalia should also be free from pressure. The patient's weight should be distributed over the thorax and pelvis, while the abdomen should be allowed to hang freely (see Fig. 25.4).

Why is it important that the abdomen hang freely?
Compression of the abdomen by the patient's body weight will increase intraabdominal pressure, which will cause engorgement of the veins of the spine, particularly the epidural venous plexus, potentially worsening surgical bleeding. Compression of the abdomen will also compress the inferior vena cava, which may lead to reduced venous return to the heart, reduced preload, and ultimately decreased blood pressure and cardiac output.

During the operation, the magnet falls off the patient's chest and onto the floor. The patient's heart rate and blood pressure drop while the surgeon begins to use electrocautery.

What is going on? What should you do?
Ask the surgeon to stop using the electrocautery while you reapply the magnet.

When the magnet became dislodged, the pacemaker changed back to DDD (i.e., synchronous mode). The pacemaker is incorrectly interpreting the electrocautery as ventricular beats. In synchronous mode, the pacemaker does not pace the ventricle when it senses the ventricle beating on its own.

Reprogramming the pacemaker to asynchronous mode instead of using a magnet to change it to asynchronous mode is advantageous in cases where it may be difficult to maintain the magnet over the device. In this case, patient positioning has made it difficult to keep the magnet over the device.

You maintain a stable plane of anesthesia using TIVA without muscle relaxation. There is bleeding throughout the case, and the mean arterial pressure is approximately 50 mm Hg throughout the operation, which lasts 10 hours. At the end of surgery, you return the patient to the supine position and extubate him. He complains that he cannot see anything out of his left eye.

TABLE 25.2 ■ Etiologies of Postoperative Vision Loss

Etiology	Comments
Retinal artery occlusion	• Caused by external compression (as in prone positioning without adequate offloading of eyes), decreased arterial supply (e.g., hypotension, embolism, thrombosis), or impaired venous drainage (e.g., jugular vein ligation) • Afferent pupillary defect
Ischemic optic neuropathy (ION)	• Anterior ION more common after cardiac surgery • Posterior ION more common after spine surgery (more commonly bilateral, but can be unilateral) • Complete visual loss or visual field deficits • Painless visual loss, afferent pupillary defect, decreased or absent color vision
Cortical blindness	• May be associated with focal neurologic deficits • Normal light reflex, hemianopia, loss of accommodation
Acute glaucoma	• Iris touches lens and blocks the flow of aqueous humor causing elevated intraocular pressure • Eye pain and redness, nonreactive pupil

What is going on?

Postoperative vision loss is a rare but known complication following anesthesia. The incidence of postoperative vision loss is higher after spinal and cardiac surgery. Risk factors include:
- Male gender
- Obesity
- Prolonged surgery (>6.5 hours)
- Significant blood loss (>45% of estimated blood volume)
- Prone positioning
- Use of a Wilson frame (see Fig. 25.4)

What are the mechanisms of postoperative vision loss?

The two most common mechanisms of postoperative vision loss after nonocular surgery are ischemic optic neuropathy (ION) and retinal artery occlusion (RAO). Etiologies of postoperative vision loss are described in Table 25.2.

What should you do?

Consult ophthalmology immediately. Administration of fluids and vasopressors to elevate the blood pressure may improve perfusion to ischemic territories.

BEYOND THE PEARLS

- Early ambulation after spine surgery is associated with improved functional outcomes.
- Etomidate and ketamine increase the amplitude of SSEP signals, unlike most other anesthetic agents.
- Dexmedetomidine does not seem to adversely affect intraoperative neuromonitoring.
- Staged spine surgery procedures (i.e., procedure performed over multiple different days) reduce risk of perioperative visual loss and should be considered in high-risk patients.
- Other complications of the prone position include airway edema, pressure injury, and accidental removal of endotracheal tube or other tubes or monitors.

- After a long operation in the prone position with large amounts of bleeding and resuscitation, airway edema is likely, and it is advisable to check a cuff leak prior to extubation (see Case 27).

References

Agerson, A. N., & Benzon, H. T. (2015). Management of acute and chronic pain. In P. G. Barash, B. F. Cullen, R. K. Stoelting, et al. (Eds.), *Clinical anesthesia fundamentals* (pp. 699–719). Philadelphia, PA: Wolters Kluwer.

Akhtar, S. (2015). Endocrine function. In P. G. Barash, B. F. Cullen, R. K. Stoelting, et al. (Eds.), *Clinical anesthesia fundamentals* (pp. 335–356). Philadelphia, PA: Wolters Kluwer.

American Society of Anesthesiologists. (2011). Practice advisory for the perioperative management of patients with cardiac implantable electronic devices: Pacemakers and implantable cardioverter-defibrillators: An updated report by the American Society of Anesthesiologists Task Force on Perioperative Management of Patients with Cardiac Implantable Electronic Devices. *Anesthesiology, 114*(2), 247–261. https://doi.org/10.1097/ALN.0b013e3181fbe7f6

Bebawy, J. F., & Koht, A. (2015). Anesthesia for neurosurgery. In P. G. Barash, B. F. Cullen, & R. K. Stoelting (Eds.), *Clinical anesthesia fundamentals* (pp. 557–579). Philadelphia, PA: Wolters Kluwer.

Breyer, K. E. W., & Roth, S. (2020). Patient positioning and associated risks. In M. A. Gropper, N. H. Cohen, L. I. Eriksson, et al. (Eds.), *Miller's anesthesia* (pp. 1079–1112). Philadelphia, PA: Elsevier.

Brull, S. J., & Claudius, C. (2015). Neuromuscular blocking agents. In P. G. Barash, B. F. Cullen, R. K. Stoelting, et al. (Eds.), *Clinical anesthesia fundamentals* (pp. 185–208). Philadelphia, PA: Wolters Kluwer.

Kiefer, J., Mythen, M., Roizen, M. F., & Fleisher, L. A. (2020). Anesthetic implications of concurrent diseases. In M. A. Gropper, N. H. Cohen, L. I. Eriksson, et al. (Eds.), *Miller's anesthesia* (pp. 999–1064). Philadelphia, PA: Elsevier.

Kindler, C. H., Evgenov, O. V., Crawford, L. C., Vazquez, R., Lewis, J. M., & Nozari, A. (2020). Anesthesia for orthopedic surgery. In M. A. Gropper, N. H. Cohen, L. I. Eriksson, et al. (Eds.), *Miller's anesthesia* (pp. 2071–2101). Philadelphia, PA: Elsevier.

Lemkuil, B. P., Drummond, J. C., Patel, P. M., & Lam, A. (2020). Anesthesia for neurologic surgery and neurointerventions. In M. A. Gropper, N. H. Cohen, L. I. Eriksson, et al. (Eds.), *Miller's anesthesia* (pp. 1868–1910). Philadelphia, PA: Elsevier.

Lin, A. P., & Schmid Biggerstaff, K. (2021). Glaucoma. In R. D. Kellerman, & D. P. Rakel (Eds.), *Conn's current therapy* (pp. 495–499). Philadelphia, PA: Elsevier.

Mahajan, A., & Neelankavil, J. P. (2020). Implantable cardiac pulse generators: Pacemakers and cardioverter-defibrillators. In M. A. Gropper, N. H. Cohen, L. I. Eriksson, et al. (Eds.), *Miller's anesthesia* (pp. 1231–1242). Philadelphia, PA: Elsevier.

Norris, M. C., & Saffary, R. (2015). General anesthesia. In P. G. Barash, B. F. Cullen, R. K. Stoelting, et al. (Eds.), *Clinical anesthesia fundamentals* (pp. 335–356). Philadelphia, PA: Wolters Kluwer.

Seubert, C. N., Mcauliffe, J. J., & Mahla, M. (2020). Neurologic monitoring. In M. A. Gropper, N. H. Cohen, L. I. Eriksson, et al. (Eds.), *Miller's anesthesia* (Chapter 39, pp. 1243–1278). Philadelphia, PA: Elsevier.

Stein, C., & Kopf, A. (2020). Management of the patient with chronic pain. In M. A. Gropper, N. H. Cohen, & L. I. Eriksson (Eds.), *Miller's anesthesia* (pp. 1604–1621). Philadelphia, PA: Elsevier.

Thackeray, E. M., & Egan, T. D. (2015). Analgesics. In P. G. Barash, B. F. Cullen, R. K. Stoelting, et al. (Eds.), *Clinical anesthesia fundamentals* (pp. 165–184). Philadelphia, PA: Wolters Kluwer.

Thompson, A., Neelankavil, J. P., & Mahajan, A. (2013). Perioperative management of Cardiovascular Implantable Electronic Devices (CIEDs). *Current Anesthesiology Reports, 3*, 139–143. https://doi.org/10.1007/s40140-013-0026-5

A 27-Year-Old Man at the Emergency Department Following a Car Accident at Highway Speed

Christian Bohringer ■ Paul Neil Frank

A 27-year-old man is transported by the paramedics to the emergency department following a car accident at highway speed. He is nonresponsive to verbal stimuli but groans and withdraws his right hand when pressure is applied to the nailbed of the middle finger. He does not open his eyes. Respirations are 16/min and irregular. He is snoring, and one out of every four breaths is completely obstructed. His left pupil is bigger than the right. He also smells of alcohol and marijuana. Vital signs show blood pressure 180/100 mm Hg and pulse 45/min. The oxygen saturation on the pulse oximeter is 92%.

What is this patient's glasgow coma scale (GCS)?

The GCS is an assessment of the patient's level of consciousness based on three categories: eye opening response, motor response, and verbal response. Table 26.1 shows the criteria for each score.

This patient does not open his eyes, even to pain, so his eye score is 1. He withdraws from painful stimuli, so his motor score is 4. He is groaning but not making words, so his verbal score is 2. His GCS score is 7. Patients with GCS of 8 or less should be intubated.

Should this patient be intubated in the emergency department, or can this wait until he arrives in the operating room?

This patient has findings consistent with elevated intracranial pressure (ICP) and should be immediately intubated in the emergency department. This will facilitate hyperventilation and diagnostic imaging. He will need a computerized tomography (CT) scan of his head prior to possible emergent craniotomy. Endotracheal intubation will also protect from aspiration of gastric contents.

Why do you believe this patient has elevated ICP?

This patient has a mechanism of injury (i.e., a high-speed motor vehicle accident) likely to result in traumatic brain injury and depressed mental status. Hypertension with bradycardia and irregular respirations, as well as asymmetric pupils, are all concerning for elevated ICP.

Hypertension, bradycardia, and irregular respirations, collectively known as Cushing triad, are a physiologic response to elevated ICP.

The finding of asymmetric pupils in the setting of traumatic brain injury is concerning for impending uncal herniation. As the uncus herniates over the tentorium, it compresses the oculomotor nerve (cranial nerve III), which is responsible for extraocular movement as well as parasympathetic innervation to the eye, which ordinarily causes miosis, or pupillary constriction. As this nerve is compressed by herniating brain tissue (see Fig. 26.1), parasympathetic tone to the eye is lost, and the pupil becomes dilated and unresponsive to light.

TABLE 26.1 ■ **Glasgow Coma Scale Score Criteria**

Best Eye Response (Up to 4 Points)	Best Motor Response (Up to 6 Points)	Best Verbal Response (Up to 5 Points)
Opens eyes spontaneously: 4	Follows commands: 6	Oriented to self (e.g., knows name): 5
Opens eyes to voice: 3	Localizes painful stimuli (e.g., uses hand to push away source of painful stimulus): 5	Confused: 4
Opens eyes to pain (e.g., sternal rub): 2	Withdraws from painful stimuli (e.g., pulls hand away when hand is pinched): 4	Inappropriate speech, but comprehensible words: 3
Does not open eyes: 1	Decorticate posturing (elbows flexed): 3	Incomprehensible sounds: 2
	Decerebrate posturing (elbows extended): 2	No verbal activity: 1
	No movement: 1	Intubated: T

Fig. 26.2 shows examples of decorticate and decerebrate posturing, both indicative of severe brain injury.

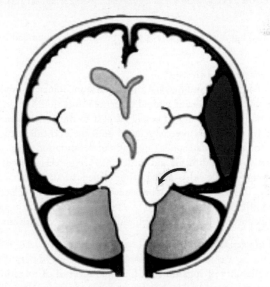

Fig. 26.1 Uncal herniation. As the uncus is forced below the tentorium, it will compress the brainstem. (Baxter, D., & Wilson, M. [2012]. The fundamentals of head injury. *Surgery, 30*(3), 116–121. Modified from Fig. 2.)

STEP 1 PEARL

The oculomotor nerve innervates the superior rectus, inferior rectus, medial rectus, and inferior oblique extraocular muscles. It is also responsible for visual accommodation via the ciliary muscle, eyelid opening via the levator palpebrae muscle (which elevates the upper eyelid), and pupillary constriction via parasympathetic fibers.

The computerized tomography (CT) scanner is ready for the patient.

Can you just give some sedation for now and intubate after the CT scan?
Sedatives should be avoided in an unconscious patient who is not intubated because they exacerbate the respiratory depression caused by the head injury. The resulting elevation of the arterial

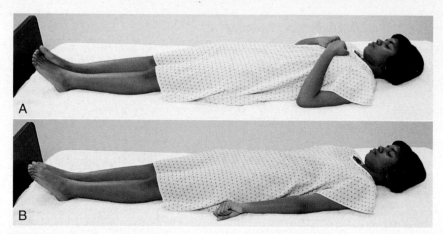

Fig. 26.2 (A) Decorticate posturing. Flexion of the elbows, wrists, and fingers. Legs are extended and internally rotated. (B) Decerebrate posturing. Arms are extended with forearms pronated. Fingers flexed. Neck and back may be arched. (Ball, J. W., Dains, J. E., Flynn, J. A., Solomon, B. S., & Stewart, R. W., [Eds.]. [2019]. Neurologic system. In *Seidel's Guide to Physical Examination* [Vol. *23*, 9th ed., pp. 567–606]. Philadelphia, PA: Elsevier. Fig. 23.25.)

carbon dioxide ($PaCO_2$) aggravates the rise in ICP produced by the head injury. This can lead to secondary brain injury.

How will you secure this patient's airway?

This patient is at risk of aspiration and may have a cervical spine injury. He should therefore be intubated with a video laryngoscope utilizing a rapid sequence intubation. The suction apparatus should be checked, and the suction device should be placed next to the patient's head prior to induction. This patient needs to be adequately pre-oxygenated until the end tidal oxygen concentration has reached 85% to allow for an extended apnea time without desaturation. This is important in case the intubation should turn out to be difficult and extra time is required to successfully place the endotracheal tube. When a low-profile video laryngoscope blade is used, the cervical collar may be left in place for the intubation. If the mouth cannot be opened with the collar in place, then the front of the collar can be removed after the administration of a neuromuscular blocking agent. Manual in-line stabilization by an assistant should then be employed to prevent neck movement during intubation.

What neuromuscular blocker should be used?

The goal is to secure the airway as quickly as possible, as a prolonged period of apnea will increase $PaCO_2$. Given the availability of sugammadex for rapid reversal of rocuronium, rocuronium has become the preferred neuromuscular blocking agent in this context. While succinylcholine causes fasciculations that may transiently elevate ICP, this is still a viable option absent some other contraindication (e.g., crush injury).

After induction, you cannot pass the endotracheal tube.

Now what?

If the endotracheal tube cannot be passed into the trachea, then a fiberoptic scope should be used to guide the endotracheal tube into the trachea. External laryngeal manipulation can be dangerous in this situation because any displacement of the underlying cervical spine can cause or exacerbate spinal cord injury.

The endotracheal tube is successfully placed.

How will you monitor this patient's carbon dioxide levels?
Continuous monitoring of end tidal carbon dioxide ($EtCO_2$) is crucial in any patient who may have raised ICP because the carbon dioxide is a major determinant of cerebral blood volume and hence ICP (see Case 23). If the $EtCO_2$ is elevated, increase minute ventilation and check the arterial blood gas (ABG) as soon as a steady state has been achieved with the new ventilation parameters to ensure that the $PaCO_2$ normal or low.

What can be done to lower the patient's ICP?
Hyperventilation to keep the arterial partial pressure of carbon dioxide ($PaCO_2$) 25-28 mm Hg can lower ICP until the brain can be decompressed in the operating room. However, this hyperventilation should be used only as a temporizing measure until the intracranial cavity can be decompressed because it is only temporarily effective and may induce cerebral ischemia. Following the decompression, the $PaCO_2$ can be allowed to rise gradually again toward normal levels (35-40 mm Hg).

An initial dose of 1 g/kg of mannitol should also be given to lower ICP and prevent further brainstem compression. Elevation of the head of the bed can also be helpful.

STEPS 1, 2, 3 PEARL

Mannitol is an osmotic diuretic. It is filtered through the glomerulus, thereby increasing the osmolarity of glomerular filtrate. This hinders the reabsorption of water by the nephron, thereby increasing free water diuresis.

What are your hemodynamic goals?
The blood pressure must be maintained at a level that maintains cerebral perfusion pressure (CPP) of at least 70 mm Hg. CPP is calculated by

$$CPP = mean\ arterial\ pressure - (either\ ICP\ or\ central\ venous\ pressure,\ whichever\ is\ greater)$$

Data from trauma registries show that transient hypotension is associated with poor outcome and that it predicts poor outcome even more strongly than transient hypoxemia.

Should you order a toxicology screen?
Yes. Many cases of trauma are associated with substance abuse, and a drug screen should be performed to check for the presence of recreational drugs like amphetamine, cocaine, alcohol, marijuana, and opioids because they may affect the amount of anesthetic required as well as the treatment that is used to control tachycardia and hypertension.

The drug screen can also be helpful for evaluating prognosis. Patients with a depressed level of consciousness due to alcohol, opioid, or benzodiazepine ingestion have a better prognosis than patients who are unconscious due to raised ICP from a severe head injury. This explains why intoxicated patients occasionally have a good neurological outcome, although their GCS was very low when they presented to the emergency room.

The CT head is shown in Fig. 26.3.

What's going on?
The patient has a large left-sided subdural hematoma with midline shift. He needs emergent craniotomy for evacuation of the hematoma to reduce ICP and restore adequate cerebral perfusion.

An expanding hematoma will increase ICP. Additionally, as the brain swells in response to injury, ICP will increase and eventually the blood vessels that perfuse the brain will be compressed. Craniotomy allows the brain more space to swell with less elevation in ICP.

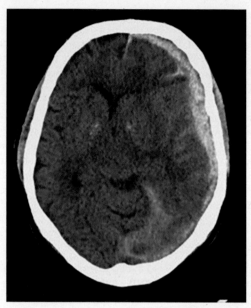

Fig. 26.3 Computerized tomography of the head showing a large left-sided subdural hematoma and midline shift. (DeCuypere, M., & Klimo, P. [2012]. Spectrum of traumatic brain injury from mild to severe. *Surgical Clinics of North America, 92*(4), 939–957. Fig. 2.)

In the operating room you check an ABG, which shows a $PaCO_2$ of 32 mm Hg. At the same time, the anesthesia machine is showing $EtCO_2$ of 22 mm Hg.

How do you explain this discrepancy?

$EtCO_2$ is the measurement of exhaled CO_2 from the entire respiratory tract. Some of the respiratory tract (e.g., alveoli) participates in gas exchange with the blood, but some of it (e.g., the trachea) does not. Parts of the respiratory tract that are ventilated but do not participate in $EtCO_2$ are known as dead space (see Case 12). By the time the exhaled CO_2 reaches the gas analyzer, it has been diluted by fresh gas that filled dead space and did not equilibrate with the blood. In healthy patients, the difference between $PaCO_2$ and $EtCO_2$ is ≤5 mm Hg.

The $PaCO_2$ should be measured as soon as steady ventilation has been established. The $PaCO_2$ should be compared to the $EtCO_2$ and the difference between the two should be calculated. There can be a significant gradient between $EtCO_2$ and $PaCO_2$ if there is increased dead space from preexisting lung disease or from sequelae of the trauma (e.g. pulmonary embolism).

What if the capnogram looks like the solid line in Fig. 26.4? Would you expect a larger or smaller difference between $PaCO_2$ and $EtCO_2$?

You would expect a larger difference. The solid line in Fig. 26.4 shows a steep upslope during phase III of the capnogram waveform. This should ordinarily have a flat plateau appearance (as in the dashed line). This suggests inhomogeneous emptying of the lung, as can be seen in obstructive pathology like bronchospasm or chronic obstructive pulmonary disease (COPD).

It is important to measure the $PaCO_2$ directly whenever there is a steep upslope during phase III, which is also known as the "plateau" phase on the capnogram tracing.

Should you apply positive end expiratory pressure (PEEP)?

PEEP increases central venous pressure because the intrapulmonary pressure is transmitted to the heart and great vessels. PEEP therefore impairs cerebral venous drainage, which will increase the

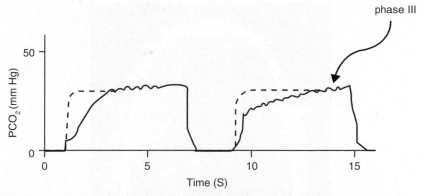

Fig. 26.4 Capnogram waveform showing a steep upslope (solid line) during phase III of the capnogram wave-form, which is a flat portion of the capnogram waveform in healthy patients *(dashed line)*. (Gravenstein, N., & Jaffe, M. B. [2021]. Capnography. In J. Ehrenwerth, J. B. Eisenkraft & J. M. Berry [Eds.], *Anesthesia Equipment* [Vol. *10*, 3rd ed., pp. 239–252]. Philadelphia, PA: Elsevier. Modified from Fig. 10.5.)

volume of blood in the cranium, contributing to elevated ICP. Therefore, the lowest amount of PEEP necessary to prevent atelectasis should be employed in patients with elevated ICP.

> The surgeon has evacuated the hematoma and decides not to replace the bone flap immediately.

Why?
Once the brain has been decompressed the neurosurgeon must decide if the bone flap can be replaced immediately or if it should be preserved and replaced after swelling has subsided. The bone flap may be stored in a freezer or temporarily implanted into a subcutaneous pocket overlying the patient's abdomen. When in doubt it is better not to replace the bone flap because this allows the brain space to swell without severely increasing ICP.

> The decision is made to store the bone flap in a freezer. You had a similar case last week where the patient's CT scan looked like the one in Fig. 26.5. In that case, the patient's bone flap was replaced immediately, and the patient did well.

Why is this different?
Fig. 26.5 shows an epidural, or extradural, hematoma. Epidural hematomas are frequently caused by an injury of a branch of the middle meningeal artery with less damage to the underlying brain. It is therefore not uncommon for a patient to make a rapid recovery following surgical decompression, and the bone flap may be replaced at the end of surgery.

Meanwhile in the case of a subdural hematoma, the bleeding usually originates from bridging veins and the damage to the underlying brain has been extensive. It is therefore much more likely that there will be persistent brain swelling and elevated ICP after decompression of a subdural hematoma than after decompressing an epidural hematoma.

STEPS 2, 3 PEARL

Epidural and subdural hematomas look different on CT scan because of the source and location of bleeding. Epidural hematomas occur above the dura, between the calvarium and the dura. The dura is attached to deep surface of the calvarium where bones meet, also called suture lines. An epidural hematoma will be bound by these areas of dural attachment, giving it a lens shape. Meanwhile, subdural hematomas occur below the dura, specifically between the brain and dura. These are not bound by suture lines. Fig. 26.6 shows an anatomic comparison of epidural and subdural hematomas.

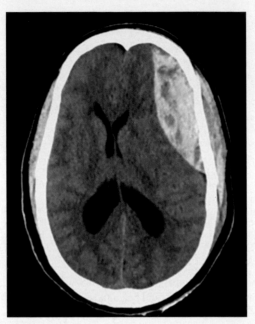

Fig. 26.5 CT head showing a left-sided epidural hematoma. Notice the lens-shape of this hematoma, as compared to the crescent-shape of a subdural hematoma. (DeCuypere, M., & Klimo, P. [2012]. Spectrum of traumatic brain injury from mild to severe. *Surgical Clinics of North America, 92*(4), 939–957. Fig. 2.)

> The surgery team placed an external ventricular drain (EVD).

What are the benefits of an EVD?

An EVD can be used to both measure ICP as well as lower ICP by draining cerebrospinal fluid. ICP needs to be monitored postoperatively, and CPP should be maintained at 70 mm Hg in adults (or 60 mm Hg in children). Vasopressor medications may be necessary to augment mean arterial pressure to achieve the desired CPP.

> You are dropping off the patient in the intensive care unit (ICU) after surgery concludes. The intensivist says they will initiate hyperosmolar therapy.

What's that? How is it helpful?

The osmolality of normal serum is 275–295 mOsm/kg. Free water is drawn from compartments of low osmolarity to compartments with high osmolarity. Higher osmolarity correlates with higher oncotic pressure. Higher plasma oncotic pressure will draw water out of neurons and into the plasma (thereby reducing cerebral swelling), whereas lower serum oncotic pressure (as in hyponatremia) will allow water to enter neurons, thereby worsening cerebral edema and further elevating ICP. Preventing hyponatremia prevents water from entering the neurons along an osmotic gradient and producing cerebral edema.

The goal of hyperosmolar therapy is to increase the patient's serum osmolality to 300–320 mOsm/kg.

How can hyperosmolarity be achieved?

Mannitol is a commonly used agent to increase serum osmolarity. However, this may lead to hypovolemia and hypotension, resulting in decreased CPP. Simultaneous administration of fluids and vasopressors is often required to mitigate the hypotensive effect of mannitol.

Epidural Hematoma- hemorrhage between skull and dura layers

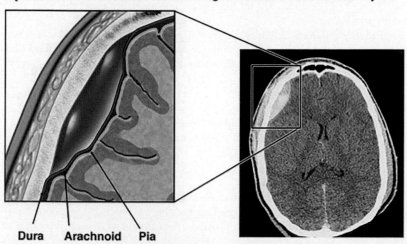

Dura   Arachnoid   Pia

Subdural Hematoma- hemorrhage between dura and arachnoid layers

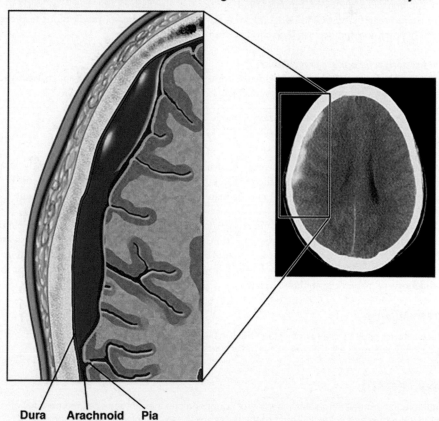

Dura   Arachnoid   Pia

Fig. 26.6 Epidural hematomas are bound by dural attachment to the calvarium, while subdural hematomas are not. This explains the different appearance on computerized tomography scan. (Freeman, W. D., & Aguilar, M. I. [2012]. Intracranial hemorrhage: Diagnosis and management. *Neurologic Clinics, 30*(1), 211–240.)

Mannitol should be given every 6 hours and serum osmolality should be checked regularly to make sure it does not rise above 320 mOsm/kg. Serum osmolality above this level has been associated with renal failure.

Normal saline (0.9% sodium chloride) can treat hypovolemia in this situation because it is more likely to preserve the normal osmolality and osmotic pressure of intravascular fluid. Sodium chloride 3% solution, known as hypertonic saline, is an alternative to mannitol and is not associated with a significant diuresis.

What about plasmalyte or ringer lactate?

Hypotonic intravenous fluids like these should be avoided in patients with elevated ICP to prevent reduction of serum osmolality. This can cause absorption of water into neurons along the osmotic gradient and exacerbate cerebral edema.

What are options for sedation for this patient?

Sedative medication decreases the cerebral metabolic rate, which reduces ICP (see Case 23). These medications will also be necessary to prevent coughing, gagging, and biting on the endotracheal tube as well as self-extubation. Care must be taken to avoid a reduction in mean arterial pressure and a drop in CPP. The ideal sedative will have a short half-life to facilitate frequent neurologic exams.

Dexmedetomidine constricts cerebral blood vessels and is frequently used for lowering ICP. Propofol, benzodiazepines, barbiturates, and opioids are alternatives, but they may need to be administered together with additional intravenous fluid and vasopressor medications to prevent arterial hypotension and decreased cerebral perfusion.

What are options for seizure prophylaxis?

Seizures are common after severe traumatic brain injury. Drugs used to prevent or treat them include levetiracetam, phenytoin, and midazolam.

Over the next 6 hours, the patient's urine output is 5 cc/kg/h.

What's going on?

Mannitol produces an immediate increase in urine output because it is filtered freely at the glomerulus and not reabsorbed from the renal tubule, thereby causing an osmotic diuresis. If the polyuria persists 20 minutes after the end of mannitol administration, it is probably caused by something other than the mannitol.

Polyuria for a prolonged period should raise concern for diabetes insipidus. A urine sample and a blood sample should be collected at the same time and the osmolality of both should be assessed. Ordinarily, if the serum osmolality is more than 310 mOsm/kg, a simultaneously collected urine sample should also exhibit a high osmolality. If, however, the urine is inappropriately dilute, then the diagnosis of diabetes insipidus is likely.

STEP 1 PEARL

The posterior pituitary gland consists of neurons with cell bodies in the hypothalamus. It releases two hormones: antidiuretic hormone and oxytocin.

STEP 1 PEARL

Antidiuretic hormone stimulates insertion of aquaporin channels into the cell membranes of the distal tubule and collecting duct of the nephron. These channels allow reabsorption of water and increased concentration of urine. Antidiuretic hormone also increases reabsorption of sodium chloride in the thick ascending limb and increases reabsorption of urea in the collecting ducts.

> **STEPS 1, 2 PEARL**
>
> There are two types of diabetes insipidus: central and nephrogenic. In central diabetes insipidus, secretion of antidiuretic hormone from the posterior pituitary gland is absent or inadequate. In nephrogenic diabetes insipidus, the kidney does not respond to antidiuretic hormone. Our patient has central diabetes insipidus.

How will you manage this patient's diabetes insipidus?

This patient should receive fluid replacement and management of electrolyte derangements as appropriate. Additionally, desmopressin-arginine vasopressin (DDAVP, a synthetic form of antidiuretic hormone) should be administered to reduce the urine output. The starting dose is 2–4 mcg, and this dose should be repeated until the urine output slows down to an acceptable level.

> **STEPS 1, 2, 3 PEARL**
>
> Nephrogenic diabetes insipidus can be caused by lithium, hypokalemia, hypercalcemia, or genetic mutations in the receptors for antidiuretic hormone. This condition is treated with hydrochlorothiazide or indomethacin. Nephrogenic diabetes insipidus will not respond to DDAVP administration.

> **STEPS 2, 3 PEARL**
>
> Patients with diabetes insipidus tend to develop hypernatremia from dehydration. If the diagnosis of diabetes insipidus is made too late then the serum sodium may be very high, and this carries the risk of osmotic demyelination syndrome within the central nervous system.

> Overnight, the patient's pupils dilate bilaterally, and the patient stops initiating breaths on pressure support ventilation. There is a period of tachycardia and hypertension followed by bradycardia and hypotension.

What's going on?

These findings are concerning for cerebral herniation. Following this biphasic hemodynamic event, there is hypothermia and low CO_2 production due to a reduction in the metabolic rate. Vasopressors will be needed to maintain mean arterial blood pressure at acceptable levels.

How is brain death diagnosed?

Begin by stopping all sedation. Adequate time needs to be allowed for sedative medications to be eliminated completely from the body prior to beginning to test for brain death. The same is true of neuromuscular blocking agents if any have been used. If residual sedative effects cannot be excluded, then cerebral blood flow studies may be necessary to confirm brain death.

Reversible metabolic or physiologic derangements must be ruled out as causes of the patient's unresponsiveness. For example, acid-base abnormalities should be identified and corrected if necessary. The patient must be normothermic (at least 36°C), and normotensive (systolic blood pressure at least 100 mm Hg).

A lack of respiratory effort is a sign of brain death. This is assessed via the apnea test. To perform the apnea test, the patient should be ventilated with FiO_2 1.0 and ventilated to a normal $PaCO_2$ prior to the beginning of apnea testing. All ventilatory support should be turned off. The $PaCO_2$ should be allowed to rise to at least 60 mm Hg (or 20 mm Hg above baseline), and it should be confirmed that the patient has no spontaneous respiratory activity.

All brainstem reflexes should be absent. Pupils should be dilated and nonreactive to light. The corneal and oculocephalic reflexes should also be absent. There should be no cough or gag in response to deep suctioning via the endotracheal tube.

STEPS 1, 2 PEARL

In the oculocephalic reflex, the patient's eyes are held open while the head is turned side to side (this test is not advisable in patients with possible or confirmed cervical spine injury). If the patient's eyes stay fixated on a point in space, brain death is ruled out, as this demonstrates a brainstem reflex.

STEPS 2, 3 PEARL

Brain death should be confirmed independently by two separate attending physicians. An intensive care physician and a neurosurgeon commonly perform these tests. A transplant surgeon who may be involved in harvesting organs from deceased donors should not be one of the physicians certifying brain death because this could be perceived as a conflict of interest.

Once the patient has been declared brain dead the process of organ donation needs to be expedited because maintaining hemodynamic stability after brain death is usually very difficult.

The patient's family has agreed to organ donation. What should be done to care for him in the meantime?
The goal here is to maintain normal physiology.

Use intravenous fluids, inotropes, and vasoactive medications to maintain normal blood pressure (mean arterial pressure 60–70 mm Hg). Patients with refractory hypotension may benefit from intravenous corticosteroids. Prevent cardiac arrhythmias by maintaining normal electrolyte and acid-base status. Treat arrhythmias with standard pharmacologic agents, cardioversion, or defibrillation if necessary.

Continue frequent pulmonary toilet, including suctioning and repositioning. Also continue strategies to prevent atelectasis, including application of PEEP.

Diabetes insipidus is common after brain death, and DDAVP may be needed to prevent polyuria. Excessive urinary volume losses can be replaced with 5% dextrose solution or sterile water.

Maintain normothermia with warming blankets and warmed, humidified inhaled gases. Continue to provide nutrition until the time of organ donation. Treat anemia and coagulopathy with blood products, as necessary.

The deceased patient is about to go to the operating room for organ donation. What is his american society of anesthesiologists (ASA) physical status?
A brain-dead patient undergoing organ removal for donation is an ASA 6.

BEYOND THE PEARLS

- The lowest possible score in each category of the GCS is one point, not zero points, and patients who are intubated cannot speak, so their verbal score is 1T. Thus, a brain-dead patient on a ventilator would have a GCS of 3T.
- When patients are unconscious due to high ICP after a head injury they may not require anesthetic drugs to prevent amnesia until after the brain has been decompressed and cerebral perfusion has been re-established. Intraoperative awareness is uncommon in emergent craniotomy and care needs to be taken not to inadvertently reduce cerebral perfusion pressure with unnecessary anesthetic drugs.
- Coagulation parameters should also be assessed in the emergency room because coagulopathy is common in head-injured patients due to the release of thromboplastin from the injured brain.

- Prolonged hyperventilation in the absence of any surgically correctable lesion should be avoided because hypocarbia will only be temporarily effective at lowering ICP and can cause cerebral ischemia.
- This brainstem compression from cerebellar herniation through the foramen magnum is often fatal because the brainstem damage is usually irreversible. Very aggressive therapy to lower ICP is therefore indicated whenever a risk of herniation exists.
- With decompression of extradural hematomas there is often a surprising improvement in neurologic state and successful extubation at the end of surgery is often possible.
- Diabetes insipidus can occur after severe head injury, brain death, or after surgery on the pituitary gland.
- During the surgery for organ donation, anesthetic drugs are usually not required as there is usually no hemodynamic response to surgical stimulation. However, neuromuscular blocking drugs are required to suppress spinal cord reflexes.
- Outcomes from severe closed-head injury can be improved significantly by preventing secondary brain injury from hypoxia, hypercarbia and hypotension, as well as early surgical decompression and maintaining an adequate cerebral perfusion pressure.

References

Abdelmalik, P. A., Draghic, N., & Ling, G. S. F. (2019). Management of moderate and severe traumatic brain injury. *Transfusion, 59*(S2), 1529–1538.

Aisiku, I. P., Silvestri, D. M., & Robertson, C. S. (2017). Critical care management of traumatic brain injury. In H. R. Winn (Ed.), *Youmans and Winn Neurological Surgery* (Vol. *349*, 7th ed., pp. 2876–2897.e8). Philadelphia, PA: Elsevier.

Bohringer, C., Duca, J., & Liu, H. (2019). A synopsis of contemporary anesthesia airway management. *Translational Perioperative and Pain Medicine, 6*(1), 5–16.

Kovacs, G., & Sowers, N. (2018). Airway management in trauma. *Emergency Medicine Clinics of North America, 36*(1), 61–84.

Marehbian, J., Muehlschlegel, S., Edlow, B. L., Hinson, H. E., & Hwang, D. Y. (2017). Medical management of the severe traumatic brain injury patient. *Neurointensive Care, 27*(3), 430–446.

McKee, A. C., & Daneshvar, D. H. (2015). The neuropathology of traumatic brain injury. In J. Grafman & A. M. Salazar (Eds.), *Handbook of Clinical Neurology* (Chapter 4, Vol. *127*, pp. 45–66). Philadelphia, PA: Elsevier.

Opdam, H. I., & D'Costa, R. (2019). Renal protection in the organ donor. In C. Ronco, R. Bellomo, J. A. Kellum & Z. Ricci (Eds.), *Critical Care Nephrology* (Vol. *132*, 3rd ed., 805–810.e3). Philadelphia, PA: Elsevier.

Otolaryngology

A 63-Year-Old Female With a Large Goiter

Paul Neil Frank ■ Quintin Kuse

A 63-year-old female with a large goiter is scheduled for total thyroidectomy. She is diaphoretic and tremulous. She complains of anxiety, 20 pounds of unintentional weight loss, diarrhea, and frequent palpitations. Her vital signs are pulse 122/min with frequent premature ventricular complexes (PVCs), blood pressure is 184/110 mm Hg, respirations 26/min, and temperature 39°C.

What is going on with this patient? Is it safe to proceed with surgery?
This presentation is concerning for severe hyperthyroidism. Because this is an elective surgery, it should be postponed until the patient has been medically stabilized. Specifically, the patient should have normal vital signs, normal volume status (euvolemic), and symptoms of hyperthyroidism should have resolved.

STEP 1 PEARL

Thyroid storm is usually precipitated by acute stress (e.g., infection, trauma, or surgery).

STEP 1 PEARL

Thyroid storm causes increased cardiac output by inducing synthesis and expression of β_1 adrenergic receptors on the heart.

STEP 1 PEARL

During thyroid storm, the serum levels of alkaline phosphatase may be elevated due to increased bone turnover.

When an elective surgery must be postponed, it is important that the anesthesiologist articulate the reason for the postponement to both the patient and the surgeon. It is equally important that the anesthesiologist be specific about what criteria must be met for the patient to safely undergo surgery in the future.

What if this were an emergent or urgent operation that could not be delayed?
If this were a case that could not be delayed (e.g., bowel obstruction, open bone fracture), the thyroid storm must be managed acutely. Give intravenous (IV) fluids to treat dehydration. Replete electrolytes as necessary. β-Blockade (e.g., esmolol) will help to normalize heart rate and blood pressure. Corticosteroids will prevent peripheral conversion of thyroid hormone. Antithyroid medications such as propylthiouracil or methimazole, as well as iodine solution, will help prevent release of thyroid hormone. Treat fever with acetaminophen and a cooling blanket.

The patient complains of a headache. Can she have an aspirin?

No. Aspirin displaces thyroid hormone from the protein that normally carries it in the blood. This increases the amount of free (unbound) thyroid hormone in the plasma and can exacerbate hyperthyroid symptoms.

STEP 1 PEARL

In primary hyperthyroidism, thyroid-stimulating hormone levels will be low in response to negative feedback exerted by high levels of thyroid hormone on the anterior pituitary gland.

STEP 1 PEARL

The thyroid gland mainly produces thyroxine (T4), which is converted into triiodothyronine (T3) by the enzyme 5′-deiodinase in peripheral tissues.

Surgery is postponed. The patient returns 3 months later after medical optimization. Today her vital signs are pulse 88/min, blood pressure 110/59 mm Hg, respirations 12/min, and temperature 36.6°C. You again notice a large goiter. A recent computed tomography (CT) of her neck is shown in Fig. 27.1.

Are there any concerns about her airway?

Yes. This tumor is causing tracheal compression and tracheal deviation. Impingement of the mass on the trachea can make intubation difficult. In patients with a mass in the neck or mediastinum, it is important to inquire about signs of airway compromise. Can the patient breathe comfortably lying flat? Have they noticed any changes in their voice? Any difficulty swallowing food? Any of these findings are concerning for significant airway impingement.

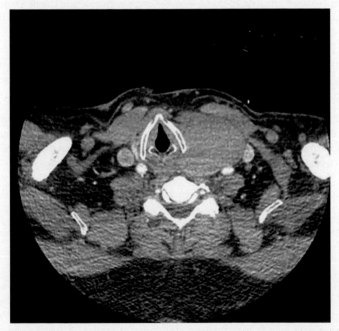

Fig. 27.1 Computed tomography (CT) scan showing a large goiter causing compression and rightward deviation of the trachea. (Modified from Keane, A., & Goldberg, D. (2020). The difficult airway and thyroid surgery. *Operative Techniques in Otolaryngology—Head and Neck Surgery, 21*(2), 138–143, Fig. 1.)

Ask the patient if they have had radiation to the head, neck, or chest. This can limit tissue mobility, even with apparently normal anatomy.

Ask about any prior neck or airway surgery.

On physical exam, check if the trachea is in the midline or if there is tracheal deviation. Check for neck range of motion and mobility of the trachea.

Review any available imaging of the neck and chest, looking for compression of the trachea or major airways.

If there is a high suspicion for airway compromise, consider a preoperative endoscopic airway exam or an awake fiberoptic intubation (see Case 24). In extreme cases, awake tracheostomy with local anesthesia and no or mild sedation may be necessary.

> The patient says she can breathe comfortably lying flat and that her voice has not changed. The surgeon says she will use a nerve integrity monitor (NIM) endotracheal tube to avoid injuring the recurrent laryngeal nerve.

How will this change your management?

A NIM endotracheal tube helps the surgeon identify the recurrent laryngeal nerve during dissection. Proper functioning of this tube relies on intact neuromuscular junctions. Therefore the patient cannot have a neuromuscular blockade in effect during surgery.

Endotracheal intubation usually involves the use of a neuromuscular blocking agent. If a NIM tube will be used during surgery, several options for intubation exist:

- Give succinylcholine for paralysis for intubation. Assuming the patient has does not have atypical pseudocholinesterase (see Case 12), the effect should wear off in minutes.

STEP 1 PEARL

Because succinylcholine is a rapid-acting depolarizing neuromuscular junction blocking agent that stimulates muscles prior to paralysis, it causes brief fasciculations, or diffuse twitching.

If paralytic is used for intubation, check for four twitches on train of four monitoring and sustained tetanus prior to the start of surgery to ensure the nerve monitoring used by the surgeon will be reliable. Notify the surgeon when neuromuscular blockade has worn off or has been fully reversed.

How does a NIM endotracheal tube work?

A NIM endotracheal tube uses electrodes on the outside of the tube against the vocalis muscle in the vocal cords (Fig. 27.2) to detect action potentials from the recurrent laryngeal nerve. The surgeon uses a sterile probe to stimulate tissue to identify the recurrent laryngeal nerve. Stimulation of the recurrent laryngeal nerve will be detected by the electrodes as a response in the vocalis muscle.

> Induction and intubation with succinylcholine are uneventful. You confirm four out of four twitches on train of four monitoring. During the operation, the patient starts moving, despite receiving 1 minimum alveolar concentration (MAC) of desflurane. The capnogram is shown in Fig. 27.3.

What can you do?

Ordinarily, neuromuscular blockade ensures that the patient will remain still during surgery. In the case where neuromuscular blocking agent cannot be used during surgery, it is necessary to maintain a greater depth of anesthesia to keep the patient still. In addition to increased concentration of anesthetic gas, opioids (e.g., fentanyl bolus, remifentanil infusion) and other IV adjuncts (e.g., propofol infusion) will help keep the patient still during surgery. Ask the surgeon to inject local anesthetic wherever possible.

The waveform on capnogram shows that the patient is breathing independently from mechanical breaths delivered by the ventilator. This is sometimes referred to as overbreathing the ventilator.

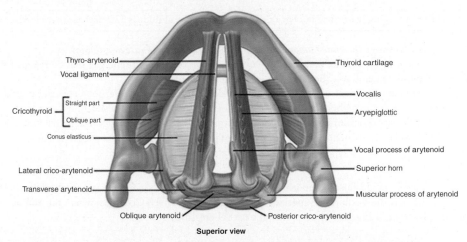

Superior view

Fig. 27.2 Vocalis muscle within the vocal cord. (R. L. Drake, A. W. Vogl, & A. W. M. Mitchell [Eds.], [2021]. Head and neck. In *Gray's atlas of anatomy* [pp. 477–610]. Philadelphia, PA: Elsevier.)

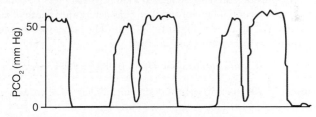

Fig. 27.3 Capnogram waveform showing the patient inspiring independently from the ventilator. (Modified from Gravenstein, N., & Jaffe, M. B. [2021]. Capnography. In: J. Ehrenwerth, J. B. Eisenkraft, & J. M. Berry [Eds.], *Anesthesia equipment* (Vol. 10, 3rd ed., pp. 239–252. Philadelphia, PA: Elsevier, Fig. 10.8.)

You touch the desflurane vaporizer and notice that it is warm.

Why does desflurane require a specialized vaporizer?

Desflurane has unique physical properties that preclude the use of a standard variable bypass vaporizer and instead require a specialized vaporizer. First, the vapor pressure of desflurane is 669 mm Hg, significantly higher than that of other anesthetic gases. Prohibitively high fresh gas flow rates would be required to output an appropriate concentration of desflurane with a variable bypass vaporizer. Second, the potency of desflurane is much lower than that of other anesthetic gases. Therefore a higher concentration of desflurane is required to achieve 1 MAC of anesthesia. Vaporization of this quantity of desflurane gas would cause cooling of a variable bypass vaporizer without an external heat source. Finally, the boiling point of desflurane is only 22.8°C, which may be encountered in an operating room. If desflurane were to boil, the output of a variable bypass vaporizer would be uncontrollable.

How does a desflurane vaporizer work?

In the commonly used desflurane vaporizer, there are two separate gas circuits: one for fresh gas and one for desflurane vapor. Desflurane is heated to 39°C, which creates a vapor pressure of 1300 mm Hg. The output of desflurane vapor is controlled based on the fresh gas flow rate and desired concentration of desflurane. This configuration is sometimes referred to as a dual-gas blender.

The surgery is being performed in Denver, Colorado, where the altitude is 5280 feet above sea level.

Do you need to change the dialed amount of desflurane to ensure adequate anesthesia?

It is important to remember that it is the *partial pressure* of an anesthetic gas that correlates to depth of anesthesia, and not the *concentration* of anesthetic gas.

The desflurane vaporizer delivers a constant concentration of desflurane, not a constant partial pressure. Therefore, at higher altitudes, lower atmospheric pressure will result in a lower partial pressure of delivered desflurane. Assuming the output of the desflurane vaporizer is set to 6.6%, at sea level, where atmospheric pressure is 760 mmHg, this corresponds to a partial pressure of

$$760 \; mm \; Hg \times 0.066 = 50.2 \; mm \; Hg$$

At sea level, the desflurane vaporizer outputs 50.2 mm Hg of desflurane vapor when the dial is set to 6.6%. If the desflurane vaporizer is set to 6.6% in Denver, Colorado, where the ambient pressure is 615 mm Hg, this corresponds to a partial pressure of

$$615 \; mm \; Hg \times 0.066 = 40.6 \; mm \; Hg$$

The desflurane vaporizer is still outputting desflurane at 6.6% of atmospheric pressure, but with lower atmospheric pressure, this corresponds to a lower partial pressure of desflurane. Again, the partial pressure—not concentration—of anesthetic gas determines depth of anesthesia.

Therefore, to increase the desflurane output to 50.2 mm Hg and ensure an adequate depth of anesthesia, the dial on the vaporizer must be increased.

$$50.2 \; mm \; Hg \, / \, 615 \; mm \; Hg = 0.082 = 8.2\%$$

A vaporizer output of 8.2% concentration of desflurane in Denver, where atmospheric pressure is 615 mm Hg, will deliver a partial pressure of 50.2 mm Hg.

What if you were using sevoflurane?

Unlike desflurane, sevoflurane is delivered via a variable bypass vaporizer. Variable bypass vaporizers deliver a constant partial pressure of anesthetic gas regardless of the atmospheric pressure. Therefore there is no need to change the dialed concentration on the variable bypass vaporizer to compensate for changes in atmospheric pressure.

Toward the end of the operation you notice the capnogram shown in Fig. 27.4.

What is going on? What should you do?

The capnogram is not returning to the baseline between breaths. This can be caused by depletion of the CO_2 absorbent or by an incompetent expiratory valve in the anesthesia machine. In either

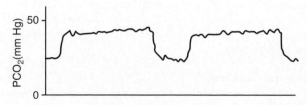

Fig. 27.4 Capnogram waveform that does not return to baseline, suggesting that the patient is rebreathing exhaled CO_2. (Modified from Gravenstein, N., & Jaffe, M. B. Capnography. In J. Ehrenwerth, J. B. Eisenkraft, & J. M. Berry [Eds.], *Anesthesia equipment* (Vol. 10, 3rd ed., pp. 239–252). Philadelphia, PA: Elsevier. Fig. 10.7.)

case, the patient is rebreathing CO_2. Increase the fresh gas flow to help displace the CO_2. Replace the CO_2 absorbent. If the capnogram waveform still does not return to the baseline between exhalations, the expiratory valve is likely incompetent.

How does CO₂ absorbent work?

CO_2 absorbent prevents rebreathing of CO_2 in the anesthesia circuit. Most CO_2 absorbents contain calcium hydroxide [$Ca(OH)_2$], which reacts with expired CO_2 to form calcium carbonate ($CaCO_3$). This reaction occurs slowly, so catalysts (e.g., sodium hydroxide, potassium hydroxide) and water are added. Absorbents vary in their capacity for CO_2 and their tendency to react with volatile anesthetics to produce potentially harmful by-products (e.g., carbon monoxide, compound A).

At the end of the operation, you want to prevent the patient from coughing during extubation.

What are your options?

Coughing, gagging, or "bucking" on the endotracheal tube creates tension on suture lines and disrupts hemostasis, particularly undesirable after operations on the head or neck. A small dose of opioid, propofol, or IV lidocaine just prior to waking up can facilitate a smoother extubation. A deep extubation can also be considered (see Case 6).

STEP 1 PEARL

The internal laryngeal nerve can be injured during surgery or damaged during food ingestion that results in food (e.g., fishbone) being trapped in the piriform fossa. Damage to this nerve can cause an impaired cough reflex and increase the risk of aspiration pneumonia.

What is a cuff leak, and why is it important?

Ordinarily, the diameter of the endotracheal tube is smaller than that of the trachea. The balloon (or cuff) of the tube is inflated to create a seal between the mucosa of the trachea and the tube. In patients with significant airway edema (e.g., after significant fluid resuscitation, or after laryngeal surgery), the internal diameter of the trachea may be the same as the outer diameter of the tube. In that case, the tube is essentially stenting open the airway. Removing the tube in this context may result in partial or complete airway closure.

In testing for a cuff leak, deflate the cuff of the endotracheal tube and be sure that you hear an air leak with positive pressure ventilation. If there is no leak with the cuff down, do not remove the tube.

What if the patient were stridorous immediately after extubation?

In the setting of recent thyroidectomy, stridor immediately after extubation is concerning for intraoperative recurrent laryngeal nerve injury. The recurrent laryngeal nerve is responsible for abduction (movement away from the midline) and adduction (movement toward the midline) of the vocal cords. Injury to this nerve (especially in bilateral operations such as total thyroidectomy) can cause the vocal cords to be stuck in the closed (median) position or the nearly closed (paramedian position). This may require emergent reintubation and possible tracheostomy.

Another possible cause of stridor postoperatively is laryngeal edema. This is most common after prolonged operations immediately around the larynx with significant bleeding and fluid resuscitation. Inhaled aerosolized racemic epinephrine can help treat stridor from laryngeal edema. Administration of heliox can improve ventilation (see Case 23). Corticosteroids may be helpful but will take hours to show benefit. Reintubation may also be necessary in this scenario as well.

There is a cuff leak, and the patient is extubated uneventfully. One hour after dropping off the patient in the postanesthesia care unit (PACU), you get a call from the bedside nurse that the patient is becoming dyspneic and stridorous.

What is going on?

In the first few hours after thyroidectomy or other neck surgery (e.g., carotid endarterectomy), new-onset stridor is concerning for bleeding causing a hematoma. Surgical bleeding within the closed space of the neck can cause airway compression.

Remove the surgical dressings and look for evidence of bleeding or swelling. Check for tracheal deviation. Call the surgeon to the bedside. Prepare to reintubate the patient. Because the hematoma may be causing airway compression, reopening the wound to release the extrinsic compression of the airway may facilitate an easier reintubation.

The patient returns to the operating room for reexploration, and hemostasis is achieved. On postoperative day 1, you are called to the bedside when the patient becomes stridorous again. This time there is no evidence of swelling of her neck. She complains of tingling of her hands and feet.

What is going on?

The presentation here is concerning for laryngospasm due to hypocalcemia. Ordinarily, the parathyroid glands help maintain calcium homeostasis. They secrete parathyroid hormone (PTH), which increases levels of serum calcium. The parathyroid glands are often intimately close to the thyroid gland, and they can be inadvertently removed during thyroidectomy.

Without PTH, serum calcium levels can drop. Hypocalcemia can cause laryngospasm (which results in stridor), neurologic sequelae (e.g., numbness and tingling of hands, feet, mouth), and cardiac arrhythmias. If the patient is still ventilating well and maintaining oxygen saturation, IV calcium chloride or calcium gluconate may improve their ventilation. If the patient is severely dyspneic or otherwise unstable, intubate them and then treat the hypocalcemia.

STEP 1 PEARL

Chief cells of the parathyroid gland sense serum calcium levels and secrete PTH in response to low serum calcium levels. PTH stimulates the kidneys to increase calcium reabsorption, decrease phosphate reabsorption, and increase production of 1,25-OH vitamin D. 1,25-OH vitamin D stimulates the intestines to increase absorption of calcium. The net effect of these mechanisms is to increase serum calcium levels.

STEP 1 PEARL

Several findings on physical exam are classically associated with hypocalcemia. Twitching of the muscles of the face in response to percussion of the facial nerve is known as *Chvostek sign*. Spasm of the muscles of the hand in response to inflation of a blood pressure cuff on the ipsilateral arm is known as *Trousseau sign*.

BEYOND THE PEARLS

- Always check for a cuff leak prior to extubation after any surgery on the neck or prolonged surgery with large fluid shifts.
- Damage to the superior laryngeal nerve can cause difficulty with voice pitch, which can be problematic for professional singers.

- Unilateral recurrent laryngeal nerve damage can result in hoarseness, ineffective cough, dysphagia and aspiration, or airway compromise. Patients who can compensate well may be completely asymptomatic.
- Treatment for unilateral cord immobility, known as medialization, can be accomplished by injection of fat, gelatin sponge, or human cadaveric collagen into the vocal cord.
- The recurrent laryngeal nerve innervates all the muscles of the larynx except the cricothyroid muscle, which is innervated by the superior laryngeal nerve.

References

Bokoch, M. P., & Weston, S. D. (2020). Inhaled anesthetics: Delivery systems. In M. A. Gropper, R. D. Miller, N. H. Cohen, L. I. Eriksson, L. A. Fleisher, K. Leslie, et al. (Eds.), *Miller's anesthesia* (Vol. 22, 9th ed., pp. 572–637.e6). Philadelphia, PA: Elsevier.

Gremillion, G., Fatakia, A., Dornelles, A., et al. (2012). intraoperative recurrent laryngeal nerve monitoring in thyroid surgery: Is it worth the cost? *Ochsner Journal, 12*(4), 363–366.

Lorenz, R. R., Couch, M. E., & Burkey, B. B. (2017). Head and neck. In C. M. Townsend, R. D. Beauchamp, B. M. Evers, K. L. Mattox (Eds.), *Sabiston textbook of surgery* (Vol. 33, 20th ed., pp. 788–818). Philadelphia, PA: Elsevier.

Patel, A. (2020). Anesthesia for otolaryngologic and head-neck surgery. In M. A. Gropper, R. D. Miller, N. H. Cohen, L. I. Eriksson, L. A. Fleisher, K. Leslie, et al. (Eds.), *Miller's anesthesia* (Vol. 70, 9th ed., pp. 2210–2235.e4). Philadelphia, PA: Elsevier.

Wissler, R. N. (2020). Endocrine disorders. In D. H. Chestnut, C. A. Wong, L. C. Tsen, W. D. N. Kee, Y. Beilin, J. M. Mhyre, et al. (Eds.), *Chestnut's Obstetric Anesthesia* (Vol. 43, pp. 1056–1087). Philadelphia, PA: Elsevier.

A 78-Year-Old Female With Recurrent Respiratory Papillomas (RRPs)

Paul Neil Frank ■ Mike Priem ■ Michelle Schiltz ■ Thomas Leland Hughes

A 78-year-old female with recurrent respiratory papillomas (RRPs) presents for laser ablation of laryngeal papillomas. She is otherwise healthy. Vital signs are within normal limits.

What are RRPs?

RRPs are benign nonkeratinizing squamous papillomas caused by human papilloma virus (HPV), typically HPV types 6 and 11. Hoarseness, stridor, and, in severe cases, respiratory distress are the most consistent signs of RRP. A vaccine exists and may result in far fewer cases in the future.

At present, there is no cure for RRP and no modality that would lead to eradication of the virus from the mucosa. Local recurrences are expected, and scarring from overly aggressive laryngeal resections may lead to permanent dysphonia, so most surgeons will accept an incomplete papilloma resection.

What are the function and innervation of the larynx?

The main functions of the larynx involve phonation, the protection and maintenance of airway patency, and the generation of Valsalva. Innervation of the airway is complex but primarily involves the glossopharyngeal nerve (cranial nerve IX) and branches of the vagus nerve (cranial nerve X). The glossopharyngeal nerve provides sensory innervation of the posterior tongue, vallecula, anterior epiglottis, and tonsils. The vagus gives rise to the superior laryngeal nerve, which further divides into the external superior laryngeal nerve and the internal superior laryngeal nerve. The internal branch of the superior laryngeal nerve provides sensation of the tongue base, epiglottis, and arytenoids. The external branch provides motor innervation to the cricothyroid muscle, which tenses the vocal cords. Injury to the superior laryngeal nerve results in voice changes but does not affect airway patency.

As the vagus nerve descends inferiorly, it gives rise to the recurrent laryngeal nerve. The left recurrent laryngeal nerve courses under the aortic arch and the right recurrent laryngeal nerve under the right subclavian artery before traveling superiorly along the trachea. The recurrent laryngeal nerves provide sensory innervation to the airway below the level of the vocal cords and motor innervation to all the intrinsic muscles of the larynx except for the cricothyroid muscle. Injury to the recurrent laryngeal nerve results in paralysis of the vocal cords and possible airway obstruction.

Laryngeal procedures may be performed to improve respiratory function, phonation, or to resect diseased tissue. A working understanding of airway innervation is necessary for awake fiberoptic intubations (see Case 24) and to predict complications of head and neck surgeries.

What are the general concerns and work up for laryngeal procedures?

Preoperative assessment includes a complete review of medical history, prior procedures and prior airway procedure notes, lab and imaging results, and videos obtained by fiberoptic airway endoscopy.

While a recent MRI or CT may be useful for planning airway management, the results may be misleading with rapidly progressing disease. Awake transnasal flexible endoscopy done on or near the day of surgery can assess the view of the glottis, axial alignment of the airway, presence and position of obstructing lesions, and vocal fold motion in the awake upright patient. However, induction of anesthesia in the supine position with loss of muscle tone may result in unexpected airway collapse and obstruction in these patients.

The patient had radiation to her neck for an unrelated malignancy 10 years ago. How might that affect her airway?

A history of radiation therapy to the neck often results in fibrosis and contractures, resulting in restricted mouth opening and poor mandibular protrusion. Induction of anesthesia and adminis-tration of neuromuscular blocking agents is unlikely to significantly improve range of motion or airway mobility.

Neck radiation therapy can also cause acute or chronic baroreceptor dysfunction (see Case 33), more commonly in patients who have had bilateral treatment. These patients may be asymptom-atic during routine activity but often exhibit labile blood pressure and heart rate during anesthesia. Chronic airway edema is frequently encountered in laryngeal surgery and contributes to a nar-rowed glottic opening. Airway masses may be friable, pedunculated, or collapsible.

As a practical matter, inhalation induction or airway maintenance via mask in patients with laryngeal masses may be very challenging and may result in cannot intubate/cannot ventilate scenarios.

What type of laser is used in this type of operation?

The carbon dioxide (CO_2) laser is utilized in the airway because scattering is minimal and the intracellular water in superficial cells absorbs virtually all the energy. Thus, vaporization of super-ficial lesions is rapid and surrounding tissue damage is negligible.

What eye protection should be worn when the CO_2 laser is in use? What about other medical lasers?

Lasers can cause ocular injury via direct exposure or a reflected beam. It is therefore critical that everyone in the operating room wears eye protection appropriate for the type of laser being used. Eye protection generally consists of goggles of an appropriate tint. Table 28.1 lists the appropriate eye protection for commonly used medical lasers.

What about protecting the patient's eyes?

In patients undergoing CO_2 laser ablation, the eyes should be closed with tape. Saline-soaked gauze should then be placed over the eyes and secured with tape, as in Fig. 28.1.

TABLE 28.1 ■ **Without Appropriate Eye Protection, Eye Injury can Occur with Less than One Second of Laser Exposure**

Laser	Appropriate Protective Goggles
CO_2	Clear glass or plastic
Potassium titanyl phosphate (KTP)	Amber-tinted
Argon	Amber-tinted
Nd:yttrium-aluminum-garnet (YAG)	Blue green-tinted or specially coated clear
Krypton	Amber orange-tinted

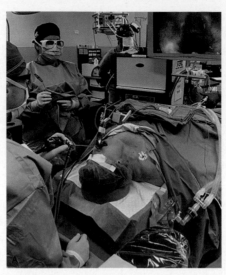

Fig. 28.1   Eye protection for a patient undergoing CO_2 laser ablation. (Reproduced from Garrett, C. G., Reinisch, L., & Fletcher, K. C. [2010]. Laser surgery: basic principles and safety considerations. *Cummings Otolaryngology: Head and Neck Surgery, 59*, 854–867.e1. Fig. 59.12.)

What can be done to protect everyone in the operating room from vaporized particles?
The smoke generated by the laser is also called the laser plume. It contains fine particles less than 1 μm in size. Depending on the laser and the lesion being ablated, viral deoxyribonucleic acid (DNA) or ribonucleic acid (RNA) may be present in the laser plume.

These fine particles can be inhaled and deposited in the alveoli of the people in the room. General surgical masks filter particles no smaller than 3 μm, so specialized laser masks may be used. A smoke evacuator should also be used at the surgical site.

What kind of endotracheal tube (ETT) should you use for this operation?
Laser-resistant endotracheal tubes reduce the risk of airway fire. These tubes have larger external diameters for a given internal diameter because of the laser resistant coating. A commonly used endotracheal tube is a specialized metal ETT that is resistant to both CO_2 and KTP lasers and has two cuffs. Both cuffs should be inflated with saline, sometimes tinted with methylene blue, to alert the clinicians to an ETT cuff rupture and possibly quench a small fire. Carefully reduce the FiO_2 to <30% prior to the activation of the laser.

The surgeon says an endotracheal tube will be in his way.

What are other options to ventilate this patient during surgery?
Table 28.2 shows other options for ventilation during surgery.

What are the potential drawbacks to natural airway anesthesia?
These techniques may not provide adequate oxygenation and ventilation in obese patients, patients with pulmonary disease, or during prolonged procedures. If high FiO_2 is used to maintain adequate oxygen saturation during natural airway anesthesia, the risk of airway fire is elevated. Additionally, the airway is not protected from aspiration of gastric contents.

TABLE 28.2 ■ Options for Ventilation for Laryngeal Surgery

Ventilation Technique	Comments
Apneic intermittent ventilation	• Ventilation via endotracheal tube followed by extubation and a period of apnea. • Allows for apneic period of 5–10 minutes in healthy patients. • Periodic reintubation for ventilation result can prolong surgery and potentially cause airway injury. • Unobstructed surgical access to the larynx. • Neuromuscular blockade allows for still field. • Inability to reliably monitor end-tidal CO_2 and FiO_2.
Jet ventilation	• Ventilation via rapid insufflation of oxygen via a narrow tube. • Minimally obstructed surgical access to the larynx—can ventilate with tube supraglottic (Fig. 28.2), infraglottic (Fig. 28.3), or transtracheal (Fig. 28.4). • Airway is not "sealed" as with traditional endotracheal intubation. • Neuromuscular blockade allows for still field. • Risk of barotrauma and pneumothorax—must ensure adequate path for gas egress from the airway. • Ventilation controlled manually or via automatic jet ventilator. • Requires total intravenous anesthesia (TIVA). • In high-frequency JV (HFJV), tidal volumes are 1–3 cc/kg, and respiratory rate is 100–300/min.
Spontaneous ventilation	• Patient sedated but breathing spontaneously. • Allows for assessment of dynamic airway function. • Surgical field moves since no neuromuscular blockade is used. • Inability reliably monitor FiO_2 and end-tidal CO_2.

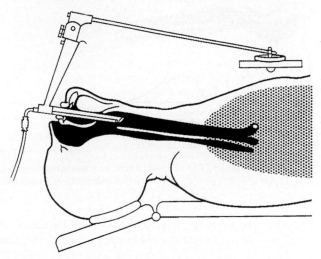

Fig. 28.2 Supraglottic JV via a suspension laryngoscope. (Reproduced from Biro, P. [2010]. Jet ventilation for surgical interventions in the upper airway. *Anesthesiology Clinics, 28*[3], 397–409. Fig. 3.)

You plan to use low-frequency JV.

What are the relative advantages and disadvantages of supraglottic and infraglottic JV?

Supraglottic JV has a lower risk of barotrauma, although it requires higher driving pressure than infraglottic JV. It also allows for a completely unobstructed view of the larynx. Supraglottic JV

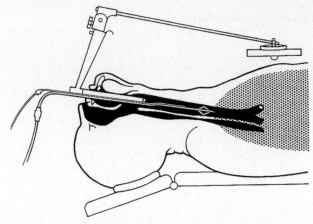

Fig. 28.3 Infraglottic JV via a catheter terminating below the vocal cords. (Reproduced from Biro, P. [2010]. Jet ventilation for surgical interventions in the upper airway. *Anesthesiology Clinics, 28*[3], 397–409. Fig. 1.)

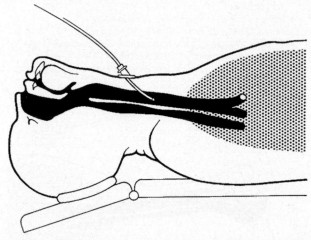

Fig. 28.4 Transtracheal JV via a catheter through the anterior neck into the trachea. (Reproduced from Biro, P. [2010]. Jet ventilation for surgical interventions in the upper airway. *Anesthesiology Clinics, 28*[3], 397–409. Fig. 4.)

usually relies on a suspension laryngoscope. Therefore, it is not available immediately after induction of anesthesia, and it is not available at the end of surgery once the laryngoscope has been removed.

Infraglottic JV creates an outwardly-directed stream of gas that prevents blood and debris from flowing past the vocal cords. Additionally, infraglottic JV reduces entrainment of ambient air, allowing for delivery of FiO_2 closer to what has been set by the anesthesiologist.

> After induction of anesthesia, the surgeon places a JV catheter (hunsacker tube) past the vocal cords, and you maintain infraglottic JV throughout the operation. The operation is uneventful, and you take the patient to the recovery room. Ten minutes later, the nurse calls you because the patient is dyspneic, with SpO_2 of 90%. Breath sounds are absent on the left side. Chest radiograph is shown in Fig. 28.5.

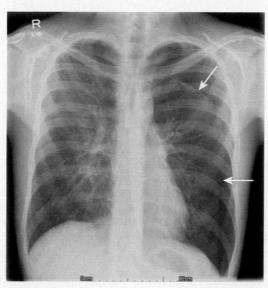

Fig. 28.5 CXR showing a left-sided pneumothorax. White arrows show the edge of the collapsed lung. (Reproduced from Hallifax, R., & Rahman, N. M. [2015]. Pneumothorax. In *Murray & Nadele Textbook of Respiratory Medicine* [Vol. *110*, 6th ed., pp. 1539–1550.e4]. Philadelphia, PA: Elsevier. Fig. 110.3.)

What's going on? What should you do?

This patient has a left-sided pneumothorax. This is likely a result of over-pressurization of the lung (i.e., barotrauma) during jet ventilation. Barotrauma can also cause tension pneumothorax (see Case 13), hypotension (likely from tension pneumothorax), and cervical or mediastinal emphysema.

Apply supplemental oxygen and continue close respiratory monitoring. The patient may require a chest tube.

> You are called emergently to another operating room, where the patient is undergoing laser laryngeal surgery with a regular endotracheal tube in place. During use of the laser, a fire erupted over the patient's face.

What's going on?

Lasers and monopolar electrosurgical units (i.e., Bovie) are implicated in airway fires, which are rare but can be catastrophic for the patient and surgical team. Facial and neck burns as well as flame and smoke airway injury occur most often in the outpatient setting, involving surgical procedures of the upper body under sedation without endotracheal intubation.

What should you do?

Stop the flow of the airway gases and remove the endotracheal tube. Pour water or saline into the patient's airway.

After the fire is extinguished, reestablish ventilation, preferably without supplemental oxygen. Check the upper and lower airways for debris and injury. The patient may require transfer to a burn center for specialized care of airway burns as well as burns involving the face and/or eyes (see Case 16).

What factors contribute to intraoperative fires?

The fire triad consists of an ignition source (e.g., electrocautery, laser), the fuel (e.g., alcohol-based surgical prep, gowns, drapes), and the oxidizer (e.g., oxygen, nitrous oxide).

How could this have been avoided?

When there is a risk of airway fire, always use the lowest possible FiO_2. Open delivery of oxygen through a direct source (e.g., nasal cannula) is the major contributor to most intraoperative fires. For procedures above the xiphoid, avoid open delivery of supplemental oxygen whenever possible. If oxygen is required, use an oxygen blender or a 5.0–6.0 endotracheal tube connector connected to the Y portion of the anesthesia circuit. No supplemental oxygen should be delivered from a 100% oxygen source such as a free-standing oxygen outlet (e.g., oxygen tank).

Minimize oxygen buildup by flushing the field with medical air, if feasible, and/or by scavenging the operating field with suction. If adequate oxygen saturation (i.e., $SpO_2 > 95\%$) cannot be maintained, secure the airway with an endotracheal tube or supraglottic airway rather than increasing $FiO_2 > 30\%$. For procedures inside the airway in an intubated patient, discontinue nitrous oxide and reduce the inspired oxygen concentration to < 30% (see Case 29). After reducing the FiO_2 by changing the controls on the anesthesia machine, be sure to allow enough time such that the fraction of expired oxygen is actually reduced to the desired safe level.

Surgeons can avoid electrosurgical ignition sources by using an alternative to monopolar electrocautery if feasible.

BEYOND THE PEARLS

- In pediatric practice, both the CO_2 laser and the microdebrider are used to treat papillomas.
- "Laser" is an acronym for Light Amplification by Stimulated Emission of Radiation.
- In the ground state, electrons orbit a nucleus at their lowest energy level occupying orbits that are closer to the nucleus. Absorption of energy causes the electrons to move to a higher orbit. As the electrons spontaneously return from the excited to the ground state, they emit photons that are reflected between mirrors in the resonant chamber, becoming further amplified as well as coherent and collimated. Since one mirror in the chamber is only partially reflective, some energy escapes as a bright, monochromatic, coherent beam of laser radiation.
- Nitrous oxide has the same oxidizing potential as oxygen if administered in the same concentrations.
- As with infraglottic JV, transtracheal JV should only be performed if there is an adequate opening for the outflow of gas out of the airway.
- In HFJV, gas exchange relies on entrainment of ambient gas, pulsatile effects of thoracic vibration and cardiac oscillation, collateral ventilation (Pendelluft), and diffusion.

References

Biro, P. (2010, September 1). Jet ventilation for surgical interventions in the upper airway. *Anesthesiology Clinics, 28*(3), 397–409.

Garrett, C. G., Reinisch, L., & Fletcher, K. C. (2005). Laser surgery: basic principles and safety considerations. In C. W. Cummings, B. H. Haughey, J. R. Thomas, & L. A. Harker (Eds.), *Cummings Otolaryngology: Head and Neck Surgery* (Vol. *59*, 4th ed., pp. 854–867. e1). Philadelphia, PA: Elsevier.

Nekhendzy, V., & Biro, P. (2018). Airway management in head and neck surgery. In C. A. Hagberg, C. A. Artime, & M. F. Aziz (Eds.), *Hagberg and Benumof's Airway Management* (Vol. *38*, 4th ed., pp. 668–691. e5). Philadelphia, PA: Elsevier.

Patel, A. (2013). Anesthesia for laser airway surgery. In C. A. Hagberg (Ed.), *Hagberg and Benumof's Airway Management* (Vol. *39*, 3rd ed., pp. 692–716. e3). Philadelphia, PA: Elsevier.

A 65-Year-Old Man Diagnosed With Severe Acute Respiratory Syndrome Coronavirus 2 and Acute Respiratory Distress Syndrome

Paul Neil Frank

This case discusses a pertinent but novel topic—Covid-19. Science and medicine are continuing to evolve in this field. Please bear this in mind as you read this case.

A 65-year-old man diagnosed with severe acute respiratory syndrome coronavirus 2 (SARS-CoV-2, commonly known as Covid-19) and acute respiratory distress syndrome (ARDS) has been intubated and mechanically ventilated for 10 days and has been unable to wean from mechanical ventilation. He has not received a Covid-19 vaccination. His oxygenation is poor. He is scheduled for a tracheostomy. Vital signs show that blood pressure is 132/67 mm Hg, pulse is 110/min, respirations are at 28/min, oxygen saturation is 84% on 100% FiO_2 and positive end expiratory pressure (PEEP) of 12 cm H_2O, and temperature is 39.2°C. A chest radiograph (CXR) is shown in Fig. 29.1.

What is Covid-19?

Covid-19 is a β coronavirus just like the virus responsible for severe acute respiratory syndrome (SARS) and Middle East respiratory syndrome (MERS). The virus was first identified in humans in 2019. The rapid worldwide spread of infections led the World Health Organization (WHO) to declare the outbreak of this virus a pandemic on March 11, 2020.

STEP 1 PEARL

Coronaviruses are enveloped viruses, meaning they are encased in a lipid layer derived from the host cell membrane. Their genetic material is single-stranded ribonucleic acid (RNA).

STEP 1 PEARL

Enveloped viruses are more sensitive to destruction by heat, drying, or detergents, and therefore are usually transmitted from person to person, as in respiratory droplets.

How does the Covid-19 virus enter cells?

Angiotensin converting enzyme 2 (ACE2) is found on the surface of alveolar epithelial cells, and it is believed that the Covid-19 virus uses these proteins to gain entry into the cells.

STEP 1 PEARL

The alveolar wall is made of two types of cells: type I pneumocytes and type II pneumocytes. Type I pneumocytes constitute 95% of the wall of the alveoli. They are simple squamous epithelial cells.

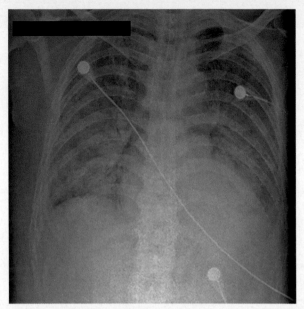

Fig. 29.1   Chest radiograph showing diffuse bilateral airspace opacification. An endotracheal tube is properly positioned in the trachea. (Modified from Coronavirus: Novel coronavirus [Covid-19] infection. Accessed December 5, 2020. Clinical Overview. Updated November 23, 2020. www.clinicalkey.com. Fig. 2B.)

> These cells facilitate gas exchange between the air space and the blood. Type II pneumocytes constitute the remaining 5% of the wall of the alveoli. These cells can divide and regenerate type I pneumocytes in response to cell damage. Type II pneumocytes also produce surfactant.

How is Covid–19 infection diagnosed?

The Centers for Disease Control and Prevention (CDC) has authorized tests that detect the genetic material (nucleic acid amplification test, NAAT) or antigens (proteins) of Covid-19. These tests can be useful in the diagnosis of acute infections, whether or not the patient has symptoms. The CDC does not recommend the use of antibody testing for the diagnosis of acute infection.

How do the Covid–19 vaccines work?

There are three clinically available Covid-19 vaccines in the United States.

The vaccine produced by Pfizer and BioNTech relies on modified RNA that encodes spike glycoprotein of the Covid-19 virus. This RNA is encapsulated in lipid nanoparticles, which facilitates its entry into host cells. This allows expression of the spike protein and generates both cellular and humoral immune responses.

The vaccine produced by Moderna works similarly to the vaccines produced by Pfizer and BioNTech. Synthetic messenger RNA encodes spike glycoprotein of the Covid-19 virus and is encapsulated in lipid nanoparticles to facilitate entry into host cells.

The vaccine produced by Johnson & Johnson and Janssen contains an adenovirus that encodes the spike protein of the Covid-19 virus. The adenovirus used is called a vector, and it cannot replicate. Once this adenovirus has entered the host cell, the spike glycoprotein of the Covid-19 virus will be expressed, resulting in cellular and humoral immunity.

> **STEP 1 PEARL**
>
> The adaptive immune response generates an antigen-specific response. It is comprised of humoral immunity and cellular immunity. Humoral immunity is implemented by B lymphocytes that secrete antibodies that bind to and cause inactivation of extracellular pathogens (e.g., viruses and bacteria). Cellular immunity is implemented by two types of T lymphocytes. Cytotoxic

T lymphocytes kill infected cells, such as those infected with a virus. Helper T lymphocytes activate macrophages to kill pathogens that have been phagocytosed by the macrophage.

What is ARDS?

ARDS is characterized by inflammation of the lungs resulting in pulmonary edema not of cardiac etiology and diffuse patchy consolidations (see Case 41). ARDS can be triggered by a primary pulmonary insult (e.g., pneumonia) or a nonpulmonary insult (e.g., trauma, sepsis).

STEP 2, 3 PEARL

ARDS is classified in terms of severity by the ratio of arterial oxygen tension to inspired oxygen concentration (PaO_2/FiO_2) where PaO_2 is expressed in mm Hg and FiO_2 is expressed as a decimal, with 100% expressed as 1.0. In mild ARDS, PaO_2/FiO_2 is 200–300. In moderate ARDS, PaO_2/FiO_2 is 100–200. In severe ARDS, PaO_2/FiO_2 is < 100.

In the morning prior to intubation, the patient complained of a loss of smell.

Is that related to Covid-19? What are the effects of Covid-19 on the neurologic system?

In patients with mild illness, neurologic symptoms are constitutional and nonspecific—headache, dizziness, and malaise are common. Patients have also endorsed losses of smell and taste.

Covid-19 has been associated with ischemic strokes. It is possible that Covid-19 induces a hypercoagulable state, which increases stroke risk. Cardiac injury and the resulting arrhythmia may also increase the risk of cardioembolic stroke (i.e., a blood clot forming in the heart and then traveling to the brain).

Encephalopathy, defined by confusion, disorientation, agitation, and somnolence, has been described in Covid-19 patients. However, these symptoms may be the result of systemic illness and treatment of systemic illness (e.g., immobility, sedation, isolation, frequent sleep disruption), rather than symptoms directly attributable to Covid-19.

What precautions should healthcare workers take when caring for a patient with Covid-19?

Healthcare workers should follow contact precautions and airborne precautions. This is particularly important when the patient is undergoing an aerosol-generating procedure (AGP), such as tracheostomy. These precautions dictate the use of personal protective equipment (PPE). PPE for this procedure includes gloves, a waterproof gown, an eye/face shield, an N95 mask, or a powered air purifying respirator (PAPR).

AGPs should be performed in negative pressure rooms.

What are other types of AGP?

Endotracheal intubation, bronchoscopy, tracheal extubation, airway surgery, noninvasive positive pressure ventilation (NIPPV), administration of nebulized medication, tracheostomy exchange, and chest compressions are all AGPs.

Should this patient receive corticosteroids?

Yes, the National Institutes of Health (NIH) recommends the administration of dexamethasone in patients who required supplemental oxygen including mechanical ventilation. If dexamethasone is not available, equivalent doses of another corticosteroid are acceptable.

What about remdesivir?

Remdesivir is an antiviral agent. It is recommended for patients with Covid-19 who are hospitalized and require supplemental oxygen, but not for patients who require mechanical ventilation, as it has not shown benefit in treating patients with advanced disease. This patient probably should not receive remdesivir.

However, there may be some benefit to administration of tocilizumab, an interleukin blocker.

Why is a tracheostomy desirable?

Prolonged endotracheal intubation carries the risks of ventilator-associated pneumonia, tracheomalacia, tracheal or laryngeal stenosis, and oral injury. Additionally, endotracheal intubation usually requires sedation for patient comfort. Prolonged sedation can lead to patient tolerance, difficulty weaning off both the ventilator and sedation, and delirium.

In patients for whom prolonged intubation is expected, a tracheostomy can improve patient mobility, oral and pulmonary hygiene, and facilitate ventilator weaning. Tracheostomy is generally tolerated better than endotracheal intubation, and patients are often more comfortable. Patients with tracheostomy can communicate more effectively via lip reading or even application of a speaking valve to the tracheostomy appliance.

Tracheostomy improves ventilation, as there is less dead space and lower resistance to gas flow, which decreases the work of spontaneous breathing. Once there is no longer a need for mechanical ventilation and the tracheostomy appliance is removed, these patients have a lower risk of aspiration from glottic incompetence.

You are reviewing the patient's chart and notice an elevated cardiac-specific troponin level.

What are the possible causes?

Covid-19 has been associated with cardiac injury due to multiple mechanisms. The differential is the same as for patients not infected with Covid-19. Table 29.1 shows the differential diagnosis.

STEP 2 PEARL

The most common finding on ECG in patients with pulmonary embolism is sinus tachycardia.

A medical student rotating on the acute care surgery service, a scrub tech in training, and an intern rotating on anesthesiology are planning to participate in the tracheostomy.

Good idea?

No, in treating COVID-positive patients, it is safest to minimize the number of people in the room. In general, the most experienced providers should be the ones in the room. Medical students, junior residents, and staff who are in training or being oriented to a new institution should not participate in the procedure unless absolutely necessary.

What about a percutaneous tracheostomy at the bedside?

Tracheostomy may be performed via open surgical technique, which usually takes place in the operating room, or percutaneous technique, which may be performed at the bedside in the intensive care unit (ICU). In the percutaneous technique, an introducer needle is advanced percutaneously through the anterior neck into the tracheal lumen, and a guidewire is threaded through the needle into the lumen. The tract is dilated, and the tracheostomy appliance is placed.

Advantages of the percutaneous technique include shorter procedure duration and the ability to perform the procedure at the bedside without the risks of patient transport to and from the operating room.

The percutaneous technique is not recommended for patients with unfavorable anatomy (e.g., obesity, history of prior tracheostomy or other neck surgery), an unstable cervical spine, an enlarged thyroid gland, or high ventilatory requirements (e.g., high FiO_2 or high-PEEP). Given this patient's poor oxygenation and high ventilatory requirements, it is safer for him to undergo surgical tracheostomy in the operating room.

How should the patient be transported to the operating room?

The goals here are to minimize transport time, minimize the number and duration of breathing circuit disconnects, and protect individuals near the patient. Staff who will be transporting the patient should don PPE outside the patient's room. Depending on the patient's neurologic and

TABLE 29.1 ■ The Differential Diagnosis of an Acute Increase in Serum Troponin Level

Diagnosis	Pathophysiology	Possible Findings
Acute coronary syndrome	Partial or total occlusion of one or more coronary arteries	• Regional wall motion abnormalities on echocardiogram • Valvular pathology (e.g., mitral regurgitation due to papillary muscle dysfunction) • Mechanical complications (e.g., ventricular septal defect, usually found days after initial insult) • ST-segment depression or elevation • Arrhythmia
Myocarditis	Direct myocyte damage	• ST-segment depression or elevation on electrocardiogram (ECG) • T wave inversion • Global ventricular dysfunction or normal wall motion, but no new focal wall motion abnormalities on echocardiogram • Arrhythmia
Acute pulmonary embolism	Right ventricular strain	• McConnell sign on echocardiography (diminished or absent motion of the right ventricular free wall with normal motion at the apex) (see Case 2) • Classically on ECG, S wave in lead I, Q wave and inverted T wave in lead III • Diagnosed on computerized tomography (CT) angiogram
Acute heart failure	Global coronary hypoperfusion	• Ventricular dysfunction on echocardiogram • Hypotension, reduced cardiac output • Cardiogenic shock
Critical illness	Oxygen supply/demand mismatch, toxicity from endogenous and exogenous inflammatory mediators	• Normal or impaired ventricular function on echocardiogram

The list here is the same as for patients not infected Covid-19. However, it should be noted that Covid-19 can precipitate these conditions.

respiratory status, it may be desirable to further sedate the patient and even give a muscle relaxant prior to transport to avoid patient agitation, ventilator dyssynchrony, or accidental extubation during transport.

The decision should be made in advance whether the patient will be transported with the ICU ventilator or with the transport ventilator. Advantages of transporting with the ICU ventilator include avoidance of circuit disconnect and maintenance of PEEP and other ventilator settings. Oftentimes, the ICU ventilator is more customizable than the transport ventilator. Disadvantages of transporting on the ICU ventilator is that this ventilator is often more difficult to transport while in use.

If the patient will be transported with the transport ventilator, the ICU ventilator should be paused and the fresh gas flow stopped. Next, the circuit should be disconnected from the patient's endotracheal tube. The transport ventilator should then be attached to the endotracheal tube, and the transport ventilator should then be activated. It is important to minimize the flow of gas through breathing circuits that are not connected to the patient. A viral filter should also be applied to the endotracheal tube during the circuit disconnect while switching ventilators if one is not already present. A tubing clamp may be applied to the endotracheal tube prior to circuit disconnect and removed prior to initiation of ventilation with the transport ventilator to avoid contamination from the endotracheal tube.

A route from the ICU to the operating room should be planned in order to minimize the length and duration of transport and to minimize exposure to surrounding individuals. If an elevator is to be used, arrangements should be made with appropriate facility staff to have an elevator ready at the desired location to minimize wait time.

In the operating room, if a circuit disconnect is necessary to connect the patient to the anesthesia machine ventilator, the same process described above for circuit disconnect and reconnect should be followed. Any staff who assisted with transport but who will not participate in the operation should leave the operating room as soon as possible.

What are the important steps of surgical tracheostomy?

After sterile prep and drape, the surgeon will dissect through the anterior neck down to the trachea. The surgeon will then enter the trachea. The anesthesiologist will then slowly withdraw the endotracheal tube, and the surgeon will place the tracheostomy appliance. The anesthesiologist will then disconnect the ventilator circuit from the endotracheal tube and connect it to the tracheostomy appliance. Communication between the surgical and anesthesiology teams is key.

> Before entering the trachea, the surgeon asks you to reduce the FiO_2 on the ventilator.

Why?

Oxygen is flammable, and electrocautery can be a source of ignition. Reducing the concentration of oxygen reduces the risk of airway fire (see Case 28).

Ideally, the surgeon should not use electrocautery when dissecting close to the trachea and when entering the trachea. This will eliminate the risk of airway fire and the need to reduce FiO_2.

Should you allow the patient to breathe spontaneously during this operation?

No, a patient coughing or exhaling will release viral particles into the surrounding air. Keep the patient fully paralyzed to minimize the risk of coughing.

> After connection of the ventilator circuit to the tracheostomy appliance, there is no end-tidal carbon dioxide (CO_2) on the capnogram.

What should you do?

Immediately notify the surgeon that there is no end-tidal CO_2 on the capnogram. Lack of end-tidal CO_2 on capnogram can be due to ventilator circuit disconnect, leak around the tracheostomy appliance (as when the cuff is only partially inflated or not inflated at all), or presence of the tracheostomy appliance in a false passage instead of the trachea. There is a risk that the tracheostomy appliance may be placed into the soft tissues between the skin and the trachea, and not inside the lumen of the trachea itself. The patient cannot be ventilated via an appliance that is not within the lumen of the trachea. The surgeon should quickly remove the tracheostomy from the false passage and replace it properly within the lumen of the trachea.

> The surgeon replaces the tracheostomy appliance, and the patient is able to be ventilated as expected. The patient returns to the ICU postoperatively. Over the next 36 hours, the patient's oxygenation status continues to worsen.

What else can be done?

Prone positioning can be helpful to improve oxygenation in patients with ARDS. By positioning the patient on their abdomen (instead of supine on their back), ventilation and perfusion are redistributed. Prone positioning recruits atelectatic segments of the lung in the dorsal parts of the lung, thereby improving ventilation and perfusion matching. It is important to ensure the tracheostomy (or endotracheal tube) is not inadvertently removed when placing the patient in the prone position.

Over the next several weeks, the patient recovers. He complains of new-onset weakness in his hands and legs that is spreading up his limbs.

What's going on?

In patients who have survived the acute phase of illness, postinfectious neurologic immune complications may manifest. These symptoms are suggestive of Guillain-Barre syndrome. A new onset of this disease has been reported after infection with Covid-19.

STEP 2 PEARL

Guillain–Barre Syndrome is an autoimmune disorder of the peripheral nerves. Symptoms present with progressive weakness starting from the hands and feet migrating toward the torso. Involvement of the diaphragm may require mechanical ventilatory support. Most patients fully recover within 1 year.

BEYOND THE PEARLS

- Oxygenation status requires context. PaO_2 of 100 mm Hg or oxygen saturation of 99% sounds fine until you learn that the patient is receiving FiO_2 1.0. Always consider FiO_2 and other ventilator settings, such as PEEP, in evaluating a patient's oxygenation status.
- Whenever possible, it is preferred to do procedures at the bedside in patients with Covid-19. This reduces risks of patient transport and the infectious risk to other individuals in the facility. Surgical and anesthesiology teams should discuss the feasibility of performing tracheostomy at the bedside.
- In prone patients, it is important to adequately pad all pressure points. There should be no pressure on the patient's eyes or on the endotracheal tube or tracheostomy appliance (see Case 25).
- According to the CDC, all individuals age 6 months and older should receive vaccination against Covid-19. This includes people who are pregnant, trying to become pregnant, and breastfeeding.

References

Abouzgheib, W., & Ross, S. E. (2019). Bedside tracheostomy in the intensive care unit. In J. E. Parrillo & R. P. Dellinger (Eds.), *Critical care medicine: Principles of diagnosis and management in the adult* (5th ed., Chapter 14, p. 193-200.e2). Philadelphia, PA: Elsevier.

Bauer, B. (2018). Immunology. In T. X. O'Connell, R. A. Pedigo, & T. E. Blair (Eds.), *Crush Step 1: The Ultimate USMLE Step 1 Review* (pp. 202–215). Philadelphia, PA: Elsevier.

Care of critically *ill patients with Covid-19*. Accessed December 14, 2020. https://www.covid19treatment-guidelines.nih.gov/critical-care.

Coronavirus: novel coronavirus (Covid-19) infection. Clinical Overview. Updated November 23, 2020. www.clinicalkey.com.

Durbin, C. G., Jr. (2005). Indications for and timing of tracheostomy. *Respiratory Care, 50*(4), 483–487.

Korff, S., Katus, H. A., & Giannitsis, E. (2006). Differential diagnosis of elevated troponins. *Heart, 92*, 987–993.

Long, B., Brady, W. J., Koyfman, A., & Gottlieb, M. (2020). Cardiovascular complications in Covid-19. *American Journal of Emergency Medicine, 38*, 1504–1507.

Reece-Anthony, R., Lao, G., Carter, C., & Notter, J. (2020). COVID-19 disease: Acute respiratory distress syndrome and prone position. *Clinics in Integrated Care, 3*, 100024.

Gold Standard, Inc. SARS-CoV-2 Virus (Covid-19) mRNA Vaccine. Drug monograph. Published March 25, 2021. www.clinicalkey.com. Accessed 6.5.2021.

Testing Overview. *Centers for Disease Control and Prevention*. Accessed September 5, 2021. https://www.cdc.gov/coronavirus/2019-ncov/hcp/testing-overview.html.

Therapeutic *management of patients with Covid-19*. Accessed September 5, 2021. https://www.covid19treat-mentguidelines.nih.gov/therapeutic-management.

Vascular

A 70-Year-Old Man With a History of Hypertension, Coronary Artery Disease With Mildly Reduced Left Ventricular Function, and a 100 Packyear Smoking History

Benjamin Morey ■ Paul Neil Frank

A 70-year-old man with a history of hypertension, coronary artery disease (CAD) with mildly reduced left ventricular function (left ventricular ejection fraction [LVEF] 45%), and a 100 pack-year smoking history is found to have a 6.1-cm abdominal aortic aneurysm (AAA) on a screening ultrasound. He is now presenting for open repair. In the preoperative holding area, his vital signs are blood pressure 163/92 mm Hg, pulse 70/min, respiration rate 12/min, oxygen saturation 95% on room air, and temperature 37.2°C.

What is an AAA, and who is at risk of developing them?

An aneurysm is a localized dilation of an artery involving all three layers of the arterial wall: intima, media, and adventitia. True aneurysms are classified as saccular (involving only a portion of the total vessel circumference), fusiform (involving the entire vessel circumference), or dissecting (the result of an arterial dissection). False aneurysms, or pseudoaneurysms, are caused by a tear in the arterial wall that leads to a collection of blood not contained by the wall of the artery but rather by surrounding tissues. Fig. 30.1 shows the anatomy of each type of aneurysm as well as a false aneurysm.

What is the most common anatomy of an AAA?

Fusiform is the most common type of AAA. The majority of AAAs are infrarenal, meaning that they do not extend above the renal arteries. However, some AAAs involve the renal arteries (juxtarenal) or even extend above them (suprarenal). When an aneurysm involves the portion of the aorta above the diaphragm, it is considered a thoracoabdominal aneurysm, the extent of which are referred to using the Crawford classification.

Computed tomography (CT) scan of the patient's abdomen, along with a three-dimensional reconstruction, is shown in Fig. 30.2.

What kind of aneurysm does he have?

The patient has a fusiform infrarenal AAA.

What are the risk factors for AAA?

Atherosclerosis is the most common etiology of AAA. Less common causes of AAA include connective tissue disorders (Marfan disease, Ehler-Danlos), vasculitis, bacterial infections (e.g., syphilis, tuberculosis), and fungal infections (i.e., mycotic aneurysms). A small subset of patients

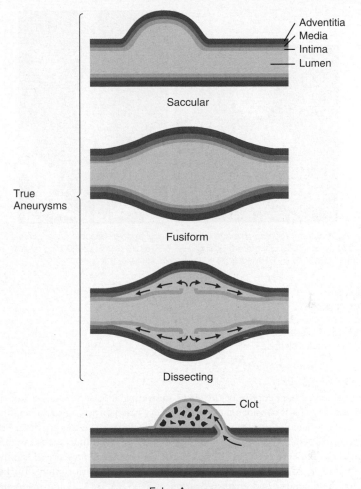

Fig. 30.1 Anatomic types of arterial aneurysms. (Data from Goodman, C. C., Fuller, K. S., & Marshall, C. [Eds.]. [2017]. *Pathology for the physical therapist assistant* [Chapter 9, pp. 245–318.e5]. Philadelphia, PA: Elsevier. Fig. 9.21.)

(3%–10% of AAAs) have "inflammatory" aneurysms, which are characterized by thickened aortic walls with surrounding fibrosis and adhesions of adjacent structures. There appears to be a stronger genetic component to these aneurysms, and patients are frequently more symptomatic than with other etiologies of AAAs. Inflammatory AAAs carry a higher surgical risk.

STEP 1, 2, 3 PEARL

The most common risk factors associated with the development of abdominal aortic aneurysms are:
- Age > 60
- Smoking
- Atherosclerosis
- Family history
- Male gender
- Hypertension

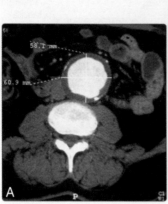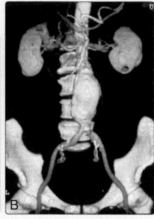

Fig. 30.2 Axial computed tomography image of an infrarenal abdominal aortic aneurysm (A) and the three-dimensional reconstruction (B). (Data from Bhangu, A., & Keighley, M. R. B. [2007]. *The flesh and bones of surgery* [Chapter 25, pp. 76–77]. Philadelphia, PA: Elsevier. Fig. 3.25.2.)

- Hyperlipidemia
- Diabetes mellitus
- Chronic obstructive pulmonary disease
- Coronary artery disease
- Peripheral vascular disease

How is an AAA diagnosed?

An AAA is defined as an aneurysm of the aorta, measuring at least 50% larger in diameter than "normal." However, what is considered normal can vary based on sex, age, and height. In general, most AAAs have a diameter greater than 30 mm. The majority of AAAs are discovered incidentally. Very rarely will AAAs be discovered on the basis of clinical findings such as vague abdominal or back pain or the presence of pulsatile mass in the abdomen. The presence of significant symptoms attributed to an AAA is an ominous sign often associated with rupture. The best imaging modalities for the diagnosis and characterization of an AAA are CT and magnetic resonance imaging (MRI). Angiography is the gold standard for diagnosis but is rarely used given its invasive nature and the reliability of CT and MRI.

The patient is nervous. He asks what could happen if he does not have the aneurysm repaired.

Rupture is the most-feared complication of an AAA and is a surgical emergency. The perioperative mortality rate in this setting is approximately 50%. However, the actual mortality rate may be significantly higher because many patients with ruptured AAAs die prior to reaching the hospital. The most common site of rupture is the posterolateral wall of the aorta, resulting in rupture into the retroperitoneal space. Patients will present with profound hemodynamic instability from acute blood loss and severe abdominal and/or flank pain. CT will demonstrate extravasation of contrast. Fig. 30.3 demonstrates a ruptured AAA on CT.

STEP 2, 3 PEARL

The presence of flank ecchymoses is called the Grey Turner sign and is associated with retroperitoneal bleeding.

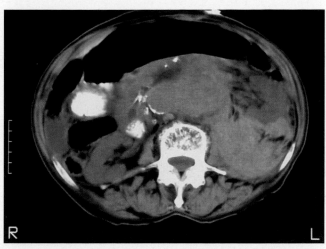

Fig. 30.3 Axial computed tomography image of a ruptured abdominal aortic aneurysm. There is a significant amount of retroperitoneal blood on the patient's left side. (Data from Kellerman, R., & Rakel, D. [2021]. *Conn's current therapy 2021* [pp. 100–104]. Philadelphia, PA: Elsevier. Fig. 2.)

When should an AAA be repaired?

The primary determining factor for surgical repair of an AAA is the risk of rupture, which is primarily influenced by the diameter of the aneurysm. The yearly risk of rupture for AAAs 5.5–6.9 cm in diameter is approximately 10%. Once larger than 7.0 cm, the annual risk of rupture increases to more than 30%. Guidelines recommend elective surgical repair of an AAA once it becomes 5.5 cm or larger. Other indications for repair include symptomatic AAAs or a rate of expansion that exceeds 0.5 cm over a 6-month period.

What are the options for repair of an AAA? What are the advantages and disadvantages of each?

There are two methods used to repair AAAs: open surgical repair and endovascular aortic aneurysm repair (EVAR). Fig. 30.4 demonstrates the basic steps involved in open surgical repair of AAAs. Open surgical approaches are used when there are anatomical hinderances to an endovascular approach. This can include factors such as a shorter aortic neck (the area between the aneurysm and the renal arteries), a more acute angle between the nondiseased portion of the aorta and that of the aneurysm, and significant atherosclerotic disease of the femoral or iliac arteries where vascular access for EVAR is obtained. In low- or intermediate-risk patients, open approach may also be preferred due to improved durability of the graft.

    EVAR is an attractive approach to the repair of AAAs given its decreased incidence of early morbidity and mortality, as well as decreased length of hospital stay when compared with open repair. There is no need for aortic cross clamp in EVAR. However, EVAR exposes patients to radiation and contrast dyes (which may be detrimental to those with preexisting renal dysfunction), is more expensive, requires increased surveillance, and is more likely to require future interventions. There is no benefit in terms of long-term mortality compared with open repair.

> The vascular surgeon says that, given the location of the aneurysm, she will have to clamp the aorta above the celiac trunk (Supraceliac).

How is this information relevant?

The largest physiologic insults that occur during an open AAA repair are the application and removal of the aortic cross clamp. The hemodynamic changes that occur are dependent on the location of clamp placement, the patient's baseline left ventricular (LV) function, the presence of CAD, intravascular volume status, degree of collateral circulation, and the anesthetic technique used.

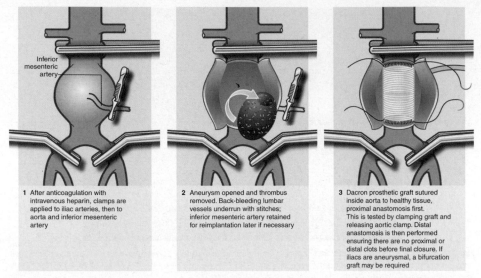

Fig. 30.4   Open surgical repair of an infrarenal abdominal aortic aneurysm. 1—Clamps are applied above and below the aneurysm. 2—The aneurysm is opened and thrombus is removed. 3—The graft is sewn to healthy aorta prior to clamp removal. (Data from Burkitt, H. G., Quick, C. R. G., & Reed, J. B. [Eds.]. [2007]. *Essential surgery: Problems, diagnosis and management* [Chapter 42, pp. 534–545]. Modified from Fig. 42.4.)

The information provided by the surgeon is important because more proximal (i.e., cephalad) levels of aortic cross-clamp application are associated with higher degrees of hemodynamic instability, cardiac stress, and risk of injury to vital organs.

Application of an aortic cross clamp results in significant increase in afterload, leading to elevated mean arterial pressure (MAP), pulmonary capillary wedge pressure (PCWP), and LV end diastolic volume. There may also be decreased LVEF and new or exaggerated cardiac wall motion abnormalities on echocardiography, especially in patients with preexisting cardiac disease. All of these changes are more pronounced with more proximal cross-clamp application. Fig. 30.5 shows the hemodynamic changes that occur with cross-clamp application at different aortic levels. Notice that the changes seen with infrarenal clamping are less severe compared with more proximal clamp application.

Aortic cross clamping can also cause an increase in venous return and hence preload. A significant amount of blood is contained within the splanchnic vasculature. When arterial flow into these vascular beds is decreased with supraceliac clamping, passive venous recoil will return much of this blood to the heart. In addition, the surge of catecholamine (e.g., epinephrine and norepinephrine) release that occurs with aortic occlusion produces systemic venoconstriction that further augments venous return.

The net result for our patient will be an increase in both afterload and preload, which can produce considerable strain on the heart. In light of the patient's CAD and reduced LVEF, he is at elevated risk for hemodynamic decompensation and permanent myocardial injury.

What other organ systems are at risk due to the application of an aortic cross clamp?
Renal, gastrointestinal, and spinal cord ischemia can produce some of the most feared complications associated with this operation. Again, more proximal application of the clamp produces greater degrees of dysfunction.

What can be done to protect the kidneys during this operation?
Mannitol and loop diuretics are commonly used to enhance renal perfusion. Mannitol enhances urine output and is thought to also increase renal blood flow (RBF) by decreasing renal vascular

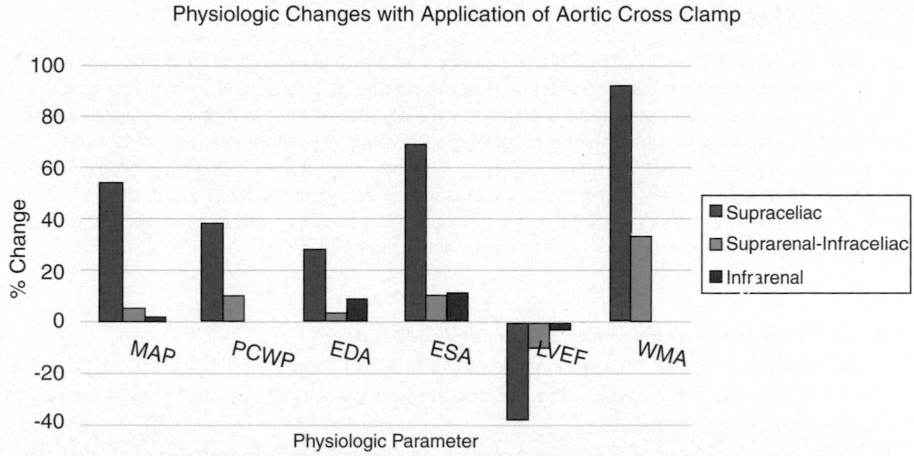

Physiologic Changes with Application of Aortic Cross Clamp

Fig. 30.5 Changes in cardiovascular variables seen with different levels of aortic occlusion Supraceliac is the most proximal cross clamp application site, while infrarenal is the most distal. *MAP*, Mean arterial pressure; *PCWP*, pulmonary capillary wedge pressure; *EDA*, LV end diastolic area; *ESA*, LV end systolic area; *LVEF*, LV ejection fraction; *WMA*, patients with wall motion abnormalities. (Data from Roizen, M. F., Beaupre, P. N., Alpert, R. A., Kremer, P., Cahalan, M. K., & Shiller, N. [1984]. Monitoring with two-dimensional transesophageal echocardiography. Comparison of myocardial function in patients undergoing supraceliac, suprarenal-infraceliac, or infrarenal aortic occlusion. *Journal of Vascular Surgery, 1*[2], 300–305.)

resistance. There is also some evidence that it acts as a free radical scavenger to attenuate damage caused by ischemic-reperfusion injury. The dopamine-1 agonist fenoldopam is also thought to be of potential benefit given its ability to preferentially dilate renal and splanchnic vasculature. Care must be taken when administering diuretics as these can precipitate hypovolemia.

While adequate perioperative urine output is reassuring, it does not reliably correlate with risk of renal injury. Currently, no pharmacologic agent has been shown to definitively prevent acute kidney injury (AKI) in patients having open AAA repair. Therefore the most effective way to prevent AKI is to maintain normal cardiac output (CO), systemic blood pressure, and volume status.

STEP 1 PEARL

Mannitol is an osmotic diuretic. It produces its diuretic effect by being freely filtered at the glomerulus without significant reabsorption. This will increase the osmotic pressure within the renal tubules, thereby drawing more free water into the tubule.

STEP 1 PEARL

Loop diuretics such as furosemide act on the thick ascending loop of Henle by blocking the $Na^+/K^+/2Cl^-$ cotransporter and interfering with the reabsorption of Na^+ and Cl^-.

AKI occurs in 3% of those cases involving infrarenal aortic cross clamping. When the clamp is applied above the renal arteries, RBF is significantly reduced, and the risk of AKI climbs to 15%. The most significant risk factor for AKI after open AAA repair is preexisting renal dysfunction, especially when baseline serum creatinine level is greater than 2 mg/dL. Other risk factors for AKI include advanced age, cross-clamp time greater than 30 minutes, preexisting cardiac dysfunction, hypovolemia, and prolonged duration of hypotension. AKI can also result from ischemic reperfusion injury, embolization of atherosclerotic debris, and surgical trauma.

STEP 1, 2, 3 PEARL

Etiologies of acute kidney injury (AKI) are classified as prerenal, intrarenal, and postrenal. AKI during open AAA repair is usually caused by acute tubular necrosis (ATN), which is a type of intrarenal AKI caused by damage to the structural elements within the kidney. Prerenal causes of AKI occur secondary to diminished renal blood flow (e.g., hypotension). However, with prolonged reductions in RBF, ischemic injury to the nephron occurs. This produces an intrinsic renal pattern of injury. Urine microscopy will classically yield granular or "muddy brown" casts with intrinsic renal causes of ARF. Table 30.1 shows the laboratory values commonly used to distinguish prerenal, intrinsic renal, and postrenal etiologies of AKI.

What can be done to protect the spinal cord during this operation?

The most reliable protective measures are hypothermia and cerebrospinal fluid (CSF) drainage. Hypothermia decreases the oxygen demand required by the spinal cord and thus decreases the amount of blood supply required.

CSF drainage via a lumbar drain augments the spinal cord perfusion pressure (SCPP), which is given by

$$SCPP = MAP - CSF \ pressure \text{ (or central venous pressure [CVP],}$$
$$\text{whichever is greater)}$$

SCPP can be augmented by increasing MAP and/or decreasing CSF pressure via CSF drainage. SCPP greater than 70 mm Hg are ideal.

Drugs such as barbiturates and glucocorticoids are commonly used in high-risk patients. Numerous other drugs, including N-methyl-D-aspartate (NMDA) receptor antagonists and the opioid antagonist naloxone, have been investigated.

Paraplegia from spinal cord ischemia is rare after open AAA repair. With higher cross-clamp application (especially for the repair of thoracoabdominal aortic aneurysms), the risk of paraplegia increases.

What is the blood supply to the spinal cord?

The arterial blood supply to the spinal cord consists of two posterior spinal arteries and one anterior spinal artery (see Fig. 30.6). The areas of the spinal cord responsible for motor function (anterior corticospinal tracts, see Case 25) are supplied by the anterior spinal artery and are susceptible to ischemia when blood flow is compromised. Patients experiencing paraplegia following aortic surgery will typically present with bilateral lower extremity weakness or paralysis.

TABLE 30.1 ■ **Laboratory Variables With Different Etiologies of Acute Kidney Injury**

Index	Prerenal	Intrinsic Renal	Postrenal
Urine osmolality (mOsm/kg)	>500	<350	<350
Urine sodium (Na⁺, mEq/L)	<20	>40	>40
Fractional excretion of Na⁺ (FE$_{Na}$)	<1%	>2%	>1%
Fractional excretion of urea (FE$_{urea}$)	<35%	>50%	Variable
Ratio of blood urea nitrogen to creatinine in the serum (BUN/Cr)	>20	<15	>20
Urine specific gravity	>1.020	<1.010	Variable

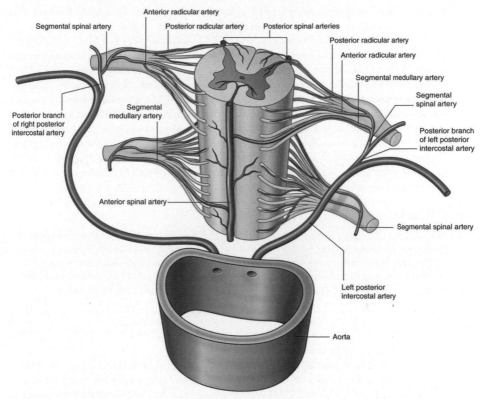

Fig. 30.6 Arterial blood supply to the spinal cord. (Data from Drake, R. L., Vogl, A. W. & Mitchell, A. W. M. (Eds.). [2020]. *Gray's anatomy for students* [4th ed., Chapter 2, 49–122.e2]. Philadelphia, PA: Elsevier. Fig. 2.55.)

STEP 1, 2, 3 PEARL

Radicular arteries feed the anterior spinal artery. The largest radicular artery is called the great radicular artery, or the artery of Adamkiewicz. Its origin is usually found between T9 and T12, but this is variable. It is responsible for the arterial supply to the anterior spinal cord. This variable location is why paraplegia can still occur after repair of infrarenal abdominal aortic aneurysms.

What are the potential gastrointestinal sequelae of aortic cross clamp?
Gastrointestinal complications arising from aortic occlusion range from mild paralytic ileus to bowel necrosis. More proximal application of the cross clamp can also cause hepatic dysfunction.

The operation will be performed under general anesthesia with an endotracheal tube and american society of anesthesiologists standard monitors.

What additional lines and monitors will you use?
Beyond ASA standard monitors, you should place an arterial catheter and ensure large-bore intravenous (IV) access. Blood pressure fluctuations are common throughout the operation, and continuous monitoring of blood pressure is vital for intraoperative management. Both severe hypertension and hypotension can occur, and it is imperative that these changes are monitored and treated. Furthermore, the ability to draw blood for laboratory analysis is key to assess the hematologic and metabolic status of the patient intraoperatively.

Open AAA repairs frequently result in large fluid shifts and blood loss. For a healthy patient with relatively few comorbidities, large-bore peripheral IV access is sufficient. For our patient with preexisting cardiac dysfunction, a central venous catheter (CVC) should be placed. A CVC will allow for rapid volume administration and administration of hemodynamic infusions such as inotropes and vasopressors. With a CVC in place, you may also opt to monitor central venous pressure (CVP) or place a pulmonary artery (PA) catheter to monitor the patient's volume status and cardiac function.

Finally, for this patient with a history of cardiac disease and CAD, it would be prudent to place a transesophageal echocardiography (TEE) probe. TEE can be a useful method to assess volume status and both global and regional cardiac function. Application of an aortic cross clamp places considerable stress on the heart. This can manifest as regional wall motion abnormalities (indicative of ischemia) or decreased LVEF. Patients with preexisting cardiac disease are more susceptible to these changes. TEE can also provide quantitative estimates of CO in addition to visual and quantitative estimates of ejection fraction.

STEP 1 PEARL

The law of Laplace applied to cardiac mechanics states that LV wall tension is proportional to intraventricular pressure and radius. It is inversely proportional to LV wall thickness. The application of an aortic cross clamp increases both preload and afterload and thus interventricular pressure and radius. This will lead to an increase in wall tension and increased myocardial oxygen demand, thus increasing the risk of ischemia and ventricular failure.

Induction and intubation are uneventful. You plan to place a PA catheter.

What are the indications for pa catheter placement?

Patients who are at risk of hemodynamic instability, and surgical procedures that cause sudden large changes in intravascular volume, preload, and/or afterload warrant the use of a PA catheter. Our patient with reduced LVEF and CAD undergoing an open AAA repair involving supraceliac cross-clamp application is in this category.

PA catheters provide a litany of hemodynamic data which is unparalleled by other less-invasive monitors (with the possible exception of TEE). In addition to PA pressure and CVP, the PA catheter can provide measurements of systemic vascular resistance (SVR), stroke volume (SV), CO/cardiac index (CO/CI), mixed venous oxygen saturation (SvO_2), and PCWP. PCWP is thought to be a reliable surrogate measurement of left atrial pressure and thus LV end-diastolic pressure (which may correlate with preload).

How is a PA catheter placed?

A PA catheter is a long sterile cable with a pressure transducer at the tip and a balloon just proximal to the tip (see Fig. 30.7). It is inserted through a specialized CVC called an introducer. A PA catheter can be inserted through any central venous access point, but it is easiest via an introducer in the right internal jugular vein. After placing and securing the introducer, the PA catheter is advanced through the introducer into the vein. Once approximately 15 cm of catheter has been inserted, the balloon should be inflated. Once the balloon is inflated, continue advancing the catheter. As the catheter is advanced, the waveform and pressure reading will change as the pressure transducer at the tip of the catheter moves from the right atrium to the right ventricle and then the PA. Fig. 30.8 shows the waveforms typically encountered as the catheter is advanced.

While you are advancing the PA catheter, the blood pressure drops, and you notice the rhythm shown in Fig. 30.9.

What is going on? What should you do?

The rhythm strip shows complete heart block. This is a known complication of PA catheter placement. Patients with preexisting left bundle branch block are at greater risk. Deflate the balloon

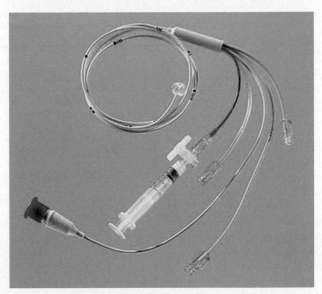

Fig. 30.7 Pulmonary artery catheter with the balloon inflated. (Data from Al-Shaikh, B., & Stacey, S. G. [2017]. *Invasive monitoring. In Essentials of equipment in anaesthesia, critical care and perioperative medicine* [Chapter 11, pp. 179–200]. Philadelphia, PA: Elsevier. Fig. 11.22.)

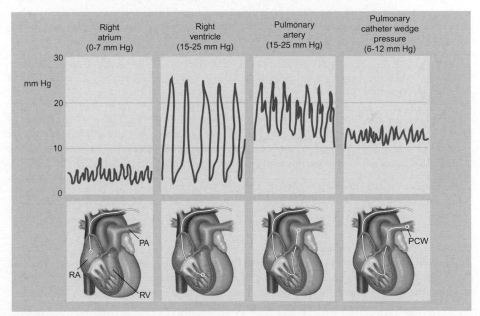

Fig. 30.8 Pressure waveforms encountered during the placement of a pulmonary artery (PA) catheter. The right atrial tracing resembles that of the central venous pressure. Upon entry into the right ventricle, systolic pressure increases dramatically with little corresponding change in the diastolic pressure. Entry into the PA produces the characteristic diastolic "step-up" whereby the diastolic pressure increases significantly. Advancing the catheter a further 3–5 cm produces a drop in the mean pressure which generally signifies the pulmonary capillary wedge pressure (PCWP). *RA*, Right atrium; *RV*, right ventricle. (Data from Henry, M., & Thompson, J. [2012]. *Clinical surgery* [Chapter 11, pp. 149–173]. Philadelphia, PA: Elsevier. Fig. 11.8.)

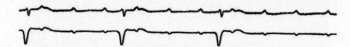

Fig. 30.9 Rhythm strip showing no consistent relationship between P waves and QRS complexes. This is consistent with complete heart block, also called third-degree heart block. (Data from Maury, P., Chilon, T., Dumonteil, N., & Fontan, A. [2008]. Complete atriovenricular block persisting after regression of infectious myocarditis. *Journal of Electrocardiology, 41*[6]. Modified from Fig. 1.)

and withdraw the catheter. It may be necessary to treat the patient with a vagolytic agent (e.g., atropine), direct chronotrope (e.g., epinephrine), or even transcutaneous pacing to achieve hemodynamic stability. Once the patient is stable, an additional attempt may be considered, depending on the necessity of the PA catheter.

What are the other potential complications of PA catheter placement?

The list of complications that can be attributed to PA catheter placement includes those associated with CVC placement (e.g., arterial puncture, hematoma formation, pneumothorax, brachial plexus injury, thrombosis, infection) in addition to several unique to PA catheters. These include: pulmonary infarction, right ventricular perforation, pulmonic or tricuspid valve damage, catheter knotting, and balloon rupture. A rare but feared complication of PA catheter placement is PA rupture. This is difficult to detect under general anesthesia, and one must have a high degree of clinical suspicion.

The use of PA catheters is relatively contraindicated in patients with known tricuspid or pulmonic stenosis or friable right atrial or right ventricular masses. Other relative contraindications are the presence of recently placed pacemaker leads, coagulopathy, and severe arrhythmias. While arrhythmias are possible with CVC placement, they are a more common complication of PA catheter placement.

> The patient stabilizes, and the second attempt at PA catheter insertion is uneventful. As the patient is being prepped and draped, the operating room nurse asks what blood products you would like to have available for this patient.

Open AAA repair has the potential for significant blood loss. You should have at least 4 units of packed red blood cells available in the room at the time of incision. Fortunately, through the use of intraoperative cell-salvage and improved surgical techniques, it is common to avoid transfusion of allogeneic blood products altogether during the repair of uncomplicated infrarenal AAAs.

> The surgeon dissects down to the aorta and applies the aortic cross clamp. The patient's blood pressure increases from 118/51 to 204/91 mm Hg. You notice new ST segment depressions on the electrocardiogram (ECG).

What is happening? How do you proceed?

Application of the aortic cross clamp increases afterload and has causes severe hypertension. This places considerable stress on the heart by increasing in LV wall tension and thus myocardial oxygen demand. In a patient with CAD, this can produce ischemia manifesting as ST segment changes or regional wall motion abnormalities. Short-acting vasodilators should be readily available to treat hypertension after cross-clamp application. It may be prudent to administer these agents prior to the application of the cross clamp to avoid extreme hypertension. Maintain blood pressure close to the patient's preoperative baseline.

There are several pharmacologic options to control hypertension during aortic occlusion. In general, short-acting agents are preferred because they are well-suited for use as infusions and can quickly be withdrawn should the patient's hemodynamic status change. If the patient is tachycardic, the β_1-selective β-blocker esmolol can help lower blood pressure by reducing heart rate. It has the additional benefit of reducing myocardial oxygen demand as well as enhancing coronary blood flow by way of increased time in diastole (vital in patients experiencing myocardial ischemia). However, in most cases of aortic occlusion, arterial vasodilation is required. This can be accomplished via deepening of the anesthetic or through direct-acting vasodilators (e.g., clevidipine, nitroprusside).

STEP 1, 2, 3 PEARL

Sodium nitroprusside is converted to nitric oxide (NO) within vascular smooth muscle cells. NO produces vasodilation via increased cyclic guanosine monophosphate (cGMP). A well-known side effect of nitroprusside is cyanide toxicity. Cyanide toxicity is more likely to occur with higher doses for longer periods of time and in patients with hepatic or renal dysfunction.

Application of an aortic cross clamp also increases preload. Counteracting this increase in venous return to the heart can limit LV dilation and the subsequent increased myocardial oxygen demand that results. Nitroglycerin is the ideal drug to do this. Its mechanism of action is similar to that of nitroprusside, but it predominantly affects the venous vasculature. This leads to blood pooling within the venous system and a decrease in venous return. Furthermore, nitroglycerin causes dilation of the coronary arteries.

You correct the hypertension, and the blood pressure is 146/67 mm Hg as the surgeon completes the remainder of the aortic anastomoses. She says she will remove the cross clamp in a few minutes.

What do you expect to happen when the cross clamp is removed? How can you best avoid hemodynamic fluctuations?

Removal of the aortic cross clamp can precipitate hypotension. Greater degrees of hypotension are encountered after clamp removal from a more proximal location. Release of the cross clamp reperfuses ischemic tissues distal to the clamp, thereby carrying byproducts of anaerobic metabolism (e.g., lactic acid, prostaglandins, adenosine, potassium) into the systemic circulation, causing vasodilation and myocardial dysfunction. Hypovolemia also contributes to hypotension following cross-clamp removal. Fig. 30.10 summarizes the complex physiologic changes that occur following cross-clamp removal.

To avoid profound hypotension following cross-clamp removal, increase the blood pressure prior to clamp removal. This can be done by titrating off any vasodilating infusions, lightening the anesthetic, and administering volume and vasopressors. Some anesthesiologists also administer calcium to augment cardiac contractility during this period. Even with a robust blood pressure prior to clamp removal, the patient may still develop significant hypotension with cross-clamp release.

The surgeon releases the cross clamp, and the blood pressure drops to 61/44 mm Hg.

What do you do next?

With an abrupt drop in blood pressure, you should administer volume, vasopressors, and inotropes. However, if the blood pressure does not respond quickly, you should ask the surgeon to reapply the clamp. This will rapidly restore the blood pressure (be careful not to overshoot with reapplication of the clamp in the setting of recently administered vasopressors). Once the blood pressure is restored, you can preemptively elevate the blood pressure prior to the next removal of the clamp. When the clamp is to be removed again, ask the surgeon to release it gradually because this will be better tolerated by the patient.

Once the cross clamp is released, maintain blood pressure with short-acting vasopressors and inotropes. Phenylephrine, norepinephrine, epinephrine, and vasopressin are good choices. It is important to maintain an appropriate intravascular volume status during this period as well by administering blood products, to replace ongoing blood loss. Be sure to replete calcium

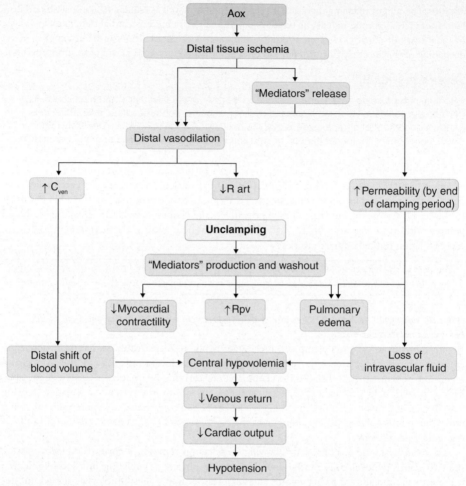

Fig. 30.10 Systemic hemodynamic response to aortic unclamping. *AoX*, Aortic cross-clamping; C_{ven}, venous capacitance; *R art*, arterial resistance; *Rpv*, pulmonary vascular resistance. (From Gelman, S. [1995]. The pathophysiology of aortic cross-clamping and unclamping. *Anesthesiology, 82,* 1026–1060.)

(an important contributor to myocardial contractility), as it may decline with the administration of blood products (see Case 13).

The surgeon may request lower blood pressures to minimize bleeding in the surgical field. In the period following cross-clamp removal, the information obtained from the PA catheter and TEE is crucial. Decreased cardiac contractility, hypovolemia, and systemic vasodilation can all be detected by these monitors. This will allow for appropriate treatment of the underlying cause of the hypotension.

STEP 1, 2, 3 PEARL

Table 30.2 shows the receptor affinity of several commonly used vasopressors and inotropes. Not included here is vasopressin which produces vasoconstriction via action at V_1 receptors in vascular smooth muscle.

TABLE 30.2 ■ **Receptor Binding of Major Vasopressor and Inotropic Drugs**

Receptor class	α1	β1	β2
Dopamine	+++	++++	++
Dobutamine	+	+++++	+++
Norepinephrine	+++++	+++	++
Epinephrine	+++++	++++	+++
Phenylephrine	+++++	0	0

Affinity for receptors is rated + to +++++. Modified from Overgaard, C. B., & Džavík, V. (2008). Inotropes and vasopressors: Review of physiology and clinical use in cardiovascular disease. *Circulation, 118*, 1047–1056.

The aortic cross clamp has been removed and the patient is hemodynamically stable. Arterial blood gas (ABG) shows pH 7.12, $PaCO_2$ 42 mm Hg, PaO_2 233 mm Hg, and bicarbonate (HCO_3-) 13 meq/l.

How do you interpret this? What should you do?

When analyzing an ABG, it is helpful to have a systematic approach. First, look at the pH. A normal pH is 7.36–7.44. Our patient is acidotic. Next, look at the $PaCO_2$ (normal value 35–45 mm Hg) and HCO_3– (normal value 22–26 mEq/L) to determine whether the acidosis is primarily metabolic or respiratory in nature. Here, with a normal $PaCO_2$ and low HCO_3–, this patient has a primary metabolic acidosis.

STEP 1 PEARL

The Winter formula is used to calculate the expected $PaCO_2$ in the setting of a metabolic acidosis in a spontaneously breathing patient.

$$PaCO_2 = (1.5 \times HCO_3^-) + 8 \pm 2$$

Thus, if the actual $PaCO_2$ in a spontaneously breathing patient were higher than predicted by the Winter formula, one would conclude that they had a concurrent respiratory acidosis.

The most common cause of metabolic acidosis in the period following aortic cross-clamp release is the washout of metabolic byproducts of anaerobic metabolism. Frequently this is a lactic acidosis (a type of anion gap metabolic acidosis). This often takes time to improve, but you can help correct it by restoring adequate perfusion by correcting hypovolemia and augmenting MAP and CO.

In cases of severe metabolic acidosis (e.g., pH < 7.2), you can consider administering sodium bicarbonate. It is important to address significant acidosis as it can lead to worsening myocardial function and impair the effectiveness of vasopressors. Make sure to increase the patient's minute ventilation after administering bicarbonate, as it is quickly converted to CO_2.

STEP 1, 2, 3 PEARL

The anion gap is calculated to further describe a metabolic acidosis and rule in or out some underlying etiologies. The anion gap is typically calculated by

$$anion\ gap = [Na^+] - [HCO_3^-] - [Cl^-]$$

Anion gap greater than 12 is considered elevated.

The mnemonic "MUDPILES" can be used to recall the differential diagnosis for anion gap metabolic acidosis.

- M—methanol
- U—uremia

- D—diabetic ketoacidosis
- P—propylene glycol, paracetamol (acetaminophen)
- I—isoniazid, iron
- L—lactate
- E—ethylene glycol
- S—salicylates

You administer blood products and fluid to replace surgical losses. The surgeon tells you that there is no longer any active bleeding. However, the patient's blood pressure is 75/52 mm Hg. Heart rate is 114/min. PCWP and CVP are elevated. The PA catheter is reading CI of 1.2 L/min/m² and mixed SvO_2 of 48%.

What are the normal values for these measurements? What is going on?

A normal CI is 2.5–4.0 L/min/m², and a normal SvO_2 is 65%–75%.

Hypotension and tachycardia—along with a low CI and SvO_2, as well as elevated CVP and PCWP—are consistent with cardiogenic shock. Elevated PCWP and CVP in the setting of significant volume administration suggest that the patient is hypervolemic as opposed to hypovolemic. In this situation you would expect to see dilation and reduced systolic function of at least one ventricle on TEE. SVR would also be elevated.

STEP 1, 2, 3 PEARL

Cardiac index is the cardiac output adjusted to the patient's body surface area (BSA). It is calculated as cardiac output (CO)/BSA. Normal values are 2.5–4.0 L/min/m².

STEP 1, 2, 3 PEARL

Systemic vascular resistance approximates afterload or the degree of vasoconstriction of the body's vasculature. It is given by

$$SVR = 80 \times [(MAP - CVP)/CO]$$

Normal values are 800–1200 dynes-sec/cm⁻⁵.

What does SvO_2 represent, and what factors cause it to change?

SvO_2 is an indicator of global tissue oxygen delivery (DO_2) and oxygen consumption (VO_2). It is a measurement of oxygen saturation of blood in the PA, and therefore it can only be measured if a PA catheter is in place. The blood in the PA is deoxygenated blood that has returned to the central circulation through the three main venous systems of the body: SVC, inferior vena cava, and coronary sinus.

STEP 1, 2, 3 PEARL

The Fick equation is used to derive SvO_2.

$$SvO_2 = SaO_2 - \frac{VO_2}{Hb \times 1.36 \times CO}$$

SaO_2 represents arterial oxygen saturation, VO_2 represents tissue oxygen consumption, Hb represents hemoglobin concentration, and CO represents cardiac output. A pulmonary artery catheter can generate a continuous output of SvO_2. This equation can be rearranged to solve for CO.

Multiple factors influence SvO_2. Factors that decrease DO_2 or increase VO_2 will decrease SvO_2. The differential diagnosis of decreased SvO_2 includes:

- Low CI: Less flow of arterial blood, as in cardiogenic or hypovolemic shock, results in decreased DO_2.
- Anemia: Low hemoglobin concentration results in decreased oxygen content of blood and decreased DO_2.
- Arterial hypoxemia: Even with appropriate DO_2 and VO_2, arterial hypoxemia, as in severe pneumonia, will cause decreased DO_2.
- Hypermetabolism: Increased rate of tissue metabolism, as in febrile patients, will increase VO_2.

In our patient, the declining SvO_2 is another indicator that they have developed cardiogenic shock. In this case, the decreased CI (and thus DO_2) is causing inadequate tissue oxygenation. However, in a case involving significant blood loss, anemia could also be a contributing factor.

What defines "Shock"? What are the different types of shock?

Shock is defined as circulatory failure that leads to insufficient DO_2. Unless reversed quickly, impaired perfusion can result in multiorgan failure. It classically presents in its initial stages as hypotension.

Shock can be classified into four categories:

- Distributive shock is characterized by widespread vasodilation. The most common cause of distributive shock is sepsis, although neurogenic and anaphylactic shock are also forms of distributive shock.
- Cardiogenic shock is caused by low-CO states, such as heart failure exacerbation.
- Obstructive shock is the result of mechanical impairment of ventricular filling or ejection. This involves a mechanical blockage of forward flow. Cardiac tamponade, large pulmonary embolism, and tension pneumothorax are causes of obstructive shock.
- Hypovolemic shock is usually caused by severe hemorrhage (e.g., after a traumatic injury or surgical blood loss).

Table 30.3 displays the hemodynamic variables associated with each type of shock.

How will you treat this patient's cardiogenic shock?

In general, the underlying causes of cardiogenic shock are decreased contractility and volume overload. The heart is overdistended and cannot squeeze well. These patients require inotropic support and oftentimes removal of volume with diuretics or hemodialysis. In some patients, afterload reduction (i.e., reducing SVR with vasodilating agents) may improve CI.

Titrate therapy to goals of MAP greater than 65 mm Hg and CI greater than 2.2 $L/min/m^2$. Follow signs of end-organ perfusion (e.g., arterial lactate level, renal function, hepatic function, mental status, SvO_2) to ensure adequate resuscitation.

If adequate MAP and CI cannot be maintained with pharmacologic support, mechanical support devices may be indicated. These include intra-aortic balloon pump (IABP), temporary

TABLE 30.3 ■ **Hemodynamic Variables Associated with Different Shock States**

Type of shock	CO	SVR	MAP	PCWP	CVP
Distributive	↑	↓	↓	= or ↓	= or ↓
Cardiogenic	↓	↑	↓	↑	↑
Obstructive	↓	↑	↓	↑	↑
Hypovolemic	↓	↑	↓	↓	↓

CO, Cardiac output; *CVP,* central venous pressure; *MAP,* mean arterial pressure; *PCWP,* pulmonary capillary wedge pressure; *SVR,* systemic vascular resistance.

or permanent ventricular assist devices (VADs), and extracorporeal membrane oxygenation (ECMO). Placement and management of these devices require a cardiac surgeon, cardiac anesthesiologist, and a perfusionist.

BEYOND THE PEARLS

- The US Preventative Service Task Force recommends a one-time screening abdominal ultrasound for AAA in men aged 65–75 years who have ever smoked.
- Due to the myriad number of factors that can affect CVP, it is a poor indicator of circulating blood volume or volume responsiveness when used alone. However, when used with other assessments of volume status, the trend in CVP can be followed to help guide management.
- TEE detection of regional wall motion abnormalities is a more sensitive indicator of myocardial ischemia compared with changes seen on ECG and PA catheters.
- PA rupture in an awake patient would characteristically present with massive hemoptysis. Airway protection is key in this situation. Classically, patients are to be placed in the lateral decubitus position with the bleeding lung (if known) downward to protect the unaffected lung.
- Fresh frozen plasma (FFP) is used to replace deficient clotting factors as it contains all clotting factors in addition to fibrinogen. Cryoprecipitate contains fibrinogen, factor VIII, factor XIII, and von Willebrand factor. It contains a higher concentration of fibrinogen compared with FFP and thus is better suited for treating hypofibrinogenemia.
- Milrinone is a phosphodiesterase-3 inhibitor. Phosphodiesterase-3 breaks down cyclic adenosine monophosphate (cAMP) within cardiac myocytes. Thus milrinone increases cAMP levels within cardiac myocytes, which subsequently increases intracellular Ca^{2+}, and thus myocardial contractility. Milrinone decreases both SVR and pulmonary vascular resistance (PVR). It also enhances lusitropy—the rate of ventricular relaxation. Its ability to augment contractility and lower PVR makes it an attractive agent in patients with right ventricular failure. However, it also can cause hypotension.
- Table 30.4 shows the normal values for intracardiac pressures, many of which can be measured with a PA catheter.
- While one would expect most shock states to present with decreased SvO_2, septic shock is the exception because it can present with elevated SvO_2. This is because sepsis causes a cellular metabolic dysfunction that prevents tissues from fully using delivered oxygen. In addition, cardiac index is usually elevated in these patients.
- IABP's are inflatable balloons that are positioned within the aorta just distal to the left subclavian artery. They are timed to inflate during early diastole and deflate in late diastole. Inflation in early diastole augments the aortic diastolic pressure (AoDP) and thus the coronary perfusion pressure (difference between AoDP and LV end-diastolic pressure). This can be extremely beneficial in patients with ischemic LV dysfunction. By deflating immediately prior to ejection in late diastole, the IABP also reduces afterload which can further augment CO.

TABLE 30.4 ■ Normal Intracardiac Pressures

Location	Mean (mm Hg)	Range (mm Hg)
Right atrium	5	1–10
Right ventricle	25/5	15–30/0–8
Pulmonary arterial systolic and diastolic pressures	23/9	15–30/5–15
Mean pulmonary arterial	15	10–20
Pulmonary capillary wedge pressure	10	5–15
Left atrial pressure	8	4–12
Left ventricular end-diastolic pressure	8	4–12
Left ventricular systolic pressure	130	90–140

Kahn, R. A., Maus, T., Salgo, I., Weiner, M. M., & Sherman, S. K. (2017). Kaplan's cardiac anesthesia. In J. A. Kaplan, G. J. T. Augoustides, G. R. Manecke, T. Maus & D. L. Reich (Eds.), *Cardiac and noncardiac surgery* (7th ed., Chapter 13, pp. 390–426). Philadelphia, PA: Elsevier. Table 13.1.

References

American Society of Anesthesiologists Task Force on Pulmonary Artery Catheterization. (2003). Practice guidelines for pulmonary artery catheterization: an updated report by the American Society of Anesthesiologists Task Force on Pulmonary Artery Catheterization. *Anesthesiology*, *99*(4), 988–1014.

Gelzinis, T. A., & Subramaniam, K. (2011). Anesthesia for open abdominal aortic aneurysm repair. K. Subramanian, K. W. Park & B. Subramaniam (Eds.), In *Anesthesia and perioperative care for aortic surgery* (pp. 301–327). New York, NY: Springer.

Maerz, L. L., & Rosenbaum, S. H. (2018). Chapter 4: Critical illness. In R. L. Hines & K. E. Marschall (Eds.), *Stoelting's anesthesia and co-existing disease* (pp. 53–78). Philadelphia: Elsevier.

Kahn, R. A., Maus, T., Salgo, I., Weiner, M. M., & Sherman, S. K. (2017). Chapter 13: Monitoring of the heart and vascular system. In J. A. Kaplan, G. J. T. Augoustides, G. R. Manecke, T. Maus & D. L. Reich (Eds.), *Kaplan's cardiac anesthesia* (7th ed., pp. 390–426). Philadelphia, PA: Elsevier.

Norris, E. J. (2015). Chapter 69: Anesthesia for vascular surgery. In R. D. Miller, L. I. Eriksson, L. A. Fleisher, J. P. Wiener-Kronish, N. H. Cohen & W. L. Young (Eds.), *Miller's anesthesia* (8th ed., pp. 2106–2157). Philadelphia, PA: Elsevier.

Overgaard, C. B., & Dzavík, V. (2008). Inotropes and vasopressors: Review of physiology and clinical use in cardiovascular disease. *Circulation*, *118*(10), 1047–1056.

Sakalihasan, N., Michel, J. B., Katsargyris, A., Kuivaniemi, H., Defraigne, J. O., Nchimi, A., et al. (2018). Abdominal aortic aneurysms. *Nature Reviews. Disease Primers*, *4*, 34.

US Preventive Services Task Force, Owens, D. K., Davidson, K. W., Krist, A. H., Barry, M. J., Cabana, M., et al. (2019). Screening for abdominal aortic aneurysm: US Preventive Services Task Force Recommendation Statement. *JAMA*, *322*(22), 2211–2218.

van Diepen, S., Katz, J. N., Albert, N. M., Henry, T. D., Jacobs, A. K., Kapur, N. K., et al. (2017). Contemporary management of cardiogenic shock: A scientific statement from the American Heart Association. *Circulation*, *136*(16), e232–e268.

Waskowski, J., Pfortmueller, C. A., Erdoes, G., Buehlmann, R., Messmer, A. S., Luedi, M. M., et al. (2019). Mannitol for the prevention of peri-operative acute kidney injury: A systematic review. *European Journal of Vascular and Endovascular Surgery: The Official Journal of the European Society for Vascular Surgery*, *58*(1), 130–140.

A 68-Year-Old Woman With Worsening Renal Function and Impending End-Stage Renal Disease

Paul Neil Frank

A 68-year-old woman with worsening renal function and impending end-stage renal disease (ESRD) due to hypertensive nephropathy is scheduled for arteriovenous (AV) fistula placement in anticipation of her beginning hemodialysis. She has never had dialysis before. She takes lisinopril, clonidine, and carvedilol for blood pressure control. In the preoperative area her vitals show blood pressure 185/90 mm Hg, heart rate 67/min, respirations 14/min, and oxygen saturation at 88% on a 4 L/min nasal cannula. She does not use oxygen at home.

STEP 1 PEARL

In healthy patients, the kidney plays a crucial role in regulation of intravascular volume and blood pressure. The kidney produces renin in response to a decreased renal blood flow or stimulation of the β1 adrenergic receptor. Renin converts angiotensinogen (produced by the liver) to angiotensin I. Angiotensin converting enzyme (ACE) in the lungs converts angiotensin I to angiotensin II. Angiotensin II causes systemic vasoconstriction and stimulates retention of sodium and water via release of aldosterone from the cortex of the adrenal glands (see Fig. 31.1). These effects all serve to increase blood pressure.

STEP 1, 2 PEARL

Lisinopril works by blocking the activity of ACE, thereby preventing the conversion of angiotensin I to angiotensin II. This blocks the hypertensive effects of angiotensin II, resulting in decreased blood pressure. Since ACE is also responsible for metabolizing bradykinin, ACE inhibitors result in elevated bradykinin levels, which can cause cough. *ACE inhibitors may also cause fetal renal agenesis and should be avoided in women of childbearing age.*

STEP 1, 2 PEARL

Clonidine is an agonist of the presynaptic α2 adrenergic receptor in the central nervous system. It's effect is to reduce activation of the sympathetic nervous system, which reduces blood pressure. Clonidine can cause bradycardia and sedation. *Abrupt cessation may result in rebound tachycardia and hypertension.*

STEP 1, 2 PEARL

Carvedilol is an antagonist of α and β adrenergic receptors. Antagonism of α1 receptors causes vasodilation. Antagonism of cardiac β1 receptors causes decreases in heart rate and inotropy, while antagonism of renal β1 receptors downregulates the production of renin.

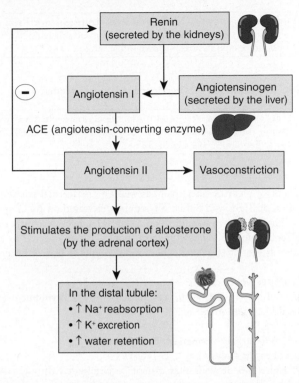

Fig. 31.1 The renin-angiotensin-aldosterone system. "Nephrology" Crush Step 1: The Ultimate USMLE Step 1 Review. (Modified from Fig. 15.14.) Pedigo, R. A. Nephrology. In T. X. O'Connell, R. A. Pedigo, & T. E. Blair (Eds.), *Crush step 1: The ultimate USMLE step 1 review* (pp. 537–579). Philadelphia, PA: Elsevier.

What chronic physiologic changes are expected in patients with ESRD?

Patients with ESRD, especially with hypertensive etiology, may develop left ventricular hypertrophy (LVH). A thick, noncompliant ventricle will require higher filling pressures and can contribute to pulmonary edema with intravascular volume overload. Patients with ESRD may also develop restrictive lung disease and premature atherosclerosis.

As the kidneys are responsible for activation of vitamin D, the loss of this function can result in hypocalcemia, eventually leading to secondary hyperparathyroidism, which causes mobilization of calcium and phosphate from bones.

STEP 1 PEARL

Vitamin D may be generated by the skin in response to exposure to the sun or ingestion from food. The liver hydroxylates vitamin D to 25(OH)-vitamin D. The kidney then activates 25(OH)-vitamin D to 1,25(OH)-vitamin D in the proximal tubule. In ESRD, filtration through the kidneys is very low, so little to no 25(OH)-vitamin D makes it to the proximal tubule. Low levels of active vitamin D result in low levels of calcium absorption from the intestine. This leads to hypocalcemia and elevated parathyroid hormone levels.

Renal failure patients are likely to be anemic, as the kidney normally secretes erythropoietin, which stimulates the production of red blood cells in bone marrow. Patients with renal failure may also result in platelet dysfunction.

Additionally, patients with renal failure may develop electrolyte and acid-base derangements.

Over the last several days, she has noticed shortness of breath at rest worse with lying down. She slept sitting up in a chair last night because she couldn't breathe comfortably lying flat. She does not use oxygen at home. Chest radiograph (CXR) is shown in Fig. 31.2.

What's going on?

The patient is volume overloaded and has developed pulmonary edema.

The patient complains of chest pain worse with deep inspiration. On auscultation of the patient's heart you appreciate a rhythmic rubbing sound. Lab tests show blood urea nitrogen (BUN) of 94 mg/dL. You obtain an electrocardiogram (ECG, Fig. 31.3).

What's going on?

The patient's complaint of pleuritic chest pain, as well as a pericardial friction rub on physical exam, marked elevation of BUN, and diffuse ST segment elevation on ECG are all suggestive of uremic pericarditis. This is a known complication of ESRD. Check serial troponin levels to rule out acute coronary syndrome. An echocardiogram should also be ordered to evaluate for pericardial effusion. If the effusion is large, the patient should undergo pericardiocentesis to drain it.

Is it safe to proceed with surgery?

No. This patient has multiple indications for urgent dialysis—she is volume overloaded and uremic. The surgery should be postponed.

What are the indications for urgent or emergent hemodialysis?

Classically, the indications for dialysis are A-E-I-O-U:

- A—Acidosis: Retention of acids that cannot be eliminated through the lungs leads to metabolic acidosis. The kidney is responsible for excreting protons and other acids that cannot be exhaled to maintain normal acid-base status. Patients with ESRD tend to become

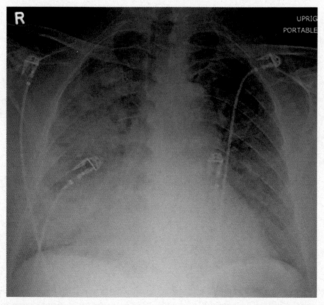

Fig. 31.2   Chest radiograph showing bilateral pulmonary edema. Notice the edema is worse in the dependent (i.e., inferior) parts of the lungs. (Data from Kimberly, H., & Stone, M. [2016]. Elderly man with acute respiratory distress. *Annals of Emergency Medicine, 67*[3], 319–331.)

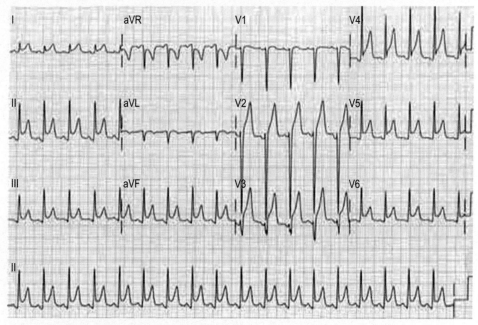

Fig. 31.3 Electrocardiogram showing diffuse ST segment elevation in leads I, II, aVF, and V3-V6. "Pericarditis." Clinical Overview. Elsevier Point of Care. 2018.

acidotic. The metabolic acidosis may have a gap (retained organic acids) and non-gap (loss of bicarbonate) component.

- E—Electrolyte disturbance: Hyperkalemia is a common electrolyte derangement in patients with renal failure. The kidney is responsible for secreting potassium. Patients with ESRD tend to retain potassium and develop hyperkalemia. These patients may also develop hypocalcemia and hyperphosphatemia.
- I—Intoxication: Toxic compounds (e.g., ethylene glycol and methanol) that have been ingested by the patient can be removed with hemodialysis.
- O—Volume overload: The kidney is responsible for maintaining euvolemia. In patients with ESRD, total body water and sodium tend to increase. This leads to intravascular volume overload, which can cause extravasation of intravascular fluid into the interstitial space (i.e., third spacing), leading to pulmonary edema and soft tissue swelling.
- U—Uremia: Elevated BUN with pericarditis, platelet dysfunction (i.e., coagulopathy), or altered mental status.

STEP 2 PEARL

Acid–base status affects potassium levels. Acidosis results in extracellular shift of potassium and hyperkalemia, whereas alkalosis results in intracellular shift of potassium and hypokalemia.

This patient needs hemodialysis urgently but she does not have any access for it.

What can be done?

Hemodialysis requires access to the patient's bloodstream. This may be accomplished via AV fistula, AV graft, or indwelling catheter. Since she does not have a fistula or graft, a temporary hemodialysis catheter must be placed.

Specialized central venous catheters can accommodate the high flow required for hemodialysis and will be ready for use immediately after placement and confirmation of proper positioning. These catheters have at least two large lumens—one for blood flow from the patient to the dialysis machine, and one for blood flow from the dialysis machine back to the patient. These can be placed in any central vein, and it is important that a sterile technique be used.

You plan to place a hemodialysis catheter in the right internal jugular vein.

How is this procedure performed?

Modern practice is to use ultrasound guidance for internal jugular central line placement. The steps for internal jugular venous catheterization are:

1. Position the patient in the Trendelenburg position (see Fig. 31.4). Ask the patient to turn their head to the contralateral side (or if the patient is anesthetized, turn their head to the contralateral side).
2. Prepare the insertion site with a sterile solution. Make circles of increasing diameter with the sterile prep stick starting over the anterolateral neck. Prepare an area at least from the ipsilateral mandible to below the ipsilateral clavicle and to the contralateral neck.
3. Don a facemask, eye protection, and hair cover. Sterilize your hands with a scrub solution. Don a sterile gown and gloves.
4. Apply a sterile drape over the anterolateral neck.
5. Prepare the central venous catheter for use by flushing all ports with saline. Arrange all of the items you will need so that they are organized and easily accessible.
6. Place a small amount of sterile ultrasound gel into the ultrasound probe sleeve. Ask an assistant to hand you the ultrasound probe into the sterile probe sleeve such that the probe sits on the ultrasound gel inside the probe sleeve. Advance the sleeve over the ultrasound probe, being careful not to contaminate yourself by touching the probe directly (see Fig. 31.5).
7. Apply a small amount of sterile ultrasound gel to the patient's anterolateral neck. Use the ultrasound to scan the neck and identify the carotid artery and internal jugular vein. You may need to ask an assistant to adjust the depth or gain on the ultrasound machine to optimize the image. The carotid artery will be round, pulsatile, and noncompressible. Meanwhile, the internal jugular vein will be irregularly shaped, nonpulsatile, and compressible. Additionally, the carotid artery is usually medial to the internal jugular vein. Scan the internal jugular vein to make sure it is patent and free from the thrombus.
8. Once you've identified both vessels, center your ultrasound probe over the internal jugular vein close to the clavicle. If the patient is awake, start by infiltrating the area overlying

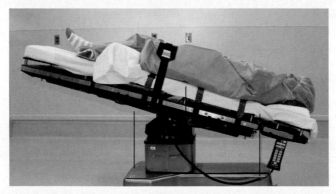

Fig. 31.4 Trendelenburg position, showing the patient supine on the operating table with the head below the level of the feet. (Data from Trendelenburg. [2020]. *AORN Journal*, 112[5], P19–P20.)

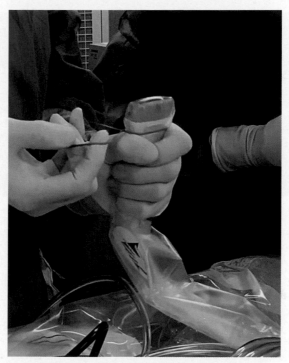

Fig. 31.5 Ultrasound probe covered by a sterile sleeve. Sterile ultrasound gel has been placed inside the sleeve. A sterile rubber band is placed near the transducer side of the probe to hold the sleeve in place. (From Martinel, V., & Fermandois-Maltes, P. [2021]. *Arthroscopic ultrasound-guided needling: An effective technique for the treatment of calcific rotator cuff tendinopathy.* Arthroscopy techniques. Arthroscopy Association of North America. Philadelphia, PA: Elsevier. Modified from Fig. 3.)

the vein with local anesthetic with a 22-gauge needle. Using an 18-gauge needle and an attached syringe, enter the skin at the center of the ultrasound probe at a 45-degree angle 1 cm cephalad from the ultrasound probe.

9. While slowly advancing the needle, withdraw on the syringe. Once the tip of the needle is in the vein, you will be able to easily draw back on the syringe, which will fill with blood.

10. Visualize the tip of your needle within the internal jugular vein on the ultrasound.

11. Put down the ultrasound probe and use the hand that was holding the probe to stabilize the needle. Remove the syringe from the needle. Dark, nonpulsatile blood should bleed from the end of the needle. *If blood is bright red and pulsatile, the needle is in an artery. In this case, remove the needle from the skin and hold pressure for 5–10 minutes.*

12. Advance the guidewire through the needle, being careful to keep the needle perfectly still. There should be little to no resistance as you advance the guidewire. Do not advance the guidewire all the way into the needle, as this can lead to a retained wire. *If you encounter resistance, withdraw the guidewire and ensure there is still blood coming from the end of the needle. If there is no longer blood coming from the end of the needle, the tip of the needle is no longer in the vessel. Attach your syringe and reposition your needle under ultrasound guidance.*

13. Once at least 20 cm of the guidewire has been advanced through the needle, leave the guidewire in place and withdraw the needle.

14. Scan the internal jugular vein with the ultrasound to confirm that the guidewire is in the vein and courses within the lumen of internal jugular vein into the chest (see Fig. 31.6).

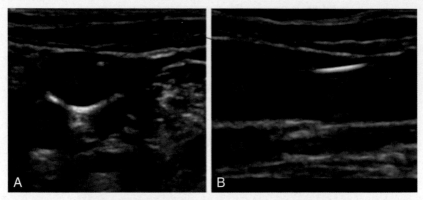

Fig. 31.6 Ultrasound of the right internal jugular vein (IJV) and carotid artery (CA) showing a guidewire (GW) properly positioned in the internal jugular vein during placement of a central venous catheter. (A) Short axis (i.e., transverse), (B) long axis (i.e., longitudinal). (Modified from Laterza, R. D., Scubb, T., & Gilliland, S. [2021] Central venous catheterization. In *Anesthesia secrets* [Chapter 23, pp. 153–160]. Philadelphia, PA: Elsevier, Fig. 23.2.)

15. Using an 11-blade scalpel, make a nick in the skin at the site where the guidewire enters the skin. In a patient of average body habitus, about half the length of the scalpel should be used to make the skin nick. *Make the skin nick such that the cutting edge of the blade is aimed anterolaterally, away from the carotid artery, which is usually medial to the internal jugular vein.*

16. Advance the dilator over the guidewire. If there is resistance, gentle twisting of the dilator can be helpful. Hold the skin taught. Do not insert more than half of the length of the dilator into the skin. Move the guidewire forward and back by 1– 2 cm to ensure it moves easily. *If the guidewire does not move easily, the guidewire may be bent. You risk injuring a blood vessel or other structure by bending the guidewire during dilation. Start by relieving pressure on the dilator. If the guidewire still does not move easily, withdraw the guidewire, hold pressure, and start over at a different site.*

17. Withdraw the dilator from the guidewire, leaving the guidewire in place. Depending on the particular central venous catheter kit being used, there may be a second, larger dilator that should be used after the first one. If so, follow step 16 as above for the second dilator.

18. Thread the catheter over the guidewire. Once the catheter is in place, withdraw the guidewire from the catheter and occlude the lumen through which the guidewire was withdrawn until a clave or another occlusive device is applied. This prevents bleeding and air embolization.

19. Ensure all ports work by aspirating blood and then flushing with saline. Always aspirate first to avoid flushing air bubbles into the patient.

20. Suture the catheter in place and apply a sterile dressing.

After obtaining consent from the patient, you place the dialysis catheter in the patient's right internal jugular vein and order a CXR to confirm proper placement. The patient's CXR is shown in Fig. 31.7.

Is that expected? What if the CXR looked like the one shown in Fig. 31.8?

Yes, Fig. 31.7 shows the expected correct position of a central venous catheter, with the tip in the superior vena cava. There is no evidence of pneumothorax or hemothorax, both of which are known complications of internal jugular vein central venous catheter placement.

If the CXR looked like the one in Fig. 31.8, the central venous catheter is likely in the arterial system and not in the venous system. The catheter shown in Fig. 31.8 was likely inadvertently placed in the internal carotid artery and courses from the carotid artery to the brachiocephalic

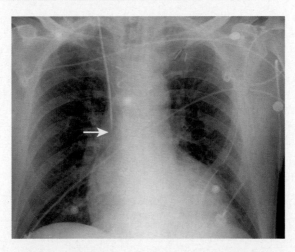

Fig. 31.7 Chest radiograph showing a properly positioned central venous catheter. The white arrow shows the tip of the catheter within the superior vena cava. (Modified from Rezaie, S. R., Coffey, E. C., & McNeil, C. R. [2019]. Central venous catheterization and central venous pressure monitoring. In J. R. Roberts, C. B. Custalow, & T. W. Thomsen [Eds.], *Roberts and Hedges' clinical procedures in emergency medicine and acute care* [7th ed., Chapter 22, pp.405–438.e3]. Philadelphia, PA: Elsevier. Modified from Fig. 22.18.)

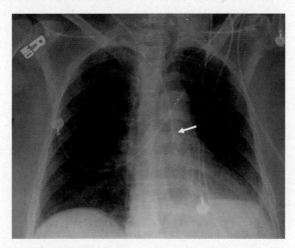

Fig. 31.8 Chest radiograph showing a central venous catheter that has been placed in an artery instead of the vein. The white arrow shows the tip overlying the descending thoracic aorta. (Data from Brixey, A., Bentz, M., & Primack, S. L. Chest radiography in the intensive care unit. In *Muller's imaging of the chest* [Chapter 69, pp. 907–928.e1] Modified from Fig. 69.29.)

artery and terminates in the thoracic aorta. *If you suspect intraarterial or extravascular placement of a central venous catheter, do not remove the catheter and do not use it.* Notify nursing staff not to use it. Consult vascular or thoracic surgery immediately.

The patient's potassium level is 6.8 mEq/L. The dialysis unit can't accommodate her for 3 Hours.

What can you do in the meantime?
The normal range for potassium is approximately 3.5–5.5 mEq/L (this varies slightly by institution), so this patient is significantly hyperkalemic. She is at risk for cardiac arrhythmia including malignant ventricular dysrhythmia (see Case 13). Administer intravenous calcium to electrically

stabilize cardiac myocyte membranes, reducing the likelihood of arrhythmia. Insulin stimulates the intracellular absorption of potassium via the sodium-potassium (Na/K) ATPase. This removes potassium from the plasma by "hiding" intracellularly, but it does not remove potassium from the body. Dextrose solution is often given along with the insulin to prevent hypoglycemia. Administration of a β agonist like albuterol (or a small dose of epinephrine) will also stimulate the intracellular uptake of potassium via the Na/K ATPase. If the patient makes urine, a dose of a loop diuretic (e.g., furosemide) may help as well.

Surgery will be rescheduled.

What is the optimal timing for surgery in ESRD patients on hemodialysis?
The patient should have surgery on the day after hemodialysis.

The patient returns one month later. She is breathing comfortably, and oxygen saturation is 98% on room air. Blood pressure is 144/77 mm Hg and Pulse is 60/minute. Her last dialysis session was yesterday.

What laboratory study should be performed prior to surgery?
It is important to check a serum potassium level prior to anesthesia.

How might ESRD affect your choice of anesthetic drugs?
The kidneys are involved in metabolism and elimination of many pharmacologic agents, including those commonly used in anesthesia. If a drug that is significantly metabolized or eliminated by the kidneys is given to a patient with ESRD, the effect of the drug will be prolonged. Metabolites of the drug may also be retained. These metabolites may have the same effect as the drug itself or they may cause toxicity.

STEP 1 PEARL

Pharmacokinetics describes what the body does to a drug. The four processes of pharmacokinetics are:
- Absorption: How the drug enters the body (e.g., oral, intramuscular, intravenous). The bioavailability of a drug describes how much of a drug administered to the patient actually enters the bloodstream. The bioavailability of drugs administered intravenously is 100%, whereas the bioavailability of orally administered drugs is lower due to destruction in the gastrointestinal tract, incomplete absorption in the intestine, and metabolism by the liver (i.e., first-pass metabolism).
- Distribution: Where the drug goes after it is absorbed. The volume of distribution (V_D) is calculated by

$$V_D = \frac{total\ amount\ of\ drug\ in\ the\ body}{plasma\ concentration\ of\ drug}$$

This is effectively a measurement of how much of the drug remains circulating in the bloodstream not bound to protein. A larger V_D indicates that a small amount of the drug stays unbound circulating in the plasma, while a lower V_D implies the opposite.
- Metabolism: How the body chemically changes a drug, also called biotransformation. Most biotransformation occurs in the liver, and there are two steps to this process. In phase I biotransformation, the drug is made more water-soluble, usually via oxidation. In phase II biotransformation, a molecule (e.g., acetyl group or glucuronide) is attached to the drug.
- Excretion: How a drug is removed from the body. This can be accomplished via renal excretion in urine or via biliary excretion in stool.

The patient's potassium level is 4.8 mEq/L, and you proceed to the operating room. You plan to use propofol and succinylcholine for induction and intubation.

Is propofol safe in ESRD patients? What about succinylcholine?
Yes and yes.

The pharmacokinetics of propofol are not altered significantly by ESRD.

An intubating dose of succinylcholine is expected to cause a transient increase in serum potassium level by 0.5 mEq/L. As long as the patient's potassium is within the normal range, and they have no other contraindication (e.g., history of stroke, burn), it is safe to give ESRD patients succinylcholine.

Would you expect a prolonged effect of succinylcholine in ESRD?
No. Succinylcholine is metabolized in the plasma by pseudocholinesterase, so ESRD should not cause a prolonged effect.

Induction and intubation are uneventful. After 10 minutes the patient has 4 twitches on train-of-four monitoring, and you want to give a non-depolarizing neuromuscular blocker.

Which non-depolarizing neuromuscular blockers will be least affected by the patient's renal failure?
Metabolism of cisatracurium is independent of the kidneys. Therefore, the duration of action should not be prolonged by ESRD. This is known as Hofmann elimination (see Case 17).

Rocuronium is primarily metabolized and eliminated by the liver. The duration of action is slightly prolonged due to a larger volume of distribution in ESRD patients. Overall rocuronium is still commonly used in patients with ESRD.

During the operation the surgeon complains that the patient is "Oozing."

What can you do to help?
Patients with ESRD may have defective platelets. This can be caused by dialysis itself, which exposes the patient's blood to anticoagulant and foreign material of the circuit, or by toxin accumulation, which can permanently poison platelets even after the toxins have been removed by dialysis. Administration of desmopressin (also known as DDAVP) will stimulate the release of factor VIII and von Willebrand factor (vWF) from endothelial cells. This can improve the function of platelets.

STEP 1 PEARL

After injury to a blood vessel, platelets adhere to the collagen of the exposed subendothelium. Additionally, vWF binds the glycoprotein Ib on the platelet surface. vWF is produced by endothelial cells and platelets.

The coagulopathy improves with administration of DDAVP. In the recovery room, the patient complains of significant pain at the surgical site. She receives morphine 5 mg intravenously. She becomes very lethargic and seizes several hours later.

What's going on?
Morphine is an opioid analgesic that is metabolized into morphine-3-glucuronide (M3G) and morphine-6-glucuronide (M6G) by the liver. In healthy patients, M3G and M6G are eliminated by the kidneys. In patients with ESRD, M3G and M6G accumulate in the blood stream. M6G is a potent μ receptor agonist that causes analgesia as well as sedation. M3G is neuroexcitatory and can cause seizures.

Would meperidine have been a better choice?
No. Meperidine is metabolized into normeperidine by the liver. Normeperidine accumulates in ESRD and can cause respiratory depression, psychosis, and seizures.

What are opioids are safest in patients with ESRD?
Fentanyl is metabolized by the liver and does not have active metabolites. It is therefore considered safe in ESRD. Remifentanil is metabolized by nonspecific esterases, a process that is independent of the kidneys, so it is also considered safe in ESRD.

What about non-opioid analgesics?
Multimodal pain control with non-opioids is always advisable.

Can the newly placed fistula be used for the patient's dialysis session tomorrow?
No. AV fistulas will be ready for use in hemodialysis 12 weeks after surgery. During this time, the vein remodels to accommodate high arterial pressures.

BEYOND THE PEARLS

- Loop diuretics (e.g., furosemide) can be useful for treating hyperkalemia, but patients who are anuric are unlikely to respond.
- Analogous metabolism of morphine to M3G, hydromorphone is metabolized by the liver into hydromorphone-3-glucuronide, which also accumulates in ESRD and can cause seizures.
- Intravenous DDAVP can cause hypotension when administered too quickly. It should be administered over at least 10 minutes.
- Estrogen may be helpful in treating uremic platelet dysfunction by increasing the amount of thromboxane A and adenosine diphosphate (ADP). It may also alter the production of clotting factors and clotting factor inhibitors.
- There are two types of dialysis: hemodialysis and peritoneal dialysis. In hemodialysis, the patient's blood is drawn into the dialysis circuit. In the circuit, blood and dialysate fluid flow in opposite directions on either side of a semipermeable membrane. Blood is then returned to the patient. In peritoneal dialysis, dialysis fluid is instilled into the peritoneal cavity and equilibrates with the patient's interstitial fluid. The fluid is then drained from the peritoneal cavity.

References

Girndt, M., & Heine, G.H. (2019). Other blood and immune disorders in chronic kidney disease. In J. Feehally, J. Floege, M. Tonelli, & R. J. Johnson (Eds.), *Comprehensive clinical nephrology* (6th ed., Chapter 83, pp. 967–978.e1). Philadelphia, PA: Elsevier.

Gold Standard Drug Database. Elsevier. Accessed December 19, 2020.

Highlights of Prescribing Information. *For Sugammadex.* Accessed December 16, 2020. https://www.access-data.fda.gov/drugsatfda_docs/label/2015/022225lbl.pdf.

Kanda, H., Hirasaki, Y., Iida, T., Kanao-Kanda, M., Toyama, Y., & Chiba, T., et al. (2017). Perioperative management of patients with end-stage renal disease. *Journal of Cardiothoracic and Vascular Anesthesia, 31*(6), 2251–2267.

Macsata, R. A., & Sidawy, A. N. (2019). Hemodialysis access: General considerations and strategies to optimize access placement. In *Rutherford's vascular surgery and endovascular therapy* (Chapter 175, pp. 2288–2288.e2). Philadelphia: Elsevier.

Malhotra, V., Malhotra, A., Pamnani, A., & Gainsburg, D. (2020). Anesthesia and the renal and genitourinary systems. In M. A. Gropper, R. D. Miller, N. H. Cohen, L. I. Eriksson, L. A. Fleisher, K. Leslie, et al. (Eds.), *Miller's anesthesia* (9th ed., Chapter 66, pp. 1929–1969.e6). Philadelphia, PA: Elsevier.

Stenvinkel, P., & Herzog, C. A. (2019). Cardiovascular disease in chronic kidney disease. In *Comprehensive clinical nephrology* (Chapter 81, pp. 942–957.e1). Philadelphia: Elsevier.

Yeun, J. Y., Young, B., Depner, T., & Chin, A. A. (2020). Hemodialysis. In A. S. L. Yu, G. M. Chertow, V. A. Luyckx, P. A. Marsden, K. Skorecki, M. W. Taal (Eds.), *Brenner and Rector's the kidney* (11th ed., Chapter 63, pp. 2038–2093). Philadelphia, PA: Elsevier.

A 75-Year-Old Woman With a History of Left-Sided Carotid Endarterectomy 2 Years Ago and Hypertension

Paul Neil Frank

A 75-year-old woman with a history of left-sided carotid endarterectomy 2 years ago and hypertension presented to the emergency department 10 days ago with new-onset left arm weakness. She was found to have an ischemic stroke and is now scheduled for right-sided carotid endarterectomy. In the preoperative holding area, her vital signs are: blood pressure 185/100 mm Hg, pulse 70/min, respiration rate 10/min, oxygen saturation 98% on room air, and temperature 36.4 degrees Celsius.

What is a stroke?
There are two types of stroke: ischemic and hemorrhagic.

Ischemic strokes are caused by the occlusion of blood supply to part of the central nervous system (CNS). The tissue supplied by the occluded blood vessel becomes ischemic and then dies. This is known as infarction. This is usually caused by the blockage of an artery, although occlusion of venous structures can also cause a stroke. Ischemic strokes are more common than hemorrhagic strokes.

Hemorrhagic strokes result from bleeding of a blood vessel in or around the brain. These may be associated with ischemic strokes that subsequently bleed (i.e., hemorrhagic transformation) or with abnormalities of the vasculature.

What are the symptoms of stroke?
The symptoms of a stroke depend on which blood vessel is disrupted and, therefore, which part of the CNS is affected. In fact, it is sometimes possible to determine what vessel is affected by a thorough history and physical examination. Fig. 32.1 shows the territory of the brain supplied by each of the major vessels.

STEP 1 PEARL

Table 32.1 shows a list of common symptoms of stroke in each vascular territory of the brain.

What is the difference between a stroke and a transient ischemic attack (TIA)?
A TIA causes a neurologic deficit that lasts less than 24 hours and then resolves. This is essentially an ischemic stroke that did not cause a permanent deficit, although there may be small infarcts visible on magnetic resonance imaging.

The patient had a stroke just 10 days ago. Should this surgery be postponed?
No. Patients with symptomatic carotid artery disease should undergo carotid endarterectomy within 2 weeks of TIA or stroke to achieve the greatest benefit.

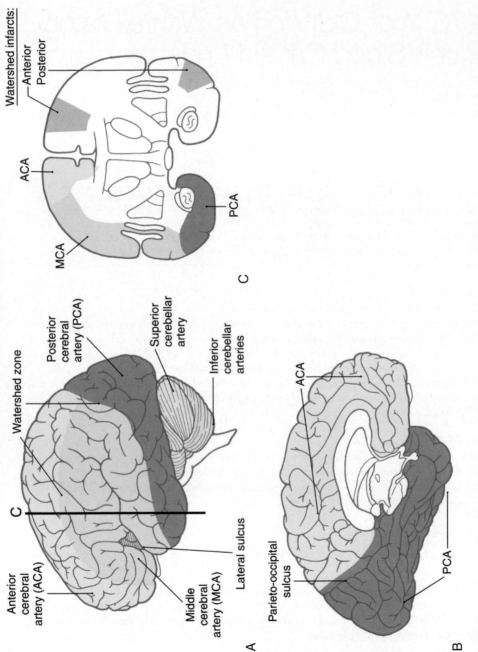

Fig. 32.1 Cerebral blood supply. Image A shows a lateral view, image B shows a medial view, and figure C shows a coronal view. Watershed infarcts are those that occur in the areas between major vascular territories. Squire, L. R., Berg, D., Bloom, F. E., Lac, S. D., Ghosh, A., & Spitzher, N. C. (Eds.). (2013). *Fundamental neuroscience* [4th ed., Chapter 8, pp. 122–137]. Philadelphia, PA: Elsevier. (Modified from Fig. 8.16.)

TABLE 32.1 ■ **Infarction of Each Vascular Territory Causes a Characteristic Constellation of Symptoms**

Territory Affected	Symptoms
Anterior cerebral artery	• Paralysis and loss of sensation of contralateral leg
Middle cerebral artery	• Paralysis and loss of sensation of contralateral face (e.g., facial droop) and arm
	• Contralateral hemianopsia
	• Aphasia (usually left side)
	• Hemineglect (nondominant side, usually right side)
Posterior cerebral artery	• Contralateral hemianopsia ("homonomous hemianopsia") with macular sparing
Penetrating artery ("lacunar")	• Contralateral paralysis (if internal capsule affected)
	• Contralateral sensory loss (if thalamus affected)
Vertebral/basilar artery	• Dizziness
	• Nausea/vomiting
	• Coma
	• Dysarthria, dysphagia
	• Paralysis of ipsilateral face, contralateral arm/leg
Anterior spinal artery	• Contralateral paralysis
	• Ipsilateral tongue deviation (if medulla affected)
Anterior/posterior inferior cerebellar artery	• Vertigo
	• Nausea/vomiting
	• Nystagmus

STEP 2, 3 PEARL

Carotid endarterectomy is indicated for most symptomatic patients with 50%–99% stenosis of the internal carotid artery and for most asymptomatic patients with low perioperative risk and 60%–99% stenosis of the internal carotid artery.

What is the blood supply to the brain?
The brain receives 80%–90% of its blood supply from the internal carotid arteries (one on each side). The remainder of the blood supply comes from the vertebral arteries, which give rise to the basilar artery. Inside the calvarium, the carotid and basilar arteries form a ring that perfuses the brain. This ring is called the circle of Willis. Fig. 32.2 shows the anatomy of the blood supply to the brain.

What are the anesthetic options for this case? What are the advantages and disadvantages of each?
A carotid endarterectomy can be performed under regional anesthesia with the patient awake or it can be performed under general anesthesia.

Regional anesthesia with an awake patient offers the advantage of a continuous real-time neurologic examination. For example, if the patient begins slurring her words during the operation, this is an indication that cerebral perfusion may be inadequate. Performing this operation under regional anesthesia also allows for greater hemodynamic stability.

The disadvantages of regional anesthesia are potential patient discomfort or claustrophobia. If the patient does not tolerate the procedure awake, it is challenging for the anesthesiologist to intubate the patient without disrupting the surgical field. Additionally, there are risks of regional anesthesia, discussed below.

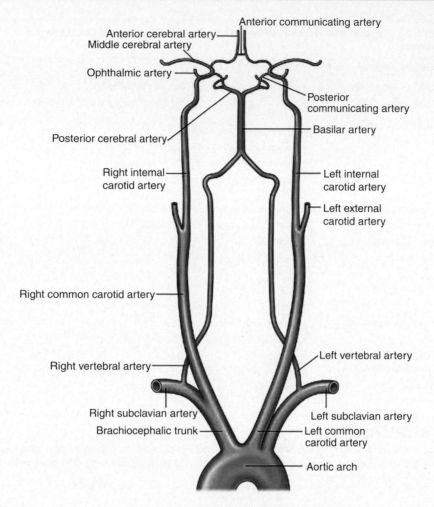

Diagram showing blood supply to brain

Fig. 32.2   The arterial supply to the brain consists of the two internal carotid arteries and the two vertebral arteries. The two vertebral arteries fuse into the basilar artery. These vessels combine to form the circle of Willis. Drake, R. L., Vogl, A.W., & Mitchell, A. W. M. (Eds.). (2021). *Gray's atlas of anatomy* [3rd ed., Chapter 8, pp. 477–610]. Philadelphia, PA: Elsevier.

The advantages of general anesthesia with endotracheal intubation include a, secure airway and better physiologic control. The disadvantage is that no intraoperative cerebral oxygenation monitor can substitute for an awake patient who will demonstrate neurologic changes in real time.

What regional anesthetic technique is required for this operation to be performed on an awake patient?

The anterolateral neck is innervated by the cervical plexus. The regional anesthetic technique for a carotid endarterectomy is a superficial cervical plexus block with or without a deep cervical plexus block. Fig. 32.3 shows proper needle placement for a superficial cervical plexus block.

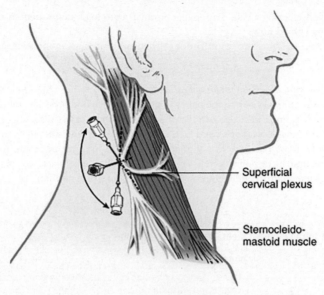

Fig. 32.3   Superficial cervical plexus block. With the patient's head turned to the contralateral side, inject local anesthetic along and deep to the posterolateral border of the sternocleidomastoid. Johnson, R. L., Kopp, S. L., Jens, K., & Gray, A.T. (2020). Peripheral nerve blocks and ultrasound guidance for regional anesthesia. In M. A. Gropper, R. D. Miller, N. H. Cohen, L. I. Eriksson, L. A. Fleisher, K. Leslie, et al. (Eds.), *Miller's anesthesia* (9th ed., Chapter 46, pp. 1450–1479e3). Philadelphia, PA: Elsevier. [Fig. 46.15].

The deep cervical plexus block carries the risk of inadvertent injection of local anesthetic into the intrathecal space or into the vertebral artery. These can result in total spinal seizures or cardiovascular collapse. This block may also anesthetize the phrenic nerve, resulting in paralysis of the ipsilateral hemidiaphragm. For these reasons, superficial cervical plexus block without deep cervical plexus block is desirable.

What are the preoperative considerations for this patient?
In addition to the standard pre-anesthetic questions (e.g., NPO time, history of anesthetic complications), the anesthesiologist should do a thorough neurologic examination and document any deficits.

If the patient has had multiple strokes in the past, it is advisable to know what symptoms are new and which are old. Patients with neurologic deficits from prior strokes should not receive succinylcholine (see Case 13). It is also crucial to know whether the patient has previously had carotid endarterectomy on the contralateral side.

A thorough cardiac history should be undertaken as well. Patients with carotid disease often have coronary artery disease. Ask about exercise tolerance and whether they have undergone any cardiac procedures in the past. Patients may be taking antiplatelet agents or other blood thinners. Patients should have a preoperative electrocardiogram and may require an echocardiogram.

Be sure to ask about a history of hypertension and/or diabetes and whether they are taking any medications for these conditions. Check the blood glucose level if the patient has diabetes. Treat with insulin to achieve a blood glucose level less than 200 mg/dL.

What are the options for intraoperative neurologic monitoring?
In awake patients having carotid endarterectomy under regional anesthesia, frequent focused neurologic exams can be performed intraoperatively, such as asking them to speak or performing a

strength test, like squeezing a ball. Any change in their neurologic exam suggests the brain is not receiving adequate blood flow.

In asleep patients, there are a multitude of neuromonitoring modalities, as described in Table 32.2.

What are the hemodynamic goals for this operation?
Careful attention should be given to the patient's preoperative blood pressure and heart rate. Since many patients undergoing carotid endarterectomy have coronary artery disease as well as intracranial artery disease, it is important to avoid tachycardia. Blood pressure should be maintained close to or even slightly above baseline. This higher pressure will improve perfusion to the ipsilateral brain through stenotic intracranial vessels. An arterial line should be placed for patients undergoing carotid endarterectomy to allow for continuous blood pressure monitoring.

TABLE 32.2 ■ **Intraoperative Cerebral Oxygenation Monitoring**

Modality	Comments
Stump pressure	• Measures blood pressure in the ipsilateral internal carotid artery after clamps are applied • Measures the perfusion pressure transmitted from the contralateral carotid and basilar artery through the circle of Willis • Minimum pressure has been reported from 25–70 mm Hg
Electroencephalogram (EEG)	• Reflects only cortical activity—does not detect ischemia in deeper structures • Requires stable anesthetic (i.e., constant level of inhaled gas, intravenous anesthetic), hemodynamics, and body temperature • Raw EEG is difficult to interpret • Processed EEG loses significant information in processing • High false negative rate (i.e., postoperative neurologic deficit without changes in EEG)
Somatosensory evoked potentials (SSEP)	• Stimulate peripheral nerve (e.g., median nerve) with electrode → detect response in corresponding territory of cortex • Measures integrity of entire dorsal column medial lemniscus pathway including deeper brain structures as well as cortex • Anesthetic gas reduces the amplitude of the SSEP signal—keep anesthetic gas concentration <0.5 mean alveolar concentration (MAC)
Jugular venous oxygen saturation (JvO$_2$)	• Sample oxygenation of blood from ipsilateral jugular vein or measure noninvasively with continuous oximeter • Determine global cerebral oxygen consumption by comparing PaO$_2$ to JvO$_2$ • Often misses small areas of ischemia or infarct
Near infrared spectroscopy (NIRS)	• Measures saturation of the entire tissue bed (i.e., arterial, venous, and capillary blood oxygen levels) • Most closely approximates venous oxygenation since most blood volume in the tissue bed is venous • Sensors placed on the forehead over frontal lobe not well-positioned to detect decreased blood flow in the middle cerebral artery (MCA)
Transcranial Doppler	• Temporal bone is acoustic window for ultrasound of MCA • Reduced velocity of blood flow in MCA may indicate the need to place a shunt • Can detect emboli in addition to measuring MCA velocity • Operator-dependent • Can interfere with surgical field • Frequent emboli in the early postoperative period predicts the development of a major neurologic deficit

The patient does not want to be awake for the operation. The operation will be performed under general anesthesia with an endotracheal tube. Somatosensory evoked potentials (SSEPs) will be used for intraoperative neuromonitoring.

How does that affect the anesthetic plan?

Inhaled anesthesia gas can affect SSEP signal quality by decreasing amplitude and increasing latency. Anesthesia gas should be used at less than 0.5 MAC. The anesthetic should be supplemented with an intravenous anesthetic.

An arterial line is placed prior to induction. After preoxygenation, the patient is induced with propofol 2 mg/kg. Her Blood Pressure Drops from 180/95 mm Hg to 70/40 mm Hg.

What's going on?

Patients with chronic severe hypertension generally have elevated sympathetic tone, resulting in elevated systemic vascular resistance (SVR). With the induction of anesthesia, SVR drops. In patients who are intravascularly volume depleted, venodilation decreases blood return to the heart (i.e., preload). Treat them quickly with volume and vasopressors.

Twenty minutes after induction but before incision, the SSEP signals show decreased amplitude bilaterally.

What could be going on?

SSEPs are most reliable with a stable level of anesthesia. Boluses of intravenous anesthetics or changing concentration of inhaled anesthetic can change the SSEP signal in a way that can confound monitoring for cerebral ischemia. In this case, it is possible that the induction medication and the initiation of inhaled anesthetic caused these changes.

Additionally, hypotension and hypoxia can cause degradation of SSEP signal quality.

Since surgery hasn't started yet, hypotension is the most likely etiology of the decreased signal quality. Hypotension is common after the induction of anesthesia prior to incision when there is very little stimulation. Treat with volume and a bolus of vasopressor.

SSEPs normalize, and surgery begins. After the vascular clamp is applied to the carotid artery, the SSEP signal shows decreased amplitude, this time only in the ipsilateral hemisphere.

What's going on? What should be done?

Decreased amplitude of the SSEP signal in the cerebral hemisphere on the same side as the carotid being clamped suggests cerebral ischemia. Increase the blood pressure to up to 20% above the patient's baseline level to improve cerebral perfusion. The surgeon may place a shunt to bypass the vascular clamps and improve cerebral blood flow.

What is a shunt?

In order to work in a bloodless field, the surgeon must apply clamps proximally and distally around the area of the carotid artery where the plaque is located. While the clamps are in place, there is no blood flow to the brain from the ipsilateral carotid artery. A shunt is a bypass for blood flow starting proximal to the proximal clamp, around the surgical field, and ending distal to the distal clamp. This allows blood flow from the ipsilateral carotid to continue while the clamps are in place. Fig. 32.4 shows the application of clamps and placement of a shunt to allow continuous blood flow to the brain while the clamps are in place.

If the patient's contralateral carotid artery is patent and their circle of Willis is intact, the ipsilateral brain will continue to receive adequate blood flow from the contralateral carotid artery through the circle of Willis. In these patients, shunting may be unnecessary. However, in some patients, stenosis of the contralateral carotid artery or an incomplete circle of Willis prevents

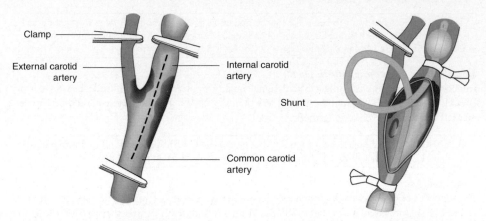

Clamp

External carotid artery

Internal carotid artery

Shunt

Common carotid artery

Fig. 32.4 Vascular clamps are applied to isolate the carotid bifurcation. A shunt allows blood to continue to flow from the common carotid artery to the internal carotid artery and up to the brain. Garden, O. J. & Parks, R. W. (Eds.). (2018). *Principles and practice of surgery* (7th ed., Chapter 21, pp. 375–408). Philadelphia, PA: Elsevier. (Modified from Fig. 21.16.)

the ipsilateral brain from receiving adequate blood flow when the clamps are in place. In these patients, shunting can prevent ischemia to vulnerable brain tissue.

> You start an infusion of phenylephrine, and the blood pressure increases to slightly above baseline. The surgeon places a shunt. SSEPs return to baseline. As the surgeon is working, the patient's heart rate drops from 68 to 30 bpm.

What's going on? What should you do?
Stimulation of the carotid sinus activates the baroreceptor reflex, which results in downregulation of the sympathetic nervous system and upregulation of the parasympathetic nervous system (see Case 33). The net effect is bradycardia and hypotension.

Ask the surgeon to stop manipulating the vessel. If the heart rate and blood pressure do not immediately improve, administer an anticholinergic agent (e.g., glycopyrrolate, atropine). The surgeon should infiltrate the area of the carotid bifurcation with local anesthetic before continuing with the operation.

What are the carotid sinus and carotid body?
The carotid sinus, also known as the carotid bulb, is a cluster of baroreceptors, or pressure-sensing cells within the wall of the carotid artery that participates in the regulation of arterial blood pressure. It is located near the bifurcation of the common carotid artery into the internal and external carotid arteries. The carotid sinus is innervated by a branch of cranial nerve IX, the glossopharyngeal nerve. When blood pressure increases, the carotid sinus sends afferent signals to the brainstem to upregulate the parasympathetic nervous system and downregulate the sympathetic nervous system. The net effect is to decrease blood pressure by slowing the heart rate, decreasing cardiac inotropy, and reducing SVR. This feedback loop is called the baroreceptor reflex.

The carotid body is a cluster of chemoreceptor cells within the wall of the carotid artery that senses arterial oxygen tension (PaO_2), carbon dioxide tension ($PaCO_2$), and pH. It is most sensitive to PaO_2. This structure is also innervated by a branch of cranial nerve IX and is located near the carotid bifurcation. At PaO_2 less than 65 mm Hg, the carotid body will send afferent signals to the brainstem to increase the respiratory drive.

What are the effects of carotid endarterectomy on the carotid sinus and carotid body?
Carotid endarterectomy can cause damage or denervation of the carotid sinus and the carotid body.

In patients who have undergone carotid endarterectomy on only one side, the baroreceptor and hypoxic respiratory drive reflexes are largely intact. However, in patients who have undergone carotid endarterectomy on both sides, there is a significant risk of postoperative hemodynamic lability and decreased ventilatory response to hypoxia.

Should you reduce ventilation in this patient to allow arterial CO₂ levels to rise?
No. In healthy patients, cerebral blood vessels dilate in response to increased $PaCO_2$. However, vasculature in areas of hypoperfused tissue (i.e., region of brain perfused by an artery with significant stenosis) are maximally vasodilated at baseline in a futile attempt to maximize blood flow. Therefore, as $PaCO_2$ rises, these blood vessels cannot dilate further. Meanwhile, blood vessels in areas that receive adequate perfusion, that are not maximally dilated at baseline will dilate in response to elevated $PaCO_2$. More blood will flow through these newly vasodilated vessels, resulting in less blood flow through the blood vessels that were maximally vasodilated at baseline. This is known as the steal phenomenon. Maintain normocapnia or slight hypocapnia during this operation.

What is considered normocapnia?
Normal arterial carbon dioxide tension ($PaCO_2$) is around 40 mm Hg.

Is that the same as an end-tidal carbon dioxide (EtCO₂) level of 40 mm Hg?
No. $PaCO_2$ is always higher than $EtCO_2$ because of dead space ventilation that dilutes exhaled carbon dioxide. Even in patients with no preexisting lung disease, $PaCO_2$ is at least 5 to 10 mm Hg greater than $EtCO_2$. Dead space increases with age (see Case 12).

STEP 1 PEARL

Patients with advanced chronic obstructive pulmonary disease (COPD) adapt to chronic hypercapnia (i.e., elevated carbon dioxide levels), and their awake baseline $PaCO_2$ will be elevated compared to patients without COPD.

During the operation, you notice new ST segment depression in the V5 lead on the rhythm strip.

What should you do?
New ST segment depression is concerning for myocardial ischemia, most likely an imbalance between myocardial oxygen demand (also called myocardial oxygen consumption) and myocardial oxygen supply. The acute management here is to decrease myocardial oxygen demand and increase myocardial oxygen supply.

Elevated preload, afterload, contractility, and heart rate all contribute to increased myocardial oxygen demand. To reduce myocardial oxygen demand, these factors should be reduced while maintaining adequate blood pressure and cardiac output. A short-acting β blocker or a centrally acting calcium channel blocker will reduce heart rate and contractility. A slower heart rate will also prolong diastole, allowing for a longer duration of myocardial perfusion. Nitroglycerin will reduce preload by increasing venous capacitance. Nitroglycerin is also a coronary vasodilator, which will increase coronary blood flow. Opioids act as sympatholytics, thereby reducing heart rate and contractility.

STEP 1 PEARL

Sublingual nitroglycerin is absorbed directly into the bloodstream and avoids first-pass metabolism (i.e., compounds absorbed through the gut are metabolized by the liver prior to entering systemic circulation). It is used for immediate relief of angina by reducing myocardial oxygen demand.

The caveat here is that elevated afterload (i.e., SVR) increases the driving pressure that perfuses the coronary arteries during diastole. *So, while elevated afterload increases myocardial oxygen demand, it also increases myocardial oxygen supply.* It also prevents tachycardia (via the baroreceptor reflex). Therefore, it is advisable to maintain or even increase afterload.

Myocardial oxygen supply is increased by augmenting delivery of oxygen to the heart. This can be accomplished by increasing coronary blood flow, hemoglobin concentration, and/or hemoglobin oxygen saturation. Check the hemoglobin level to rule out anemia, and make sure the patient is adequately oxygenated. Coronary blood flow can be elevated by slowing heart rate to prolong diastole, increasing diastolic blood pressure (i.e., afterload or SVR), or by coronary vasodilation (see Case 19).

STEP 1 PEARL

The left ventricle is only perfused via coronary arteries during diastole. During systole, the contraction of the myocardium compresses the coronary arteries and prevents blood flow. Diastolic blood pressure (primarily based on systemic vascular resistance, afterload) is the driving force pushing blood through the coronary arteries.

STEP 1 PEARL

The oxygen content of blood is given by

$$CaO_2 = 1.34 \times Hb \times SaO_2 + 0.003 \times PaO_2$$

Where Hb is the hemoglobin concentration, SaO_2 is the arterial oxygen saturation, and PaO_2 is the arterial oxygen tension.

Therefore, to treat this patient with new ST segment depression and suspected myocardial supply-demand mismatch, reduce heart rate and contractility, ensure adequate hemoglobin concentration and hemoglobin oxygen saturation, and, if necessary, consider increasing afterload with a vasopressor. The net effect of these interventions will be to reduce oxygen demand and increase oxygen supply.

You administer a beta blocker to slow the heart rate and start a phenylephrine infusion to augment afterload. The ST segment depressions resolve. The operation concludes, and the patient is extubated. While still in the operating room, a neurologic examination shows rightward deviation on tongue protrusion.

What's going on?

This is most likely due to intraoperative hypoglossal nerve (cranial nerve XII) injury. The marginal mandibular nerve (branch of cranial nerve VII), recurrent and superior laryngeal nerves (cranial nerve X), as well as the hypoglossal nerve, are at risk for injury during carotid endarterectomy. Fortunately, most cranial nerve injuries are transient.

STEP 1, 2, 3 PEARL

Cranial nerve VII is responsible for motor control of the face, including eyelid closing. Injury to the marginal mandibular branch of this nerve causes drooping of the ipsilateral lower lip. The effect here is primarily cosmetic.

STEP 1, 2, 3 PEARL

The superior laryngeal branch of cranial nerve X divides into the internal and external branches. The internal branch provides sensory innervation to the mucosa of the oropharynx from the epiglottis to the vocal cords. Injury to the internal branch can cause diminished mucosal sensation above the vocal cords. The external branch provides motor innervation to the cricothyroid muscle, which tenses the vocal cords. Injury to the external branch can cause weakness or paralysis of the cricothyroid muscle, resulting in voice weakness and difficulty with generating high pitches, a problem of particular concern to singers.

STEP 1, 2, 3 PEARL

Cranial nerve XII provides motor innervation to the tongue. Damage to this nerve causes ipsilateral weakness on tongue protrusion. Assuming the contralateral nerve is intact, the tongue will deviate to the side of the damaged nerve on protrusion.

On postoperative day 2, the patient develops a headache and then seizes. What's going on?

This patient should undergo emergent head computerized tomography (CT). This is concerning for intracranial hemorrhage. This may be due to cerebral hyperperfusion syndrome, a condition believed to arise from a sudden increase in cerebral blood flow after carotid endarterectomy that is associated with inadequate cerebral autoregulation and brain edema. Cerebral hyperperfusion syndrome may manifest with headache, seizures, focal neurologic deficits, and intracerebral hemorrhage. If there is evidence of significant intracranial hemorrhage on CT, emergent neurosurgical evaluation is indicated.

BEYOND THE PEARLS

- In 15% of patients, the circle of Willis is not a complete ring.
- Contraindications to regional anesthesia for carotid endarterectomy include patient refusal, language or communication barriers, and challenging anatomy, and a high carotid bifurcation, which would require significant mandibular traction. Patients who are claustrophobic or anxious are also poor candidates for this technique.
- Patients with carotid disease often have chronic hypertension, and a "normal" blood pressure may not be enough to perfuse the brain through a stenotic carotid artery. Maintain blood pressure at or above baseline at all times. (see Case 23)
- Patients who have had bilateral carotid endarterectomies have diminished respiratory drive. Use narcotics sparingly.
- At least 40% of patients undergoing carotid endarterectomy have symptomatic coronary artery disease. Myocardial infarction is responsible for up to 50% of deaths in the perioperative period after carotid endarterectomy.

References

Akhtar, S. (2022). Ischemic heart disease. In R. L. Hines, & S. B. Jones (Eds.), *Stoelting's anesthesia and co-existing disease* (8th ed., Chapter 5, pp. 79–106). Philadelphia, PA: Elsevier.

Arnold, M., & Perler, B. A. Carotid endarterectomy. In *Rutherford's vascular surgery and endovascular therapy* (Chapter 91, pp. 1194–1214).

Cassella, C. R., & Jagoda, A. (2017). Ischemic stroke: Advances in diagnosis and management. *Emergency Medicine Clinics of North America, 35*(4), 911–930.

Shalabi, A., & Chang, J. (2020). Anesthesia for vascular surgery. In M. A. Gropper, R. D. Miller, N. H. Cohen, L. I. Eriksson, L. A. Fleisher, K. Leslie, et al. (Eds.), *Miller's anesthesia* (9th ed., Chapter 56, pp. 1825–1867). Philadelphia, PA: Elsevier.

Urology

A 75-Year-Old Man With Benign Prostatic Hypertrophy

Paul Neil Frank

A 75-year-old man with benign prostatic hypertrophy (BPH) is scheduled for transurethral resection of the prostate (TURP) for relief of urinary obstruction. He takes terazosin daily. In the preoperative area, vital signs are blood pressure 134/77 mm Hg, pulse 80/min, respirations 12/min, oxygen saturation 96% on room air, and temperature 36.7°C.

What is terazosin? How might it affect anesthetic management?

Terazosin is a competitive antagonist of α_1 adrenergic receptors and is used to improve the symptoms of BPH. These receptors are found in the bladder neck, urethra, and prostate. Stimulation of these receptors causes smooth muscle contraction in the urethra, which increases resistance to urinary outflow, essentially exacerbating the symptoms of BPH. Blockade of these receptors causes smooth muscle relaxation, thereby reducing resistance to urinary outflow.

α_1 receptors are also found on vascular smooth muscle throughout the body. As in the urethra, stimulation of these receptors causes smooth muscle contraction. In vascular smooth muscle, contraction increases systemic vascular resistance, which increases blood pressure. Conversely, blockade of these receptors causes vascular smooth muscle relaxation, thereby reducing systemic vascular resistance. This can cause hypotension, which may be exacerbated by anesthetic agents administered during surgery.

STEP 1 PEARL

The α_1, α_2, β_1, and β_2 adrenergic receptors, as well as muscarinic receptors, are all G protein–coupled receptors (GPCRs).

STEP 2 PEARL

BPH can cause urinary hesitancy, frequency, urgency, and nocturia. Complications include acute urinary retention, urinary tract infections, hydronephrosis, and kidney injury, which may progress to kidney failure.

How is a TURP performed?

A resectoscope is placed through the urethra, and the prostate is resected with electrocautery or laser. Fluid is used to distend the bladder and to wash away blood and dissected tissue.

What are the anesthetic options for this case?

TURP is generally performed under spinal anesthesia. Spinal anesthesia allows the patient to remain awake during the procedure, which allows the anesthesiologist to continuously monitor

TABLE 33.1 ■ **Each Type of Irrigation Solution May Cause Potential Side Effects with Systemic Absorption**

Solution	Side Effects
Glycine	• Inhibitory neurotransmitter that can cause transient blindness • Hypotonic to plasma • Metabolized to ammonia
Mannitol	• Rapidly expands intravascular volume
Distilled water	• Very hypotonic to plasma (0 mOsm/kg) • Can cause hemolysis
Lactated Ringer, 0.9% sodium chloride	• Electrically conductive, cannot use with monopolar resection
Sorbitol	• Can cause hyperglycemia and lactic acidosis

for changes in neurologic or respiratory status. If the patient is not a candidate for neuraxial anesthesia or refuses neuraxial anesthesia, the procedure can be performed under general anesthesia.

What spinal level is ideal for a TURP?
A spinal level of T10 will provide adequate anesthesia to the prostate and bladder neck, as well as blocking the sensation of bladder distention.

Higher spinal levels will block the sensation of abdominal or shoulder pain that may indicate bladder perforation. In the event of bladder perforation, irrigation fluid leaks through a hole in the bladder and fills the peritoneum, which irritates the diaphragm. The patient may perceive this as shoulder pain. Bladder perforation can be caused by direct injury or overdistention.

STEP 1 PEARL

Sympathetic innervation to the bladder and urethra comes from T11 through L2 nerve roots via the hypogastric plexus. Parasympathetic innervation to the bladder and urethra comes from nerve roots S2 through S4 via the pelvic parasympathetic plexus, which joins the hypogastric plexus. The prostate is also innervated via the hypogastric plexus.

The surgeon says he will use glycine irrigation solution.

What are the options for irrigation solution? What are the potential complications of each?
Table 33.1 shows possibilities for irrigation solutions during TURP and the potential complications of each.

What are the criteria for the ideal irrigation fluid?
Irrigation fluid should be transparent, electrically inert (so as not to disperse current from electrocautery), isotonic with plasma, nontoxic, nonhemolytic, and easy to sterilize. Unfortunately, no solution fulfills all these criteria.

STEP 1 PEARL

The osmolality of normal human plasma is 275–295 mOsm/kg. It is approximated by

$$osmolality = 2 \times [Na] + \frac{[glucose]}{18} + \frac{[BUN]}{2.8}$$

where [Na] is the serum sodium concentration in mEq/L, [glucose] is the serum glucose concentration in mg/dL, and [BUN] is blood urea nitrogen concentration mg/dL.

Why does the choice of irrigation solution matter? Won't the irrigation solution just be in the bladder and urethra?
No. The prostate contains a rich blood supply, including large venous sinuses. During TURP, these large venous sinuses may be violated, and irrigation solution can enter systemic circulation through these sinuses.

How much irrigation fluid is absorbed during a TURP?
Irrigation fluid can be absorbed at a rate of 10–30 cc/min.

What determines how much irrigation solution is absorbed?
Factors that influence the amount of fluid absorption include:
- Height of the bag of irrigation solution: A larger difference in height between the bag of irrigation solution and the patient means greater hydrostatic pressure gradient, which drives more irrigation fluid into the venous system.
- Amount of bladder distention: Again, greater pressure of irrigation fluid within the bladder will drive more fluid into the venous system.
- Extent of opened venous sinuses: More opened venous sinuses means more opportunity for irrigation fluid to enter the venous system.
- Duration of surgical resection: The longer the operation, the more time irrigation solution can flow into the venous system.

The surgeon allows the first-year resident to get some experience operating. After 75 minutes of surgery, your patient is cold.

What is going on?
Use of room temperature irrigation solution can cause hypothermia. Spinal anesthesia ablates thermoregulatory vasoconstriction at and below the level of the spinal placement. In addition, elderly patients tend to have a reduced ability to maintain their body temperature.

Recommend that the surgeon use warmed irrigation fluids, apply a forced air warming blanket, and warm the room.

The patient's blood pressure has gradually increased to 180/106 mm Hg and his pulse has decreased to 44/min.

What is going on?
A significant volume of irrigation solution has likely been absorbed through the prostatic venous sinuses, which can rapidly increase intravascular volume. This can cause hypertension and reflex bradycardia.

What is reflex bradycardia, and how does it happen?
The body regulates arterial blood pressure through a negative feedback loop called the baroreceptor reflex. Specialized cells called stretch receptors embedded in the walls of the aortic arch and

carotid arteries (specifically the carotid sinus) transmit signals to the brainstem. When blood pressure is too high, the stretch receptors sense an increase in stretch of the arterial wall, and afferent signaling (i.e., to the brainstem) increases. As a result, sympathetic (i.e., efferent) signaling is downregulated, and parasympathetic signaling is upregulated. The net effect is to decrease heart rate, contractility, and systemic vascular tone.

STEP 1 PEARL

The stretch receptors in the carotid sinus are innervated by the glossopharyngeal nerve (cranial nerve IX). The stretch receptors in the aortic arch are innervated by the vagus nerve (cranial nerve X).

The patient also complains of shortness of breath, and you notice the pulse oximeter is reading 92% on room air. The patient becomes restless and confused. He then seizes.

What is going on?

The respiratory symptoms and drop in oxygen saturation are concerning for pulmonary edema, likely from circulatory overload. As intravascular volume increases rapidly from absorption of irrigation fluid, hypervolemia may lead to pulmonary edema.

Mental status changes and seizure are concerning for hyponatremia and hypoosmolality. As hypotonic irrigation solution enters the blood stream, the cells of the brain absorb free water, resulting in cerebral edema and possibly elevated intracranial pressure. This can result in altered mental status, seizure, and coma.

The patient's symptoms are consistent with TURP syndrome.

What should you do?

Notify the surgeon, and tell them that surgery needs to end as expeditiously as possible. Treat seizures with benzodiazepines and magnesium if necessary. The patient will require endotracheal intubation. Give intravenous (IV) furosemide or mannitol to treat volume overload and pulmonary edema.

Once the patient has stabilized, send laboratory studies for serum sodium, serum osmolality, and hemoglobin level.

STEP 1 PEARL

Furosemide is a diuretic that works by inhibiting sodium-potassium-chloride (Na-K-2Cl) symporter in the loop of Henle in the nephron. It also causes acute venodilation.

Labs show serum sodium level of 118 mEq/L.

What should you do?

A normal serum sodium level is 135–145 mEq/L, and a serum sodium level of 118 mEq/L is dangerously low. Give IV 3% sodium chloride, known as hypertonic saline, to correct hyponatremia. In severely hyponatremic and symptomatic patients such as this, consider giving a bolus of 100 mL of 3% saline to improve neurologic status and quickly raise serum sodium levels by 2–3 mEq/L.

Start an infusion of 3% saline at a rate of 1 mL/kg/h with a goal of increasing the serum sodium concentration by 1 mEq/L/h for the first 4 hours but not by more than 10 mEq/L in the first 24 hours of treatment. Serum sodium levels should be checked every 2 hours.

Why should you correct hyponatremia slowly?
Rapid correction of hyponatremia risks central pontine myelinolysis (CPM).

What is CPM?
After rapid correction of hyponatremia, patients develop encephalopathy, cranial nerve palsies, and quadriplegia within several days.

STEP 2, 3 PEARLS

Patients with acute hyponatremia are at greatest risk from cerebral edema if the hyponatremia is not corrected. Meanwhile, patients with chronic hyponatremia are at greatest risk from CPM if hyponatremia is corrected too quickly.

You notice that the patient is slowly bleeding from IV sites and from his nose.

What is going on? What should you do?
Abnormal bleeding is a known complication of TURP. This may be due to dilution of platelets and clotting factors from absorption of irrigation fluid, primary fibrinolysis from release of plasminogen activator from the prostate, or disseminated intravascular coagulopathy (DIC) from systemic absorption of thromboplastin in prostate tissue.

Send coagulation studies including thromboelastography (TEG, see Case 20) and replace clotting factors, platelets, and fibrinogen as needed. Maintain adequate hydration and hemodynamics. Consider giving ε aminocaproic acid.

What is ε aminocaproic acid? How does it work?
ε aminocaproic acid is an antifibrinolytic agent.

Ordinarily, plasminogen circulates in the blood until it is activated to plasmin by tissue plasminogen activator (tPA), which is found bound to fibrin on the surface of blood clots. Plasmin then cleaves fibrin on clots. This process is highly regulated, and because tPA is generally found only on clots, this process occurs in a very localized fashion.

If plasminogen activator from the prostate is absorbed into systemic circulation, plasminogen will be activated to plasmin throughout the body, leading to systemic primary hyperfibrinolysis. ε aminocaproic acid works by inhibiting plasminogen.

BEYOND THE PEARLS

- During TURP, a decrease in the rate of return of irrigation solution can be an early sign of bladder perforation.
- Volume overload is more likely in TURP when the surgery lasts more than 1 hour, when the bag of irrigation fluid is more than 40 cm above the patient, when hypotonic irrigation fluid is used, and when the bladder pressure is greater than 15 cm H_2O.
- The baroreceptor reflex is not functional at an arterial blood pressure less than of 50 mm Hg.
- The severity of symptoms of hyponatremia are correlated with how quickly the serum sodium level falls.
- Severe hyponatremia, with serum sodium level less than 115 mEq/L may also manifest with QRS widening, ventricular ectopy, and ST segment elevation.
- Coagulopathy after TURP is more common when more than 35 g of prostatic tissue is resected.
- There is a risk of bacteremia and sepsis after TURP.
- Newer techniques for TURP include use of laser resection, plasma vaporization, photoselective vaporization, microwave thermotherapy, and aquablation. These allow for precise resection and less bleeding.

References

Berl, T., & Sands, J. M. (2019). Disorders of water metabolism. In J. Feehally, J. Floege, M. Tonelli, & R. J. Johnson (Eds.), *Comprehensive clinical nephrology* (6th ed., pp. 94–110.e1). Philadelphia, PA: Elsevier.

Huddleston, L. L., & Liu, L. L. (2018). Hemostasis. In M. C. Pardo, & R. D. Miller (Eds.), *Basics of anesthesia* (7th ed., pp. 377–394). Philadelphia, PA: Elsevier.

Malhotra, V., Malhotra, A., Pamnani, A., et al. (2020). Anesthesia and the renal and genitourinary systems. In M. A. Gropper, R. D. Miller, N. H. Cohen, L. I. Eriksson, L. A. Fleisher, K. Leslie, et al. (Eds.), *Miller's anesthesia* (9th ed., pp. 1929–1969.e6). Philadelphia, PA: Elsevier.

Schonberger, R. B. (2018). Fluid, electrolyte, and acid–base disorders. In R. L. Hines, & K. E. Marschall (Eds.), *Stoelting's anesthesia and co-existing disease* (7th ed., pp. 407–424). Philadelphia, PA: Elsevier.

Sun, L. S., & Davis, N. A. (2020). Cardiac physiology. In M. A. Gropper, R. D. Miller, N. H. Cohen, L. I. Eriksson, L. A. Fleisher, K. Leslie, et al. (Eds.), *Miller's anesthesia* (9th ed., pp. 384–402.e2). Philadelphia, PA: Elsevier.

An 86-Year-Old Female With History of von Willebrand Disease Type I

Sean Lam ■ Paul Neil Frank

An 86-year-old female with history of von Willebrand disease (vWD) type I presents from a nursing home with fever, new-onset confusion, and abdominal pain radiating to the groin over the past 24 hours. She received 2 L of normal saline and a dose of ceftriaxone in the emergency department. Computed tomography (CT) reveals an obstructive kidney stone causing hydronephrosis. She will undergo urgent ureteroscopic lithotripsy and ureteral stent placement. Vital signs show a blood pressure of 76/43 mm Hg, pulse 128/min, respirations 18/min, oxygen saturation 95% on 4 L/min nasal cannula, and temperature 39.2°C. Lactate level is 5.4 mmol/L.

> **STEP 1 PEARL**
>
> Ceftriaxone is a third-generation cephalosporin that works against primarily gram-negative bacteria. Cephalosporins are β-lactam agents that inhibit synthesis of bacterial cell walls.

> **STEP 1 PEARL**
>
> There are four types of kidney stones, each with their own predisposing factors, as in Table 34.1.

Why groin pain?

Sympathetic nerves of the ureters originate from the T10 through L2 spinal levels. Nociceptive fibers course with sympathetic fibers. Ureteral pain can therefore be referred to the T10–L2 distribution, which corresponds to the lower back, flank, ilioinguinal region, and scrotum or labia.

How would you describe this patient's hemodynamic state?

This patient is hypotensive and refractory to fluid resuscitation. Her lactate is elevated. She has a likely source of infection (obstructing ureteral stone). The patient is in septic shock.

Where does lactate come from? Why would you check a lactate level here?

In septic shock, there is a defect in oxygen utilization known as cytopathic hypoxia. Hypoperfusion may result in decreased oxygen delivery as well. This leads to anaerobic metabolism and the production of lactate. Glucose metabolism in the generation of adenosine triphosphate (ATP) results in production of pyruvate, which can either undergo aerobic or anerobic metabolism to produce energy. In sepsis, decreased oxygen utilization results in accumulation of pyruvate, which is converted to lactate.

Studies have shown that the probability of survival is linked to initial lactate level and the time required for normalization of an elevated lactate level. An initial level of 4 mmol/L or greater and/or persistently elevated lactate level requiring 48 hours or more to normalize were associated with increased mortality.

TABLE 34.1 ■ Types of Kidney Stones

Type of Stone	Risk Factors	Comments
Calcium oxalate	• Hypercalcemia, as in hyperparathyroidism and some cancers • Ethylene glycol ingestion • Inflammatory bowel disease • Vegan diet • Poor hydration	• Most common type of kidney stone
Magnesium ammonium phosphate (struvite)	• Infection with urease-positive organisms (e.g., *Proteus*)	• Associated with high urinary pH • Can fill entire renal pelvis (i.e., "staghorn calculi")
Uric acid	• Gout • High cell turnover (e.g., leukemia)	• Treat with allopurinol, which inhibits xanthine oxidase and prevents uric acid production
Cysteine	• Cystinuria (autosomal recessive)	• Treat by alkalinizing urine

How should you stabilize this patient prior to surgery?

Treatment of sepsis involves early aggressive fluid resuscitation, antibiotic administration, and source control. In the first 3 hours, the patient should receive at least 30 cc/kg crystalloid. Obtain blood cultures and a serum lactate level, and administer empiric antibiotics. If the patient does not respond to fluid boluses (mean arterial pressure persistently less than 65 mm Hg), then vasopressors (e.g., norepinephrine, phenylephrine, vasopressin) are indicated. Infusions of vasopressors are best administered into the central venous system; therefore a central venous catheter should be placed. In addition, invasive blood pressure monitoring via an arterial catheter is helpful.

STEP 1 PEARL

Mechanism of action of common pressors:
- Norepinephrine stimulates α_1, α_2 adrenergic receptors resulting in peripheral vasoconstriction and β_1 resulting in increased chronotropy and inotropy although the beta effect is much less significant than the alpha effect.
- Phenylephrine stimulates α_1 adrenergic receptors resulting in peripheral vasoconstriction.
- Vasopressin stimulates V_{1a} receptor on vascular smooth muscle cells resulting in peripheral vasoconstriction.

What are empiric antibiotics?

Empiric administration of antibiotics is indicated when the exact cause of an infection is unknown. Empiric antibiotics are usually broad spectrum and represent an educated guess as to the type of pathogen causing the infection. Once blood cultures identify the causative organism, empiric antibiotics can be replaced by antibiotics narrowly tailored to treat this organism.

If possible, blood cultures should be drawn prior to administration of antibiotics so that the causative organism can be identified.

What is vWD?

vWD is the most common inherited coagulation disorder and results in a qualitative and/or quantitative deficiency of the glycoprotein (GP) known as von Willebrand factor (vWF). There are multiple types of vWD with different inheritance patterns and characteristics. Patients with vWD have impaired platelet adhesion thus impaired hemostasis. This can present as easy bruising or bleeding with even minor trauma.

STEP 1 PEARL

vWF is secreted by endothelial cells, platelets, and megakaryocytes. vWF acts as a carrier for factor VIII. Without vWF, factor VIII would be cleared from the plasma, and there would be a deficiency of factor VIII. For this reason, patients with vWD also tend to have decreased levels of factor VIII.

What is the inheritance pattern of vWD?

Most types of vWD are inherited in an autosomal dominant fashion. However, type 3 vWD is more often inherited in an autosomal recessive fashion. Type 1 vWD often demonstrates variable expression and incomplete penetrance.

STEP 1 PEARL

Autosomal dominant inheritance means individuals with even one copy of the mutated gene (i.e., one from either parent) are affected. Autosomal recessive inheritance means that only individuals with two copies of the mutated gene (i.e., one from each parent) are affected.

STEP 1 PEARL

Variable expression means that there are varying degrees of phenotypic manifestation of a given genotype. For example, two patients with the same abnormal alleles may have different levels of disease severity. Incomplete penetrance means that some individuals with a disease genotype will not manifest the disease, while others will.

What is primary hemostasis?

Primary hemostasis leads to the formation of a platelet plug.

In primary hemostasis, there is vasoconstriction of the injured blood vessel. vWF attaches to the exposed subendothelial collagen and binds platelets via the platelet GP Ib receptor, thereby recruiting platelets to the site of injury. Receptor binding activates platelets, resulting in a shape change and release of factors that promote further platelet aggregation, such as adenosine diphosphate (ADP), thromboxane A2, and serotonin. In addition, the platelet GPIIb/IIIa receptor undergoes a change in conformation, thereby increasing its affinity for fibrinogen.

What is secondary hemostasis?

Secondary hemostasis is the stabilization of the platelet plug and fibrin crosslinking. Serine proteases become activated with the goal of generating thrombin. Thrombin is required to cleave fibrinogen to fibrin. Fibrin crosslinks platelets to form a stable thrombus.

STEP 1 PEARL

Despite their names, primary and secondary hemostasis are interdependent and occur simultaneously.

What abnormalities on coagulation studies would you expect for this patient?

Laboratory findings in patients with vWD include increased bleeding time, increased partial thromboplastin time (PTT), and a normal prothrombin time (PT).

TABLE 34.2 ■ Types of vWD and Treatment of Each. vWF Concentrate May be Given Directly or in Combination with Other Factors, Particularly Factor VIII

Type	Qualitative or Quantitative Deficiency of vWF	Treatment
1	Quantitative	Desmopressin
2 A	Qualitative and quantitative	Desmopressin (partially effective); vWF concentrate
2B	Qualitative and quantitative	vWF concentrate; *avoid desmopressin as it may cause thrombocytopenia*
2M	Qualitative	Desmopressin
3	Quantitative (low or undetectable levels of vWF)	vWF concentrate

vWD, von Willebrand disease; *vWF*, von Willebrand factor.

You intubate the patient, and the operation begins. The urologist complains that there is more mucosal bleeding than expected.

What can you do to help?
Keeping in mind that this patient has vWD type 1, administration of desmopressin may be helpful in treating coagulopathy. Desmopressin is an effective treatment for some types of vWD (Table 34.2). It works by increasing the release of vWF from endothelial cells.

Antifibrinolytic agents (e.g., tranexamic acid, aminocaproic acid) and platelet transfusion may be helpful as well.

STEP 1 PEARL

Desmopressin is a synthetic analog of vasopressin. Vasopressin is synthesized in the hypothalamus and stored in the postpituitary gland.

STEP 1 PEARL

The largest reservoir of vWF is contained in Weibel-Palade bodies of endothelial cells. vWF is also found in the α-granules of platelets.

What is meant by quantitative deficiency of vWF? Qualitative deficiency of vWF?
In a *quantitative deficiency*, the amount or concentration of a compound is low. For example, patients with type 3 vWD have much a lower concentration of vWF than do healthy individuals.

In a *qualitative deficiency*, the amount or concentration of a compound may be normal, but its function is poor. For example, patients with vWD type 1 may have a normal level of vWF, but the vWF does not function normally.

Should patients with vWF receive vWF concentrate prior to surgery?
Patients with vWD type 3, as well as patients with vWD types 1 or 2 who do not respond to desmopressin and who are undergoing surgery, should receive vWF with or without factor VIII. The goal is to demonstrate normal levels of vWF and factor VIII activity. Levels of vWF and factor VIII activity should be checked postoperatively, and additional vWF and/or factor VIII should

be given as needed. For major surgery, monitoring and treatment may continue for up to 10 days postoperatively.

> The procedure is uneventful, and the patient is extubated. In the recovery area she is barely arousable. You look at the medication administration record, and you notice that she received a large dose of lorazepam in the emergency department for back pain.

What is the mechanism of action of benzodiazepines?

γ-Aminobutyric acid (GABA) is an inhibitory neurotransmitter. Benzodiazepines enhance the opening of the GABA-activated chloride channels through an allosteric mechanism, resulting in neuronal hyperpolarization of the limbic, thalamic, and hypothalamic regions of the brain. Benzodiazepines are commonly used in anesthesia as an amnestic, anxiolytic, sedative, and hypnotic. They also function as anticonvulsants.

What can you do to wake her up?

Flumazenil can be used to reverse the sedative effects of benzodiazepines.

> You give the patient flumazenil 0.2 mg Intravenously, and she wakes up.

What is the mechanism of action of flumazenil?

Flumazenil is a competitive antagonist of the benzodiazepine receptor. The onset is rapid and peaks within 1–3 minutes. Flumazenil is given in doses of 0.2–0.5 mg, up to 3 mg in incremental doses.

> You check back on the patient 40 minutes later, and she is sleepy once again. She has not received any additional medication.

What is going on?

The dose of flumazenil has likely worn off, while the effect of lorazepam persists. Flumazenil is rapidly metabolized in the liver, so the reversal of sedation caused by benzodiazepines is short lived. The plasma half-life of flumazenil is 1 hour, whereas the half-life of lorazepam is 12 hours. The duration of reversal depends on the benzodiazepine used, and surveillance after administration is highly recommended. If recurrent sedation occurs, then either repeated administrations or a continuous infusion is required until the effect of the benzodiazepine wears off.

BEYOND THE PEARLS

- Parasympathetic innervation of the ureters arises from the S2 to S4 spinal levels.
- Extracorporeal shock wave lithotripsy (ESWL) relies on repetitive high-energy shockwaves focused on the ureteral stone. First-generation ESWL required submersion of the patient in a water bath. Newer generations do not require submersion and rely on piezoelectric crystals or electromagnetic generators.
- Contraindications to ESWL include pregnancy, active urinary tract infection, and untreated bleeding disorders.
- Females with vWD frequently present with menorrhagia. Up to 20% of patients who present with menorrhagia are diagnosed with vWD.
- Rapid administration of desmopressin can cause hypotension and flushing. It should be administered over 30 min.
- Flumazenil is contraindicated in patients with active cyclic antidepressant overdose with cardiac conduction abnormalities (e.g., widened QRS complex, arrhythmia), anticholinergic toxicity (e.g., hyperthermia), or motor symptoms (e.g., rigidity).
- Flumazenil may cause seizures in patients with benzodiazepine dependence.

References

Berliner, N. (2020). Leukocytosis and leukopenia. In L. Goldman, & A. I. Schafer (Eds.), *Goldman-Cecil Medicine* (26th ed., p. 1094–1103.e2). Philadelphia, PA: Elsevier.

Gold Standard, Inc. Flumazenil. Drug monograph. Published October 24, 2019. www.clinicalkey.com. Accessed 6.5.2021.

Leebeek, F. W. G., & Eikenboom, J. C. J. (2016). Von Willebrand's Disease. *The New England Journal of Medicine, 375*(21), 2067–2080.

Gold Standard, Inc. Lorazepam. Drug monograph. Published March 24, 2021. www.clinicalkey.com. Accessed 6.5.2021.

Huddleston, L. L., & Liu, L. L. (2018). Hemostasis. In M. C. Pardo, & R. D. Miller (Eds.), *Basics of anesthesia* (pp. 377–394). Philadelphia, PA: Elsevier.

Malhotra, V., Malhotra, A., Pamnani, A., & Gainsburg, D. (2020). Anesthesia and the renal and genitourinary systems. In M. A. Gropper, R. D. Miller, N. H. Cohen, L. I. Eriksson, L. A. Fleisher, K. Leslie, et al. (Eds.), *Miller's anesthesia* (9th ed., pp. 1929–1959.e6). Philadelphia, PA: Elsevier.

Miller, R., Eriksson, L., Fleisher, L., Wiener-Kronish, J., Cohen, N., & Young, W. (2014). *Miller's anesthesia* (8th ed., Vol. 2). Philadelphia, PA: Elsevier.

Pedigo, R. A., & Thomas, E. B. (2017). Nephrology. In *Crush step 1: The ultimate USMLE step 1 review* (pp. 537–579). Philadelphia, PA: Elsevier.

Rhodes, A., Evans, L. E., Alhazzani, W., Levy, M. M., Antonelli, M., Ferrer, R., et al. (2017). Surviving sepsis campaign: International guidelines for management of sepsis and septic shock: 2016. *Intensive Care Medicine, 43*(3), 304–377. https://doi.org/10.1007/s00134-017-4683-6.

Non-Operating Room Anesthesia (NORA)

A 71-Year-Old Man With 30 Pounds of Unintentional Weight Loss and Abdominal Discomfort

Paul Neil Frank

A 71-year-old man with 30 pounds of unintentional weight loss and abdominal discomfort over the last 6 months is scheduled for magnetic resonance imaging (MRI) with sedation. He has a history of claustrophobia and takes alprazolam daily for sleep. He underwent a left knee replacement 3 years ago and has no other past medical history. His body mass index (BMI) is 22 kg/m². In the pre-anesthesia area, vital signs are blood pressure 130/60 mm Hg, pulse 67/min, respirations 12/min, oxygen saturation 100% on room air, and temperature 36°C.

How is non-operating room anesthesia (NORA) different from anesthesia in the operating room?
The equipment in remote locations is often different than what is used in the main operating room, sometimes due to space constraints or due to environmental constraints (e.g., MRI magnet). Similarly, there may be a smaller or different selection of anesthetic drugs immediately available. Always arrive early and familiarize yourself with the equipment and drugs available to you. If necessary, bring desired drugs or equipment from the main operating room area to the remote location.

Proceduralists in remote locations may also be less familiar with working with anesthesiologists. Here, communication is key. Ask the proceduralist how they will perform the procedure, including details like the level of anticipated pain, patient positioning, and whether any patient cooperation will be required. For example, some computerized tomography (CT)-guided studies and procedures require a temporary cessation of patient respiration, which requires a patient awake enough to cooperate or general anesthesia with endotracheal intubation and muscle relaxation. Many proceduralists are not part of the primary care team responsible for the patient and may not have fully reviewed the chart. Share with the proceduralist any concerns you have regarding the patient's comorbidities and the proposed procedure.

NORA locations are frequently far from the main operating room area. Therefore, assistance usually takes longer to arrive once it is requested. Staff in remote locations (e.g., MRI, GI lab) may be less familiar with the equipment and sequence of events of anesthesiology. If you anticipate a challenging anesthetic, it is worthwhile to have an assistant present prior to starting the case.

How does an MRI machine work?
MRI machines use a very strong magnet and radiofrequency pulsations to generate images. Hydrogen ions of the body are all spinning around axes much like the way planet Earth spins around its axis. Ordinarily, these axes are oriented in random directions. In the presence of a strong magnetic field, some of these axes line up in the same direction as the magnetic field. A radiofrequency signal is then turned on, which deflects the direction of the axes of rotation by

some amount. When the radiofrequency is turned off, the axes return to their original orientation in response to the magnetic field, and in so doing they emit a new electromagnetic signal.

> One of the new staff members is worried about radiation exposure.

What do you tell her?
While the MRI does generate radiofrequency electromagnetic radiation, this is not ionizing radiation, and it is not known to be harmful. This is in contrast to CT and x-ray imaging, which generate ionizing radiation.

> You've got some spare time before the patient will be ready.

Can you roll a desk chair into the scanner room and read on your laptop while the scanner is off?
No. *The magnet is always on.* Anyone who enters the area around the scanner must remove all metal objects from their body. Common items to be removed include money clips, hearing aids, jewelry, hairpins, belt buckles, and keys. Metal objects may become missiles in the strong magnetic field of the MRI machine.

Are all metals dangerous around MRI?
No. Aluminum, titanium, copper, bronze, and silver are not magnetic, and are therefore safe around the MRI. MRI-compatible equipment (e.g., specialized infusion pumps) is made with these metals.
Nickel has magnetic properties and is not MRI compatible.

Can you bring your anesthesia machine into the scanner room? What about the anesthesia cart?
Standard anesthesia machines and anesthesia carts contain metal components that have magnetic properties and are therefore unsafe to have near the MRI machine. Every piece of equipment including patient monitors, tubing, cables, gas cylinders, IV poles, and infusion machines *must be MRI compatible*. It is important to familiarize yourself with this equipment before caring for a patient in the MRI suite.

What special screening needs to be done before the patient enters the scanner?
There is a long list of items for which patients should be screened prior to entering the MRI scanner:
- Cardiac pacemaker, implantable defibrillator
- Internal wires or electrodes (e.g., pacing wires, deep brain stimulator)
- Vascular stent or inferior vena cava (IVC) filter
- Aneurysm clips
- Implanted or external drug pump (as for chemotherapy, pain medicine, or insulin)
- Intravenous access (e.g., port-a-cath, pulmonary artery catheter with thermodilution coil)
- Implanted surgical hardware (e.g., orthopedic pins, rods, screws, plates)
- Artificial joints
- Cochlear implant, hearing aids
- Removable dental appliances
- Retained bullet or other metals
- Shunt (e.g., ventriculoperitoneal shunt) with programmable valve
- Spinal cord stimulator
- Breast tissue expander
- Penile implant
- Intrauterine device (IUD)
- Radiation seeds (for cancer treatment)
- Body piercings
- Wig or hair implants

If the patient has any of these items, the item may need to be removed if feasible (as in body piercing) or confirmed to be MRI compatible (as some pacemakers are). If the object cannot be removed and cannot be confirmed to be MRI compatible, the patient should not undergo an MRI.

It is confirmed that the patient's prosthetic knee is MRI compatible.

What other precautions should be taken for patient safety?
The MRI is quite loud. It can be uncomfortable for awake patients and can damage hearing. Patients should be given earplugs or earmuffs.

The patient had an omelet and potatoes for breakfast at 8 AM this morning. It's now 1 PM. The radiology technician says they are running ahead of schedule and asks if we can start this patient's scan early.

What do you say?
The same *nil per os* (NPO) guidelines that apply in the operating room apply in other clinical areas. This patient had a heavy meal only 5 hours ago. The guidelines advise that patients not undergo anesthesia for elective procedures or studies for 8 hours after a large meal. Therefore, you should wait until 3 PM to safely anesthetize this patient. Beware, however, that the NPO guidelines are just that—guidelines—and that patients with comorbidities such as gastroesophageal reflux disease (GERD) or intraabdominal pathology may still have food in their stomach 8 hours after ingesting it. These patients may require rapid sequence intubation regardless of their NPO status.

What other adjustments does the anesthesiologist need to make for taking care of a patient having an MRI?
Aside from familiarizing yourself with different equipment and screening the patient for any objects that may be a contraindication to an MRI, you will not even be in the same room as the patient when they are under anesthesia; you will not have easy and immediate access to the patient's airway. It is important to have the American Society of Anesthesiologists (ASA) standard monitors easily visible at all times. Continuous monitoring of expiratory carbon dioxide (CO_2) is crucial.

It should also be noted that patient tables in the MRI and other non-operating room locations are much less mobile than those in the operating room. These tables cannot be positioned in Trendelenburg or reverse Trendelenburg, and your access to the patient's airway may be limited by other equipment such as an MRI scanner or C-arm for fluoroscopy.

You are planning moderate sedation for this patient.

What's that? What are the common levels of sedation?
Table 35.1 describes the continuum of depth of anesthesia from lightest to deepest.

What about monitored anesthesia care (MAC)?
Although the term MAC is frequently used to describe sedation that is not general anesthesia, MAC does not describe a specific depth of anesthesia. Rather, MAC describes a specific anesthesia service performed by a qualified anesthesia provider for a diagnostic or therapeutic procedure. MAC is indicated when sedation beyond moderate sedation is required or may be required.

The patient undergoes MRI with sedation without complication. After the patient has left the scanner, a new anesthesia technician brings a non-MRI compatible oxygen cylinder into the scanner, and it flies into the scanner and gets stuck.

Now what?
Thankfully nobody was hurt. The only way to turn off the magnet is to quench it. The magnet is normally maintained at extremely cold temperature, near absolute zero. This temperature is

TABLE 35.1 ■ **Levels of Sedation**

Depth of Sedation	Description
Minimal sedation ("anxiolysis")	Patient responds normally to verbal commands. Airway reflexes, as well as respiratory and cardiovascular function, remain intact.
Moderate sedation ("conscious sedation")	Patient responds to verbal commands, possibly accompanied by gentle tactile stimulation. Airway reflexes and respirations remain intact without intervention. Cardiovascular stability is usually maintained.
Deep sedation	Patient responds to repeated or painful stimulation. Airway protective reflexes are impaired, and may require assistance (i.e., jaw thrust, oropharyngeal airway) to maintain a patent airway. Respiratory function is impaired, and may require positive pressure ventilation. Cardiovascular stability is usually maintained.
General anesthesia	Patient does not respond to painful stimulation. Patient requires support maintaining a patent airway and adequate ventilation. Cardiovascular stability may be impaired, requiring support as appropriate.

maintained by liquid helium. In quenching the magnet, the helium is vented outside away from the magnets. As the magnets quickly heat, the magnetic field dissipates. Quenching the magnet may damage the MRI machine, so this should only be done as a last resort.

The patient's MRI Is concerning for pancreatic cancer, and he is scheduled for endoscopic retrograde cholangiopancreatography (ERCP).

What is ERCP?
ERCP uses fluoroscopy to visualize the biliary and pancreatic ducts with contrast injected through an endoscope into the duodenal papilla. Fig. 35.1 shows the relevant anatomy.

STEP 1, 2 PEARLS

Most pancreatic malignancies occur at the head of the pancreas and are adenocarcinoma. Common symptoms include abdominal pain radiating toward the back, weight loss, and obstructive jaundice.

STEP 1, 2, 3 PEARLS

Trousseau sign of malignancy, also known as migratory thrombophlebitis, is recurrent blood clots in multiple superficial veins and is classically associated with pancreatic adenocarcinoma, although it can be seen in other malignancies as well.

STEP 1, 2 PEARLS

Courvoisier sign is a palpable but nontender gallbladder. Again, this is classically associated with pancreatic cancer.

What safety concerns do you have?
ERCP uses fluoroscopy, which is based on x-ray imaging. The risk of exposure to ionizing radiation is high. It is important for everyone in the procedure room to wear lead that covers the chest, abdomen, and pelvis, as well as a thyroid shield and lead goggles.

What are the anesthetic options for this case?
During ERCP, the patient is usually prone on the fluoroscopy table. This makes spontaneous ventilation difficult and the airway relatively inaccessible to the anesthesiologist. ERCP can be a complex procedure with a duration of several hours. Some interventions performed during ERCP

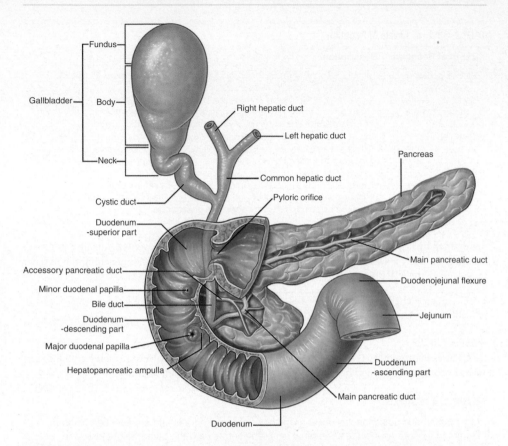

Fig. 35.1 Anatomy of the duodenum, pancreas, and biliary tree. The common bile duct and the pancreatic duct drain into the duodenum via the major duodenal papilla. Drake, R. L., Vogl, A. W., & Mitchell, A. W. M. (Eds.). (2021). Abdomen. In *Gray's atlas of anatomy. Pancreas and gallbladder* (3rd ed.). Philadelphia, PA: Elsevier.

can be painful. Additionally, the stomach is insufflated for the procedure, sometimes with CO_2. As with laparoscopic procedures, CO_2 is continuously absorbed into the systemic circulation, resulting in significant hypercapnia if ventilation is inadequate. Finally, the procedure failure rate for ERCP is twice as high when the procedure is done under sedation, as opposed to general anesthesia. Given these considerations, ERCP is frequently done under general anesthesia with endotracheal intubation, although ERCP can also be performed with a specialized laryngeal mask airway (LMA) that accommodates the duodenoscope, or under conscious sedation with a natural airway (i.e., no airway device in place).

> Induction and intubation are uneventful. The patient is positioned prone, and the procedure begins. The endoscopist complains that she cannulate the duodenal papilla.

How can you help?

Administration of glucagon causes temporary relaxation of the smooth muscles of the gastro-intestinal tract. This relaxes the sphincter of Oddi, which increases the diameter of the duode-nal papilla. Administration of secretin stimulates pancreatic secretion, which will drain into the duodenum via the duodenal papilla. Identification of the source of drainage will help localize the duodenal papilla.

BEYOND THE PEARLS

- MRI machines with stronger magnets produce images of higher quality than do machines with weaker magnets.
- Anytime a patient will have anesthesia but will not be intubated (as in sedation or LMA), have supplies and drugs ready to emergently intubate the patient.
- Administration of gadolinium contrast for MRI in patients with poor kidney function (GFR <30 mL/min/1.73 m^2) carries the risk of nephrogenic systemic fibrosis, a potentially life-threatening complication.
- Other drugs that can relax the sphincter of Oddi include somatostatin, nitroglycerin, calcium channel blockers, nalbuphine, and naloxone. Conversely, opioids tend to provoke spasms of the sphincter of Oddi.

References

American Society of Anesthesiologists. *Position on monitored anesthesia care.* https://www.asahq.org/standards-and-guidelines/position-on-monitored-anesthesia-care. (Accessed July 27, 2022).

Canard, J. M., Lennon, A. M., Létard, J. C., Etienne, J., & Okolo, P. (2011). Endoscopic retrograde cholangiopancreatography. In J. M. Canard, J. C. Letard, L. Palazzo, I. Penman, A. M. Lennon (Eds.), *Gastrointestinal Endoscopy in Practice* (Chapter 10, 370–465). Philadelphia, PA: Elsevier.

Chung, M., & Vazquez, R. (2020). Non-operating room anesthesia. In M. A. Gropper, R. D. Miller, N. H. Cohen, L. I. Eriksson, L. A. Fleisher, K. Leslie K, et al. (Eds.), *Miller's anesthesia* (9th ed., Chapter 73, pp. 2284–2312.e3). Philadelphia, PA: Elsevier.

Continuum of Depth of Sedation: Definition of General Anesthesia and Levels of Sedation/Analgesia. Committee on Quality Management and Departmental Administration. American Society of Anesthesiologists. https://www.asahq.org/standards-and-guidelines/continuum-of-depth-of-sedation-definition-of-general-anesthesia-and-levels-of-sedationanalgesia. (Accessed August 4, 2021).

UCLA Health System MRI *Safety Screening Questionnaire (Outpatients).* https://www.uclahealth.org/radiology/workfiles/referralforms/MRI-safety-screening-questionnaire-outpatient.pdf. (Accessed December 9, 2020).

A 51-Year-Old Man With Major Depressive Disorder

Nancy Suliman Saied ■ Michelle Elyse Meshman ■ Paul Neil Frank

A 51-year-old man with major depressive disorder (MDD), including chronic suicidal ideation, presents for electroconvulsive therapy (ECT) after multiple unsuccessful attempts at medication therapy. He is otherwise healthy. Vital signs show a blood pressure of 125/78 mm Hg, pulse of 70/min, respiratory rate 11/min, and oxygen saturation of 99% on room air.

What is MDD?

The specific Diagnostic and Statistical Manual of Mental Disorders, Text Revision (DSM-5TR) criteria for MDD include at least five of the symptoms listed in Table 36.1 within a 2-week period. The American Psychiatric Association publishes the DSM-5TR, which is a collection of diagnostic criteria for men0tal health disorders. The goal of DSM-5TR is to elucidate and classify mental disorders in order to improve diagnoses, treatment, and research.

What is ECT?

ECT is one of the most effective treatments in psychiatry. ECT uses a small electric current to cause a grand mal seizure and alter the brain's neurochemistry, providing relief for certain psychiatric diseases. Electrodes are placed on the patient's scalp, and a brief electrical charge of 100–600 micro-coulombs lasting ≤2 ms is administered.

TABLE 36.1 ■ **Diagnostic Criteria for Major Depressive Disorder**

- Sleep disturbances (insomnia or hypersomnia)
- **Diminished interest or loss of pleasure in activities (anhedonia)**
- Guilt or feelings of worthlessness
- Fatigue or loss of energy
- Diminished ability to concentrate
- Significant weight or appetite changes
- Psychomotor agitation or retardation
- Recurrent thoughts of death, suicidal ideation, suicide attempt, or specific plan for committing suicide
- **Depressed mood**

Diagnosis of major depressive disorder requires that at least five of these criteria be met, and at least one of the symptoms must be diminished interest/pleasure or depressed mood (**bolded**).

> **STEP 2 PEARL**
>
> Seizures can be classified based on whether they affect a single part of the brain or the whole brain.
> - Partial seizure: Begin in one region of brain and produce symptoms that can be traced to a particular region of the brain (i.e., focal deficits). This is the most common type of seizure.
>   - Simple partial seizure: Consciousness intact and seizure is localized.
>   - Complex partial seizure: Consciousness is impaired, and a postictal confused state often occurs.
> - Generalized seizure: Causes a loss of consciousness and involves disruption of electrical brain activity.
>   - Tonic-clonic (grand mal) seizure: Sudden loss of consciousness with bilateral extremity movements. During the tonic phase, the body is rigid, and the trunk and limbs are extended. Subsequently, the patient becomes flaccid until resumption of consciousness. Patient will have a postictal confusion and drowsiness. Incontinence, tongue biting, and emesis can occur.
>   - Absence (petit mal) seizure: Impaired consciousness without loss of postural tone or continence. No postictal confusion. Involves school-age children who disengage, then return to normal activity several seconds later. May be confused as day-dreaming. Episodes are brief but can be frequent (up to 100 times per day). May have minor clonic activity (e.g., eye-blinking or head-nodding).

How long does the seizure last during ECT?
Seizures for ECT usually last 15–70 seconds.

How many ECT treatments does a patient typically receive?
The number of treatments in an ECT course varies based on patient response. A typical course could include 3 treatments per week for a total of 6–20 treatments.

Which patients are candidates for ECT?
ECT is indicated for symptoms of severe mental illness, including psychosis, mania, catatonia, and depression. ECT may be considered after failure of medication therapy or for those patients requiring rapid intervention, such as those who are acutely suicidal, catatonic, or nutritionally compromised.

What are the contraindications to ECT?
Contraindications to ECT include:
- Pheochromocytoma
- Unstable cervical spine
- Recent intracranial surgery (<3 months)
- Recent cerebrovascular accident (<3 months)
- Intracranial aneurysm
- Severe aortic stenosis
- Coronary artery disease including recent myocardial infarction or angina
- Retinal detachment
- Glaucoma
- Congestive heart failure
- Severe pulmonary disease
- Major bone fracture

The patient is nervous and asks about the risks of ECT.

ECT is considered a safe procedure. Common side effects include nausea, headache, and muscle ache. Cognitive impairment is also common, and usually manifests as temporary antegrade amnesia (cannot learn new information) or retrograde amnesia (cannot recall previously learned information) that lasts up to several days.

What kind of anesthesia is required for ECT?
ECT is performed under general anesthesia. Therefore, patients must adhere to standard *nil per os* (NPO) guidelines.

What special anesthesia setup is required?
In addition to American Society of Anesthesiologists (ASA) standard monitors (see Case 14), electroencephalogram (EEG) leads are placed on the scalp to monitor the seizure. Then, stimulating electrodes will be applied to the patient's scalp (either unilaterally or bilaterally) to generate the seizure, and a bite block may be placed in the patient's mouth. A second blood pressure cuff may be applied to a distal extremity, most commonly above the ankle.

Of course, emergency drugs, defibrillator, and airway supplies should always be immediately available.

Why would a second blood pressure cuff be used?
One blood pressure cuff is used to monitor blood pressure as per ASA standard monitoring. The second blood pressure cuff acts as a tourniquet that will be inflated just prior to administration of neuromuscular blocking agent. It will stop blood flow beyond the cuff to the distal part of the extremity, thereby preventing the neuromuscular blocking agent from reaching the neuromuscular junctions distal to the blood pressure cuff. When the seizure starts, tonic-clonic activity may be observed only distal to the second blood pressure cuff, as the remainder of the body's neuromuscular junctions will have been exposed to the neuromuscular blocking agent.

What neuromuscular blocking agent will you use?
Succinylcholine is frequently used because it is fast-acting and has a short duration of action. Rocuronium may also be used, as it is relatively fast-acting and can be reversed quickly with sugammadex.

Will you intubate this patient?
Patients undergoing ECT generally are not intubated. The anesthesiologist supports the patient's airway and provides mask ventilation.

Patients with a high risk of aspiration (e.g., pregnant beyond first trimester, history of esophagectomy) or those with a known difficult airway require endotracheal intubation for ECT.

Since you are not intubating the patient, why are you administering neuromuscular blocking agent?
Grand mal seizures cause tonic-clonic jerking movements. These rapid and unpredictable movements pose a danger to the patient and staff. Neuromuscular blockade prevents these movements.

The psychiatrist says the patient's seizure was too short during his last ECT session.

What drug should you use for induction?
Etomidate may prolong the duration of seizures.

What are the side effects of etomidate?

Common side effects of etomidate include:
- Pain on injection
- Thrombophlebitis
- Postanesthetic nausea and vomiting
- Myoclonus, hiccups, and other involuntary movements
- Inhibition of 11-β-hydroxylase that results in decreased cortisol and aldosterone synthesis (i.e., adrenal suppression)

STEP 1 PEARL

Three important hormones are produced in the cortex of the adrenal glands. These hormones are synthesized from cholesterol in specialized parts of the adrenal cortex. Aldosterone, a mineralocorticoid, is produced in the zona glomerulosa, which is the outermost layer of the adrenal cortex. Cortisol, a glucocorticoid, is produced in the zona fasciculata. Meanwhile, the zona reticularis, the innermost layer of the adrenal cortex, produces androgens.

Describe the pharmacokinetics of etomidate.

Pharmacokinetics is what the body does to a drug. It can be described by absorption, distribution, metabolism, and excretion.

Etomidate is given intravenously and mainly protein-bound in the bloodstream. It is metabolized by ester hydrolysis in the liver and then excreted primarily via the urine.

Describe the pharmacodynamics of etomidate.

Pharmacodynamics is what the drug does to the body at a molecular, cellular, and physiologic level.

Etomidate works by facilitating stimulation of γ-aminobutyric acid (GABA) receptors, as do most commonly used anesthetic agents. GABA type A receptors are the major inhibitory ion channels of the brain. Upon ligand binding, there is an increase in chloride ion conduction that leads to neuronal hyperpolarization and depression of the reticular activating system, which normally mediates consciousness.

Etomidate is a rapid-acting hypnotic agent. It lacks analgesic properties. In the central nervous system, it decreases cerebral metabolic activity. It also causes the activation of seizure foci that can be seen on EEG as fast activity. This may cause myoclonus. Etomidate is used in ECT because it generates a longer seizure duration than either propofol or methohexital.

From both a respiratory and cardiovascular standpoint, etomidate offers relative stability. It causes less respiratory depression than barbiturates, such as thiopental. It also causes minimal changes in blood pressure, heart rate, and cardiac output.

Could methohexital be used for induction?

Yes, methohexital could also be given here. Methohexital is a barbiturate that lowers the seizure threshold, although it does not change the duration of seizure. It is also relatively short-acting. Methohexital can cause hypotension and myocardial depression, and it tends to blunt the sympathetic response to ECT. It causes pain and myoclonus when injected. It can also trigger an exacerbation of acute intermittent porphyria (AIP).

STEP 1, 2 PEARL

AIP is a condition of defective heme synthesis. This leads to accumulation of the heme precursor. In AIP, activity of the enzyme porphobilinogen deaminase is approximately half that of healthy patients, which leads to accumulation of porphobilinogen and δ-aminolevulinic acid (ALA). Exacerbation of AIP can be triggered by alcohol, medications, and starvation. Patients will present with abdominal pain, dark urine, psychological disturbances, and polyneuropathy. Treatment focuses on inhibiting the enzyme ALA synthase, which is the first enzyme in the cascade of heme synthesis. This can be accomplished by giving the patient glucose, dextrose, or heme.

Shortly after administration of succinylcholine, the patient fasciculates and then stops. The scalp electrodes are then activated, and the patient seizes. The patient's heart rate drops from 74/min to 20/min.

What is going on?

After initiation of the seizure, there is a parasympathetic response that can cause severe bradycardia or even asystole.

What should you do?

Treat bradycardia with atropine. However, the bradycardic response is usually followed by a sympathetic discharge that causes hypertension and tachycardia. Caution should be taken regarding the treatment of bradycardia as the patient will likely become tachycardic soon after the subsequent sympathetic discharge.

STEP 1, 2 PEARL

Atropine is a competitive antagonist of postganglionic muscarinic acetylcholine receptors in the autonomic nervous system. It does not affect cholinergic signaling at neuromuscular junctions (remember, the acetylcholine receptors at neuromuscular junctions are nicotinic, not muscarinic).

The patient's heart rate quickly normalizes. The seizure has lasted over 2 minutes.

What should you do?

Give a small dose of propofol or benzodiazepine to terminate the seizure.

In the recovery room the patient's blood pressure is 180/104 mm Hg, and his pulse is 105/min.

What should you do?

An intravenous dose of labetalol will reduce heart rate and blood pressure. It is one of the first-line drugs used to treat hypertension after ECT.

The nurse pages you 15 minutes later that the patient is confused and yelling.

What should you do?

Postoperative delirium is known to occur after ECT. If verbal reorientation and deescalation are unsuccessful, haloperidol, dexmedetomidine, midazolam, or even propofol (in small doses) may be used to calm the patient.

BEYOND THE PEARLS

- Although etomidate is considered to maintain relative hemodynamic stability, it can cause hypotension, particularly when given in large doses to patients who are chronically ill or hypovolemic.
- Consider giving the patient glycopyrrolate preprocedurally to prevent severe bradycardia.
- Propofol may be given for induction for ECT, but raises the seizure threshold.
- Ketamine may be given for induction for ECT, but it may exacerbate the sympathetic surge and postoperative delirium.
- Antiepileptic drugs and benzodiazepines may shorten seizure duration. These may be tapered or discontinued prior to ECT in consultation with the psychiatrist.
- Pregnant patients can safely undergo ECT after consultation with an obstetrician or a maternal-fetal medicine specialist. A nonparticulate antacid should be given preoperatively, and continuous fetal heart rate monitoring used. It is prudent to intubate these patients for ECT.
- Patients with implanted pacemakers or defibrillators can safely undergo ECT after consultation with a cardiologist. It may be necessary to apply a magnet or reprogram the device (see Case 25).

References

American Psychiatric Association, (2013). *Diagnostic and statistical manual of mental disorders* (5th ed.). Washington, DC: American Psychiatric Association.

Avramov, M. N., Husain, M. M., & White, P. F. (1995). The comparative effects of methohexital, propofol, and etomidate for electroconvulsive therapy. *Anesthesia and Analgesia, 81*(3), 596–602.

Atlee, J. L. (2006). *Complications in anesthesia* (2nd ed., pp. 903–904). Philadelphia, PA: Elsevier.

Bains, N., & Abdijadid, S. (2021). Major depressive disorder: *StatPearls [Internet]*. Treasure Island, FL: StatPearls Publishing. https://www.ncbi.nlm.nih.gov/books/NBK559078.

Bokoch, M. P., & Eilers, H. (2018). Intravenous anesthetics: *Basics of Anesthesia* (pp. 117–118) (7th ed.). Philadelphia, PA: Elsevier.

Chawla, N. (2020). Anesthesia for electroconvulsive therapy. *Anesthesiology Clinics, 38*(1), 183–195.

Cui, W., & Lee, C. Z. (2018). Anesthesia for procedures in non-operating room locations: *Basics of Anesthesia* (pp. 670–671) (7th ed.). Philadelphia, PA: Elsevier.

Sear, J. W. (2011). Clinical pharmacology of intravenous anesthetics. In A. S. Evers, M. Maze, & E. D. Kharasch (Eds.), *Anesthetic Pharmacology* (2nd ed., pp. 420–443). New York, NY: Cambridge University Press.

Fragen, R. J., Shanks, C. A., Molteni, A., & Avram, M. J. (1984). Effects of etomidate on hormonal responses to surgical stress. *Anesthesiology, 61*, 652–656.

Holtan, E. E. (2014). Etomidate. In B. S. Freeman & J. S. Berger (Eds.), *Anesthesiology Core Review* (pp. 155–156). New York, NY: McGraw-Hill Education Medical.

Kirkgoz, T., & Guran, T. (2018). Primary adrenal insufficiency in children: Diagnosis and management. *Best Practice & Research. Clinical Endocrinology & Metabolism, 32*(4), 397–424.

Le, T., Bhushan, V., Kallianos, K., Mehlman, M., Sochat, M., & Sylvester, P. (2015). *Neurology: First aid for the USMLE Step 1*. New York, NY: McGraw Hill Medical.

Dershwitz, M., & Rosow, C. (2012). Pharmacology of intravenous anesthetics. In D. E. Longnecker, D. L. Brown, M. F. Newman, & W. M. Zapol (Eds.), *Longnecker Anesthesiology* (2nd ed., Chapter 41). New York, NY: McGraw Hill.

Morel, J., Salard, M., Castelain, C., Bayon, M. C., Lambert, P., Vola, M., et al. (2011). Haemodynamic consequences of etomidate administration in elective cardiac surgery: A randomized double-blinded study. *British Journal of Anaesthesia, 107*(4), 503–509.

Saatcioglu, O., & Tomruk, N. B. (2011). The use of electroconvulsive therapy in pregnancy: A review. *The Israel Journal of Psychiatry and Related Sciences, 48*(1), 6–11.

Vuyk, J., Sitsen, E., & Reekers, M. IV anesthetics. In *Miller's Anesthesia* (8th ed., pp. 850–854). Philadelphia, PA: Elsevier.

Critical Care

A 57-Year-Old Woman With Altered Mental Status

Stefano Iantorno ■ Joon Choi ■ Patrick Chan ■ Raj Dasgupta

A 57-year-old woman with a past medical history of poorly controlled diabetes, cirrhosis due to chronic hepatitis C infection, and hypothyroidism was brought to the emergency department by her family for altered mental status. The patient had been in her usual state of health until 3 days prior, when she bumped her left leg against the edge of the bed at home. The patient had been complaining of worsening left lower extremity pain since then, but over the 24 hours prior to presentation, she started to feel more unwell and acting more confused.

In the emergency department, the patient was uncomfortable appearing but able to answer most questions appropriately and was found to be alert and oriented to person and place. The patient denied any infectious prodromal symptoms such as fevers, chills, cough, shortness of breath, abdominal pain, nausea, vomiting, flank pain, dysuria, or changes in urinary frequency. The patient described the pain as starting from the thigh, radiating down the leg, and exacerbated by movement. She denied any numbness, weakness, or paresthesias associated with the pain. The patient reported a long-standing history of diabetes mellitus and had been taking insulin for a number of years, as well as lactulose for hepatic encephalopathy and furosemide and spironolactone for medical management of her ascites.

Initial vitals were concerning for hypotension, with blood pressure of 75/30 mm Hg, heart rate of 103 beats per minute, and oxygen saturation of 96% on room air. Her physical exam was notable for diffuse erythema and swelling of the left lower extremity, which was extremely tender to palpation. Lung and heart exam were without abnormal findings other than tachycardia.

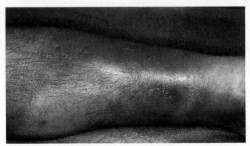

Fig. 37.1 Example of cellulitis. (From Gawkrodger, D. J., and Ardern-Jones, M. R. (2021). Dermatology an Illustrated Colour Text. Elsevier.)

What is the definition of sepsis and septic shock?

According to the Sepsis-3 guidelines, released in 2016, sepsis was defined as organ dysfunction caused by dysregulated response to infection. In a clinical setting, organ dysfunction can be determined by a sequential sepsis-related organ failure assessment (SOFA) score of 2 or higher, with a higher score correlating to a higher chance of mortality. The SOFA score is a scoring system that evaluates 6 organ systems (respiratory, cardiovascular, liver, renal, coagulopathy, and neurologic) on an individual 0 to 4 scale to arrive at a composite score from 0 to 24 to assess patient's severity of sepsis. This score can be cumbersome to calculate during the acute setting; therefore, to expedite evaluation and treatment of patients with sepsis at higher risk of mortality, a quickSOFA (qSOFA) score can be calculated, especially for patients who are not in the ICU. The qSOFA score involves three components: the patient's respiratory rate, mental status, and systolic blood pressure. A point is given if patient's respiratory rate is greater than or equal to 22 breaths per minute, Glasgow Coma Scale is less than 15, or systolic blood pressure is less than or equal to 100 mm Hg. A qSOFA score of 2 or 3 corresponds to high risk for in-hospital mortality. This enables rapid identification of patients who have life-threatening dysregulation of the host response to infection. This appears to be a more sensitive and specific approach than the previous definition used in Sepsis-2 guidelines with systemic inflammatory response syndrome (SIRS) criteria. Septic shock can be clinically identified as those patients having a vasopressor requirement to maintain a minimum mean arterial pressure (MAP) of 65 mm Hg and a serum lactate of 2 mmol/L (18 mg/dL) or greater in the absence of hypovolemia.

A bedside ultrasound revealed a collapsible inferior vena cava and hyperdynamic left ventricular function. A chest radiograph had no significant focal opacities, and an electrocardiogram revealed sinus tachycardia without ischemic changes. Lactate levels and blood cultures were drawn. A 2 liter fluid bolus was started, and the patient was started empirically on vancomycin, ceftriaxone, and clindamycin.

What is adequate intravenous fluid resuscitation when septic shock is suspected?
Patients with suspected septic shock should be fluid resuscitated with at least 30 mL/kg of ideal body weight within 3 hours from presentation. Several retrospective trials showed that failure to achieve this goal was associated with increased mortality, increased length of intensive care unit (ICU) stay, and delayed resolution of hypotension.

CLINICAL PEARL—STEP 2/3

Lactate can be a marker of poor tissue perfusion; therefore, trending lactate levels can be useful in sepsis. However, there are other etiologies for elevated lactate levels. Therefore, resuscitation should be individualized based on the patient's clinical scenario.

What fluids should be used in septic shock?
In terms of fluids, there has been a paradigm shift regarding the use of chloride-rich solution such as normal saline versus a balanced solution such as lactated Ringer's solution. With recent studies and meta-analyses, a balanced crystalloid solution has shown reduction in mortality and reduction in the need for renal replacement therapy when compared with normal saline.

CLINICAL PEARL—STEP 2/3

Fluid resuscitation should be with a balanced crystalloid solution, such as lactated Ringer's solution.

In terms of colloid versus crystalloid, there have been several studies that do not show clear benefit when using colloid solutions compared with crystalloid solutions; therefore the routine use of colloid solution such as albumin is not recommended.

Significant lab findings included normal white blood cell (WBC) count on arrival, normocytic anemia to 8.1, thrombocytopenia to 37, anion gap metabolic acidosis of 10 with gap 26, and low chloride to 99. Glucose was low to 61, and lactate was elevated to 14.2 but decreased to 11 after administration of 2 liters of intravenous fluids. The initial labs were also notable for acute kidney injury with serum creatinine of 1.94 and worsening transaminases, bilirubinemia, and prothrombin time/international normalized ratio from baseline. C-reactive protein was elevated to 117. Urinalysis showed proteinuria but was negative for pyuria, hematuria, leukocyte esterase, or nitrites.

The patient continued to be hypotensive despite intravenous fluid resuscitation, so a central venous line was placed, and the patient was started on intravenous norepinephrine and vasopressin and transferred to the ICU. Antibiotics were broadened from ceftriaxone to piperacillin-tazobactam, while vancomycin and clindamycin were continued. A computed tomography (CT) scan of the chest, abdomen, and pelvis with intravenous contrast was ordered, as well as a CT scan of the left lower extremity.

CLINICAL PEARL—STEP 2/3

Vancomycin and piperacillin-tazobactam when used in conjunction has been associated with acute kidney injury. Caution should be exercised if both antibiotics are used, and if no methicillin resistant *Staphylococcus aureus* is isolated, vancomycin should be discontinued.

When are blood cultures obtained in sepsis?

Typically, blood cultures should be obtained on admission or as soon as sepsis is suspected, ideally before initiation of empiric antibiotics. Additional cultures from specific body sites such as skin abscesses, pleural fluid, cerebrospinal fluid, or ascitic fluid can be collected after empiric antibiotic initiation.

When should antibiotics be initiated? What is appropriate antibiotic therapy for septic shock?

Empiric broad-spectrum antibiotic coverage should be initiated within 1 hour of presentation if shock is present; however, antimicrobials can be delayed up to 3 hours if shock is absent, allowing time for further evaluation of likelihood of sepsis. If blood cultures are not obtained prior to the 1 hour mark in the setting of shock (or 3 hour mark if shock is absent), antibiotics should be administered regardless given increased mortality with delay in antibiotics. Broad-spectrum antibiotics should include gram-positive coverage and gram-negative coverage.

CLINICAL PEARL—STEP 2/3

Patients who are at high risk for multidrug-resistant gram-negative infections can be covered with double gram-negative coverage until speciation and sensitivities result.

CLINICAL PEARL—STEP 2/3

For patients at high risk for fungal infections, empiric antifungal therapy is warranted (see Table 37.1).

TABLE 37.1 ■ **Common Risk Factors for *Candida* Infection**

Candida colonization at multiple sites
Neutropenia
Chronic immunosuppression
Gastrointestinal perforation
Long intensive care unit stay
Presence of central venous catheters
Use of broad-spectrum antibiotics

Aside from antibiotics, what other important principle must be addressed in sepsis to prevent persistent infection?

One important principle in treating sepsis is source control. Appropriate source control is the cornerstone in the management of sepsis. Interventions may include incision and drainage, percutaneous drainage, debridement, or removal of infected devices.

CLINICAL PEARL—STEP 2/3

Intravenous devices or catheters are often overlooked sources of infection in the intensive care unit setting. Therefore, duration and indication of devices or catheters should be reviewed daily to prevent CLABSI (central line associated bloodstream infection).

On examination upon transfer to the medical ICU, the patient is found to not be alert or oriented to person, place, or time. She appears agitated and uncomfortable, moaning nonsensical words, and is unable to answer questions or follow commands. The patient is intubated for airway protection, and an arterial line is placed for hemodynamic monitoring. CT imaging did not reveal any intrathoracic or intraabdominal sources of infection, but CT of the left lower extremity appears to have soft tissue stranding involving the lower leg and tracking to the medial thigh, without any gas or edema in the deep fascial layers, with overall findings suggesting cellulitis. Epinephrine is added given rising pressor requirements overnight.

What vasopressors should be used in septic shock?

A very well studied first-line agent recommended by the Surviving Sepsis guidelines is norepinephrine, which functions via α_1 and β_1 agonism (see Table 37.2). Vasopressin, which acts on both V1 and V2 receptors, is added as a second-line agent despite absence of proven mortality benefit, although when used in synergy with norepinephrine, it has been shown to achieve goal MAPs with lower norepinephrine dose. Epinephrine can also be added as a second-line agent, especially in the presence of cardiac dysfunction given strong effects on β_1. Phenylephrine is recommended when tachyarrhythmias are present, given its peripheral vasoconstriction effects. Although dopamine was previously considered a first-line agent, as shown in multiple studies, this vasopressor agent has been shown to have increased mortality and higher incidence of arrhythmias compared with norepinephrine. However, it can be used in highly selected patients who have absolute or relative bradycardia and a low risk of tachyarrhythmias. Angiotensin II agonist is a reasonable addition for refractory septic shock.

TABLE 37.2 ■ **Common Vasopressors and Mechanism of Action**

Vasopressor	Mechanism of action
Norepinephrine	α_1, β_1 agonist
Vasopressin	V1 and V2 receptors
Epinephrine	α_1, β_1, β_2 agonist
Phenylephrine	α_1 agonist

What is the recommended MAP goal?

The MAP should target 65 mm Hg. The rationale to maintain a MAP goal is for adequate organ and tissue perfusion.

CLINICAL PEARL—STEP 2/3

Avoid targeting higher MAP goals as studies have not shown clear benefit; however, there is increased risk of vasopressor side effects, such as digital ischemia or mesenteric ischemia, with higher MAP goals.

On the second hospital day, blood cultures resulted positive for *Streptococcus pyogenes* with susceptibilities. The patient was noted to have worsening leukocytosis with increased bandemia despite appropriate intravenous antibiotic therapy. On repeat examination, the patient is noted to have worsening erythema tracking along the medial surface of the left leg, with many large hemorrhagic bullae and underlying desquamation of the skin, without crepitus on palpation. Given the concern for necrotizing fasciitis, the patient underwent surgical debridement and was confirmed by pathologic findings of dermal and subcutaneous mixed inflammation and fat necrosis.

Given rising pressor requirements, phenylephrine was added for pressor support. Stress dose hydrocortisone was started.

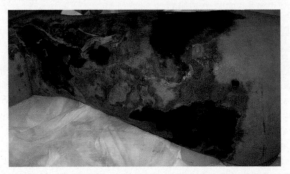

Fig. 37.2 Necrotizing soft tissue infection of the left lower extremity. (Smuszkiewicz, P., Trojanowska, I., & Tomczak, H. (2008). Late diagnosed necrotizing fasciitis as a cause of multiorgan dysfunction syndrome: A case report. *Cases Journal, 1*(1), 125. https://doi.org/10.1186/1757-1626-1-125.)

What is the role of stress dose steroids in septic shock?

Sepsis and septic shock are thought to be states of relative adrenal insufficiency in which the body's demand driven by increased metabolic rates exceeds adrenal gland glucocorticoid production. However, experimental measurements of cortisol and other serum hormonal intermediates have been shown to be poorly descriptive of true adrenal state given profound metabolic disarray in sepsis and the lack of well-established physiologic ranges under these conditions. In several studies, hydrocortisone with or without fludrocortisone did not result in significant mortality benefit, but it did decrease time to resolution of shock. As such, current guidelines recommend hydrocortisone in shock unresponsive to initial intravenous fluid resuscitation and broad-spectrum antibiotics.

CLINICAL PEARL—STEP 2/3

The dose of hydrocortisone for septic shock is 200–300 mg total daily dose, divided into three or four times per day.

Nephrology was consulted for worsening kidney function with a serum creatinine level of 2.28, decreasing urine output, and worsening acidosis with pH 7.16. The patient was started on a sodium bicarbonate drip, and continuous renal replacement therapy was initiated. The serum lactate level worsened to 14. Blood cultures and wound cultures taken on the day of surgical debridement confirmed *S. pyogenes*.

CLINICAL PEARL—STEP 2/3

There is conflicting evidence regarding sodium bicarbonate therapy in patients with acidosis. However, in one randomized clinical trial, in the cohort that received bicarbonate therapy, there was decreased composite outcome of mortality at day 28 or the presence of at least 1 organ failure at day 7 in patients with pH less than 7.20 and acute kidney injury. Thus, an argument can be made for sodium bicarbonate therapy in this patient population.

The initial Laboratory Risk Indicator for Necrotizing Fasciitis (LRINEC) score was 8. Given the pathology findings from the initial intraoperative debridement, the patient was diagnosed with necrotizing fasciitis. The patient was taken to the operating room again for reexploration and possible amputation given increased mottling of the left lower extremity and rising serum creatine kinase. Intravenous immunoglobulin was administered. The patient was noted to have increasing oxygen requirements on the ventilator in order to maintain oxygen saturations greater than 90%. After discussion with family, patient was transitioned to comfort measures only, given the lack of response despite maximal therapy.

What is the LRINEC score? How is it interpreted?

The LRINEC score is used as a screening tool for patients who are at risk of having necrotizing fasciitis and may benefit from operative debridement (see Table 37.3). It takes into account serum measurements of C-reactive protein, WBC count, hemoglobin, sodium, creatinine, and glucose. Any score greater than 6 is considered positive.

TABLE 37.3 ■ **LRINEC Score**

Criteria	Value	Points
C-reactive protein	≥150 mg/L	+4
White blood cell count	15–25 K/μL, >25 K/μL	+1, +2
Hemoglobin	11–13.5 g/dL, <11 g/dL	+1, +2
Sodium	<135 mEq/L	+2
Creatinine	>1.6 mg/dL	+2
Glucose	>180 mg/dL	+1

From Wong, C. H., Khin, L. W., Heng, K. S., Tan, K. C., & Low, C. O. (2004). The LRINEC (Laboratory Risk Indicator for Necrotizing Fasciitis) score: a tool for distinguishing necrotizing fasciitis from other soft tissue infections. *Critical Care Medicine*, 32(7), 1535–1541.
LRINEC, Laboratory Risk Indicator for Necrotizing Fasciitis.

What is the prognosis of sepsis and septic shock?
Studies have shown that mortality increases with severity of the presentation. Different models, such as SOFA, have been developed to predict disease severity. Lactate is a well-validated predictive marker that has been associated with restoration of adequate perfusion, with levels greater than 4 mmol/L being associated with worse prognosis. According to some studies, septic shock can have a mortality of more than 40%, with patients younger than 44 years of age and without significant comorbidities having overall better prognosis. With the introduction of early goal-directed therapy and ICU bundles as part of the Surviving Sepsis campaign, mortality has decreased over time; however, there is still significant mortality and more research is needed to better understand how to best treat patients with sepsis. Different organisms may influence outcomes as well: bloodstream infections of gram-negative organisms have been associated with worse outcomes before shock develops, but outcomes were similar after onset of shock. Following successful recovery, up to 10% of patients will experience readmission.

Case Summary

- **Complaint/History:** 57-year-old woman presenting initially with left leg pain.
- **Findings:** Left leg erythema, hypotensive, tachycardic, in shock.
- **Lab Results/Test:** Elevated WBC, inflammatory markers, blood cultures with *S. pyogenes*.

Diagnosis: Necrotizing soft tissue infection secondary to *S. pyogenes*.

- **Treatment:** Intravenous antibiotics, surgical debridement, intravenous immunoglobulin.

BEYOND THE PEARL

1. Patients at risk for fluid overload such as end-stage renal disease or heart failure patients should still receive the 30 mL/kg ideal body weight initial fluid resuscitation within the first 3 hours. A retrospective study showed increased mortality when failing to reach the benchmark of 30 mL/kg within the first 3 hours, regardless of comorbid conditions, specifically including heart failure and end-stage renal disease. However, with that being said, subsequent fluid resuscitation should be tailored to patient's comorbidities and clinical scenario.
2. Dynamic assessment of fluid responsiveness is gaining favor to guide subsequent fluid resuscitation. Dynamic parameters include response to passive leg raise via stroke volume, stroke volume variation, pulse pressure variation, or echocardiography.
3. Starch-containing solutions should not be used for fluid resuscitation.

4. Daily reassessment of antimicrobials and appropriate deescalation help to prevent development of multidrug-resistant organisms and avoid side effects of medications.
5. Clindamycin can be used in necrotizing fasciitis and toxic shock syndrome due to its antitoxin effects.
6. Intravenous immunoglobulin has been associated with improved outcomes in select patients in the setting of necrotizing fasciitis associated with group A streptococcal infection.
7. Strict glucose control is important in patients with sepsis, with goal glucose level of 140–180 mg/dL.

References

Singer, M., Deutschman, C. S., Seymour, C. W., Shankar-Hari, M., Annane, D., & Bauer, M., et al. The third international consensus definitions for sepsis and septic shock (sepsis-3). *JAMA*, 315(8), 801–810. https://doi.org/10.1001/jama.2016.0287.

Rhodes, A., Evans, L. E., Alhazzani, W., Levy, M. M., Antonelli, M., Ferrer, R., et al. (2017). Surviving sepsis campaign: International guidelines for management of sepsis and septic shock: 2016. *Intensive Care Medicine*, 43(3), 304–377.

Cinel, I., Kasapoglu, U. S., Gul, F., & Dellinger, R. P. (2020). The initial resuscitation of septic shock. *Journal of Critical Care*, 57, 108–117.

Gazmuri, R. J., & de Gomez, C. A. (2020). From a pressure-guided to a perfusion-centered resuscitation strategy in septic shock: Critical literature review and illustrative case. *Journal of Critical Care*, 56, 294–304.

Annane, D., Sébille, V., Charpentier, C., Bollaert, P. E., François, B., & Korach, J. M., et al. (2002). Effect of treatment with low doses of hydrocortisone and fludrocortisone on mortality in patients with septic shock. *JAMA*, 288(7), 862–871.

Sprung, C. L., Annane, D., Keh, D., Moreno, R., Singer, M., & Freivogel, K., et al. (2008). Hydrocortisone therapy for patients with septic shock. *The New England Journal of Medicine*, 358(2), 111–124.

Keh, D., Trips, E., Marx, G., Wirtz, S. P., & Abduljawwad, E., et al. (2016). Effect of hydrocortisone on development of shock among patients with severe sepsis: The HYPRESS randomized clinical trial. *JAMA*, 316(17), 1775–1785.

Venkatesh, B., Finfer, S., Cohen, J., Rajbhandari, D., Arabi, Y., Bellomo, R., & et al. (2018). Adjunctive glucocorticoid therapy in patients with septic shock. *The New England Journal of Medicine*, 378(9), 797–808.

Annane, D., Renault, A., Brun-Buisson, C., Megarbane, B., Quenot, J. P., & Siami, S., et al. (2018). Hydrocortisone plus fludrocortisone for adults with septic shock. *The New England Journal of Medicine*, 378, 809–818.

Jaber, S., Paugam, C., Futier, E., Lefrant, J. Y., Lasocki, S., & Lescot, T., et al. (2018). Sodium bicarbonate therapy for patients with severe metabolic acidaemia in the intensive care unit (BICAR-ICU): A multicentre, open-label, randomised controlled, phase 3 trial. *Lancet*, 392(10141), 31.

Kadri, S. S., Swihart, B. J., Bonne, S. L., Hohmann, S. F., Hennessy, L. V., & Louras, P., et al. (2017). Impact of intravenous immunoglobulin on survival in necrotizing fasciitis with vasopressor-dependent shock: A propensity score-matched analysis from 130 US hospitals. *Clinical Infectious Diseases*, 64(7), 877–885.

Lee, C. C., Chi, C. H., Lee, N. Y., Lee, H. C., Chen, C. L., Chen, P. L., et al. (2008). Necrotizing fasciitis in patients with liver cirrhosis: Predominance of monomicrobial gram-negative bacillary infections. *Diagnostic Microbiology and Infectious Disease*, 62(2), 219–225.

Vignon, P., Begot, E., Mari, A., Silva, S., Chimot, L., Delour, P., et al. (2018). Hemodynamic assessment of patients with septic shock using transpulmonary thermodilution and critical care echocardiography: A comparative study. *Chest*, 153(1), 55–64.

Smuszkiewicz, P., Trojanowska, I., & Tomczak, H. (2008). Late diagnosed necrotizing fasciitis as a cause of multiorgan dysfunction syndrome: A case report. *Cases Journal*, 1(1), 125. https://doi.org/10.1186/1757-1626-1-125.

A 66-Year-Old Man Presenting With Palpitations and Shortness of Breath

Rastko Rakočević ■ Moses Koo ■ Raj Dasgupta

A 66-year-old man presented to the emergency department with generalized discomfort, palpitations, and shortness of breath. He has a medical history significant for obesity, hyperlipidemia (HLD), and uncontrolled hypertension (HTN). His home medications are rosuvastatin, amlodipine, and losartan for many years. Two weeks ago, he noted an upper respiratory illness and worsening shortness of breath to the point of being symptomatic even at rest. He also complains of occasional tightness in his chest that is exertional and resolves after rest. He has been compliant with all of his medications. On physical examination, he is afebrile, body mass index (BMI) is 38, blood pressure is 80/60 mm Hg, heart rate is 102 beats per minute, respiratory rate is 25 breaths per minute, and oxygen saturation is 92% on room air. Physical exam is notable for obesity, diaphoresis, moderate lower extremity edema with overlying erythema, and cool extremities. Pulse was weak with palpable pulsus alternans. He has regular tachycardia with occasional ectopic heartbeats, distant S1/S2 with no additional heart sounds heard, and bilateral crackles with expiratory wheeze. His neck is obese and the jugular vein is hard to examine. His abdomen is soft and nontender. The remainder of the exam is normal. A chest radiograph is obtained showing enlarged cardiac silhouette with evidence of pulmonary vascular congestion.

This patient appears to be in shock. What clues in the history and presentation point toward the etiology of the shock?
A patient who presents with signs of hemodynamic instability must be evaluated for signs of shock. Differentiating between cardiogenic from other etiologies of shock can often be difficult. There are several clues in the patient's presentation that indicate a cardiac etiology. The patient is presenting with shortness of breath, palpitations, and chest tightness. These are all symptoms that can be consistent with a cardiac etiology. In regards to his history, he has several cardiac risk factors, including obesity, hyperlipidemia, and hypertension. These cardiac risk factors help risk stratify the likelihood of cardiac disease in this individual.

CLINICAL PEARL—STEP 2/3

Viral myocarditis should be on the differential in patients with cardiac dysfunction who have had a recent history of viral upper respiratory illness.

What is the definition of cardiogenic shock?
Cardiogenic shock is defined broadly as cardiac dysfunction that results in the inability of the current cardiac output (CO) to keep up with the body's needs. The landmark SHOCK Trial proposed objective cutoffs for diagnosis of cardiogenic shock which include:
1. Systolic blood pressure (SBP) less than 90 mm Hg for greater than 30 min or inotropes/vasopressors needed to maintain SBP greater than 90 mm Hg

2. Evidence of end organ perfusion (urine output less than 30 mL/h or cool extremities)
3. Cardiac Index (CI) less than or equal to 2.2 and Pulmonary Capillary Wedge Pressure greater than or equal to 15 mm Hg.

BASIC SCIENCE PEARLS—STEP 1

Cardiac output (CO) is the volume of blood a heart ejects per minute and is a product of stroke volume (SV) and heart rate (HR) (CO = SV × HR). SV is dependent on the three major factors: preload (end-diastolic volume of blood or pressure in ventricles); afterload (pressure or resistance against which ventricles must strain to eject blood) and ventricular contractility (inotropy). The Frank-Starling Law is an interplay between preload and cardiac contractility. In general, as more myocardial fibers stretch during diastole, the greater the contractility will be during the systole. This is true up to a point when myocardial fibers are stretched to their maximum tension, and further filling volume will not increase and may actually decrease cardiac contractility. Patients with severe ventricular dysfunction will reach this state faster, with markedly increased preload and insufficient contractility, leading to increased pulmonary and systemic congestion.

What are some clues in the physical exam that would be consistent with cardiogenic etiology of shock?
Classic physical exam findings that would point towards cardiogenic shock or heart failure include lower extremity edema, elevated jugular venous distension, and crackles on lung exam (See Table 38.1).

TABLE 38.1 ■ List of Physical Exam Findings That Can be Commonly Found in Patients with Cardiogenic Chock

Neurologic exam	Encephalopathy
Cardiac Exam	S3, weak heart sounds, weak pulses, pulsus alternans, narrow pulse pressure, jugular venous distension, slow capillary refill
Pulmonary Exam	Increased work of breathing, pulmonary rales, crackles, complete absence of breath sounds (effusion)
Abdominal Exam	Ascites with congestive hepatopathy/cirrhosis
Extremity Exam	Cold and mottled, clammy skin, edema

BASIC SCIENCE PEARL—STEP 1

Pulse pressure is the difference between systolic and diastolic blood pressures. In cardiogenic shock, there is a narrow pulse pressure, which is a reflection of decreased CO and increased vascular resistance respectively. This is in contrast with septic shock where a widened pulse pressure is observed.

What other tests can you order to further support your diagnosis?
Diagnostic measures can range from noninvasive to invasive. Noninvasive would include a electrocardiograms (ECG), point of care ultrasound (POCUS), and laboratory tests; invasive would include pulmonary artery catheterization (PAC) as well as left heart catheterization to evaluate for coronary artery disease, which is one of the most common etiologies of cardiogenic shock.

Given the concerns for cardiogenic shock, you recall that an acute coronary syndrome (ACS) could be the most time sensitive etiology for cardiogenic shock. You decide to obtain an ECG to evaluate for evidence of cardiac ischemia. You do not note any ST elevations or depressions; however, you do note T wave inversions (TWI), most pronounced in V2 and V3, which might be suggestive of Wellen's syndrome (Fig. 38.1).

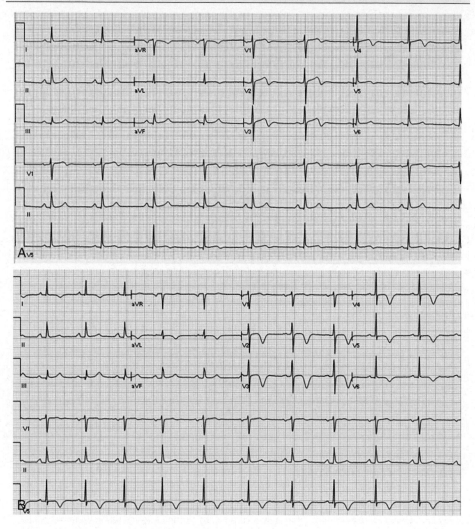

Fig. 38.1 Examples of Wellens syndrome. (A) With biphasic T waves in V2 and V3. (B) With deeply inverted T waves in V2 and V3. (*The American Journal of Emergency Medicine, 30*[1].)

CLINICAL PEARL - STEP 2/3

Wellen's syndrome is an ECG finding that is highly specific for proximal left anterior descending artery (LAD) stenosis. There are two types, Type I and Type II. Type I is characterized by biphasic T waves in V2 and V3. Type II is characterized by deeply inverted TWI in V2 and V3.

What are different ECG findings that are concerning for ischemia?

If there is a concern for cardiogenic shock, an ECG is warranted to evaluate for cardiac ischemia. If there are signs of cardiac ischemia, interventions must be taken to temporize and prevent further cardiac myocyte injury. Classic ECG findings associated with ischemia are ST segment elevations, ST segment depressions, T wave inversions, pathologic Q waves, or new left bundle branch block (LBBB).

BASIC SCIENCE PEARL—STEP 1

ST elevations occur when there is an acute complete occlusion of a coronary artery, which results in transmural infarction of the myocardium. On the other hand, ST depressions and T wave inversions are secondary to subtotal or partial occlusion of a coronary artery, resulting in subendocardial infarction that does not extend through the entire thickness of the myocardium.

CLINICAL PEARL—STEP 2/3

ST-elevation myocardial infarction (STEMI) is a medical emergency as there is an acute total occlusion of a coronary artery, most often due to atherosclerotic plaque rupture. This requires immediate intervention as cardiac myocyte injury occurs within minutes of complete occlusion.

CLINICAL PEARL—STEP 2/3

A new LBBB can be a manifestation of ischemia or infarction. Old ECGs are helpful in this scenario to determine if the LBBB is new or pre-existing.

As you review the ECG changes, you realize that your patient does not have an STEMI, but you are concerned that the TWI represent ischemic changes. You know that regardless of the ECG finding, high concern for acute coronary syndrome (ACS) warrants urgent medical and possible invasive intervention. Since there is no contraindication, you order heparin drip, aspirin, and a statin. You call a cardiology consultation, order serial ECGs and troponins, and evaluate the patient with a bedside ultrasound.

How is point of care ultrasound used in the evaluation of cardiogenic shock?

Although a thorough echocardiography (ECHO) usually requires a trained technician and cardiologist to interpret the study, a point of care ultrasound (POCUS) is a quick and effective tool to differentiate the etiology of shock, especially when cardiogenic shock is suspected. In the setting of cardiogenic shock, the most critical information to gain is the left ventricular ejection fraction (LVEF). Evaluation is done through four standard ECHO views: parasternal long axis (PLAX), parasternal short axis (PSAX), apical 4 chamber (A4C), and subcostal view, which all evaluate heart chambers from different views to give an overall assessment of their function.

CLINICAL PEARL—STEP 2/3

The left ventricle should be assessed in several different views to determine most accurate LVEF.

Cardiac POCUS views were difficult but did show minimal pericardial effusion, tricuspid annular plane systolic excursions (TAPSE), of 17 mm (Fig. 38.2), visually decreased LVEF with no obvious regional wall motion abnormalities, and E-point septal separation (EPSS) of 14.5 mm (Fig. 38.3).

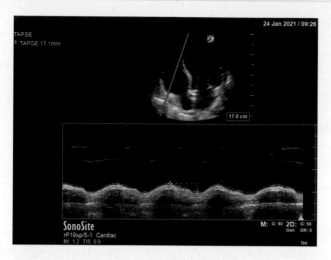

Fig. 38.2   A4C view, TAPSE 17 mm. (Courtesy of Rastko Rakocevic, MD.)

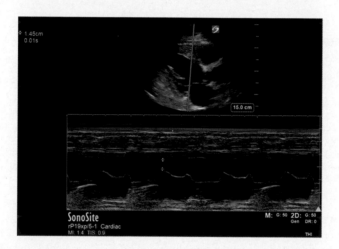

Fig. 38.3   PLAX view with EPSS showing 14.5 mm. (Courtesy of Rastko Rakocevic, MD.)

What does all of this mean in regard to your patient?

In critically ill patients, quick estimations of the left ventricular (LV) and right ventricular (RV) contractility are made via calculating E-point septal separation (EPSS) and tricuspid annular plane systolic excursions (TAPSE), respectively. EPSS measures the distance between the interventricular septum and mitral valve leaflet during its maximal excursion in early diastole via M-mode in the PLAX view, with a value greater than 7 mm correlating with LVEF less than 50%. M-mode is a specific mode that displays motion along a chosen ultrasound line over time. TAPSE is done by measuring the length of the tricuspid valve annulus movement during systole via M-mode in the A4C view, with a value less than 17 mm correlating with RV systolic dysfunction.

The EPSS of 14.5 mm suggests that the patient likely has reduced cardiac function. The TAPSE of 17 mm, although borderline, suggests that the right ventricle is functioning normally. However, you decide to obtain more information to support your diagnosis of cardiogenic shock.

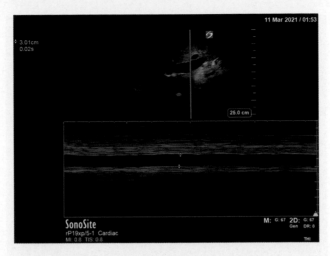

Fig. 38.4   Ultrasound view of IVC with minimal variability, IVC size 3 cm. (Courtesy of Rastko Rakocevic, MD.)

What other information can you obtain with bedside POCUS?
Besides bedside cardiac ultrasonography, an assessment of the inferior vena cava (IVC) as well as lung ultrasonography can further support your diagnosis of cardiogenic shock by evaluating for evidence of volume overload. The IVC ultrasound is performed by evaluating the IVC diameter and its collapsibility with breathing via M-mode just distal to the junction of the hepatic vein and IVC. This measurement correlates with the right atrial (RA) pressures. The lung ultrasound is performed by evaluating for the presence of artifacts throughout your lung view.

> You find that your patient's IVC is 3.0 cm in diameter and has no respiratory variations (Fig. 38.4). While performing the lung ultrasound, you see vertical white (hyperechoic) lines propagating through the whole depth of your ultrasound window, which move synchronously with lung movement.

How should you interpret your findings?
Interpreting IVC ultrasonography findings are most useful in non-intubated patients with nonlabored breathing. In this setting, IVC diameter of less than 2.1 cm with greater than 50% collapsibilty with inspiration correlates with a right atrial (RA) pressure of less than 5 mm Hg, which is normal. Conversely, an IVC diameter of greater than 2.1 cm with less than 50% collapsibility with respiration correlates with a RA pressure of 10-20 mm Hg, which would be consistent with volume overload state.

Lung ultrasonography can also be useful in setting of cardiogenic shock. Vertical "comet-tail" artifacts (also known as "B-lines"), which span from the pleural line all the way to the end of the ultrasound field, represent pleural changes after they become thickened from excess interstitial volume, resulting in increased echogenicity. In the appropriate clinical setting, this can represent pulmonary edema. See video 38.1 for an example of lung ultrasound demonstrating B-lines.

CLINICAL PEARL—STEP 2/3

It is acceptable to see 1–2 B-lines in the posterior-basilar fields (gravity-dependent) even in some euvolemic patients (Fig. 38.5).

> The troponin you ordered earlier returned slightly elevated. However, at the time, you were astute enough to order several other labs to evaluate your patient's cardiogenic shock.

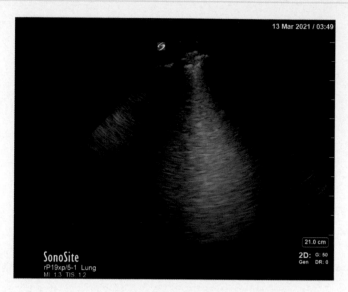

Fig. 38.5 Ultrasound view of B-lines. (Courtesy of Rastko Rakocevic, MD.)

What are important lab findings that are important to monitor with cardiogenic shock?
Important lab findings can be broken up into two main categories, cardiac specific markers and markers of end organ perfusion. For cardiac specific markers, we look at proBNP (precursor to B-natriuretic peptide [BNP]) and troponin. For markers of end organ perfusion, we look at lactate (for tissue perfusion), liver function tests (for congestive hepatopathy), and renal function (for renal perfusion and congestion).

BNP and proBNP are peptides released by overstretched myocardium. These markers are elevated in the setting of decompensated heart failure or cardiogenic shock. They have high sensitivity and a strong negative predictive value.

Troponin is an enzyme released by damaged cardiomyocytes and its rise is positively correlated with the extent of cardiac damage. As such, it is an important marker to check given that the majority of acute cardiogenic shock is likely ischemic in origin. It is important to note that, while an individual measurement may be important, trending troponin value until its peak gives valuable information in regards to the extent of myocardial injury.

BASIC SCIENCE PEARL—STEP 1

Troponin I, as opposed to Troponin-T, is more cardiac-specific. Troponin I levels start rising 4–8 hours after the initial insult; it will peak at 12 hours. Troponin levels are often trended every few hours until their peak.

Blood urea nitrogen (BUN), creatinine (Cr), and urine output can serve as surrogate of renal organ perfusion in the setting of cardiogenic shock. It is important to note that renal dysfunction in cardiogenic shock can happen via two independent pathophysiological processes. One mechanism is decreased cardiac contractility and output causing low forward flow and renal hypoperfusion. The other is increased venous stasis due to the back up of fluid, causing renal venous congestion.

Similarly, congestion can occur in the liver as well, causing a rise in the liver function tests (LFTs); bilirubin usually rises first, followed by a delayed hepatocellular pattern, which is characterized by rise in aspartate aminotransferase (AST) and alanine aminotransferase (ALT) values.

An exception is if the patient develops "shock liver", in which case, a severe, but isolated, hepatocellular pattern can be seen on lab values.

Tissue hypoperfusion and high peripheral tissue oxygen demand during cardiogenic shock will cause rising lactic acid levels due to dependence on anaerobic metabolism.

> Your other labs finally return and are concerning for elevated Cr, elevated lactate, and elevated liver function tests. The patient is not making urine, and the pro-BNP is elevated. You conclude based on the above findings that your patient's cardiogenic shock is associated with fluid overload and congestion and that you would like to diurese the patient even though the blood pressure is low.

Why is volume overload a complicating factor in cardiogenic shock?
Patients with cardiogenic shock or heart failure are prone to excessive stretch of the myocardial fibers, resulting in less effective contractility, further propagating decompesation. This is the basis for the Frank-Starling curve (Fig. 38.6).

> However, while discussing the case with other physicians on call, there is ongoing debate and disagreement regarding the etiology of shock, as patient had erythema in lower extremities which might be suggestive of cellulitis.

What other modalities do you have to evaluate for cardiogenic shock?
The main form of invasive evaluation is a pulmonary artery catheter (PAC or Swan-Ganz catheter) (Table 38.2). The main use of PAC is in patients with unclear etiology of shock or mixed

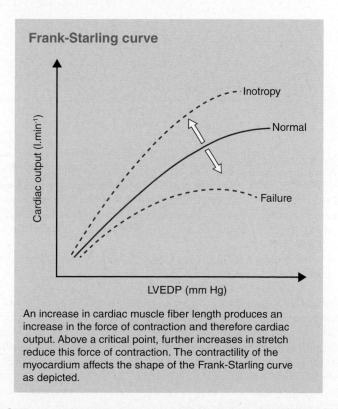

An increase in cardiac muscle fiber length produces an increase in the force of contraction and therefore cardiac output. Above a critical point, further increases in stretch reduce this force of contraction. The contractility of the myocardium affects the shape of the Frank-Starling curve as depicted.

Fig. 38.6   Frank-Starling curve. (*Anaesthesia and Intensive Care Medicine, Vol. 19.* Elsevier.)

TABLE 38.2 ■ The Standard Ranges for Pressures Measured Via Swan-Ganz Catheter

Measurements	Normal Range	Significance
Central Venous Pressure	2–10 mm Hg	Elevated values indicate either volume overload or right-sided obstructive process
Pulmonary Arterial Pressure	15–25 mm Hg	Elevated values indicate either volume overload, pulmonary hypertension, or left-sided heart failure
Capillary Wedge Pressure	6–15 mm Hg	Surrogate number for left ventricular end diastolic pressure. Elevations indicate volume overload or left-sided failure
Cardiac Output	Variable	Calculated via thermodilution versus Fick method to approximate stroke volume and heart rate calculation
Cardiac Index	2.5–4.2 L/min/m^2	Cardiac output divided by body surface area which helps normalize the values. Decreased values indicate heart failure, severe valvular regurgitation, or pulmonary hypertension

TABLE 38.3 ■ Pulmonary Artery Catheterization Interpretation

	CVP	PAP	PAWP	CO	SVRI
Hypovolemic	↓	↓	↓	↓	↑
Cardiogenic	↑	↑	↑	↓	↑
Distributive	↓	↓	↓	↑	↓
Obstructive					
— PE	↑	↑	↓	↓	↑
— Tamponade	↑	↑	↑	↓	↑

CO, Cardiac output; *CVP*, central venous pressure; *PAP*, pulmonary artery pressure; *PAWP*, pulmonary artery wedge pressure; *SVRI*, systemic vascular resistance index

shock (i.e., cardiogenic and septic shock). This catheter can measure the central venous pressure (CVP), right atrial pressures (RAP), pulmonary artery pressure (PAP), and pulmonary artery wedge pressure (PAWP), which is an approximation of the left atrial pressure. The PAC is useful because it can also obtain information regarding the cardiac output (CO) and cardiac index (CI), either by utilizing the Fick's method (calculated based on the difference between arterial and mixed venous blood oxygen) or thermodilution (calculated through differences in temperature of infused saline) (Table 38.3).

It should be noted that the main objective of PAC evaluation is not diagnosis but clarification of etiology of shock.

A PAC is placed and cardiogenic shock is higher on the differential given the hemodynamic measurements. What are the next steps in management in regard to this patient's cardiogenic shock?

In this scenario, with elevated troponins and new cardiogenic shock, patient was diagnosed with a NSTEMI (non ST elevation acute coronary event). The initial management includes stabilization of the patient, which includes aspirin and heparin for antiplatelet and anticoagulation for antithrombotic therapy, nitroglycerin for pain, diuresis for volume optimization, and he should undergo coronary angiogram within 24 hours.

CLINICAL PEARL—STEP 2/3

In the setting of a STEMI, the management is different. The goal is to revascularize as soon as possible. The goal is for percutaneous intervention (PCI) within a 120-minute window. If PCI is unavailable and the patient presents within 12 h of initial symptoms, thrombolytics should be given within 30 minutes from presentation, and then the patient should be transferred to a PCI capable center.

The patient is taken for coronary angiogram, which showed three vessel coronary artery disease. No PCI was performed, and patient was referred for possible coronary artery bypass graft (CABG). However, in the meantime, despite the initial aggressive diuretic use, our patient continued to have decreased urine output.

There is a concern for continued cardiogenic shock. What is the next best intervention?
Patients may not recover adequate tissue perfusion even after initial supportive care. If the patient has continued cardiogenic shock, starting vasopressors or inotropes is crucial to restore adequate tissue perfusion. The first-line agent for patients in shock is norepinephrine as it has both α_1 (vasoconstriction) and β_1 (inotropic) activity. However, in the setting of cardiogenic shock with decreased cardiac output, inotropes should be initiated to support the cardiac function. The most common agents include dobutamine and milrinone. These two agents act via different mechanisms; however, the net effect is that there is increase in β_1 activity as well as vasodilatory effect, which results in decreased afterload. Another agent that is often used is epinephrine, which is a potent β_1 agonist. Epinephrine does, however, provide some vasoconstriction, which may increase afterload.

Dobutamine and epinephrine are both added and titrated up; however, despite this, patient's lactate continue to rise and urine output is still low.

At this time, what other modalities do we have to support this patient in the setting of cardiogenic shock?
If the above interventions are not sufficient to stabilize the patient, temporary mechanical devices could be used. The most basic mechanical device is an intra-aortic balloon pump (IABP), which is favorable given its familiarity with its widespread use. The main advantages of IABP are a decrease in the left ventricular afterload and improvement of coronary artery and brain perfusion. The balloon is inserted via an artery (most commonly femoral) and advanced upstream to be positioned in the proximal portions of the descending aorta. The balloon inflation is synchronized with cardiac rhythm and inflates during diastole, displacing the blood both distally towards abdominal organs and lower extremities but, more importantly, proximally towards the coronary arteries and brain. Subsequently, it deflates during the systole and reduces the left ventricular afterload. It is estimated that it provides around 0.5 to 1.0 L/min of support to the CO.

The IABP is perfect to increase coronary perfusion; however, as mentioned earlier, its support in terms of CO is quite minimal. If more support is needed, an impella device can be considered.

Impella is another mechanical device commonly used in patients with cardiogenic shock. In simplistic terms, it is a catheter that is positioned with one part in the left ventricle and the other part in the ascending aorta. The portion in the left ventricle has an inlet that draws blood and propels it out through the outlet that is sitting in the ascending aorta. It has variable amount of support depending on the size, with Impella CP providing 2.5-4 L/min cardiac output whilst the Impella 5.0/5.5 can provide up to 5.0 or 6.0 L/min flow. The advantage of the Impella is the ability to generate significant cardiac output to augment a failing heart. There are considerable drawbacks to an Impella, including necessitating anticoagulation given the high risk of thrombosis, hemolysis, and stroke. Sometimes, an Impella is contraindicated (LV thrombus) or there is continued cardiogenic shock despite Impella support. In these scenarios, patients can be placed on veno-arterial extracorporeal membrane oxygenation devices (ECMO). ECMO is a form of cardiopulmonary bypass that is achieved via large cannulas that draw blood from the patient, circulate through a membrane oxygenator to perform gas exchange, and ultimately return back to the patient through the arterial system. ECMO is often used as a bridge to more durable left ventricular assist devices or even heart transplantation.

Our patient was eventually placed on mechanical circulatory support with an intra-aortic balloon pump. He was optimized from a volume standpoint via diuresis, responding well with a continuous infusion of loop diuretic. Afterwards, he was successfully weaned off IABP, and he underwent CABG for his coronary artery disease. He was eventually discharged and followed up with cardiothoracic surgery and cardiology as an outpatient.

Case Summary

- **Complaint/History:** A 66-year-old man presented to the emergency department with, generalized discomfort, palpitations, and shortness of breath.
- **Findings:** Clinical signs of cardiogenic shock, TWI on ECG, decreased left ventricular function on point of care ultrasound
- **Lab Results/Tests:** elevated troponin, elevated lactic acid, triple vessel disease on coronary angiogram

Diagnosis: Cardiogenic shock due to ischemic cardiomyopathy

- **Treatment:** Initial inotropic and vasopressor support, diuresis, eventual upgrade to mechanical support with IABP, and ultimately bridged to three vessel CABG.

BEYOND THE PEARLS

- Early presentation of left main coronary artery (LMCA) stenosis syndrome can present with specific ECG findings: ST elevation in aVR ≥1 mm; ST depression in leads I, II, aVL, and V4-6; ST elevation in aVR ≥V1.
- Unlike ST elevations, ST depressions are less specific and cannot be used to localize infarcts.
- In patients presenting with **prior** LBBB on ECG or paced rhythm with suspicion for ischemia, Modified Sgarbossa Criteria should be used:
  a) ≥1 lead with ≥1 mm of concordant ST elevation (STE in the same direction as the QRS complex)
  b) ≥1 lead of V1–V3 with ≥1 mm of concordant ST depression
  c) ≥1 lead anywhere with ≥1 mm proportionally excessive discordant STE, as defined by ≥25% of the depth of the preceding S-wave
- Although not discussed in this case, one etiology of cardiogenic shock can be acute valvular compromise, such as acute mitral valve regurgitation, which requires surgical intervention. A cardiothoracic surgery consultation should be obtained.
- Bedside POCUS can also identify a pericardial effusion in most views but is best appreciated in the PLAX. Large effusions or quick accumulation of pericardial fluid can cause tamponade physiology and shock.
- Using the POCUS we can also approximate CO by using continuous-wave Doppler. This technique, (called LVOT/VTI measurement) uses transaortic flow on A4C and aortic root diameter on PLAX to approximate the stroke volume (and CO when multiplied with HR).
- Any clinical scenario that causes elevated intrathoracic/intra-abdominal pressures, or backward blood flow/pressure directed towards the IVC, could cause false results in an

evaluation of the IVC (i.e. tricuspid or pulmonary valve regurgitation, portal hypertension, pulmonary hypertension, high positive pressure mechanical ventilation).
- There are many false positive and false negative etiologies for the BNP or ProBNP. Patients with severe pulmonary disease, renal dysfunction, supraventricular arrhythmias, and advanced age can have elevated and "smoldering" BNP values. Patients taking sacubitril/valsartan, a first-line agent for heart failure treatment, will also have elevated BNP levels (but not proBNP) as sacubitril inhibits the enzyme that cleaves BNP. Finally, obese patients may present with falsely decreased BNP levels.
- Hyponatremia is a poor prognosticating factor in patients with heart failure.
- Despite low blood pressure in cardiogenic shock, certain vasopressors should be used with caution. For example, a pure α_1 agonist such as phenylephrine would be a suboptimal choice, as vasoconstriction will increase afterload, which worsens cardiogenic shock.

References

Al-Khalisy, H., Nikiforov, I., Jhajj, M., Kodali, N., & Cheriyath, P. (2015). A widened pulse pressure: A potential valuable prognostic indicator of mortality in patients with sepsis. *Journal of Community Hospital Internal Medicine Perspectives*, 5(6), 29426. Published 2015 Dec 11.

Avolio, A. P., Kuznetsova, T., Heyndrickx, G. R., Kerkhof, P. L., & Li, J. K. J. (2018). Arterial flow, pulse pressure and pulse wave velocity in men and women at various ages. *Advances in Experimental Medicine and Biology*, 1065, 153–168. https://doi.org/10.1007/978-3-319-77932-4_10. PMID: 30051383.

Basir, M. B., Schreiber, T., Dixon, S., Alaswad, K., Patel, K., Almany, S., et al. (2018). Feasibility of early mechanical circulatory support in acute myocardial infarction complicated by cardiogenic shock: The Detroit cardiogenic shock initiative. *Catheterization and Cardiovascular Interventions*, 91(3), 454–461.

Bradley, T. D., Holloway, R. M., McLaughlin, P. R., Ross, B. L., Walters, J., & Liu, P. P. (1992). Cardiac output response to continuous positive airway pressure in congestive heart failure. *The American Review of Respiratory Disease*, 145(2 Pt 1), 377–382.

Charlesworth, M., & Knowles, A. (2018). Control of cardiac function *Anaesthesia and Intensive Care Medicine* (19, pp. 308–313). Elsevier.

Çinar, T., Hayiroglu, M. I., Seker, M., Dogan, S., Çiçek, V., Öz, A., et al. (2019). The predictive value of age, creatinine, ejection fraction score for in-hospital mortality in patients with cardiogenic shock. *Coronary Artery Disease*, 30(8), 569–574.

De Backer, D., Biston, P., Devriendt, J., Madl, C., Chochrad, D., Aldecoa, C., et al. (2010). Comparison of dopamine and norepinephrine in the treatment of shock. *New England Journal of Medicine*, 362(9), 779–789.

Dhawan, I., Makhija, N., Choudhury, M., & Choudhury, A. (2019). Modified tricuspid annular plane systolic excursion for assessment of right ventricular systolic function. *Journal of Cardiovascular Imaging*, 27(1), 24–33. https://doi.org/10.4250/jcvi.2019.27.e8.

Dünser, M. W., Mayr, A. J., Ulmer, H., Knotzer, H., Sumann, G., Pajk, W., et al. (2003). Arginine vasopressin in advanced vasodilatory shock: A prospective, randomized, controlled study. *Circulation*, 107(18), 2313–2319.

Fincke, R., Hochman, J. S., Lowe, A. M., Menon, V., Slater, J. N., Webb, J. G., et al. (2004). SHOCK Investigators. Cardiac power is the strongest hemodynamic correlate of mortality in cardiogenic shock: A report from the SHOCK trial registry. *Journal of the American College of Cardiology*, 44(2), 340–348.

Furtado, S., & Reis, L. (2019). Inferior vena cava evaluation in fluid therapy decision making in intensive care: Practical implications. Avaliação da veia cava inferior na decisão de fluidoterapia em cuidados intensivos: Implicações práticas. *Revista Brasileira de terapia intensiva*, 31(2), 240–247. https://doi.org/10.5935/0103-507X.20190039.

Garg, P., Morris, P., Fazlanie, A. L., Vijayan, S., Dancso, B., Dastidar, A. G., et al. (2017). Cardiac biomarkers of acute coronary syndrome: From history to high-sensitivity cardiac troponin. *Internal and Emergency Medicine*, 12(2), 147–155.

Hochman, J. S. (2003). Cardiogenic shock complicating acute myocardial infarction: Expanding the paradigm. *Circulation*, 107, 2998–3002.

Jacobs, A. K., French, J. K., Col, J., Sleeper, L. A., Slater, J. N., Carnendran, L., et al. (2000). Cardiogenic shock with non-ST-segment elevation myocardial infarction: A report from the SHOCK Trial Registry. *Journal of the American College of Cardiology*, 36(3S1), 1091–1096.

Jäntti, T., Tarvasmäki, T., Harjola, V. P., Parissis, J., Pulkki, K., Sionis, A., et al. (2017). Frequency and prognostic significance of abnormal liver function tests in patients with cardiogenic shock. *The American Journal of Cardiology*, *120*(7), 1090–1097.

Kubiak, G. M., Ciarka, A., Biniecka, M., & Ceranowicz, P. (2019). Right heart catheterization—background, physiological basics, and clinical implications. *Journal of Clinical Medicine*, *8*(9), 1331.

Lambrechts, L., & Fourie, B. (2020). How to interpret an electrocardiogram in children. *BJA Education*, *20*(8), 266–277. https://doi.org/10.1016/j.bjae.2020.03.009.

Levitov, A., Frankel, H. L., Blaivas, M., Kirkpatrick, A. W., Su, E., Evans, D., et al. (2016). Guidelines for the appropriate use of bedside general and cardiac ultrasonography in the evaluation of critically ill patients—part II: Cardiac ultrasonography. *Critical Care Medicine*, *44*(6), 1206–1227. https://doi.org/10.1097/CCM.0000000000001847.

Masip, J., Peacock, W. F., Price, S., Cullen, L., Martin-Sanchez, F. J., Seferovic, P., et al. (2018). Indications and practical approach to non-invasive ventilation in acute heart failure. *European Heart Journal*, *39*(1), 17–25.

McKaigney, C. J., Krantz, M. J., La Rocque, C. L., Hurst, N. D., Buchanan, M. S., & Kendall, J. L. (2014). E-point septal separation: A bedside tool for emergency physician assessment of left ventricular ejection fraction. *The American Journal of Emergency Medicine*, *32*(6), 493–497. https://doi.org/10.1016/j.ajem.2014.01.045.

Menon, V., Slater, J. N., White, H. D., Sleeper, L. A., Cocke, T., & Hochman, J. S. (2000). Acute myocardial infarction complicated by systemic hypoperfusion without hypotension: report of the SHOCK trial registry. *The American Journal of Medicine*, *108*(5), 374–380. https://doi.org/10.1016/S0002-9343(00)00310-7.

Moon, J. C., Perez De Arenaza, D., Elkington, A. G., Taneja, A. K., John, A. S., Wang, D., et al. (2004). The pathologic basis of Q-wave and non-Q-wave myocardial infarction: A cardiovascular magnetic resonance study. *Journal of the American College of Cardiology*, *44*(3), 554–560.

Mueller, C., McDonald, K., de Boer, R. A., Maisel, A., Cleland, J. G., Kozhuharov, N., et al. (2019). Heart Failure Association of the European Society of Cardiology practical guidance on the use of natriuretic peptide concentrations. *European Journal of Heart Failure*, *21*(6), 715–731.

Myhre, P. L., Vaduganathan, M., Claggett, B., Packer, M., Desai, A. S., Rouleau, J. L., et al. (2019, March 26). B-type natriuretic peptide during treatment with sacubitril/valsartan: The PARADIGM-HF trial. *Journal of the American College of Cardiology*, *73*(11), 1264–1272. https://doi.org/10.1016/j.jacc.2019.01.018.

Nativi-Nicolau, J., Selzman, C. H., Fang, J. C., & Stehlik, J. (2014). Pharmacologic therapies for acute cardiogenic shock. *Current Opinion in Cardiology*, *29*(3), 250–257.

Nguyen, H. B., Banta, D. P., Stewart, G., Kim, T., Bansal, R., Anholm, J., et al. (2010). Cardiac index measurements by transcutaneous Doppler ultrasound and transthoracic echocardiography in adult and pediatric emergency patients. *Journal of Clinical Monitoring and Computing*, *24*(3), 237–247.

O'gara, P. T., Kushner, F. G., Ascheim, D. D., Casey, D. E., Chung, M. K., De Lemos, J. A., et al. (2013). 2013 ACCF/AHA guideline for the management of ST-elevation myocardial infarction: A report of the American College of Cardiology Foundation/American Heart Association Task Force on Practice Guidelines. *Journal of the American College of Cardiology*, *61*(4), e78–e140.

Parikh, K. S., Agarwal, R., Mehrotra, A. K., & Swamy, R. S. (2012). Wellens syndrome: A life-saving diagnosis. *The American Journal of Emergency Medicine*, *30*(1), 255.e3–3255.e5. https://doi.org/10.1016/j.ajem.2010.10.014

Picano, E., Frassi, F., Agricola, E., Gligorova, S., Gargani, L., & Mottola, G. (2006). Ultrasound lung comets: A clinically useful sign of extravascular lung water. *Journal of the American Society of Echocardiography*, *19*(3), 356–363.

Polyzogopoulou, E., Arfaras-Melainis, A., Bistola, V., & Parissis, J. (2020). Inotropic agents in cardiogenic shock. *Current Opinion in Critical Care*, *26*(4), 403–410.

Ponikowski, P., Voors, A. A., Anker, S. D., Bueno, H., Cleland, J. G. F., Coats, A. J. S., et al. (2016). 2016 ESC guidelines for the diagnosis and treatment of acute and chronic heart failure: The Task Force for the diagnosis and treatment of acute and chronic heart failure of the European Society of Cardiology (ESC). Developed with the special contribution of the Heart Failure Association (HFA) of the ESC. *European Heart Journal*, *37*(27), 2129–2200.

Prondzinsky, R., Unverzagt, S., Lemm, H., Wegener, N. A., Schlitt, A., Heinroth, K. M., et al. (2012). Interleukin-6, -7, -8, and -10 predict outcomes in acute myocardial infarction complicated by cardiogenic shock. *Clinical Research in Cardiology*, *101*(5), 375–384.

Rahulkumar, H. H., Bhavin, P. R., Shreyas, K. P., Krunalkumar, H. P., Atulkumar, S., & Bansari, C. (2019). Utility of point-of-care ultrasound in differentiating causes of shock in resource-limited setup. *Journal of Emergencies, Trauma, and Shock, 12*(1), 10.

Rakočević, R., Thomas, R., & Oriscello, R. G. (2020, February 28). Clinical dilemma—cardiac memory vs myocardial ischemia. *Cureus, 12*(2), e7129. https://doi.org/10.7759/cureus.7129.

Rovai, D., Di Bella, G., Rossi, G., Lombardi, M., Aquaro, G. D., L'Abbate, A., et al. (2007). Q-wave prediction of myocardial infarct location, size and transmural extent at magnetic resonance imaging. *Coronary Artery Disease, 18*(5), 381–389.

Sen, F., Ozeke, O., Kirbas, O., Burak, C., Kafes, H., Tak, B. T., et al. (2016). Classical electrocardiographic clues for left main coronary artery disease. *Indian Heart Journal, 68*(Suppl 2), S226–S227. https://doi.org/10.1016/j.ihj.2016.03.025.

Sequeira, V., & van der Velden, J. (2015). Historical perspective on heart function: The Frank-Starling Law. *Biophysical Reviews, 7*(4), 421–447.

Smith, S. W., Dodd, K. W., Henry, T. D., Dvorak, D. M., & Pearce, L. A. (2012, December). Diagnosis of ST-elevation myocardial infarction in the presence of left bundle branch block with the ST-elevation to S-wave ratio in a modified Sgarbossa rule. *Annals of Emergency Medicine, 60*(6), 766–776. https://doi.org/10.1016/j.annemergmed.2012.07.119. Erratum in: (2013). *Annals of Emergency Medicine, 62*(4), 302.

Thygesen, K., Alpert, J. S., & Jaffe, A. S. (2012, October 16). Third universal definition of myocardial infarction. *Circulation, 126*(16), 2020–2035. https://doi.org/10.1161/CIR.0b013e31826e1058.

Vahdatpour, C., Collins, D., & Goldberg, S. (2019). Cardiogenic shock. *Journal of the American Heart Association, 8*(8), e011991. https://doi.org/10.1161/JAHA.119.011991.

van Diepen, S., Katz, J. N., Albert, N. M., Henry, T. D., Jacobs, A. K., Kapur, N. K., et al. (2017). Contemporary management of cardiogenic shock: A scientific statement from the American Heart Association. *Circulation, 136*(16), e232–e268.

Wellens, H. J. J., & Conover, M. B. (1992). *The ECG in emergency decision making* (pp. 32). St Louis: WB Saunders Company.

A 53-Year-Old Man With Two Weeks of Progressive Abdominal Pain

Ammar Dahodwala ■ Ben Cantrill ■ Patrick Chan ■ Raj Dasgupta

A 53-year-old man presents to the emergency department with two weeks of progressive abdominal pain, which is located above his umbilicus. The pain is sharp, nonradiating, 8/10 intensity, and without any known alleviating or exacerbating factors. He also endorses lightheadedness, shortness of breath with exertion, and dark stools. He has not seen a physician in over 20 years and is unaware of any medical conditions he has. He reports a fall a few weeks ago that has left him with unrelenting left knee pain for which he takes several tablets of ibuprofen multiple times per day. He also drinks 6–10 cans of beers daily. On physical examination, pulse rate is 134 beats per minute, blood pressure is 76/51 mm Hg, respiration rate is 32 breaths per minute, and oxygen saturation is 92% on 3 L/min nasal cannula. There is diffuse tenderness to palpation over the epigastrium and digital rectal examination reveals melanotic stool. The remainder of exam is normal. Pertinent laboratory values include hemoglobin of 5.1 g/dL, platelet count of 53,000/μL, sodium of 125 mEq/L, creatinine of 3.4 mg/dL, total bilirubin of 3.2 mg/dL, and international normalized ratio (INR) of 1.69.

What type of shock is this patient presenting with?

The four major categories of shock are distributive, cardiogenic, obstructive, and hypovolemic. The patient in this case has likely hypovolemic hemorrhagic shock. Hemorrhagic shock is classified into four different classes based on the stages of hemorrhagic shock, which is described in Table 39.1. It allows the physician to triage the severity of the patient's volume loss and provide appropriate targeted therapy. Significant parameters to note are vital signs such as heart rate and blood pressure, as well as parameters of end-organ perfusion, which manifests clinically with urine output and mental status.

CLINICAL PEARL—STEP 2/3

Tachycardia can be one of the first signs of hemorrhagic shock. It is the body's compensatory mechanism for hypovolemia to maintain cardiac output.

How should this patient initially be managed?

If visible, direct pressure should be applied to the area of bleeding. If bleeding is not visible, then a Focused Assessment with Sonography in Trauma (FAST) exam should be performed to identify internal bleeding. The FAST exam includes (1) right upper quadrant view of the abdomen between the kidney and liver, (2) left upper quadrant view of the abdomen between the kidney and spleen, (3) suprapubic view, and (4) subxiphoid cardiac view. The extended FAST (eFAST) exam includes lung windows to assess for pneumothorax as well as hemothorax. An example of a FAST exam is shown in Fig. 39.1, demonstrating free fluid in the abdomen, which is abnormal. Next, two large-bore intravenous (IV) lines (16 gauge or larger) should be placed immediately for

TABLE 39.1 ■ **Classes of Hemorrhagic Presentations Per American College of Surgeons Advanced Trauma Life Support (ATLS)[4]**

	Class I	Class II	Class III	Class IV
Blood loss (mL)	Up to 750	750–1000	1500–2000	>2000
Blood loss (% blood volume)	Up to 15%	15–30%	30–40%	>40%
Pulse rate (bpm)	<100	100–120	120–140	>140
Systolic blood pressure (mm Hg)	Normal	Normal	Decreased	Decreased
Pulse pressure (mm Hg)	Normal or increased	Decreased	Decreased	Decreased
Respiratory rate	14–20	20–30	30–40	>35
Urine output (mL/h)	>30	20–30	5–15	Negligible
Mental status	Slightly anxious	Mildly anxious	Anxious, confused	Confused, lethargic

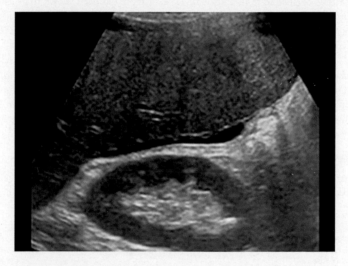

Fig. 39.1 Example of positive FAST with fluid in the hepatorenal recess (also known as Morrison pouch) (*Radiology of Infectious Diseases*, April 10, 2018.)

the administration of volume replacement. Larger lumen diameter and shorter catheter length IVs allow for faster infusion rates.

BASIC SCIENCE PEARL—STEP 1

Poiseuille's law in fluid dynamics is the basis for large diameter and shorter catheters for rapid infusions. The law states that flow through a cylindrical pipe is proportional to the radius to the fourth power and inversely proportional to the length.

CLINICAL PEARL—STEP 2/3

It is vital to remember that retroperitoneal bleeds are not readily identifiable with a FAST exam. A computed tomography (CT) scan must be obtained instead.

In regard to targets for resuscitation, patients should be resuscitated to a goal hemoglobin level of 7 g/dL. If the patient is hemodynamically unstable or copious bleeding continues, transfusion goals can be increased. In a landmark trial of relatively hemodynamically stable patients with an upper gastrointestinal bleed, those randomized to a lower transfusion threshold of 7 g/dL compared to 9 g/dL had improved mortality at 6 weeks. Patients with cirrhosis (Child-Pugh Class A and B) in particular had improved mortality.

CLINICAL PEARL—STEP 2/3

For patients in acute hemorrhage, hemoglobin levels may not be reflective as it takes time to equilibrate. Thus, for a hemodynamically unstable patient for which there is high suspicion of hemorrhage, transfusions should be given empirically until the patient has been stabilized. Frequent laboratory checks may be necessary to confirm the suspicion for hemorrhage.

As this patient is presenting with hemorrhagic shock, he should be resuscitated with blood products. Healthcare providers must be cautious with resuscitation via crystalloid solutions as these solutions can exacerbate bleeding by diluting out the patient's clotting factors. In the emergency department setting, crystalloid resuscitation of 1.5 L or more has been shown to be associated with increased mortality in trauma patients. The foundation of massive transfusion protocols (MTP) is to administer packed red blood cells (PRBCs), platelets, and fresh frozen plasma (FFP) in equivalent ratios. Typical MTPs will utilize a 1 PRBC:1 FFP:1 platelet ratio.

Given the risk of coagulopathy, what laboratory studies are available to assess coagulopathy?
The standard measurements of coagulopathy include measuring the prothrombin time (PT), partial thromboplastin time (PTT), and fibrinogen level. If the PT and PTT are prolonged, FFP may be administered to correct coagulopathy. If the fibrinogen level is low, cryoprecipitate, which contains only certain concentrated factors, may be administered.

BASIC SCIENCE PEARL—STEP 1

PT measures the extrinsic pathway for coagulation, which is dependent on factor VII. PTT measures the intrinsic pathway for coagulation, which measures factors XII, XI, VIII, and IX.

BASIC SCIENCE PEARL—STEP 1

Factors I, II, V, and X are part of the common pathway for coagulation.

BASIC SCIENCE PEARL—STEP 1

Von Willebrand factor, factor VIII, fibrinogen, and factor XIII are components that make up cryoprecipitate.

Furthermore, in addition to measuring coagulation factors, thromboelastography (TEG) has emerged as an alternative method to analyze clotting ability in the critically ill patient. In particular, TEG measures clot strength, clot formation, and fibrinolysis simultaneously. TEG uses either a rotating pin (old) or vibration frequencies (new) to determine elasticity and strength of clotting, which is then depicted in a graphical format, as shown in Fig. 39.2.

There are several important measured parameters with TEG: reaction time to initiation of fibrin clot (R time), clot formation time (K time), alpha (α) angle, maximum amplitude (MA), and lysis time at 30 minutes (LY-30).

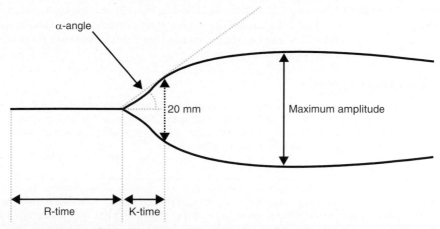

Fig. 39.2 A sample thromboelastography tracing. R-time is reaction time to initiation of a fibrin clot, clot formation time (K-time), alpha (α) angle (rate of fibrin cross-linking), maximum amplitude (MA, the maximum strength of the clot), and lysis time at 30 minutes (LY-30) (*International Journal of Obstetric Anesthesia, U.S. National Library of Medicine.*)

Clinically, a long R-time implies that it is taking a long time to initiate the fibrin clot, which is dependent on the clotting factors. Thus, plasma should be considered in patients with high R-time. Alpha angle and K value are surrogates for a rate of clot formation after the clotting process has initiated, which reflects the function of fibrinogen, as fibrinogen cross-linking is necessary to stabilize the clot. If the alpha angle is low or the K value is high, cryoprecipitate should be administered as it contains concentrated fibrinogen. The MA, which represents the strength of the clot, is dependent on platelet count and function. If the MA is low there is a platelet deficiency or decrease in platelet function, preventing the formation of a "strong" clot. In that scenario, platelets and desmopressin (DDAVP) should be considered. LY-30 is a measurement of clot breakdown or fibrinolysis. For patients with high LY-30, there is concern for hyperfibrinolysis or increased clot breakdown. To decrease clot lysis, an antifibrinolytic such as tranexamic acid or aminocaproic acid should be considered.

CLINICAL PEARL—STEP 2/3

One randomized trial of 111 patients with either TEG-directed transfusion or conventional coagulation assay-directed transfusion found that the risk of death was lower in the TEG-directed transfusion group (19.6%) versus standard conventional coagulation assay directed transfusion (36.4%) at 28 days.

What is your differential diagnosis for hemorrhagic shock?

The differential diagnosis for a patient presenting with hemorrhagic shock is wide. It is important to consider all possibilities prior to narrowing your differential based on the patient's history and physical exam. Common etiologies for hemorrhagic shock include medication use, coagulopathies, gastrointestinal bleeding, obstetric or gynecologic bleeding, pulmonary hemorrhage, ruptured aneurysms, retroperitoneal bleeding, and trauma. In this case, the patient's history and exam can focus the differential diagnosis on medication use and gastrointestinal bleeding. Medication use in this patient encompasses his recent non-steroidal anti-inflammatory drugs (NSAID) use secondary to his left knee pain. This patient also has significant drinking history; therefore, bleeding esophageal varices is also on the differential. Gastrointestinal bleeding in this patient can be subdivided into upper gastrointestinal bleeding (UGIB) and lower gastrointestinal bleeding (LGIB). In the setting of melena, UGIB is more likely. As such, specific etiologies for UGIB include: esophageal varices, esophagogastric mucosal tears (Mallory-Weiss), peptic ulcer disease, gastritis, and gastric/esophageal malignancy.

CLINICAL PEARL—STEP 2/3

In patients with bright red blood per rectum, it can be difficult to differentiate from brisk upper gastrointestinal bleeding versus lower gastrointestinal bleeding. In this setting, if there is hemodynamic instability, the concern for brisk upper gastrointestinal bleeding increases significantly and prompt evaluation should be performed.

After initial resuscitation in the emergency department, the patient is admitted to the medical intensive care unit (ICU) with a diagnosis of hemorrhagic shock. He received an MTP where he was transfused 6 units packed RBC, 6 units of FFP, and 6 units of platelets. Repeat hemoglobin level at 7.6 g/dL. He undergoes an emergent endoscopy with the on-call gastroenterology team. They found an actively bleeding gastric ulcer for which 2 clips were deployed endoscopically to achieve hemostasis. Characteristic images are seen in Fig. 39.3.

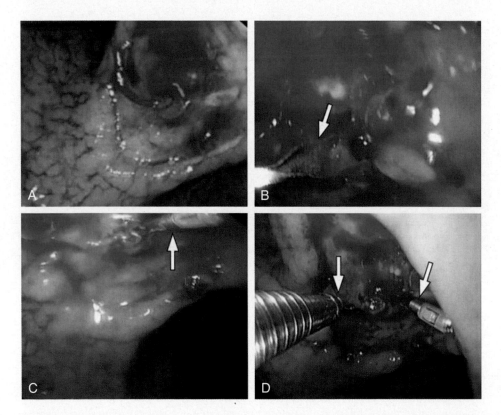

Fig. 39.3 Endoscopy of bleeding gastric ulcer. (A) A bleeding gastric ulcer at the angular notch. (B) An endoscopic clip was applied tangentially. (C) The first clip secured hemostasis, which stopped bleeding. (D) A second clip was then added. The clips are indicated by the white arrows. (*Lancet (London, England), U.S. National Library of Medicine.*)

Following the endoscopic intervention, the patient's hemoglobin begins to rise and stabilize. The ICU team deems him medically stable to transfer to the floors the following morning. While on the General Internal Medicine service, a right upper quadrant ultrasound reveals advanced cirrhosis.

Which patient populations are at higher risk of developing coagulopathy?

After clinical stabilization, it is important to identify the underlying etiology of the patient's non-traumatic hypovolemic hemorrhagic shock in order to provide targeted therapy and prevent a recurrence. There are numerous etiologies for coagulopathy that have been identified. They are divided into inherited and acquired causes. Inherited causes for coagulopathy include genetic disorders such as Von Willebrand disease or hemophilia. Examples of acquired causes of coagulopathy include chronic liver disease, chronic kidney disease, disseminated intravascular coagulopathy, vitamin K deficiency, medication-induced, and the development of circulating anticoagulants. In all of these examples, there is a shared dysfunction of platelets and/or the clotting cascade. In this case, the patient presents with two risk factors for developing coagulopathy. His NSAID use prevents the patient from forming a stable platelet plug and the patient's cirrhosis predisposes him to thrombocytopenia and decreased circulating clotting factors. Both of these acquired risk factors contribute to the patient's initial hemorrhagic shock presentation.

CLINICAL PEARL—STEP 2/3

There are other medications that contribute to platelet dysfunction or coagulopathy that should be reversed during acute hemorrhage. Table 39.2 below lists common etiologies and notable reversal agents.

On hospital day #2, the patient begins to endorse shortness of breath at rest. You obtain a bedside chest x-ray with the findings shown in Fig. 39.4.

Which patient populations are at higher risk of developing complications from aggressive fluid resuscitation?

In patients who are presenting with hemorrhagic shock, the primary objective is to locate the bleed while at the same time maintaining intravascular volume. However, care must be taken with intravascular volume resuscitation in certain patient populations. These populations include but are not limited to patients with chronic liver disease, heart failure, and chronic kidney disease. In each of these disease states, the patient is unable to regulate their intravascular volume to the same degree as the general population. In this context, these patients are more vulnerable to over-resuscitation.

Consequences of over-resuscitation include pulmonary edema, lower extremity edema, exacerbation of heart failure, or even abdominal compartment syndrome.

TABLE 39.2 ■ **Common Drugs Involved in Hemorrhage and Reversal Agents**

Drug	Reversal Agent
Aspirin	Desmopressin (DDAVP)
Coumadin	Fresh frozen plasma, 3 or 4 factor prothrombin complex concentrate (PCC), Vitamin K
Anti-factor Xa inhibitors, such as rivaroxaban, apixaban	Andexanet alfa
Dabigatran	Idarucizumab

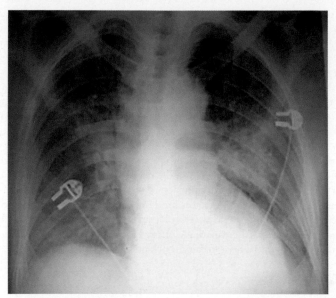

Fig. 39.4   Chest x-ray showing pulmonary edema. (*Radiologic Clinics of North America, Elsevier, September 24, 2008.*)

With IV diuresis, he returns to his baseline state of health. Patient was also concomitantly diagnosed with cirrhosis based on laboratory findings and imaging findings. He is discharged from the hospital with a diagnosis of hemorrhagic shock secondary to NSAID use complicated by cirrhosis. During his outpatient follow-up appointment 2 weeks postdischarge, he reports adherence to his medication regimen, no further bleeding episodes, and a desire to explore strategies toward sobriety.

Case Summary

- **Complaint/History:** 53-year old male with abdominal pain presenting with melena
- **Findings:** Hypotensive, tachycardic, in shock
- **Lab Results/Test:** Hemoglobin 5.1 g/dL, endoscopy with bleeding gastric ulcer

Diagnosis: Hemorrhagic shock secondary to bleeding gastric ulcer, course complicated by pulmonary edema from fluid resuscitation

- **Treatment:** Massive transfusion protocol, endoscopic clipping

BEYOND THE PEARLS

1. In the setting of trauma, there is a clinical triad of hypothermia, coagulopathy, and acidosis. Each component is interrelated, and when all of the findings are present, this results in progressive coagulopathy which results in further hemorrhage, ultimately leading to increased morbidity and mortality.
2. If the patient is in hemorrhagic shock but there is no obvious source of bleeding, one often overlooked area is the lower extremities, especially the thighs.
3. Blood products often contain citrate as an anticoagulant. With repeated transfusions, the citrate can bind to calcium, causing hypocalcemia. Serial calcium levels should be checked and repleted as necessary.

4. In patients with active hemorrhage, an empiric antifibrinolytic, such as tranexamic acid, can be given, especially if given early in the clinical course.
5. If a patient starts developing a distended, tense abdomen with little to no urine output after aggressive resuscitation, there should be high suspicion of abdominal compartment syndrome.
6. In a patient who has cirrhosis and has gastrointestinal bleeding, octreotide drip, proton pump inhibitor, and IV antibiotics should be initiated.
7. An introducer sheath, which is a short, wide diameter, single-lumen central venous catheter, is preferred for large volume transfusions given the ability of rapid infusion.
8. In a patient with a positive FAST, a diagnostic peritoneal lavage may be necessary to rule out intra-abdominal source of bleeding.

References

Rossaint, R., Bouillon, B., Cerny, V., Coats, T. J., Duranteau, J., Fernández-Mondéjar, E., et al. (2016). The European guideline on management of major bleeding and coagulopathy following trauma: fourth edition. *Critical Care, 20*(1), 100. https://doi.org/10.1186/s13054-016-1265-x.

Villanueva, C., Colomo, A., Bosch, A., Concepción, M., Hernandez-Gea, V., Aracil, C., et al. (2013). Transfusion strategies for acute upper gastrointestinal bleeding. *New England Journal of Medicine, 368*(24), 2341. https://doi.org/10.1056/nejmx130015.

Ley, E. J., Clond, M. A., Srour, M. K., Barnajian, M., Mirocha, J., Margulies, D. R., et al. (2011). Emergency department crystalloid resuscitation of 1.5 L or more is associated with increased mortality in elderly and nonelderly trauma patients. *Journal of Trauma: Injury, Infection & Critical Care, 70*(2), 398–400. https://doi.org/10.1097/ta.0b013e318208f99b.

Gutierrez, G., Reines, H. D., & Wulf-Gutierrez, M. E. (2004). Clinical review: Hemorrhagic shock. *Critical Care, 8*(5), 373. https://doi.org/10.1186/cc2851.

Gonzalez, E., Moore, E. E., Moore, H. B., Chapman, M. P., Chin, T. L., Ghasabyan, A., et al. (2016, June). Goal-directed hemostatic resuscitation of trauma-induced coagulopathy: A pragmatic randomized clinical trial comparing a viscoelastic assay to conventional coagulation assays. *Annals of Surgery, 263*(6), 1051–1059.

Kumar, K. R. D., & Halawar, R. S. (2018, April 10). Comparative study of ultrasound findings in seropositive pediatric and adult patients with dengue fever. *Radiology of Infectious Diseases*, No Longer Published by Elsevier. https://www.sciencedirect.com/science/article/pii/S2352621117300293.

Chow, L., Carr, A., MacKenzie, L., Walker, A., Archer, D., & Lee, A. (2016). The effect of dalteparin on thromboelastography in pregnancy: An in vitro study. *International Journal of Obstetric Anesthesia, 28*, 22–27. U.S. National Library of Medicine. https://pubmed.ncbi.nlm.nih.gov/27717636/.

Lau, J. Y., Barkun, A., Fan, D. M., Kuipers, E. J., Yang, Y. S., Chan, F. K. (2013). Challenges in the management of acute peptic ulcer bleeding. *Lancet (London, England), 381*(9882), 2033–2043. U.S. National Library of Medicine.

Bonomo, L., Larici, A. R., Maggi, F., Schiavon, F., & Berletti, R. (2008, September 24). Aging and the respiratory system. *Radiologic Clinics of North America, 46*(4), 685–702.

A 71-Year-Old Female With Dyspnea on Exertion

Curtis Maehara ■ Patrick Chan ■ Stuart Schroff ■ Raj Dasgupta

A 71-year-old female presents to the emergency department with 2 weeks of progressive weakness, dyspnea on exertion, and lower extremity edema. She denies any cough, hemoptysis, syncope, or diaphoresis. She lives in a board and care facility that provides assisted living. Her past medical history is significant for human immunodeficiency virus (HIV) on antiretroviral therapy (ART); hypothyroidism controlled by levothyroxine; atrial fibrillation on daily diltiazem, but not on home anticoagulation; chronic kidney disease stage 3B; hypertension; and diet-controlled type 2 diabetes mellitus. On physical examination, blood pressure is 109/66 mm Hg, pulse rate 68 beats per minute, respiration rate 17 breaths per minute, and oxygen saturation 99% on room air. Of note, the patient has been chronically debilitated and is now wheelchair-dependent. She has been noticing left greater than right lower extremity edema.

What are some causes of dyspnea?

Dyspnea is one of the most common chief complaints on presentation to the hospital. There are a multitude of infectious and noninfectious causes of dyspnea. Many infectious causes are generally associated with fever, leukocytosis, and possibly hemodynamic changes. These causes include bacterial, viral, or even subacute etiologies, such as fungal or mycobacterial infections. At the same time, noninfectious causes should be explored, including chronic obstructive pulmonary disease, interstitial lung disease, acute respiratory distress syndrome, chronic heart failure, and pulmonary emboli.

In general, when should you consider pulmonary embolism as a diagnosis?

Pulmonary embolism (PE) is a venous thromboembolism (VTE) causing blockage in the pulmonary arteries of the lungs. It requires a high index of suspicion in patients with the right risk factors to make the diagnosis. Patients often only present with dyspnea as their primary symptom. Occasionally, they can have associated chest pain, lower extremity edema, palpitations, lightheadedness, or dizziness. Patients can also develop more severe symptoms of hemoptysis and/or pleural rub, which are complications of pulmonary infarction.

History and physical exam should always be performed prior to diagnostic testing. Symptom onset can be acute or even subacute, depending on the severity and progression of disease. Once there is high suspicion for PE, a Wells' score can be utilized to assess the pretest probability for PE (Table 40.1). Wells' scores of greater than 4 were classified in the "likely" group and ≤4 in the "unlikely" group, with an overall incidence of PE of 37.1% and 12.1%, respectively. If PE is initially suspected, but the patient falls in the "unlikely" group, D-dimer should be ordered. If the D-dimer is positive, then a computed tomography pulmonary angiography (CTPA) should be obtained. If the D-dimer is negative, then consider stopping evaluation for PE given low pretest probability. If a patient falls in the "likely" group, a CTPA should be obtained for more accurate testing.

TABLE 40.1 ■ Original Wells' Score (Points) for Pulmonary Embolism

Clinical Characteristic	Score
Clinical signs of lower-extremity deep vein thrombosis	3
Alternative diagnosis less likely than pulmonary embolism	3
Heart rate > 100 beats/min	1.5
Surgery or immobilization within 4 weeks	1.5
Previously objectively diagnosed pulmonary embolism or deep vein thrombosis	1.5
Hemoptysis	1
Active cancer	1
Classification	
Pulmonary embolism unlikely	≤4
Pulmonary embolism likely	>4

CLINICAL PEARL—STEP 2/3

CTPA is minimally invasive and provides direct visualization of the pulmonary arteries, providing high sensitivity and specificity.

How do you categorize the severity of a pulmonary embolism?
PE is usually divided into three categories: low, intermediate, and high risk based on the likelihood for developing cardiovascular compromise, shock, or need for cardiopulmonary resuscitation. Patients can develop tissue hypoperfusion, hypoxia, metabolic or lactic acidosis, altered mental status, oliguria, or other signs of end organ damage. Hemodynamic compromise for massive PE includes a systolic blood pressure less than 90 mm Hg or a blood pressure drop of greater than 40 mm Hg lasting longer than 15 minutes or requiring vasopressors. However, it should be noted that other causes of hypotension should be ruled out. Patients with submassive PE usually have normal blood pressure, but they present with evidence of right ventricular (RV) dysfunction. RV changes can also be noted on electrocardiogram (ECG), transthoracic echocardiography (TTE), or computed tomography (CT) imaging. ECGs contribute to the diagnosis with new changes, such as an S1, Q3, T3 pattern. Right bundle-branch block or right-axis deviation, however, are more prominent in massive embolism but are also nonspecific. Other lab tests include cardiac biomarkers, such as cardiac troponin and brain natriuretic peptide (BNP), which can represent ventricular stretching with RV strain in the setting of a pulmonary embolism.

CLINICAL PEARL—STEP 2/3

Massive PE is defined as pulmonary embolism causing hemodynamic instability. Submassive PE is defined as PE without hemodynamic instability but with evidence of RV dysfunction or myocardial injury.

CLINICAL PEARL—STEP 2/3

Acute RV dysfunction is a life-threatening condition. In the setting of acute PE, the RV can become stressed, leading to RV dysfunction. If this occurs, the RV will have decreased cardiac output leading to hypotension and hypoperfusion of the RV, which further contributes to RV dysfunction. This cyclical decompensation eventually leads to RV failure and cardiac arrest (Fig. 40.1).

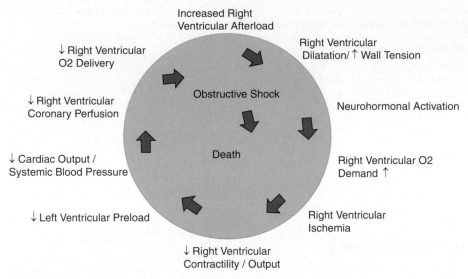

Fig. 40.1   Diagram of pathophysiology of acute right heart failure.

What is the best way to establish the diagnosis of pulmonary embolism?

CTPA is sensitive and specific for detecting emboli in pulmonary arteries. Contrast is adminis-tered, and the CT scan is timed such that the pulmonary arteries are opacified. If there is a PE within the pulmonary arteries, there will be a filling defect, which is an area that is not opacified by the contrast. Other imaging modalities include a ventilation-perfusion scan (V/Q scan). V/Q scan is not usually the first choice of imaging but can be utilized for patients with contraindications to contrast (eg, anaphylaxis or renal failure) or radiation (eg, pregnancy). Baseline chest radiography should ideally be normal; otherwise V/Q scan interpretation can be more difficult. A normal lung perfusion can effectively rule out an acute PE but can also be nonspecific. Transthoracic echocar-diography (TTE) can also be utilized to assess right heart strain to support findings of PE. On TTE, right to left ventricle ratio greater than 1.0, tricuspid annular plane excursion (TAPSE) less than 1.7 cm, or McConnell's Sign (RV hypokinesis with sparing of apical motion) can all suggest PE with 94%–100% specificity. Lower extremity Dopplers are also used as adjuncts for PE. They have a high sensitivity and high specificity for detecting a lower extremity deep venous thrombo-embolism (DVT) and a sensitivity of 44% for detection of PE in critically ill patients.

CLINICAL PEARL—STEP 2/3

A V/Q scan is a two-part scan that uses a radioactive tracer inhaled to assess ventilation while also employing an injected tracer intravenously to assess perfusion. Thus, a PE will show a perfusion defect without a corresponding ventilation defect, which is also known as a mismatched defect. It is important to have a ventilation scan, as areas of lung that have little baseline ventilation will have compensatory hypoxic vasoconstriction to preserve V/Q matching, resulting in a matched defect.

A CTPA scan of the chest was obtained and (Fig. 40.2) demonstrates the pulmonary embolism.

What are some causes of pulmonary embolism?

PE is a type of VTE that occurs due to a variety of acquired risk factors, hereditary risk factors, and mixed or idiopathic reasons, most commonly postsurgical or malignancy-associated, which

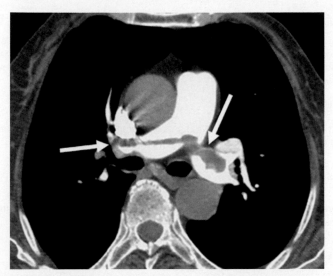

Fig. 40.2   Acute saddle pulmonary embolism on CTPA (Courtesy of Curtis Maehara).

TABLE 40.2 ■ **VTE Risk Factors**

Acquired Risk Factors	Hereditary Risk Factors	Mixed/Unknown
Bed rest	Antithrombin deficiency	High levels of factor VIII
Travel	Protein C deficiency	High levels of factor IX
Immobilizer or cast	Protein S deficiency	High levels of factor XI
Trauma/spinal cord injury	Factor V Leiden	High levels of factor fibrinogen
Major surgery	Prothrombin gene	Activated Protein C resistance in
Orthopedic surgery	mutation	absence of Factor V Leiden
Malignancy	Dysfibrinogenemia	Hyperhomocysteinemia
Oral contraceptives	Plasminogen deficiency	High levels of plasminogen activator
Hormonal replacement therapy		Elevated levels of lipoprotein (a)
Antiphospholipid syndrome		Low levels of tissue factor pathway
Myeloproliferative disorders		inhibitor
Polycythemia vera		
Central venous catheters		
Age		
Obesity		
Pregnancy/postpartum period		

are summarized in Table 40.2. It is estimated that a majority of pulmonary embolisms usually originate from deep vein thrombosis.

How do you manage someone with an acute pulmonary embolism?
The immediate first step in the management of a patient with acute PE is resuscitation and supplemental oxygenation as needed. If patients are hypotensive, vasopressors or inotropes should be initiated, and a strong consideration should be made for systemic thrombolytic therapy. If supplemental oxygen is insufficient, endotracheal intubation should be performed for respiratory faliure.

CLINICAL PEARL—STEP 2/3

Systemic thrombolytic therapy is indicated in massive PE. Thrombolytics have the strongest data for hemodynamically unstable PE. Studies have shown that thrombolytics in this population have a reduction in the composite outcome of decreased mortality and recurrent PE.

CLINICAL PEARL—STEP 2/3

Caution must be taken when intubating patients with acute PE as they can hemodynamically decompensate with induction medications for intubation.

After stabilization, the next step should be addressing and managing the PE. Patients should receive empiric anticoagulation unless contraindicated. In the ICU, patients are generally treated with unfractionated heparin (UFH) or low-molecular-weight heparin (LMWH) unless there are major contraindications.

CLINICAL PEARL—STEP 2/3

If there is a high index of suspicion for PE but difficulty in obtaining CT imaging due to resources, renal function, or other barriers, empiric anticoagulation should be initiated pending diagnostic studies.

CLINICAL PEARL—STEP 2/3

If patient has contraindication to anticoagulation, the patient should be considered for a retrievable inferior vena cava filter to prevent recurrent pulmonary emboli.

Although anticoagulation is the mainstay therapy for PE, there are several advanced therapies that are used for specific populations. These include systemic thrombolysis, catheter-directed thrombolysis, and embolectomy. Patients should be risk-stratified into low, intermediate, or high risk for hemodynamic compromise to help assess if advanced therapies are warranted. This assessment takes into account a scoring system called the pulmonary embolism severity index (PESI), biochemical markers of RV dysfunction (troponin level, pro-BNP level), and cardiac imaging to assess for RV dysfunction.

In regards to the PESI score, patients can be stratified into 5 severity classes for 30 day mortality rates. This table is simplified into low risk for class I or II and intermediate to high risk for classes III to V (Table 40.3).

Patients stratified into classes I or II have low risk features for PE, and some of these patients can even be treated as outpatients. For those in classes III to V, further stratification should be made to determine which patients are at higher risk of decompensation and considered for possible advanced therapy. Patients with an intermediate to high PESI score who have both biochemical and imaging evidence of RV dysfunction are classified as intermediate to high risk. Patients with intermediate to high PESI score who have only one of either biochemical or imaging evidence of RV dysfunction or no evidence of RV dysfunction are classified as low to intermediate risk.

In patients with intermediate- to high-risk PE, data for thrombolytics (systemic and catheter-directed) is less supportive than when compared to patients with massive PE; however, thrombolytics should still be considered. Despite weaker data, there are some data to support decreased risk of hemodynamic collapse with the use of thrombolytics; however, this has to be weighed against the risk of major bleeding and intracranial hemorrhage. There are significant bleeding risks with systemic thrombolytic therapy, with approximately 10% of patients having major bleeding and

TABLE 40.3 ■ Pulmonary Embolism Severity Index (PESI)

Pulmonary Embolism Severity Index (PESI)

Age	+1 for each year of age
Sex	+10 for Male
History of malignancy[a]	+30
History of heart failure	+10
History of chronic lung disease	+10
Pulse rate ≥110 beats per minute	+20
Systolic blood pressure <100 mm Hg	+30
Temperature <36°C	+20
Respiratory rate ≥30/min	+20
Arterial oxyhemoglobin saturation <90%	+20
Altered mental status	+60

PESI Score	Class	Risk 30 Day Mortality
0–65	I	0.0%–1.6%
66–85	II	1.7%–3.5%
86–105	III	3.2%–7.1%
106–125	IV	4.0%–11.4%
≥ 125	V	10%–24.5%

[a]Any diagnosis of cancer other than basal cell or squamous cell carcinoma within the past 6 months, any treatment of cancer in the past 6 months or recurrent or metastatic cancer.

TABLE 40.4 ■ Contraindications to Thrombolytic Therapy

Absolute Contraindications	Relative Contraindications
Neurological surgery or head trauma within 3 weeks	Cancer
Prior hemorrhagic strokes	Age >75–80
Ischemic stroke within prior 3 months	Oral anticoagulant therapy
Central nervous system neoplasm or arteriovenous malformations (AVMs)	Noncompressible punctures
	Traumatic resuscitation
Gastrointestinal bleeding within 1 month	Refractory hypertension
Active bleeding, excluding menses	Advanced liver disease
	Major non-CNS surgery within 3 weeks
	Pregnancy or within 1 week postpartum

approximately 1%–3% having intracranial hemorrhage. Given risk of bleeding, systemic thrombolysis has several absolute contraindications, the most notable being ischemic stroke in the past 3 months, recent head surgery, active bleeding, and history of hemorrhagic strokes (Table 40.4). In the setting of relative contraindications, use of half-dose systemic thrombolysis has been utilized with similar efficacy and lower bleeding risk.

Catheter-directed thrombolysis is a minimally invasive technique that has gained popularity in recent years. The concept is to have thrombolytics continuously infusing directly into the pulmonary artery via a percutaneous catheter. The benefit of such a modality is lower dose of thrombolytics, which can theoretically have decreased risk of bleeding and complications. It is still being investigated based on case series, but some have shown a number of favorable survival outcomes.

In the setting of significant proximal clot burden, failed thrombolysis, or absolute contraindication to thrombolysis, percutaneous thrombectomy or surgical embolectomy can be considered. In this situation, the clot is surgically or percutaneously removed from the pulmonary circulation.

CLINICAL PEARL—STEP 2/3

Given the complex management of PE, a multidisciplinary management team consisting of interventional radiologists, cardiologists, surgeons, pulmonologists, and intensivists should be utilized as part of a PE response team (PERT) to discuss the management of patients with PE.

Our patient was diagnosed with intermediate- to high-risk submassive PE. She was taken for right heart catheterization showing mildly elevated right sided pressures. Percutaneous thrombectomy of the left and right pulmonary arteries were performed (See Fig. 40.3 and Fig. 40.4). Patient was placed on brief heparin infusion and was transitioned to rivaroxaban for a minimum 3–6 months given provoked VTE and prolonged immobility. Further discussion of continuation of anticoagulation was deferred to subsequent outpatient follow-up visits.

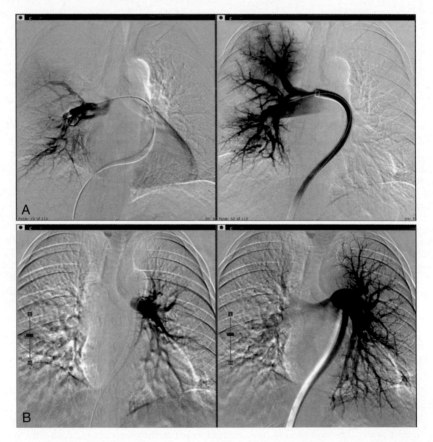

Fig. 40.3 Image (A) with selective right pulmonary angiogram; left image showing filling defect consistent with right main pulmonary artery embolism; right image showing resolution of pulmonary embolism with brisk distal filling after thrombectomy. Image (B) with selective left pulmonary angiogram. Left image showing filling defect consistent with left main pulmonary artery embolism; right image showing resolution of pulmonary embolism with brisk distal filling after thrombectomy. (Image courtesy of Justin Cheng, MD.)

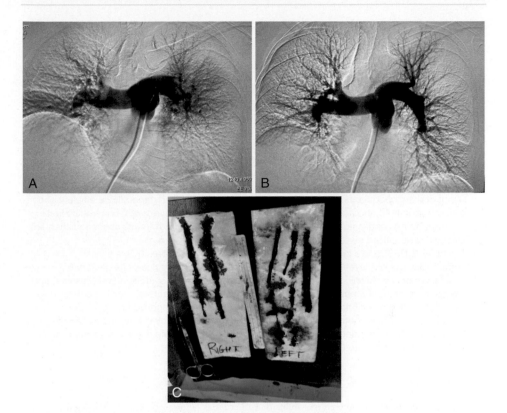

Fig. 40.4 Image (A) is a prethrombectomy pulmonary angiogram. Image (B) is a postthrombectomy pulmonary angiogram with improved distal filling. Image (C) is an image of the clots that were retrieved with thrombectomy. (Image courtesy of Stuart Schroff, MD.)

Case Summary

- **Complaint/History:** A 71-year-old female presents with 2 weeks of progressive weakness, dyspnea, and subjective chills with lower extremity swelling.
- **Findings:** Oxygen saturation is 99% on room air; physical exam reveals nonpitting lower extremity swelling.
- **Labs/Tests:** Labs reveal elevated D-dimer, pronatriuretic brain peptide and troponins; CTPA reveals PE in bilateral pulmonary arteries; a right-heart catheterization confirms PE with elevated right-sided heart pressures.

Diagnosis: Submassive PE

- **Treatment:** The patient had percutaneous thrombectomy performed with therapeutic unfractionated heparin for 24 hours, then transitioned to rivaroxaban for 3–6 months in the setting of provoked venous thromboembolism.

BEYOND THE PEARLS

- ECG findings with ST-T changes (TW inversions, ST depressions and even ST elevations) in right-sided leads (particularly lead III, precordial leads in V1–V3, and sometimes V4) can indicate right heart strain.
- When RV failure is present and central venous pressure is increased, intravenous fluids should be avoided to prevent worsening right heart failure.
- One caveat to bedside TTE is that the sensitivity for ruling out PE is variable at 50%–70%. With the addition of bedside lower extremity Doppler, sensitivity can increase to 70%–80%. However, this should not deter bedside ultrasonographic evaluation for VTE; bedside ultrasonography should be performed on all patients suspected of PE or DVT.
- A rare mimicker of PE is a pulmonary artery sarcoma, which is a rare tumor that originates from the pulmonary arteries.
- Direct oral anticoagulants, such as rivaroxaban or apixaban, can generally be efficient and safe to use in mild and moderate chronic kidney disease; however, warfarin remains first-line treatment in end-stage renal disease. Decisions to use or not to use anticoagulation are strictly individualized given high risks with bleeding.
- A simplified PESI score can be used instead of the full PESI score. This is a less complicated scoring system consisting of six parameters that include age, history of cancer, history of chronic cardiopulmonary disease, heart rate, systolic blood pressure, and oxygen saturation. If a patient is positive for any one of these factors, they are categorized as high risk. If a patient has none of these factors, they are categorized as low risk.
- In regards to percutaneous reperfusion therapies, catheter-directed thrombolysis tends to be favored over percutaneous thrombectomy if there are multiple distal pulmonary emboli that are not amenable to thrombectomy.

References

Aujesky, D., Obrosky, D. S., Stone, R. A., Auble, T. E., Perrier, A., Cornuz, J., et al. (2005). Derivation and validation of a prognostic model for pulmonary embolism. *American Journal of Respiratory and Critical Care Medicine, 172*(8), 1041–1046. https://doi.org/10.1164/rccm.200506-862OC.

Ceylan, N., Tasbakan, S., Bayraktaroglu, S., Cok, G., Simsek, T., Duman, S., & Savas, R. (2011). Predictors of clinical outcome in acute pulmonary embolism. *Academic Radiology, 18*(1), 47–53. https://doi.org/10.1016/j.acra.2010.08.024.

Kiser, T. H., Burnham, E. L., Clark, B., Ho, P. M., Allen, R. R., Moss, M., et al. (2018). Half-dose versus full-dose alteplase for treatment of pulmonary embolism. *Critical Care Medicine, 46*(10), 1617–1625. https://doi.org/10.1097/CCM.0000000000003288.

Konstantinides, S. V., Meyer, G., & Diaconu, N. (2020). 2019 ESC Guidelines for the diagnosis and management of acute pulmonary embolism developed in collaboration with the European Respiratory Society (ERS). *European Heart Journal, 41*(4), 543–603. https://doi.org/10.1093/eurheartj/ehz405.

Marshall, P. S., Mathews, K. S., & Siegel, M. D. (2011). Diagnosis and management of life-threatening pulmonary embolism. *Journal of Intensive Care Medicine, 26*(5), 275–294. https://doi.org/10.1177/0885066610392658.

Marti, C., John, G., Konstantinides, S., Combescure, C., Sanchez, O., Lankeit, M., et al. (2015). Systemic thrombolytic therapy for acute pulmonary embolism: a systematic review and meta-analysis. *European Heart Journal, 36*(10), 605–614. https://doi.org/10.1093/eurheartj/ehu218.

Modi, S., Deisler, R., Gozel, K., Reicks, P., Irwin, E., Brunsvold, M., et al. (2016, June 8). Wells criteria for DVT is a reliable clinical tool to assess the risk of deep venous thrombosis in trauma patients. *World Journal of Emergency Surgery: WJES, 11*, 24. https://doi.org/10.1186/s13017-016-0078-1.

Piazza, G., & Goldhaber, S. Z. (2006). Acute pulmonary embolism: part II: treatment and prophylaxis. *Circulation, 114*(3), e42–e47. https://doi.org/10.1161/CIRCULATIONAHA.106.620880.

Tapson, V. F. (2008). Acute pulmonary embolism. *The New England Journal of Medicine, 358*(10), 1037–1052. https://doi.org/10.1056/NEJMra072753.

Wells, P. S., Anderson, D. R., Rodger, M., Stiell, I., Dreyer, J. F., Barnes, D., et al. (2001). Excluding pulmonary embolism at the bedside without diagnostic imaging: management of patients with suspected pulmonary embolism presenting to the emergency department by using a simple clinical model and d-dimer. *Annals of Internal Medicine, 135*(2), 98–107. https://doi.org/10.7326/0003-4819-135-2-200107170-0001.

A 61-Year-Old Male With Shortness of Breath

Justine Ko ■ Anna Grzegorczyk ■ Raj Dasgupta

A 61-year-old male with history of B-cell acute lymphoblastic leukemia (ALL) presents to the hospital from the hematology clinic with shortness of breath. The patient reports he had shortness of breath, cough, and dyspnea for 2 days. A rapid response is called due to hypoxia with a pulse oximetry reading of 68%.

On physical exam, the patient is tachypneic with a respiratory rate of 40 breaths per minute, tachycardic with a heart rate of 110 beats per minute, blood pressure of 120/74 mm Hg, and afebrile with a temperature of 36.9°C. On pulmonary exam, he is noted to have diffuse crackles in bilateral lungs. He is started on supplemental oxygen via high-flow nasal cannula ; however, he continues to decompensate, and he is shortly intubated afterwards and transferred to the intensive care unit. His initial arterial blood gas (ABG) showed 7.46/42/82 on an fraction of inspired oxygen (FiO$_2$)of 70%.

Chest x-ray and computed tomography (CT) scan of the chest is obtained and shows bilateral infiltrates with diffuse ground glass opacities in dependent lung zones that were not seen on imaging 1 month ago (Fig. 41.1 and Fig. 41.2).

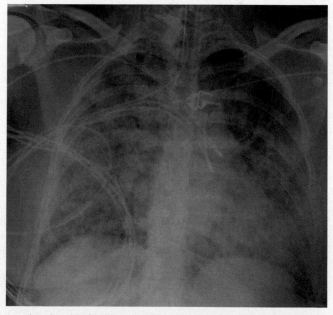

Fig. 41.1 Chest x-ray imaging showing bilateral, patchy infiltrates. (*Clinical Chest Medicine*, 2014.)

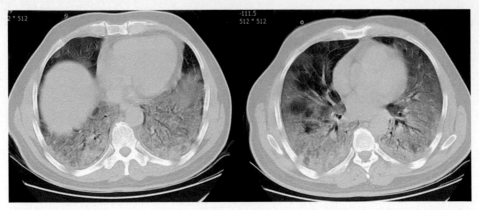

Fig. 41.2 Computed tomography imaging showing dense consolidative opacities with diffuse ground glass opacities, more predominant in the dependent position. (*Radiología (English Edition)*, vol. 63 (4), 2021.)

What is the differential for diffuse ground glass opacities on chest imaging?
The differential for diffuse bilateral infiltrates on chest x-ray and diffuse ground glass opacities on CT imaging is broad.

- Infection
  - Multifocal bacterial pneumonia
  - Fungal infection with blastomycosis, histoplasmosis, coccidioidomycosis, cryptococcus
  - Mycobacterial infection
  - If immunosuppressed, can consider *Pneumocystis jirovecii* pneumonia (PCP) and cytomegalovirus (CMV)
  - Viral infection with COVID-19
- Inflammatory conditions
  - Cryptogenic organizing pneumonia, pulmonary vasculitis, acute eosinophilic pneumonia, and acute interstitial pneumonitis
  - Diffuse alveolar hemorrhage
  - Pulmonary alveolar proteinosis
- Malignancy
- Acute cardiogenic pulmonary edema
- Graft versus host disease
- Fat embolism syndrome
- Medication-induced pneumonitis
- Acute respiratory distress syndrome (ARDS)
- Near drowning

Infectious diseases and hematology specialists were consulted. Patient underwent a bronchoscopy with bronchoalveolar lavage. The studies returned negative for bacterial, fungal, and acid fast bacilli (AFB) stains and cultures. PCP direct fluorescent antibody test, CMV polymerase chain reaction (PCR), and COVID-19 PCR tests were also negative. Interferon-gamma release assay was negative. Transthoracic echocardiogram shows normal cardiac function with an ejection fraction of 55%.

The patient remains hypoxic, and labs are significant for an elevated alveolar-arterial (A-a) oxygen gradient. The patient was diagnosed with ARDS.

What is ARDS?

As the name suggests, ARDS is a clinical syndrome characterized by acute respiratory failure secondary to inflammation within the lungs. The hallmark of this disease is due to fluid accumulation within the lungs secondary to capillary leak from diffuse inflammation.

The initial definition of ARDS was developed by the American-European Consensus Conference in 1994. However, due to limitations in this first definition, an international panel of experts revised it and developed what is now recognized as the "Berlin definition" in 2012. This definition of ARDS is recognized by both the American Thoracic Society (ATS) and the Society of Critical Care Medicine (SCCM).

The Berlin definition categorizes ARDS by the severity of hypoxemia as measured by the PaO_2/FiO_2 ratio (Table 41.1). The PaO_2 is the partial pressure of oxygen as measured by an arterial blood gas. The FiO_2 is the fraction of inspired oxygen, which is the concentration of oxygen. Other criteria in the Berlin definition include timing from insult to injury, etiology of edema, and radiographic findings. If there is no known risk factor for ARDS, cardiac etiology should be ruled out with an echocardiogram.

CLINICAL PEARL—STEP 2/3

The Berlin definition of ARDS includes timing from insult to injury, radiographic findings, origin of edema, and severity of hypoxemia as measured by the PaO_2/FiO_2 ratio.

CLINICAL PEARL—STEP 2/3

Cardiogenic etiology must be excluded for the definition of ARDS. This can be done non-invasively with an echocardiogram.

What are some triggers for ARDS?

ARDS can be caused by direct (epithelial) injury such as pneumonia, aspiration, smoke inhalation, near drowning, pulmonary contusion, embolism, re-expansion injury or reperfusion injury or indirect (vascular) modes of injury such as sepsis, trauma and burns, pancreatitis, transfusion-related acute lung injury, stem cell transplants, drug toxicity, cardiothoracic surgery, and shock.

Patients with ARDS are generally hypoxic and have an elevated A-a oxygen gradient. This is calculated by subtracting the alveolar oxygen pressure (P_AO_2) from the arterial oxygen pressure (PaO_2).

TABLE 41.1 ■ **Berlin Definition of Acute Respiratory Distress Syndrome**

Timing	Within 1 week of known clinical insult or new or worsening respiratory symptoms
Chest imaging (chest x-ray or CT scan)	Bilateral opacities not explained by effusions, lobar/lung collapse or nodules
Origin of edema	Not fully due to cardiac failure or fluid overload Obtain transthoracic echocardiogram to exclude cardiogenic etiology
Oxygenation	Mild: 200 mm Hg < PaO_2/FiO_2 ≤300 mm Hg with PEEP ≥5 Moderate: 100 mm Hg < PaO_2/FiO_2 ≤200 mm Hg with PEEP ≥5 Severe: PaO_2/FiO_2 ≤100 mm Hg with PEEP ≥5

CT, Computed tomography; *PEEP,* positive end expiratory pressure.

BASIC SCIENCE PEARL—STEP 1

The P_AO_2 is calculated by the following equation, $(P_{atm}-P_{H_2O}) \times FiO_2-PaCO_2/RQ$. P_{atm} is the atmospheric pressure, which is influenced by altitude and temperature. The P_{H_2O} is the atmospheric pressure of water, which is fixed at 47 mm Hg. $PaCO_2$ is the partial pressure of carbon dioxide. RQ is the respiratory quotient, which is defined as the volume of carbon dioxide released over the volume of oxygen absorbed during respiration at the cellular level. This is a constant value of 0.8.

CLINICAL PEARL—STEP 2/3

ARDS is an acute process that occurs within 1 week of a known clinical insult.

What is the pathophysiology behind ARDS?
After an insult, alveolar macrophages release cytokines. Polymorphonuclear cells are activated and become sequestered in the pulmonary microcirculation. These cells degranulate, releasing inflammatory mediators, proteolytic enzymes, and toxic oxygen metabolites which damage the capillary walls of the lungs. This leads to increased alveolar-capillary permeability. Injury to the pneumocytes causes impaired transport of sodium, chloride, and water from alveoli and decreased surfactant production and function. Exudate that is protein-rich fluid that contain fibrin, red blood cells (RBC), and platelets accumulate into the lung interstitium and alveoli, obliterating the distal airspaces. Inflammation and filling of the lung with this proteinaceous material decreases lung compliance causing it to become "stiff", and the collapse of alveoli causes shunt-like physiology. The destruction of the capillary bed leads to increased dead space. In the most severe cases, this cytokine response ultimately leads to multiorgan failure (Figs. 41.3–41.7).

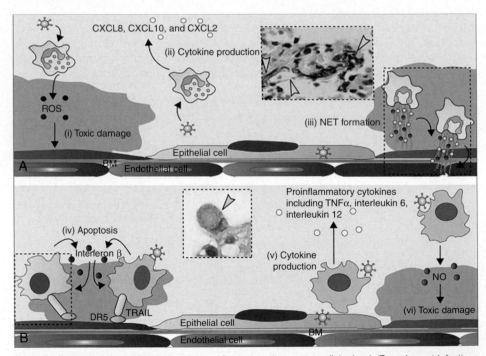

Fig. 41.3 Pathophysiology of acute respiratory distress syndrome at a cellular level. (From *Lancet Infectious Diseases*, 2014.)

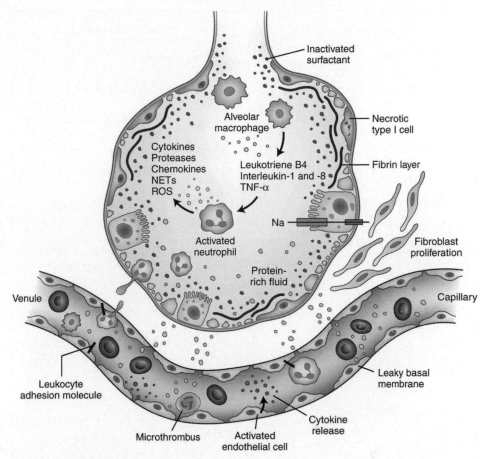

Fig. 41.4 Pathophysiology of acute respiratory distress syndrome at a cellular level. (*Fuhrman and Zimmerman's Pediatric Critical Care, 2022.*)

CLINICAL PEARL—STEP 2/3

The inflammation within the lungs causes a capillary leak, which in turn causes fluid, protein, and other substances to shift into the alveoli.

BASIC SCIENCE PEARL—STEP 1

Remember that oxygen is diffusion-limited. When there is a capillary leak in ARDS, the thickness of the alveolar-capillary membrane increases and the surface area of the alveoli in contact with the capillary decreases, leading to a decrease in the diffusion of oxygen. This is a clinical application of Fick's law of diffusion, whose structural properties are based on surface area and thickness.

What are the stages of ARDS?

ARDS is categorized into three pathologic stages (Table 41.2).

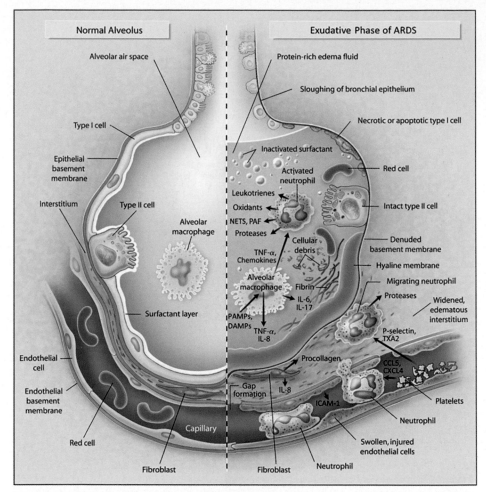

Fig. 41.5 The normal alveolus (*left*) and an alveolus during the exudative phase of acute respiratory distress syndrome (*right*). (*New England Journal of Medicine*, 2000.)

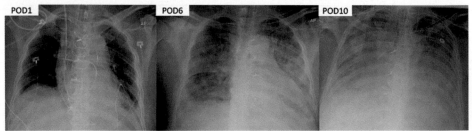

Fig. 41.6 Progression of acute respiratory distress syndrome imaging on chest x-ray over a period of 10 days following thoracic surgery. (*Journal of Thoracic and Cardiovascular Surgery*, 2020.)

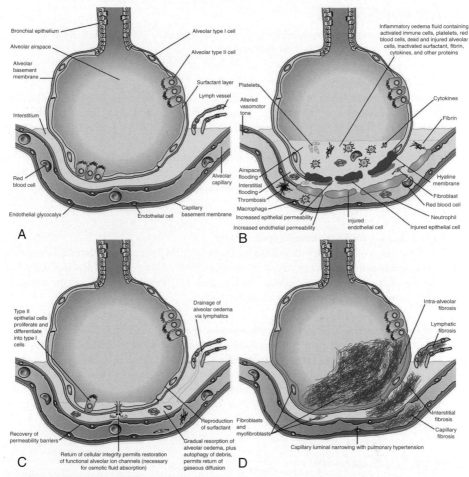

Fig. 41.7 Normal alveolus (A) as compared to the exudative (B), proliferative (C), and fibrotic (D) phases in the pathogenesis of acute respiratory distress syndrome. (*Lancet (London, England)*, 2016.)

TABLE 41.2 ■ Pathologic Stages of Acute Respiratory Distress Syndrome

Stage	Timing	Characteristics
(1) Early Exudative Stage	First 7–10 days	• nonspecific reaction to lung injury • interstitial edema • acute/chronic inflammation • type 2 pneumocyte hyperplasia • hyaline membrane formation
(2) Fibroproliferative Stage	After 7–10 days (can last 2–3 weeks)	• resolution of pulmonary edema • proliferation of type 2 pneumocytes • squamous metaplasia • interstitial infiltration by myofibroblasts • early deposition of collagen
(3) Fibrotic Stage	After 3 weeks	• obliteration of normal lung architecture • fibrosis • cyst formation • can vary from mild to severe

---

CLINICAL PEARL—STEP 2/3

Not everyone with ARDS will progress through all the stages of ARDS, especially if the underlying cause can be identified and addressed early.

What is the clinical presentation of ARDS?

Patients will present with primary respiratory complaints, namely shortness of breath and inability to breathe. Depending on the severity, they will have increased work of breathing. The presentation is acute, often suddenly occurring or rapidly progressing. Imaging will have findings concerning for diffuse airspace disease.

In regard to other symptoms or associated findings, these are most commonly secondary to the underlying condition that triggered the ARDS. For example, patients with pneumonia can have a fever with leukocytosis, while patients with pancreatitis may present with abdominal pain with a history of recent alcohol use.

What are the imaging findings consistent with ARDS?

Chest X-ray imaging of patients with ARDS is nonspecific. The appearance is often bilateral diffuse alveolar opacities that are not explained by effusions, lobar or lung collapse, or nodules. Earlier on during the clinical course, these findings can be subtle. CT imaging often shows ground glass opacities or dense consolidations in dependent lung zones.

What is the most important principle in the management of an intubated ARDS patient?

Patients with ARDS are vulnerable to ventilator-induced lung injury (VILI) because the lung injury is heterogeneous. This results in regional differences in lung compliance. Stiff, noncompliant lungs are difficult to ventilate and are associated with high airway pressures. These high pressures contribute to VILI, which is also thought to contribute to cytokine release and further lung injury. Therefore, lung protective ventilation strategy with low tidal volume is the most important intervention for intubated patients with ARDS.

CLINICAL PEARL—STEP 2/3

In ARDS, the two interventions that have shown mortality benefit are lung protective ventilation strategy with low tidal volumes and early proning.

One important paradigm in the management of ARDS is that the interventions are aimed at providing supportive care while minimizing further lung injury, especially from mechanical ventilation. This strategy is to buy time for the initial insult that caused ARDS to resolve, and for the inflammatory process within the lungs to hopefully improve. This framework provides the basis for the recommended interventions in ARDS.

Lung protective strategy: A protective ventilation strategy requires a fine balance between alveolar recruitment through maintaining positive end expiratory pressure (PEEP) and preventing VILI through volutrauma (too much volume) or barotrauma (too much pressure) Fig. 41.8.

According to the ARDSNet trial, lung protective ventilation strategy included low tidal volume, with recommended volumes of 4-8 mL/kg of predicted body weight (PBW) with a goal of 4-6 mL/kg of PBW if possible, and a plateau pressure goal of less than 30 cm H_2O.

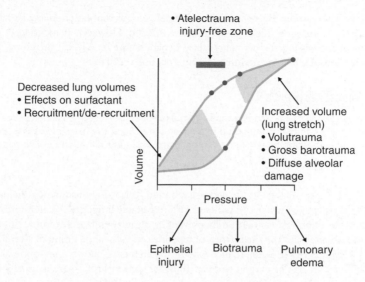

Fig. 41.8 Acute respiratory distress syndrome protective ventilation. (*Foldman-Cecil Medicine*, 2020 26e, 97, 635–641.)

CLINICAL PEARL—STEP 2/3

The ARDSNet protocol started patients off at 6 mL/kg of PBW initially. A plateau pressure was subsequently measured. If plateau pressures were greater than 30 cm H_2O, then the tidal volume was decreased by 1 mL/kg of PBW until plateau pressures were less than 30 cm H_2O. If patients were unable to tolerate lower tidal volume due to hypercapnia, then tidal volumes could be increased by 1 mL/kg of PBW up to a maximum of 8 ml/kg of PBW.

CLINICAL PEARL—STEP 2/3

A plateau pressure is measured by recording the pressure after performing a half-second pause at the end of an inspiratory breath.

CLINICAL PEARL—STEP 2/3

Common PBW formulas are as follows:
- male: 50 + [2.3 × (height in inches − 60)]
- female: 45.5 + [2.3 × (height in inches − 60)]

CLINICAL PEARL—STEP 2/3

Barotrauma, which is lung injury due to elevated pressures, can lead to complications such as pneumothorax, pneumomediastinum, pneumoperitoneum, and subcutaneous emphysema.
   Clues for a pneumothorax include:
   - unilateral breath sounds
   - acutely elevated peak pressures
   - hemodynamic instability (if tension physiology)

Permissive hypercapnia: Because of the low tidal volume ventilation, many patients would have resultant CO_2 retention due to low minute ventilation. However, as mentioned previously, the paradigm of preventing further lung injury is paramount in ARDS; therefore, permissive hypercapnia is allowed while maintaining low tidal volume ventilation.

CLINICAL PEARL—STEP 2/3

Acceptable permissive hypercapnia ranges from a pH of 7.15–7.25. If pH is below this range, the respiratory rate can be increased up to a maximum of 35. If the pH is still less than the acceptable range, then the tidal volume can be increased in this situation to prevent severe acidosis.

PEEP: PEEP is the pressure at the end of expiration. This is the pressure that helps maintain the patency of already open alveoli. In patients with recruitable lung, PEEP can improve oxygenation and promote improved ventilation by preventing alveolar collapse/decruitment and therefore decreases atelectrauma (the shear stress of repetitive opening and closing of alveoli). As such, maintaining a level of PEEP helps reduce oxygen requirements, allows more optimal ventilator settings, and decreases risk of oxygen toxicity. Thus, for a given FiO_2, there is usually a range of PEEP that is targeted to maintain recruitment of alveoli (Table 41.3).

CLINICAL PEARLS—STEP 2/3

Goal ventilator settings include PEEP ≥5 cm H_2O (to prevent atelectrauma), plateau pressure <30 mm H_2O (to prevent barotrauma), and tidal volumes of 4–6 mL/kg of PBW (to prevent volutrauma), as well as PaO_2 between 55 mm Hg–80 mm Hg (to prevent oxygen toxicity).

What is prone positioning, and how does it help in ARDS?

Prone positioning places the patient in a prone (face down) position. The PROSEVA trial demonstrated mortality benefit in patients with severe ARDS who underwent prone positioning. In this trial, there were several key points. (1) Patients included in the trial were those who had a P/F ratio <150, FiO_2 >60%, and PEEP ≥5. (2) Patients were proned early in the course of their disease (<36 hours after intubation). (3) Patients were proned for a goal of 16 hours.

The rationale for prone positioning can be explained via the schematic below. In the supine position, the heart contributes to compressive changes in the bases. However, in the prone position, the heart is resting mostly on the sternum as opposed to the lung parenchyma, allowing maximal recruitment of alveoli to assist in ventilation and oxygenation (Figs. 41.9 and 41.10).

CLINICAL PEARL—STEP 2/3

The prone position allows for the recruitment of more alveoli. This allows for optimization of ventilator settings to achieve the ARDSNet parameters mentioned earlier in the chapter, which in turn reduces the risk of VILI.

TABLE 41.3 ■ **Sample Positive End Expiratory Pressure Table for Acute Respiratory Distress Syndrome**

FiO_2	0.4	0.5	0.6	0.7	0.8	0.9	1.0
PEEP (cmH_2O)	5–8	8–10	10	10–14	14–16	16–18	18–24

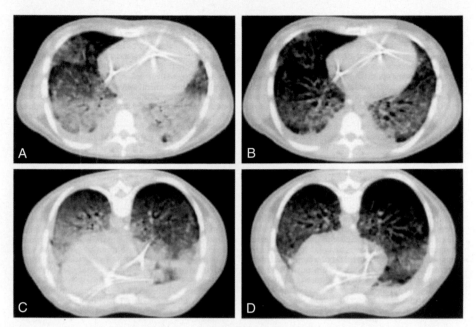

Fig. 41.9 Changes on chest imaging with prone positioning. (A) CT image of the lung parenchyma in supine position at end exhalation. (B) CT image of the lung parenchyma in supine position at end inspiration. (C) CT image of the lung parenchyma while in prone position at end exhalation. (D) CT image of lung parenchyma while in prone position at end inspiration. (*Respiratory Care*, 2015.)

CLINICAL PEARL—STEP 2/3

Patients are usually proned for 16–18 hours a day.

CLINICAL PEARL—STEP 2/3

Prone positioning for patients who are mechanically ventilated does come with risks that providers need to monitor for, including dislodgement of endotracheal tubes and access lines, development of pressure injuries, and facial edema.

What are some adjuncts in the management of ARDS?
Aside from mechanical ventilation and supportive care, research has investigated the role of several other therapeutic interventions, such as fluid management, paralysis, and steroids.

Fluid status: As mentioned earlier, one characteristic of ARDS is noncardiogenic pulmonary edema. Conservative fluid management was shown to shorten ventilator duration and had improved lung function via the FACTT trial. This can be achieved via the use of diuretics and reduced fluid administration and intake.

Paralytics: Ventilator dyssynchrony can make it difficult to properly oxygenate or ventilate the patient who requires ventilator support. However, the use of paralytics in patients with moderate to severe ARDS is still being debated as multiple, large studies have had conflicting results on utility as well as adverse events such as risk of myopathy with paralysis. For that reason, if a paralytic is used, it is advised to use the lowest effective dose for the shortest amount of time as medically necessary. Administration with concomitant corticosteroids should be avoided.

Supine position	**Prone position**
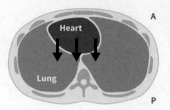	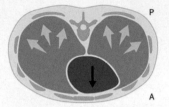
Gravitational pressure of heart and mediastinum on the lungs.	Decreased gravitational pressure of heart and mediastinum on the lungs.
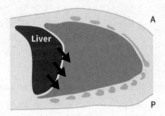	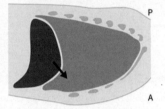
Compressive effects of the abdominal organs on the lungs.	Decreased compressive effects of the abdominal organs on the lungs.
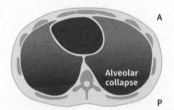	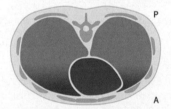
Expansion of the chest wall and overall less homogeneous chest wall compliance.	More homogeneous chest wall compliance due to restriction of anterior chest wall movement.

Fig. 41.10 Explanation of prone imaging. (*Canadian Medical Association Journal*, 2020-11-23, Volume 192, Issue 47, Pages E1532–E1537, 2020 Joule.)

CLINICAL PEARL—STEP 2/3

Cisatracurium was the neuromuscular blockade that was studied in ARDS trials, ACURASYS and ROSE.

Steroids: The use of steroids in the management of ARDS has had mixed results and is not routinely used. One exception is in the setting of the novel coronavirus disease 2019 (COVID-19) infection. In this clinical context, the RECOVERY trial found a role for steroids as a primary intervention in patients requiring invasive and noninvasive oxygenation.

Other medications and interventions: Medications including beta blockers, statins, and therapies targeting the pathophysiology of ARDS have been trialed for their antiinflammatory effects. However, no pharmaceutical agents have been found to be effective and some, such as the use of keratinocyte growth factor, have been found to be harmful. Other interventions not considered standard of care for the management of ARDS include inhaled nitric oxide and extracorporeal membrane oxygenation (ECMO).

CLINICAL PEARL—STEP 2/3

The EOLIA trial was a randomized trial in severe refractory ARDS patients comparing venovenous ECMO with conventional mechanical ventilation. There was no mortality benefit with ECMO; however, there was a significant cross-over from the control group, making it difficult to interpret the results.

CLINICAL PEARL—STEP 2/3

Patient factors to consider for ECMO selection include reversible cause, no major comorbidities, and no contraindications to anticoagulation.

CLINICAL PEARL—STEP 2/3

Risks of ECMO include bleeding, heparin-induced thrombocytopenia, and vessel injury from cannulation.

After the patient was intubated, he was placed on lung protective ventilation strategy as mentioned above. The patient progressed to severe ARDS, met the criteria for proning, and was proned for several days in succession. Despite the above interventions, the patient's course was complicated by multiorgan failure as well as sepsis from ventilator-associated pneumonia. Due to the progression of multiorgan failure, the patient's family decides to pursue comfort measures only, and the patient passed shortly after compassionate extubation.

What is the prognosis for ARDS?
ARDS has a high mortality rate with the worst prognosis for those with severe ARDS. The hospital mortality rate of ARDS can range from 35–50% depending on initial severity. The attributable mortality is less known, but those who survive severe ARDS often have pulmonary, cognitive, and physical deficits as well as emotional distress due to their illness that can affect overall longevity.

What is the most common cause of death in patients with ARDS?
Sepsis is the most common cause of mortality. Multiorgan failure frequently results due to both a cytokine response as well as sepsis and can be seen in up to 70% of patients. Pulmonary dysfunction is also a common primary cause of death.

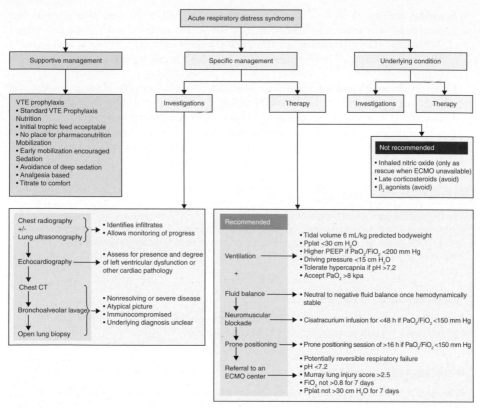

Fig. 41.11 Flowchart for identifying and managing acute respiratory distress syndrome. (*Lancet (London, England)*, 2016.)

Case Summary

- **Complaint/History:** A 61-year-old male with B-cell ALL presents with shortness of breath.
- **Diagnostic Findings:** New bilateral airspace opacities, diffuse ground glass opacities on CT chest, normal echocardiogram.
- **Labs:** P/F ratio 117, negative infectious work up.

Diagnosis: Severe ARDS.

- **Treatment:** Intubation, lung protective ventilation, proning.

BEYOND THE PEARLS

- ARDS is a life-threatening condition characterized by poor oxygenation and noncompliant lungs as a response to various etiologies. Early recognition is essential.
- Driving pressure is a parameter that may be more predictive of appropriate pressures to prevent VILI. The driving pressure is defined as the plateau pressure minus the PEEP. Given

that ARDS is a heterogenous disease, a fixed mL/kg per PBW may be overestimating appropriate volumes and pressures.
- Unfortunately, no drug has been proven to be effective in preventing or managing ARDS. The treatment strategy is supportive care and focuses on (1) reducing shunt fraction, (2) increasing oxygen delivery, (3) decreasing oxygen consumption, and (4) avoiding further lung injury.
- Complications from ARDS include barotrauma, nosocomial infections including ventilator associated pneumonia, central venous catheter-associated infections, and urinary tract infections, and multiorgan failure.
- Morbidity amongst survivors includes cognitive, psychological, and physical impairments that may last for months to years following their acute illness.
- Many patients with ARDS require a tracheostomy (due to prolonged mechanical ventilation) and a percutaneous feeding tube in the recovery phase.
- ARDS management stems from several landmark trials.
  - Low tidal volume ventilation: ARDSNet trial, 2004. This is sometimes also referred to as the ARMA trial.
  - Fluid management: FACTT trial, 2005.
  - Prone positioning: PROSEVA trial, 2013.
  - Paralysis: ACURASYS trial, 2010. ROSE trial, 2016.
  - Steroids: COVID-19: RECOVERY trial, 2020.
  - ECMO: CESAR trial, 2009. EOLIA trial, 2017.
- Despite not being standard of care for ARDS, inhaled nitric oxide and ECMO can be rescue therapies for ARDS in refractory cases. Patients should be selected on a case-by-case basis.

References

Annane, D., Pastores, S.M., Rochwerg, B., Arlt, W., Balk, R.A., & Beishuizen, A., et al. Guidelines for the diagnosis and management of critical illness-related corticosteroid insufficiency (CIRCI) in critically ill patients (part I): Society of Critical Care Medicine (SCCM) and European Society of Intensive Care Medicine (ESICM) 2017. *Intensive Care Medicine*, 43(12), 1751–1763. https://doi.org/10.1007/s00134-017-4919-5.

Diamond, M., Peniston, H. L., Sanghavi, D., & Mahapatra, S. (2022, January). Acute Respiratory Distress Syndrome: *StatPearls [Internet]*. Treasure Island, FL: StatPearls Publishing. Retrieved from. https://www.ncbi.nlm.nih.gov/books/NBK436002/.

Fan, E., Brodie, D., & Slutsky, A. S. (2018). Acute respiratory distress syndrome: Advances in diagnosis and treatment. *JAMA*, *319*(7), 698–710. https://doi.org/10.1001/jama.2017.21907.

Ketcham, S. W., Sedhai, Y. R., Miller, H. C., Bolig, T. C., Ludwig, A., Co, I., et al. (2020). Causes and characteristics of death in patients with acute hypoxemic respiratory failure and acute respiratory distress syndrome: A retrospective cohort study. *Critical Care*, *24*(1), 391. https://doi.org/10.1186/s13054-020-03108-w.

Kidson, K. M., Ayas N.T., & Henderson, W. R. (2022). Respiratory system mechanics and energetics. In *Murray & Nadel's Textbook of Respiratory Medicine, 2-Volume Set* (Chapter 11, pp. 140–153.e3). Elsevier.

Steinberg, K. P., Hudson, L. D., Goodman, R. B., Hough, C. L., Lanken, P. N., Hyzy, R., et al. (2006). Efficacy and safety of corticosteroids for persistent acute respiratory distress syndrome. *New England Journal of Medicine*, *354*(16), 1671–1684.

Pham, T., & Rubenfeld, G. D. (2017). Fifty years of research in ARDS. The epidemiology of acute respiratory distress syndrome. A 50th birthday review. *American Journal of Respiratory and Critical Care Medicine*, *195*(7), 860–870. https://doi.org/10.1164/rccm.201609-1773CP.

Slutsky, A. S., & Villar, J. (2019). Early paralytic agents for ARDS? Yes, no, and sometimes. *The New England Journal of Medicine*, *380*(21), 2061–2063. https://doi.org/10.1056/NEJMe1905627.

Sweeney, R. M., & McAuley, D. F. (2016). Acute respiratory distress syndrome. *Lancet (London, England)*, *388*(10058), 2416–2430. https://doi.org/10.1016/S0140-6736(16)00578-X.

Umbrello, M., Formenti, P., Bolgiaghi, L., & Chiumello, D. (2016). Current concepts of ARDS: A narrative review. *International Journal of Molecular Sciences*, *18*(1), 64. https://doi.org/10.3390/ijms18010064.

Venus, K., Munshi, L., & Fralick, M. (2020). Prone positioning for patients with hypoxic respiratory failure related to COVID-19. *CMAJ: Canadian Medical Association Journal*, *192*(47), E1532–E1537.

Ashtari, S., Vahedian-Azimi, A., Shojaee, S., Pourhoseingholi, M. A., Jafari, R., Bashar, F. R., et al. (2021). Computed tomographic features of coronavirus disease-2019 (COVID-19) pneumonia in three groups of Iranian patients: A single center study. *Radiología (English Edition), 63*(4), 314–323. https://doi. org/10.1016/j.rxeng.2021.03.003.

Casey, J. D., & Ware, L. B. (2020). What are the pathologic and pathophysiologic changes that accompany ARDS? In. *Evidence-based practice of critical care*. Elsevier.

Goodman, L. R. (2022). *Felson's Principles of Chest Roentgenology: A Programmed Text*. Elsevier.

Janz, D. R., & Ware, L. B. (2016). Approach to the patient with the acute respiratory distress syndrome. *Clinics in Chest Medicine, 35*(4), 685–696.

Kallet, R. H. (2015). A comprehensive review of prone position in ARDS. *Respiratory Care, 60*(11), 1660–1687.

Zimmerman, J. J., & Rotta, A. T. (2022). *Fuhrman and Zimmerman's Pediatric Critical Care*. Elsevier.

Salna, M., Polanco, A., Bapat, V., George, I., Argenziano, M., & Takeda, K. (2020). A case of coronavirus disease 2019 (COVID-19) presenting after coronary artery bypass grafting. *Journal of Thoracic and Cardiovascular Surgery, 160*(4), e193–e195.

Short, K. R., Kroeze, E., Fouchier, R., & Kuiken, T. (2014). Pathogenesis of influenza-induced acute respiratory distress syndrome. *Lancet Infectious Diseases, 14*(1), 57–69.

Sweeney, R. M., & McAuley, D. F. (2016). Acute respiratory distress syndrome. *Lancet, 388*(10058), 2416–2430. https://doi.org/10.1016/S0140-6736(16)00578-X.

Ware, L. B., & Matthay, M. A. (2000). The acute respiratory distress syndrome. *The New England Journal of Medicine, 342*, 1334–1349.

Venus, K., Munshi, L., & Fralick, M. (2020). Prone positioning for patients with hypoxic respiratory failure related to COVID-19. *CMAJ: Canadian Medical Association Journal, 192*(47), E1532–E1537.

Hudson, L., & Slutsky, A. (2020). Mechanical ventilation: *Goldman-Cecil medicine* (26th ed., Chapter 97, pp. 635–641). Elsevier.

A 32-Year-Old Man Presenting With Shortness of Breath

Ashil Panchal ■ Joon Choi ■ Patrick Chan ■ Raj Dasgupta

A 32-year-old man was admitted to the hospital with shortness of breath. His past medical history was significant for human immunodeficiency virus (HIV) with a recent CD4 count of 54. His initial vital signs were temperature of 35°C, heart rate (HR) of 90 beats per minute, blood pressure (BP) 104/53 mm Hg, respiratory rate (RR) of 36 breaths per minute, and oxygen saturation of 90% on a non-rebreather mask. His chest radiograph (CXR) showed interstitial and patchy airspace opacities concerning for Pneumocystis pneumonia (Fig. 42.1). The patient was started empirically on intravenous sulfamethoxazole and trimethoprim, prednisone, as well as antibiotics to cover community-acquired pneumonia. He was subsequently intubated for acute hypoxic respiratory failure and transferred to the intensive care unit (ICU).

What are the common ventilator modes? What is a basic description of each mode?

The most common ventilator modes are volume assist control (AC), pressure AC, pressure support (PS), volume synchronized intermittent mandatory ventilation (SIMV), and pressure SIMV.

An assist control mode (either volume or pressure) is a mode in which a mandatory breath is delivered at set intervals. The volume or pressure designation in this instance is simply a notation of which variable is fixed. For example, in volume assist control, a set tidal volume (TV) breath is delivered at fixed intervals, depending on the set RR. Likewise, in pressure assist control, a set pressure is delivered with each breath, again, at fixed intervals depending on the RR. However, the ventilator is dynamic and able to not only deliver breaths at a set rate in this mode, but also deliver a breath when the patient initiates a breath. If the patient does initiate a breath, the delivered breath will be the same breath as the set breath on the ventilator.

On the flip side, PS mode is a mode in which there is no mandatory breath at all (no set RR); all breaths have to be patient-initiated. The volume and length of breath is determined by the patient's own respiratory effort. This mode provides support to the patient by maintaining a set pressure on inspiration after the patient initiates a breath. This is considered a spontaneous mode of ventilation.

SIMV is best understood as a hybrid mode that combines assist control and PS. This mode has a set breath that is delivered at fixed intervals, as in assist control. The set breath can be volume or pressure. However, when a patient initiates a breath on top of the set rate, the ventilator delivers a PS breath instead the set breath, allowing the patient to breathe spontaneously for these self-triggered breaths.

What initial ventilator settings should you place the patient on?

There is no one superior mode of mechanical ventilation. Each mode of mechanical ventilation has its own strengths and weaknesses. However, given that the patient was intubated for a primary

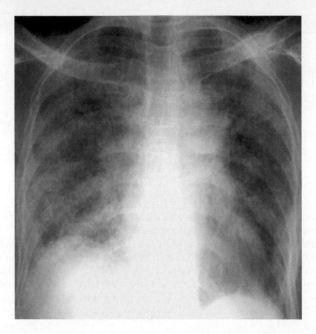

Fig. 42.1   Chest Radiograph showing bilateral interstitial and patchy airspace opacities. (*Imaging of the Chest.* Saunders/Elsevier, 2008.)

pulmonary etiology, and since there is a concern for acute respiratory distress syndrome (ARDS), low TV ventilation strategy should be used for its mortality benefit (as previously addressed in the ARDS chapter). Therefore, volume assist control may be preferable in this scenario.

For volume assist control, the main variables that are set by the provider are the TV, RR, positive end expiratory pressure (PEEP), fraction of inspired oxygen (FiO_2), and flow rate. The TV is the desired volume that is delivered to the patient with each breath. The RR is the total number of breaths per minute. The PEEP is the pressure that the ventilator maintains in the airway during expiration. The FiO_2 is the percent of oxygen that is delivered via the ventilator. The flow rate determines how fast the TV is delivered to the patient, usually expressed in units of liters per minute.

In this scenario, 6 mL/kg ideal body weight was calculated for the TV, RR set to 26 breaths per minute, PEEP at 10 cm H_2O, and FiO_2 at 100%.

CLINICAL PEARL—STEP 2/3

A high RR is usually set in critically ill patients, such as in the setting of sepsis. This is due to the high metabolic demand, resulting in increased CO_2 production, requiring higher CO_2 elimination.

The patient appeared to be stabilized with the above settings. Overnight, as the resident physician on call, you are notified that this patient's ventilator's peak alarm is being triggered. A nurse calls you to the bedside to evaluate the patient.

What is a peak pressure alarm?
A peak pressure alarm is an alarm that is triggered when the ventilator senses pressures at or above the set limit by the user. Conventional peak alarms are typically set at 40 cm H_2O. Thus, the

alarm was designed to warn providers that elevated pressures are being delivered to the patient, necessitating an evaluation of the etiology. Of note, when a peak pressure alarm is triggered, the ventilator immediately cuts off flow and terminates the breath. This is a protective mechanism to prevent high pressures and barotrauma.

CLINICAL PEARL—STEP 2/3

Although not discussed in this chapter, pressure assist control is a mode in which the pressure being delivered is set at a constant pressure for a specified inspiratory time. Therefore, peak pressure alarms in pressure assist control are less meaningful, as the ventilator already sets a limit for pressure being delivered.

How do you evaluate the etiology of this alarm? What is the differential diagnosis for elevated peak pressures?
To build a differential diagnosis for a ventilator peak alarm, we must review the factors that can impact how much pressure the ventilator must generate to deliver a specified breath.

The determinants of this pressure can be broken up into three main parts, the pressure related to the airway circuit, the pressure related to lung compliance, and the PEEP. The PEEP is often set on the ventilator, and only in specific clinical scenarios does the total PEEP value change intrinsically without changing the setting on the ventilator. Thus, the two main variable components that contribute to changes in pressure are usually from the airway circuit and lung compliance.

BASIC SCIENCE PEARL—STEP 1

Lung compliance is expressed as the change in volume over the change in pressure. Thus, a more compliant lung is one that allows a greater change in volume over a set change in pressure. A less compliant lung is one that only allows a smaller change in volume over a set change in pressure.

In regards to airway circuit, this includes the ventilator tubing, the endotracheal tube, the trachea, and the bronchi. These components contribute to airway pressure by causing increased pressure from increased airway resistance.

CLINICAL PEARL—STEP 2/3

This pressure that is due to the airway circuit is best understood by Ohm's law, which is used for electrical circuits, but the concept can still be applied here. Per Ohm's law, $V = IR$, where V is the potential difference, I is the flow, and R is the resistance. In regards to mechanical ventilation, V is akin to the pressure difference or change in pressure, I is the flow rate, and R is the resistance of the entire airway circuit. Thus, when there is flow (I), the change in pressure is proportional to the resistance of the circuit.

The other contribution to the pressure is lung compliance. In a closed space, when volume is added, pressure must increase. Thus, in the thoracic cavity, when volume, or air, is delivered via a ventilator, the pressure within the lungs must increase as well. The amount of pressure increased depends on the expandability or compliance of the lung.

Thus, to summarize the concepts above, a change in pressure detected on the ventilator can be due to airway circuit resistance or lung compliance.

What maneuver can you do to help narrow your differential diagnosis?

In a patient on volume assist control mode with an elevated peak pressure, the next step would be to measure a plateau pressure via an end inspiratory hold maneuver. An end inspiratory hold is a maneuver in which a pause (usually 0.5 seconds) is initiated at the end of an inspiratory breath. During this pause, there is no airflow or movement, and the pressure is recorded as a plateau pressure. The plateau pressure is a surrogate for the pressure within the alveoli, which reflects lung compliance. As mentioned above, airway circuit resistance only contributes to pressure when there is flow through the circuit. At the time when there is no flow, the pressure due to airway resistance becomes zero. Thus, the plateau pressure measures pressure contribution only from lung compliance.

CLINICAL PEARL—STEP 2/3

If a plateau pressure cannot be measured, two common reasons are due to ventilator alarms and patient-initiated breaths. As a safety feature, if a ventilator alarm is triggered, most ventilators will not perform an advanced maneuver, such as an inspiratory hold. Similarly, ventilators may not allow an advanced maneuver during a patient-initiated breath.

How do you interpret your plateau pressure?

The plateau pressure should be interpreted in conjunction with the peak pressure. If the peak pressure is elevated out of proportion to the plateau pressure (greater than 5 cm H_2O difference between peak and plateau), this suggests an increased airway circuit resistance. Etiologies include tubing issues such as kinked tubing or biting down of the endotracheal tube (ETT), mucus plugging, or bronchospasm.

If the peak pressures are not elevated out of proportion to the plateau pressure, this suggests the increase in pressure is due to a lung compliance issue. This can be broken into categories, such as issues with lung compliance, increased abdominal pressure, restrictive chest wall disorders, mainstem intubation, or pleural space diseases (See Table 42.1).

TABLE 42.1 ■ **Causes of Elevated Peak Pressures**

High Peak, Low Plateau	High Peak, High Plateau
Tubing issues	Parenchymal lung pathology
- Kinked tubing	- ARDS
- Patient biting on endotracheal tube	- Pulmonary edema, pneumonia
- Excess condensed fluid in the tubing	
- Clogged filter	
Mucus plugging	Abdominal pathology
	- Abdominal compartment syndrome
	- Ascites
Bronchospasm	Chest wall pathology
	- Circumferential chest wall burn
	- Obesity
	Mainstem intubation
	Pleural space disease
	- Pleural effusion
	- Pneumothorax

The nurse informs you that the peak pressures were previously 25 cm H_2O with plateau pressures of 22 cm H_2O. However, at the time the nurse called you, the peak pressures were 40 cm H_2O while the plateau pressure remained the same at 22 cm H_2O. You proceed to check the ventilator tubing and the endotracheal tube. You attempt to pass the suction catheter through the endotracheal tube; however, you meet some resistance. After relaxing the patient's jaw manually, a repeat plateau and peak pressure were measured, which are improved but still elevated. At this point, you are able to pass the suction catheter and suction out some secretions. After this, the peak pressures return to 25 cm H_2O.

Over the next few days, the patient improves and is on minimal ventilator settings. You are covering the night shift again and get called regarding elevated peak pressures.

As you show up at the bedside, the nurse informs you that the peak pressures are again 40 cm H_2O; however, the plateau pressures are now 38, despite the same set TV.

What would you do next?

Given the elevated plateau pressure and elevated peak pressure, this is an issue with lung compliance. As such, one should evaluate the different etiologies for a sudden decreased lung compliance. which include ETT malpositioning, pneumothorax, pleural effusion, flash pulmonary edema, and abdominal compartment syndrome.

A quick physical exam is performed. There are absent breath sounds on the left side. The abdomen is soft, and nondistended. A bedside ultrasound is performed that is suggestive of pneumothorax. A chest radiograph (CXR) is ordered, which confirms pneumothorax (Fig. 42.2).

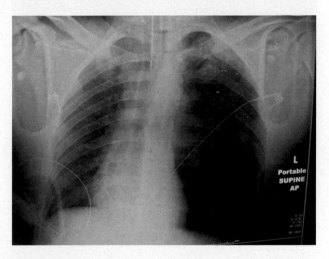

Fig. 42.2   Left-sided pneumothorax in intubated patient. (*Rosen's Emergency Medicine: Concepts and Clinical Practice*. Elsevier, 2018.)

CLINICAL PEARL—STEP 2/3

Bedside ultrasonography is a sensitive adjunct to evaluate for pneumothorax. The presence of lung sliding effectively rules out pneumothorax. However, the absence of lung sliding has poor specificity for pneumothorax (See Table 42.2). A pneumothorax should be confirmed with a chest radiograph unless the patient is hemodynamically unstable.

TABLE 42.2 ■ Causes of False-Positive Bedside Ultrasound for Pneumothorax

Causes of Absent Lung Sliding in Bedside Ultrasound
Right mainstem intubation
Mucus plug
Severe ARDS
Severe pneumonia
Lung fibrosis
History of pleurodesis
History of pneumonectomy
Severe hyperinflation

A surgical consult was requested and an emergent left-sided surgical chest tube was placed with adequate re-expansion of the lung (Fig. 42.3).

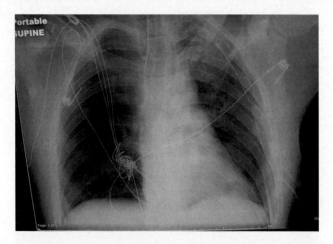

Fig. 42.3 Interval placement of left-sided surgical chest tube. Adequate re-expansion of lung. (*Rosen's Emergency Medicine: Concepts and Clinical Practice.* Elsevier, 2018.)

With the above care, the patient continued to improve throughout his ICU stay and the ventilator was weaned to a PEEP of 5 cm H_2O and FiO_2 of 40%.

Now that the patient is on minimal ventilator settings, how do you assess a patient's readiness for extubation?

There are no strict criteria to evaluate a patient for readiness for extubation. However, there are several parameters that are often assessed as a screening tool, and if a patient meets most of the parameters, then the patient should be considered for a spontaneous breathing trial.

These parameters include, but are not limited to, the following:

- Improving disease process that resulted in intubation
- FiO_2 less than 40%–50%, PEEP < 8 cm H_2O
- RR < 35
- Stable cardiovascular status, HR < 140, minimal to no pressors

> **CLINICAL PEARL—STEP 2/3**
>
> Before considering a spontaneous breathing trial, patients should be clinically improving from their disease process, be on minimal ventilator settings, and be hemodynamically stable.

What is a spontaneous breathing trial?
As the name suggests, a spontaneous breathing trial (SBT) is a test to assess if a patient can potentially be liberated from a ventilator. The ventilator settings are changed to a spontaneous mode, such as PS mode, with minimal or no ventilator support.

> **CLINICAL PEARL—STEP 2/3**
>
> In PS ventilation mode, as mentioned previously, the patient must breathe spontaneously. In this mode, a PS pressure is set, and the PEEP is set. During a patient-initiated breath, the ventilator will provide the PS pressure as long as the patient continues to inhale. Once the ventilator senses that the flow of air is decreasing (suggesting that the patient is done taking their breath), it will terminate the PS pressure and switch to PEEP pressure for exhalation.

A true spontaneous breathing trial is one in which there is minimal support provided by the ventilator; therefore, a PS of 5–8 cm H_2O is usually set with a PEEP of 5 cm H_2O. This is typically carried out for at least 30 minutes, but no longer than 120 minutes due to the potential for patient fatigability.

> **CLINICAL PEARL—STEP 2/3**
>
> The PS that is set during pressure support ventilation mode is the amount of pressure above the PEEP level that is set. Therefore, if a patient is on a pressure support of 7 cm H_2O over a PEEP of 5 cm H_2O, when the patient initiates a breath, they receive a total of 5 + 7 cm H_2O during the breath. At the end of the breath, the pressure returns back to the PEEP level, which would be 5 cm H_2O in this case.

> **CLINICAL PEARL—STEP 2/3**
>
> A spontaneous breathing trial is usually performed in conjunction with a spontaneous awakening trial in which sedation is turned off to allow the patient to wake up.

When does someone pass a spontaneous breathing trial?
A patient will have passed a spontaneous breathing trial if they are able to tolerate minimal PS settings for at least 30 minutes, but no longer than 120 minutes, without meeting any of the termination criteria listed below.

When does someone fail a spontaneous breathing trial?
A patient will have failed a spontaneous breathing trial if there is evidence of fatigue, hypoxia, or hemodynamic instability. Examples of criteria that would result in the termination of a spontaneous breathing trial are listed below.
- $PaO_2 \leq 50–60$ mm Hg on $FiO_2 \geq 50\%$ or $SaO_2 \leq 90\%$
- RR > 35
- HR > 140
- Cardiac arrhythmias
- Hemodynamic instability
- SBP > 180 mm Hg or increased by $\geq 20\%$

When can you repeat a spontaneous breathing trial after a patient has failed?
The frequency of spontaneous breathing trials is not yet well defined; however, they should generally be performed at least once daily. If the clinical condition of a patient changes, it may be reasonable to attempt the trial again on the same day. However, due to the necessity for nursing and respiratory therapists to be available during a spontaneous awakening and spontaneous breathing trial, it is often difficult to perform this trial multiple times throughout the day.

What are some weaning parameters that are sometimes used as adjuncts to assess for extubation?
There are several different weaning parameters that can be obtained; however, there is debate regarding their usefulness as there is no one parameter that is able to predict successful liberation from the ventilator. The most extensively studied parameter is the Rapid Shallow Breathing Index, or the RSBI.
  • It is defined as the RR divided by the TV, where RR is in breaths per minute, and TV is in liters. Patients with RSBI greater than 105 are more likely to fail extubation
There are several other parameters, such as the negative inspiratory force, maximal inspiratory pressure, and total minute ventilation. These parameters are less well studied.

What type of patients are at high risk for post extubation stridor?
The following risk factors are considered high risk factors for post extubation stridor
  • traumatic initial intubation
  • intubation for more than 6 days
  • large endotracheal tube
  • female
  • reintubation after unplanned extubation
Only patients who are at high risk for post extubation stridor should have their cuff leak checked. Otherwise, it is not recommended to check cuff leak for other types of patients as its interpretation is less meaningful.

If your patient is determined to be at high risk for post extubation stridor and they have no cuff leak, what is the next step in management?
Systemic steroids should be administered at least 4 hours prior to planned extubation. Repeat cuff leak should not be routinely performed.

The patient was ultimately extubated a couple of days later, initially to a high-flow nasal cannula. The chest tube was eventually clamped and discontinued without re-expansion of pneumothorax. He completed a 21-day course of sulfamethoxazole and trimethoprim with a prednisone taper. He was also started on antiviral therapy for his HIV and discharged with outpatient follow-up.

Case Summary

  ■ **Complaint/History:** 32-year-old man with HIV presenting with shortness of breath.
  ■ **Findings:** Found to have respiratory distress and hypoxia, intubated for respiratory failure
  ■ **Lab results/Tests:** Bilateral infiltrates on chest radiograph

---

Diagnosis: Pneumocystis pneumonia, complicated by pneumothorax

---

  ■ **Treatment:** Sulfamethoxazole and trimethoprim, steroids, surgical chest tube

BEYOND THE PEARLS

- When a peak pressure alarm is triggered, the ventilator will terminate the breath as a safety mechanism. Thus, no further volume will be delivered to the patient in that scenario. As such, patients can receive less volume than specified when the peak pressure alarm is triggered.
- A PS breath is terminated after a significant drop in the inspiratory flow.
- If the patient is fighting against the ventilator to breathe (also termed ventilator dyssynchrony), this can cause elevated peak pressures, hypoxia, and poor ventilation.
- Oxygen toxicity occurs with prolonged high FiO_2; therefore, the FiO_2 should be weaned if high levels of oxygen are not needed.
- One contributor to increased peak pressures includes auto-PEEP, which is PEEP that is intrinsically generated, usually from the inability to completely exhale due to obstructive lung disease.
- If there is no lung sliding or B-lines on an intubated patient on the left side, one important differential is right mainstem intubation.
- Pneumocystis pneumonia is called pneumocystis because of its propensity to cause cysts in the lungs, which are at high risk for rupture, resulting in pneumothorax.
- For patients who are high risk extubations, they can be extubated directly to non-invasive positive pressure ventilation, such as high flow nasal cannula or bilevel positive airway pressure ventilation.
- If a patient is hemodynamically unstable or significantly hypoxic and the ventilator is alarming, it is prudent to remove the ventilator from the equation. Disconnect the patient from the ventilator and perform manual bag valve ventilation until the underlying etiology is identified.
- Although peak and plateau pressures cannot always be reliably measured in pressure assist control, the expiratory flow loop can give valuable information in regards to the change in compliance or airway resistance.

References

Boles, J. -M., Bion, J., Connors, A., Herridge, M., Marsh, B., Melot, C., et al. (2007). Weaning from mechanical ventilation. *European Respiratory Journal, 29*(5), 1033–1056. https://doi.org/10.1183/09031936.00010206.

Fan, E., Del Sorbo, L., Goligher, E. C., Hodgson, C. L., Munshi, L., Walkey, A. J., et al. (2017). An official American Thoracic Society/European Society of Intensive Care Medicine/Society of Critical Care Medicine clinical practice guideline: mechanical ventilation in adult patients with acute respiratory distress syndrome. *American Journal of Respiratory and Critical Care Medicine, 195*, 1253.

Girard, T. D., Alhazzani, W., Kress, J. P., Ouellette, D. R., Schmidt, G. A., Truwit, J. D., et al. (2017). An official American Thoracic Society/American College of Chest Physicians Clinical Practice Guideline: liberation from mechanical ventilation in critically ill adults. Rehabilitation protocols, ventilator liberation protocols, and Cuff Leak Tests. *American Journal of Respiratory and Critical Care Medicine, 195*(1), 120–133. https://doi.org/10.1164/rccm.201610-2075st.

Girard, T. D., et al. "Spontaneous Awakening and Breathing Trials – SCCM." *Society of Critical Care Medicine*, https://www.sccm.org/getattachment/86464100-4b13-4da5-b3d1-39a9a4cceb64/Spontaneous-Awakening-and-Breathing-Trials.

Müller, N. L., & Silva, C. I. S. (2008). *Imaging of the Chest*. Philadelphia: Saunders/Elsevier.

Slutsky, A.S., & Brochard, L. Mechanical ventilation. In L. Goldman & A. Schafer (Eds.), *Goldman–Cecil Medicine* (pp. 635–641). Philadelphia: Elsevier.

Walls, R., Hockberger, R., & Gausche-Hill, M. (2018). *Rosen's Emergency Medicine: Concepts and Clinical Practice*. Philadelphia: Elsevier.

A 62-Year-Old Male With Altered Mental Status in the Intensive Care Unit

Dominic Engracia ▪ Patrick Chan ▪ Raj Dasgupta

A 62-year-old male has been admitted to the intensive care unit (ICU) after being found with acute encephalopathy and covered in melena on the street. He has a past medical history of hypertension, major depressive disorder, and myopia. His social history is significant for homelessness and polysubstance abuse including alcohol, meth, and cocaine. He was intubated for airway protection and sedated for esophagogastroduodenoscopy (EGD) and colonoscopy in the ICU. His hospital course has been complicated by septic shock and acute renal failure. Fentanyl, propofol, and midazolam have been used for analgesia and sedation. On hospital day five, his sedation is weaned and he is put on a spontaneous breathing trial. While appearing intermittently awake, he rarely follows commands for weaning parameters for extubation and has periods of agitation requiring physical restraints. He is left intubated, and sedation is restarted at half dose. He continues to have altered mental status. Laboratory evaluation was unremarkable, including chemistry panel and thyroid studies. Computed tomography (CT) scan of the head revealed no abnormalities.

What is ICU delirium?

Delirium is an acute state of brain dysfunction and confusion defined by fluctuating mental status, inattention, and either disorganized thinking or an altered level of consciousness. This disturbance in mental status can fluctuate throughout the day and may occur in addition to baseline disease (e.g., dementia). The pathophysiology behind the development of delirium is thought to be related to the imbalance of neurotransmitters that modulate cognition, behavior, and mood. Delirium is subcategorized based on its presenting psychomotor symptoms such as hyperactive, hypoactive, or mixed. The incidence of delirium appears to be highest in the ICU, with up to 80% of mechanically ventilated patients having delirium. Delirium only identifies a collection of signs indicating an altered mental state; it does not suggest or elucidate an etiology.

CLINICAL PEARL—STEP 2/3

Hypoactive delirium is more common and is associated with worse outcomes compared to those patients with hyperactive delirium. This subtype is characterized by withdrawal, flat affect, apathy, lethargy, and decreased responsiveness. Due to the apparent quiet and negative symptomatology, it is often underdiagnosed.

How is delirium diagnosed in the ICU?

The standard for delirium diagnosis is evaluation by using criteria from The Diagnostic and Statistical Manual of Mental Disorders, Fifth Edition (DSM-5), although this is not always feasible in the clinical setting. Delirium is often diagnosed clinically using validated screening tools such as the Confusion Assessment Method for the Intensive Care Unit (CAM-ICU) or the Intensive Care Delirium Screening Checklist (ICDSC). The Confusion Assessment Method

(CAM) was developed and validated for diagnosing delirium, although this was designed for patients who were able to communicate verbally. To assist with diagnosis in nonverbal, mechanically ventilated patients, the CAM was adapted into the CAM-ICU (Fig. 43.1). This abbreviated version assesses four cardinal features—acute changes/fluctuations in mental status, inattention, disorganized thinking, and an altered level of consciousness. The presence of the first two, plus either the third or fourth feature, indicates a diagnosis of delirium. It should be noted that this diagnostic tool cannot be used when patients are heavily sedated, such as those on −4 and −5 on the Richmond Agitation-Sedation Scale (RASS). The ICDSC assesses eight diagnostic features of delirium over an entire nursing shift (altered level of consciousness, inattention, disorientation, psychosis, altered psychomotor activity, inappropriate speech/mood, sleep disturbance, and symptom fluctuation), with the presence of four or more of the listed features indicating the presence of delirium.

What predisposing and precipitating risk factors for delirium did this patient have?
Risk factors for delirium are numerous and can be classified into two categories: predisposing (baseline characteristics) and precipitating (hospital-related or iatrogenic) (Table 43.1). This patient has multiple baseline risk factors that have been consistently found to increase the risk of delirium, including advanced age, alcohol and drug use, depression, and a high severity of illness. He also has multiple precipitating factors such as mechanical ventilation, sepsis, and deep sedation involving the use of benzodiazepines and opioids.

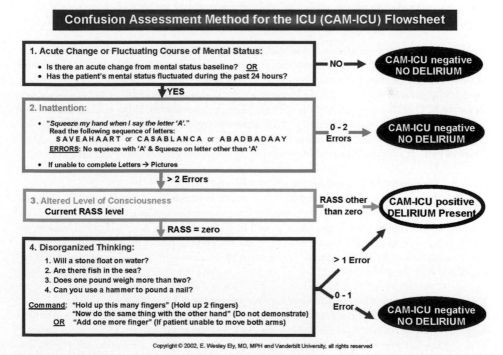

Fig. 43.1 Confusion Assessment Method for the Intensive Care Unit.

TABLE 43.1 ■ Risk Factors for Delirium

Predisposing Risk Factors (baseline characteristics)
Advanced age
Baseline cognitive impairment (e.g., dementia)
Frailty
Alcohol and drug abuse
Severity of illness on hospital admission

Precipitating Risk Factors (hospital-related or iatrogenic)
Metabolic disturbances
Sepsis
Mechanical ventilation
Sleep disturbances
Poor pain control
Prolonged restraint use and immobility
Head trauma
Medications (benzodiazepines, opioids, propofol)
Deep sedation
Anticholinergics
Steroids
Surgery

CLINICAL PEARL—STEP 2/3

Benzodiazepines should not be used as first-line for sedation or agitation. Benzodiazepines can actually precipitate worsening mental status and worsening delirium. Currently, propofol and dexmedetomidine are recommended over benzodiazepines for sedation in critically ill, mechanically ventilated adults.

How can delirium be prevented in critically ill patients?
It is important to identify modifiable risk factors that could lead to delirium for critically ill patients in the ICU. Precipitating risk factors represent an area of potential modification and intervention for delirium prevention and treatment. Medications are perhaps the most prevalent modifiable risk factor for ICU delirium, specifically the use of analgesics and sedatives. Using nonbenzodiazepine sedatives (propofol or dexmedetomidine) over benzodiazepines has been shown to decrease the incidence of delirium in ICU patients. Other important modifiable factors that providers should be aware of include adequate pain control, good sleep hygiene, and early mobility and exercise.

What are the outcomes of delirium in critically ill patients?
Delirium has a high prevalence in the ICU, and multiple studies have shown that this problem is associated with many poor outcomes. Studies have shown the presence of ICU delirium to be associated with higher reintubation rates as well as higher ICU and hospital costs. Delirium in the ICU has not consistently been shown to be associated with higher mortality rates. However, it is strongly associated with cognitive impairment up to 12 months after discharge and may be associated with longer hospital stays.

What are ways in which we can assess and monitor pain in the ICU?
Patients in the ICU have been found to have heightened pain experiences compared to healthier subjects. This pain at rest typically involves the back and lower extremities, and is often difficult to recognize in those who are intubated and sedated. When patients are able to self-report, the Numerical Rating Scale can be used for pain assessment, with 0 indicating no pain and 10 for maximum pain. If there is an inability to report, validated scales in the ICU include the Behavioral Pain Scale and the Critical-Care Pain Observation Tool (CPOT). The CPOT uses indicators in

nonverbal patients to evaluate the presence of pain: facial expressions, body movements, muscle tension, and compliance with the ventilator (or vocalization in extubated patients).

What analgesic medications can we use and how should we use them to manage pain in these patients?

Opioids continue to be the mainstay for analgesia in the ICU (Table 43.2), but a multi-modal approach with nonopioid analgesics should be considered. Even in the critically ill patient, acetaminophen is a good first-line choice. Ketamine at low doses can provide pain relief without neurological side effects. It also does not cause hypotension or suppress respiratory drive. Gabapentin can also be used for those with a history of neuropathic pain. Certain agents should be used cautiously or avoided at all if possible. Most recent guidelines do not recommend routine use of nonsteroidal antiinflammatory drugs (NSAIDs), such as ibuprofen and ketorolac. Response to these medications should be assessed periodically and adjustments can be made to both dose and frequency. An important focus should be kept on de-escalating opioid use when appropriate.

CLINICAL PEARL—STEP 2/3

While opioids continue to be the front-line agents for pain control in the ICU, attention should be given to common side effects, especially with prolonged use. These include respiratory depression, decreased gastric motility, and opioid dependence and withdrawal.

CLINICAL PEARL—STEP 2/3

Methylnaltrexone can be used for opioid-induced constipation.

How should sedation be utilized in the ICU?

Critically ill patients in the ICU, specifically those receiving mechanical ventilation, require analgesia and sedation to provide comfort and prevent self-harm (e.g., self-extubation, ventilator dyssynchrony) (Table 43.3). In addition to the identification and modification of predisposing and precipitating factors that lead to anxiety, pain, and delirium, validated sedation and delirium scales should be used to regularly monitor patients. Multiple sedation scales have been developed and validated for use in the ICU, including the RASS (Table 43.4). For a more objective approach, bispectral index monitors (BIS), which are based on the processing of electroencephalographic signals, are currently being investigated, although not currently widely used. When using sedatives, a structured, patient-focused approach should be used to ensure responsible use while attempting

---

TABLE 43.2 ■ Analgesic Options in the ICU

Drug	Onset/Duration	Advantages	Disadvantages
Morphine Sulfate	5–10 min/2–4 h	Reduces tachypnea	↓BP, respiratory depression, accumulation in hepatic/renal failure
Fentanyl	1–2 min/2–4 h (longer in liver failure)	Less hypotension than morphine	3A4 inhibitors may increase fentanyl; fever will increase fentanyl patch levels by 30%
Hydromorphone	5–10 min/2–4 h	May work if patient is tolerant to morphine or fentanyl	Respiratory depression, caution in nonventilated patient; highly addictive

ICU, Intensive care unit.

TABLE 43.3 ■ Sedative Options in the ICU

Drug	Onset/Duration	Advantages	Disadvantages
Propofol	30–50 s/ approximately 3–10 min (dose dependent)	Short acting	↓BP, increased serum triglyceride, pancreatitis, propofol infusion syndrome, zinc depletion
Dexmedetomidine	Immediate/ approximately 6 min (longer in liver failure)	Very short duration; has some analgesic properties	↓BP, ↓HR; not approved for use 24 h, some studies use longer
Lorazepam (Ativan)	5–20 min/6–8 h; up to 24–72 h in elderly/ cirrhosis/ ESRD	Inexpensive, longer half-life	Propylene glycol toxicity at high doses (anion gap metabolic acidosis, renal insufficiency)
Midazolam (Versed)	5–10 min/1–4 h (longer in ESRD/ CHF/liver failure)	Shorter acting if preserved organ function; fast onset	Many drug interactions, may increase midazolam levels, active metabolite accumulates in renal failure
Ketamine	30 s/5–10 min	Does not cause hypotension, bronchodilator, anti-convulsant effects	Can cause hallucinations or psychosis, may cause laryngospasm (rare), should be avoided in patients with a history of ischemic heart disease

CHF, congestive heart failure; *ESRD*, End-Stage Renal Disease, defined as glomerular filtration rate (GFR) less than 15 mL/min; *ICU*, Intensive care unit.
↓BP, hypotension.
↓HR, bradycardia.
Sessler et al., Estrad et al.

TABLE 43.4 ■ Richmond Agitation-Sedation Scale

Score	Term	Description
+4	Combative	Overtly combative or violent; immediate danger to staff.
+3	Very agitated	Pulls on or removes tube(s) or catheter(s) or has aggressive behavior toward staff.
+2	Agitated	Frequent nonpurposeful movement or patient-ventilator dyssynchrony.
+1	Restless	Anxious or apprehensive but movements not aggressive or vigorous.
0	Alert and calm	
−1	Drowsy	Not fully alert, but has sustained (more than 10 s) awakening, with eye contact, to voice.
−2	Light sedation	Briefly (< 10 s) awakens with eye contact to voice.
−3	Moderate sedation	Any movement (but no eye contact) to voice.
−4	Deep sedation	No response to voice, but any movement to physical stimulus.
−5	Unarousable	No response to voice or physical stimulation.

Sessler et al.

to de-escalate therapy. Inappropriate and prolonged use of sedatives has been associated with poor outcomes, including prolonged duration of mechanical ventilation, length of ICU admission, and length of hospital admission. Maintaining light levels of sedation in critically ill patients is recommended by current society guidelines and is associated with a shorter time to extubation and reduced tracheostomy rates. Daily sedation interruptions, defined by a period of time each day during which sedation is completely discontinued and a patient is allowed to achieve arousal/ alertness, have been shown to be effective in maintaining light levels of sedation.

BASIC SCIENCE PEARL—STEP 1

Propofol primarily binds to GABA-A receptors and produces sedative and amnestic effects, but no analgesia is provided. Dexmedetomidine is a selective α_2-adrenoceptor agonist with anesthetic and sedative properties, and provides mild analgesia. Ketamine is primarily a non-competitive NMDA receptor antagonist that provides dissociative sedation.

Can antipsychotic medications be used in the ICU?
The most recent recommendations from the 2018 Pain, Agitation, Delirium, Immobility, and Sleep Guidelines from the Society of Critical Care Medicine recommend against the use of halo-peridol or atypical antipsychotics to prevent or treat delirium in critically ill patients.

What approach should we take to treat this patient's delirium?
Currently, there is a great absence of strong evidence for the use of pharmacologic agents in the treatment of delirium. The Clinical Practice Guidelines for the Prevention and Management of Pain, Agitation/Sedation, Delirium, Immobility, and Sleep Disruption in Adult Patients in the ICU (PADIS), most recently updated in 2018, have a few recommendations regarding delirium treatment. Use of dexmedetomidine is recommended for mechanically ventilated patients when agitation precludes weaning or extubation.

Nonpharmacologic, multicomponent interventions are instead recommended to reduce or shorten delirium (e.g., reorientation, cognitive stimulation, sleep improvement, immobility reduction, visual/hearing impairment reduction).

CLINICAL PEARL—STEP 2/3

When agitation precludes the weaning of sedation and extubation, dexmedetomidine is a useful agent to utilize. It does not depress ventilation, and studies have shown benefit over benzodiazepines in regards to time to extubation and overall sedation duration.

The patient is assessed and diagnosed with delirium using the CAM-ICU. Dexmedetomidine is started, and the patient becomes calmer. Restraints are removed and nurses start to focus on keeping the patient oriented while minimizing sleep interruptions. The remaining analgesic and sedative medications are weaned and the patient is successfully extubated on dexmedetomidine. Dexmedetomidine is discontinued 2 days later when the patient is transferred to the floor. Appropriate eye glasses are provided to the patient and the hospital social worker assists with homelessness and polysubstance abuse issues prior to discharge.

Case Summary

- **Complaint/History:** A 62-year-old male currently intubated and sedated in the ICU, unable to follow commands with periods of agitation.
- **Findings:** On physical exam, alert and oriented to name only, no other abnormal focal neurological deficits.

■ **Lab Results/Test:** No abnormal labs on chemistry panel. CT head negative.

Diagnosis: ICU delirium.

■ **Treatment:** Non-pharmacologic approach (early mobilization, uninterrupted sleep, orientation), dexmedetomidine can be considered when agitation precludes weaning or extubation.

BEYOND THE PEARLS

- It is well described that the circadian rhythm is abolished in critically ill, sedated patients. Studies have attempted to describe the potential effectiveness of nighttime dexmedetomidine for maintaining a natural sleep-wake cycle as it is thought to naturally promote non-rapid eye movement (NREM) sleep. One study showed that nightly infusion improved sleep by increasing sleep efficiency and modifying the sleep pattern to mainly at night. Another study showed a similar effect but found a disturbed sleep architecture without evidence of rapid eye movement (REM) sleep.
- Propofol has been associated with a life-threatening side effect called propofol infusion syndrome. This syndrome is caused by impairment of mitochondrial activity, resulting in multisystem organ dysfunction. Common findings include elevated triglyceride levels, pancreatitis, rhabdomyolysis, acute renal failure, and cardiac failure. Green urine can be present and is a unique side effect due to metabolites but is transient and benign.
- Ketamine and its unique properties can make it a useful alternative compared to other medication options. It has been found to lower airway resistance, which may have benefits in patients with status asthmaticus. It has also been shown to suppress electroencephalogram discharges in patients with seizures, suggesting an anticonvulsant effect. Finally, although concerns have been raised about its potential effects on increasing intracranial pressure, this association has not been found in a recent systematic review.
- Fentanyl is often not detected in a routine urine drug screen.
- ICU delirium bundle protocols have improved sleep in hospitalized patients and reduced the incidence of delirium.

References

Pun, B. T., & Ely, E. W. (2007). The importance of diagnosing and managing ICU delirium. *Chest, 132,* 624–636.

Levy, J. H. (2016). Intensive care unit delirium. *Anesthesiology, 125,* 1229–1241.

Ely, E. W., Inouye, S. K., Bernard, G. R., Gordon, S., Francis, J., May, L., et al. (2001). Delirium in mechanically ventilated patients: Validity and reliability of the confusion assessment method for the intensive care unit (CAM-ICU). *JAMA, 286*(21), 2703–2710.

Devlin, J. W., Skrobik, Y., Gélinas, C., Needham, D. M., Slooter, A., Pandharipande, P. P., et al. (2018). Clinical practice guidelines for the prevention and management of pain, agitation/sedation, delirium, immobility, and sleep disruption in adult patients in the ICU. *Critical Care Medicine, 46*(9), e825–e873.

Chanques, G., Sebbane, M., Barbotte, E., Viel, E., Eledjam, J. J., & Jaber, S. (2007). A prospective study of pain at rest: Incidence and characteristics of an unrecognized symptom in surgical and trauma versus medical intensive care unit patients. *Anesthesiology, 107*(5), 858–860.

Gélinas, C., Fillion, L., Puntillo, K. A., Viens, C., & Fortier, M. (2006). Validation of the critical-care pain observation tool in adult patients. *American Journal of Critical Care, 15*(4), 420–427.

Sessler, C. N., & Varney, K. (2008). Patient-focused sedation and analgesia in the ICU. *Chest, 133*(2), 552–565.

Kollef, M. H., Levy, N. T., Ahrens, T. S., Schaiff, R., Prentice, D., & Sherman, G. (1998). The use of continuous i.v. sedation is associated with prolongation of mechanical ventilation. *Chest, 114*(2), 541–548.

Sessler, C. N., Gosnell, M. S., Grap, M. J., Brophy, G. M., O'Neal, P. V., Keane, K. A., et al. (2002). The Richmond Agitation-Sedation Scale: Validity and reliability in adult intensive care unit patients. *American Journal of Respiratory and Critical Care Medicine, 166*(10), 1338–1344.

Alexopoulou, C., Kondili, E., Diamantaki, E., Psarologakis, C., Kokkini, S., Bolaki, M., et al. (2014). Effects of dexmedetomidine on sleep quality in critically ill patients: A pilot study. *Anesthesiology*, *121*(4), 801–807. https://doi.org/10.1097/ALN.0000000000000361.

Oto, J., Yamamoto, K., Koike, S., Onodera, M., Imanaka, H., & Nishimura, M. (2012). Sleep quality of mechanically ventilated patients sedated with dexmedetomidine. *Intensive Care Medicine*, *38*(12), 1982–1989. https://doi.org/10.1007/s00134-012-2685-y.

Erstad, B. L., & Patanwala, A. E. (2016). Ketamine for analgosedation in critically ill patients. *Journal of Critical Care*, *35*, 145–149. https://doi.org/10.1016/j.jcrc.2016.05.016.

A 34-Year-Old Female With Blood Tinged Sputum

Ara Vartanyan ■ Nathan Lim ■ Patrick Chan ■ Michelle Koolaee ■ Raj Dasgupta

A 34-year-old female presents to the emergency department with complaints of fevers, chills, night sweats, and a progressive productive cough for 2 months. Her sputum is blood-tinged and has been getting progressively bloodier. She has no significant past medical history and is not taking any medications. On physical examination, her blood pressure is 100/60 mm Hg, heart rate is 100 beats per minute, respiration rate is 28 breaths per minute, and oxygen saturation is 90% on room air. There are decreased breath sounds with diffuse crackles bilaterally. The remainder of the exam is normal. A chest radiograph (CXR) reveals bilateral diffuse airspace opacities (Fig. 44.1).

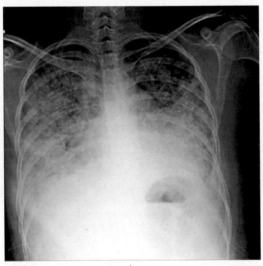

Fig. 44.1 Chest x-ray with diffuse bilateral airspace opacities. (Reproduced from: *Reumatología Clínica (English Edition)*, vol. 14, no. 5, 2018.)

It appears that the patient is having hemoptysis. Prior to doing a full evaluation for hemoptysis, what are some other disease processes that can be confused for hemoptysis?
Hemoptysis, by definition, is coughing up blood, usually from bleeding from the lung or airway. However, other sites of bleeding can mimic hemoptysis, such as bleeding from the nose, throat, or

even the gastrointestinal tract. As such, reasonable attempts should be made to differentiate true hemoptysis from these other sources of bleeding.

After a brief physical exam and review of systems, patient's presentation is consistent with hemoptysis. How do we quantify the hemoptysis?
Previously, massive hemoptysis was defined by a specific amount of expectorated blood within a particular period of time. For example, prior definitions of massive hemoptysis suggested either 100 mL over 1 hour or even as little as 150 mL over 24 hours. However, there has been a shift towards the characterization of the hemoptysis based on the briskness of the bleed or the effect of the bleed on the patient's ability to protect one's airway.

CLINICAL PEARL—STEP 2/3

In terms of outcomes, previous studies have estimated that life-threatening hemoptysis can occur in 5% to 15% of patients who present with hemoptysis.

What is the initial evaluation of massive hemoptysis?
For patients who are presenting with life-threatening hemoptysis, the first step involves stabilizing the patient and establishing airway protection. The next step involves localizing the site and determining the cause of the bleeding, and finally, the last step would be the treatments aimed at stopping or preventing recurrent bleeding.

The patient was placed on supplemental oxygen given her low oxygen saturation and high likelihood of decompensation. Despite supplemental oxygen, she continued to have hemoptysis and further desaturations, eventually resulting in endotracheal intubation with an 8.5 mm endotracheal tube (ETT). A central line was placed for resuscitation.

What is on the differential diagnosis?
The differential for hemoptysis is broad. The top three major categories include primary pulmonary processes, infections, and autoimmune etiologies. Within each category, there are numerous etiologies that could cause hemoptysis. However, the most common primary pulmonary etiologies for hemoptysis include bronchiectasis or malignancy, which cause erosion into the bronchial arteries, resulting in airway bleeding. Common infections include tuberculosis, fungal infections such as aspergillus, and necrotizing pneumonias. Autoimmune conditions such as systemic lupus erythematosus and antineutrophil cytoplasmic antibody (ANCA) associated vasculitis are common etiologies of hemoptysis. In addition to these categories, there are other etiologies, which are summarized below (Table 44.1).

How would you work-up this patient?
For patients with hemoptysis, a broad work-up should be initiated. To help narrow the differential, if not already obtained, a simple CXR should be obtained to determine the extent of the bleed.

Routine labs such as complete blood count (CBC), complete metabolic panel (CMP), coagulation studies, and type and screen should be among the initial labs that are drawn.

CLINICAL PEARL—STEP 2/3

Reversal of coagulopathy can be life-saving in massive hemoptysis.

TABLE 44.1 ■ Etiologies of Hemoptysis

Pulmonary
1. Bronchiectasis
2. Malignancy
3. Pulmonary embolism and infarction

Infectious
1. Aspergillosis and other fungal infections
2. Necrotizing pneumonia and lung abscess
3. Tuberculosis
4. Parasites

Rheumatologic
1. ANCA-associated vasculitis
2. Systemic lupus erythematosus
3. Goodpasture syndrome
4. Behçet disease
5. Cryoglobulinemia

Cardiac
1. Congestive heart failure
2. Mitral stenosis

Vascular
1. Arteriovenous malformation
2. Pulmonary artery aneurysm

Coagulopathy
1. Von Willebrand disease
2. Hemophilia
3. Disseminated intravascular coagulation

Iatrogenic
1. Airway erosion from airway stent
2. Mediastinal or lung radiation therapy
3. Lung laceration from chest tube placement or thoracentesis
4. Coagulopathy from thrombolytic therapy or medications
5. Tracheoinnominate artery fistula in patients with tracheostomy
6. Complication from bronchoscopy, transthoracic needle aspiration, or lung biopsy
7. Swan-Ganz catheterization

Miscellaneous
1. Foreign body aspiration
2. Trauma

Source: Davidson, K., & Shojaee, S. (2020). Managing massive hemoptysis. *Chest, 157*(1), 77–88. https://doi.org/10.1016/j.chest.2019.07.012.

CLINICAL PEARL—STEP 2/3

Patients with active bleeding should always have an active type and screen for the possibility of blood transfusions in the near future.

Given concern for infection, sputum cultures and acid-fast bacilli stain and cultures should also be obtained. Autoimmune etiologies should be considered. An antinuclear antibody panel, ANCA panel, erythrocyte sedimentation rate, C-reactive protein level, and complement levels should be obtained. A urinalysis to look for proteinuria or red cell casts to suggest glomerulonephritis can also be especially helpful in this scenario.

CLINICAL PEARL—STEP 2/3

Autoimmune diseases can present as a pulmonary-renal syndrome, which is characterized by rapidly progressive glomerulonephritis and diffuse alveolar hemorrhage. This syndrome carries high morbidity and mortality; early recognition can significantly improve outcomes.

If the patient is stable enough, a CT chest should also be obtained to better elucidate the location of the bleed.

You decide to send the above work up, and the relevant labs return below. What is your interpretation of the results?

Laboratory	Results
Leukocyte count	17,000/μL (17 ×10⁹/L)
Hematocrit	25%
Platelet count	550,000/μL (550 ×10⁹/L)
Serum creatinine	1.2 mg/dL
Urinalysis	Normal, no protein, no RBCs
Erythrocyte sedimentation rate	75 mm/h
C-reactive protein	186 mg/L
c-ANCA	Positive
p-ANCA	Negative
Antiproteinase-3 (PR3) antibodies	Positive
Antimyeloperoxidase (MPO) antibodies	Negative

Given the constellation of symptoms, the patient was diagnosed with ANCA-associated vasculitis, more specifically, granulomatosis with polyangiitis (GPA) given c-ANCA and antiproteinase 3 antibody positivity.

CLINICAL PEARL—STEP 2/3

The presentation of GPA can be highly variable, ranging from milder disease limited to the upper airway tract such as sinusitis, saddle nose deformity or tracheal stenosis and cutaneous lesions such as palpable purpura to severe life-threatening manifestations with pulmonary and renal involvement.

What is the management of massive hemoptysis?

If the side of bleeding is known, immediate lateralization by moving the patient into a decubitus position, with the bleeding side down, is the first step. This maneuver is performed to prevent the hemorrhage from spilling over onto the other side. Additional temporizing interventions include nebulized tranexamic acid, which is a synthetic antifibrinolyic agent. However, these interventions are often insufficient, and intubation for airway protection is typically required for life-threatening hemoptysis.

Generally, intubation with a larger diameter ETT (≥8.5 mm inner diameter) is preferred, as this will allow for more advanced bronchoscopic interventions, such as bronchial blockers or cryotherapy. There are also double-lumen ETTs, which can provide single lung ventilation and isolation of the bleeding side. However, its use is not recommended in massive hemoptysis because the narrower lumens do not permit efficient evacuation of clots or use of larger flexible bronchoscopes to manage hemoptysis.

What is the role of bronchoscopy in massive hemoptysis?

Flexible bronchoscopy is a useful diagnostic and therapeutic tool in the setting of massive hemoptysis, especially if the patient is already intubated. It can be used to localize a bleed when the area of bleeding is unknown. Sometimes, a CT scan cannot reliably identify the area of bleeding. However, with a bronchoscope, the airway is sequentially examined, and blood is suctioned to identify the area of bleed. If the area of bleed is localized, a bronchial blocker may be placed to confine the bleed to that lobe or segment.

CLINICAL PEARL—STEP 2/3

If bronchial blockers are not available, Fogarty balloons are sometimes used to occlude the airway that is bleeding.

Advanced bronchoscopic interventions can also include cryoablation and argon plasma coagulation (APC), which are used for hemostasis.

CLINICAL PEARL—STEP 2/3

For bleeding of either the left or right upper lobes, bronchial blocker placement is often unsuccessful because the blocker has a high likelihood of migrating. Therefore, selective intubation of the left or right mainstem bronchus is sometimes preferred.

The patient received a bronchoscopy after intubation. Upon entering the airway, there were blood-tinged secretions noted from the bilateral main stem bronchi. The blood was suctioned out, and the area of bleeding could not be identified. However, the rate of accumulation of blood in the airway was not life-threatening. A bronchoalveolar lavage (BAL) was performed with serial lavages to evaluate for diffuse alveolar hemorrhage (DAH). Upon serial lavage, there was increase in bloody return, suggesting DAH (Figs. 44.2 and 44.3).

What is DAH?

DAH is a syndrome characterized by bleeding into the alveolar spaces of the lungs and is due to the disruption of the alveolar capillary basement membrane. It is recognized by the clinical constellation of hemoptysis, anemia, diffuse radiographic pulmonary infiltrates, and hypoxemic respiratory failure. While all causes of DAH have the common denominator of an injury to the alveolar microcirculation, there are several histologic subtypes. The most common underlying histology of DAH is of a small vessel vasculitis known as pulmonary capillaritis. The diagnosis of DAH is made with flexible bronchoscopy with BAL with serial aliquots in the same locaiton. Alveolar hemorrhage is confirmed when lavage aliquots are progressively more hemorrhagic.

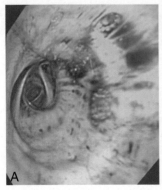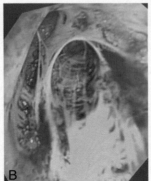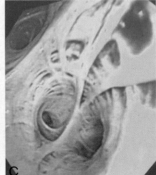

Fig. 44.2 Bronchoscopy images with residual blood in the airway but no active hemorrhage or significant oozing. (A) Image A shows the bronchus intermedius, (B) Image B shows the right upper lobe bronchus, and (C) Image C is the left lower lobe bronchus. (Courtesy of Patrick Chan, MD.)

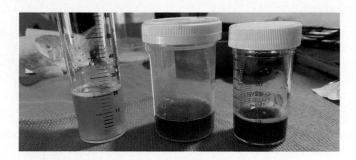

Fig. 44.3 Serial lavage showing progressively more bloody return, suggestive of diffuse alveolar hemorrhage. (Courtesy of Anna Grzegorczyk, MD.)

CLINICAL PEARL—STEP 2/3

While the presence of hemoptysis is a cardinal sign of DAH, it may be absent in some cases.

In general, if there was persistent life-threatening hemoptysis despite endobronchial interventions, what would be the next step?

Bronchial artery embolization (BAE) was first introduced in 1974 and is highly effective in controlling hemoptysis. Using a percutaneous approach, an arteriogram can be used to locate the bronchial arteries, which typically originate at the level of T5 and T6 from the thoracic aorta. Active extravasation is only found in a minority of cases. However, other visible abnormalities such as tortuosity, arteriovenous malformations, aneurysms, and dilation may be suggestive of a recent bleed. After the culprit vessel is located, an embolic material is injected into the vessel, occluding flow to achieve hemostasis.

CLINICAL PEARL—STEP 2/3

Although uncommon, the most feared complication of embolization is spinal cord ischemia due to embolism of the anterior spinal arteries.

CLINICAL PEARL—STEP 2/3

For DAH, BAE is not commonly used; treatment should instead be focused on treating the underlying cause.

If BAE is unsuccessful or unavailable, what other options are available for massive hemoptysis?

For refractory hemoptysis, a thoracic surgery consultation for lung resection is the next best option. The role of surgery is assessed on a case by case basis, as many factors contribute to operative risk in these patients. However, if the bleeding is localized to a structural problem or localized to one area of lung, surgical intervention may be more favorable. Examples include tracheoinnominate fistula, arteriovenous malformations, recurrent bleeding from mycetoma or bronchiectasis, as well as chest trauma.

CLINICAL PEARL—STEP 2/3

With the advent of BAE, surgical intervention for hemoptysis has declined due to higher morbidity and mortality with emergent surgical intervention versus elective surgical intervention. Thus, BAE is preferred for emergent stabilization of patients with acute, active hemoptysis.

CLINICAL PEARL—STEP 2/3

Common complications after thoracic surgery include empyema and bronchopleural fistula.

How do we manage this patient's GPA in this setting?

Initial therapy consists of high-dose oral or intravenous steroids. In a critically ill patient, pulse dose steroids are often administered with IV methylprednisolone 500 to 1000 mg daily for up to 5 days. The dose of steroids is then decreased and transitioned to an oral form once appropriate. Soon after the initiation of IV steroids, induction therapy with steroid-sparing agents is begun, with either cyclophosphamide or rituximab. Prolonged treatment with cyclophosphamide can be complicated by hemorrhagic cystitis and malignancy risk. Another anticipated effect of cyclophosphamide is an expected nadir of white blood cell counts; oftentimes neutropenic precautions would need to be taken.

CLINICAL PEARL—STEP 2/3

Data suggest that rituximab is equally as effective as cyclophosphamide. Rituximab is a monoclonal antibody targeted to CD20, which is found primarily on B cells, thus depleting B cell count. Induction rituximab typically consists of weekly infusions for 4 weeks. A thorough infectious work up should be performed prior to the initiation of these immunosuppressants.

CLINICAL PEARL—STEP 2/3

Ovarian protection should be discussed if the patient is to receive cyclophosphamide. The risk of ovarian failure increases with older age and the higher cumulative dose received. Rates of malignancy are also increased with cyclophosphamide use.

Plasmapheresis, the extracorporeal removal of abnormal cells or substances in the blood, is another option for critically ill patients with the aim of removing disease-causing autoantibodies. Plasma exchange is usually performed with seven sessions over 2 weeks, depending on patient response. There are numerous complications, including catheter-related complications, coagulopathy, hypocalcemia, and reactions to blood product exposure. Furthermore, recent data may suggest less benefit of plasma exchange, especially in the setting of ANCA vasculitis. However, plasma exchange still remains as a potential therapeutic option for the critically ill.

What are the general maintenance management strategies for GPA?

Management of GPA involves chronic immunosuppression with a combination of glucocorticoids and steroid-sparing therapy. Glucocorticoids are an important backbone in the initial management of GPA. Given the myriad of adverse side effects associated with long-term steroid use, it is recommended for gradual tapering as tolerated based on symptoms. However, with that being said, recent data suggest that a more rapid taper of steroids is non-inferior to a prolonged steroid course.

As for steroid-sparing maintenance therapy, options include rituximab, azathioprine, and methotrexate. Rituximab maintenance typically consists of infusions every 6 months. Recent studies have suggested that rituximab maintenance therapy is superior to azathioprine. However, azathioprine remains a mainstay of maintenance therapy, especially given its oral formulation, favorable side effect profile, and relative safety in pregnancy.

Other medications can be considered for maintenance, such as leflunomide, and mycophenolate mofetil.

The duration of maintenance therapy is less well defined, with general consensus being at least 2 to 3 years after most recent life-or organ-threatening episode. However, therapy beyond this time frame involves shared decision making between the patient and provider.

BASIC SCIENCE PEARL—STEP 1

A thiopurine methyltransferase (TPMT) activity level should be checked prior to azathioprine use. TPMT is involved in metabolism of thiopurine drugs such as azathioprine, and decreased TPMT levels with azathioprine use can lead to enhanced bone marrow toxicity.

CLINICAL PEARL—STEP 2/3

ANCA titer values may not be reflective of disease activity. Increases in immunosuppression or changes to therapy should be made based on clinical signs and symptoms rather than ANCA titers.

What routine screening is recommended for patients with GPA?

After recovery, regular monitoring with pulmonology and rheumatology is important to ensure continued stability of the patient. Evaluation for other sequelae of GPA should be pursued, such as interstitial lung disease, renal involvement, cutaneous involvement, and neuropathy.

Routine laboratory evaluation of serum creatinine, urinalysis, and urine protein can provide crucial information about the development of glomerulonephritis.

The development of treatment-induced infection is also a significant risk factor, as the patient will be on chronic immunosuppression. Providers and the patient should be aware of infectious symptoms, as infection may also trigger vasculitis flare. For prolonged courses of glucocorticoid use, appropriate prophylaxis with antibiotics should be used, along with therapies to mitigate osteoporotic risk if indicated.

CLINICAL PEARL—STEP 2/3

Prophylaxis against *Pneumocystis jirovecii* should be given in patients receiving significant doses (equivalent to 20 mg/day prednisone or greater) of glucocorticoid therapy for prolonged periods of time (1 month or greater).

In terms of our patient, she received 1 g of methylprednisolone daily for 3 days. She was also started on rituximab concurrently. The patient improved on methylprednisolone and rituximab, and was successfully extubated a few days later. The patient opted for an oral regimen instead of rituximab infusions. Therefore the patient was discharged with azathioprine and an outpatient steroid taper.

Case Summary

- **Complaint/History:** 34-year-old female with new-onset hemoptysis.
- **Findings:** Shortness of breath with diffuse bilateral airspace opacities on chest radiography.
- **Lab Results/Test:** Elevated erythrocyte sedimentation rate (ESR), C-reactive protein (CRP), c-ANCA and PR3 antibody positivity. Bronchoscopy with worsening hemorrhage on serial lavages.

Diagnosis: Diffuse alveolar hemorrhage from GPA vasculitis.

- **Treatment:** Pulse dose steroids, rituximab.
- **Maintenance:** Prednisone taper, azathioprine for patient preference for oral therapy.

BEYOND THE PEARLS

- Drug-induced ANCA-associated vasculitis has been reported with methimazole, hydralazine, and levamisole-contaminated cocaine.
- ANCA positivity is seen in 90% of patients with active generalized GPA, which means that 10% of patients have negative ANCA. Although GPA is typically associated with PR3, up to 10%–20% of patients with GPA can have MPO antibodies. In serology-negative cases, biopsy can provide a definitive diagnosis.
- Leukopenia and thrombocytopenia are uncommon in ANCA vasculitis. Their presence may help to distinguish GPA from other autoimmune etiologies.
- False positive ANCAs can also occur in bacteremia and other infections.
- Patients who receive multiple courses of rituximab may be at risk of hypogammaglobulinemia and may require intravenous immunoglobulin for replacement.
- Avacopan was a recently FDA-approved oral medication, which can be used as an adjunct for ANCA-associated vasculitis, to reduce the dose of glucocorticoids and control disease.
- Extracorporeal membrane oxygenation (ECMO) is sometimes used as rescue therapy in severe hypoxemic respiratory failure; however, in the setting of DAH, its use is controversial due to the necessity for anticoagulation while on ECMO, resulting in worsening alveolar hemorrhage.

References

Aguilera-Pickens, G., & Abud-Mendoza, C. (2018). Pulmonary manifestations in systemic lupus erythematosus: Pleural involvement, acute pneumonitis, chronic interstitial lung disease and diffuse alveolar hemorrhage. *Reumatología Clínica (English Edition)*, *14*(5), 294–300. https://doi.org/10.1016/j.reumae.2018.03.001.

Campos, J. H. (2003). An update on bronchial blockers during lung separation techniques in adults. *Anesthesia & Analgesia*, *97*, 1266–1274. https://doi.org/10.1213/01.ane.0000085301.87286.59.

Davidson, K., & Shojaee, S. (2020). Managing massive hemoptysis. *Chest*, *157*(1), 77–88. https://doi.org/10.1016/j.chest.2019.07.012.

Guillevin, L. (2015). Rituximab or azathioprine maintenance in ANCA-associated vasculitis. *New England Journal of Medicine*, *372*(4), 385–387. https://doi.org/10.1056/nejmc1414728.

Ibrahim, W. H. (2008). Massive haemoptysis: The definition should be revised. *European Respiratory Journal*, *32*(4), 1131–1132. https://doi.org/10.1183/09031936.00080108.

Kathuria, H., Hollingsworth, H. M., Vilvendhan, R., & Reardon, C. (2020). Management of life-threatening hemoptysis. *Journal of Intensive Care*, *8*, 23. https://doi-org.libproxy1.usc.edu/10.1186/s40560-020-00441-8.

Lara, A. R., & Schwarz, M. I. (2010). Diffuse alveolar hemorrhage. *Chest*, *137*(5), 1164–1171. https://doi.org/10.1378/chest.08-2084.

Stone, J. (2010). Rituximab versus cyclophosphamide for ANCA-associated vasculitis. *New England Journal of Medicine*, *363*(21), 2072–2074. https://doi.org/10.1056/nejmc1009101.

Walsh, M. (2020). Plasma exchange and glucocorticoids in severe ANCA-associated vasculitis. *New England Journal of Medicine*, *382*(22), 2168–2169. https://doi.org/10.1056/nejmc2004843.

A 48-Year-Old Male With Dyspnea on Exertion, Weakness, and Fatigue

Deanna Lo ■ Patrick Chan ■ Raj Dasgupta ■ Justin Tiulim

A 48-year-old male presents to the emergency department with 3 days of dyspnea on exertion, weakness, and fatigue. He also reports associated bleeding from his gums and easy bruising of his extremities. He denies fever, chills, night sweats, weight loss, sore throat, cough, nausea, vomiting, abdominal pain, dysuria, or diarrhea. He has no significant past medical history and no prior surgical history. He currently takes no medications. He also denies use of tobacco, alcohol, or illicit drugs.

On the physical exam, the temperature is 37.7°C, blood pressure is 124/78 mm Hg, pulse rate is 130 beats per minute, respiration rate is 25 breaths per minute, and oxygen saturation is 96% on room air. The patient appears fatigued, nontoxic, has slight bleeding around the gums, and has several ecchymotic lesions on extremities with petechiae. The remainder of the physical exam is normal (Fig. 45.1).

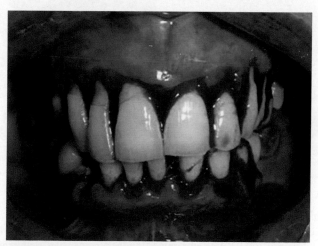

Fig. 45.1 Image of gingival bleeding. (Reproduced from Khan, S., Afaf, Z., Gupta, N. D., & Bey, A. [2012]. Acute gingival bleeding as a complication of falciparum malaria: A case report. *Oral Surgery, Oral Medicine, Oral Pathology and Oral Radiology, 113*[5]. https://doi.org/10.1016/j.oooo.2011.10.016.)

Laboratory studies are significant for a white blood cell count of 2.3 K/mm^3, hemoglobin of 8.6 g/dL, and platelets of 23 K/mm^3. The differential is notable for 15% promyelocytes. Other coagulation studies are notable for elevated prothrombin time (PT) of 42.3 seconds, elevated international normalized ratio (INR) of 2.3, elevated partial thromboplastin time (PTT) of 46.7 seconds, reduced fibrinogen level of 92 mg/dL, and elevated D-dimer of 16 mcg/mL. The remainder of the laboratory studies include sodium of 136 mmol/L, potassium of 4.4 mmol/L, and creatinine of 0.94 mg/dL. The rest of the complete metabolic panel including calcium, phosphorus, liver enzymes, total protein, and albumin is within normal limits.

Electrocardiogram notes sinus tachycardia with no evidence of ischemic changes. Chest radiograph shows no evidence of an acute cardiopulmonary process.

The patient is subsequently admitted to the intensive care unit for further management. Further diagnostics are obtained, including a peripheral smear with findings notable for many large atypical blasts with large nuclei, cytoplasmic Auer rods, and positive staining for myeloperoxidase. Fluorescence in situ hybridization (FISH) is sent for the promyelocytic leukemia 1-retinoic acid receptor (PML-RAR)-alpha gene (Fig. 45.2).

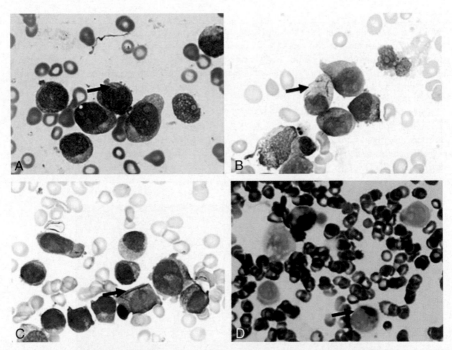

Fig. 45.2   Acute myeloid leukemia with Auer rods (A, B, C). Myeloperoxidase stain-positive (D). (Reproduced from Raj, K. [2013]. Acute leukaemia. *Medicine, 41*[5], 269–274. https://doi.org/10.1016/j.mpmed.2013.03.011.)

What is the most likely diagnosis in this patient?

Based on the clinical history and diagnostics as described above, this patient likely has acute promyelocytic leukemia (APML), with labs suggesting the presence of disseminated intravascular coagulation (DIC).

What is the underlying pathology?

APML is a hematologic malignancy that involves a genetic mutation in which there is a translocation of the PML gene on chromosome 15 and the RAR-alpha gene (RAR-alpha) on chromosome 17, resulting in the fusion gene PML-RAR-alpha. The resulting fusion oncoprotein has a high affinity for genes in hematopoietic cells involved in retinoic acid induced maturation. Ultimately, this results in the arrest of maturation and differentiation of myeloblasts. Promyelocytes fill the bone marrow and normal hematopoiesis is disrupted. Patients subsequently present with signs and symptoms related to overcrowding from immature cells (Fig. 45.3).

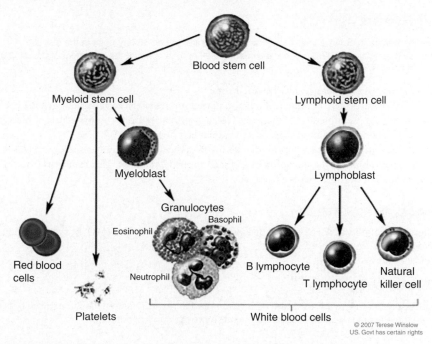

Blood stem cell

Myeloid stem cell

Lymphoid stem cell

Myeloblast

Lymphoblast

Granulocytes

Basophil

Eosinophil

Red blood cells

Neutrophil

B lymphocyte

T lymphocyte

Natural killer cell

Platelets

White blood cells

© 2007 Terese Winslow
US. Govt has certain rights

Fig. 45.3 Myeloid and lymphoid cell lineages. (Reproduced from Brody, Tom. *Clinical Trials: Study Design, Endpoints and Biomarkers, Drug Safety, FDA and ICH Guidelines*. Elsevier/AP, 2012.)

BASIC SCIENCE PEARL—STEP 1

APML involves the translocation of genes from chromosome 15 and 17.

What is the epidemiology of this disease?

APML accounts for less than 10% of acute myeloid leukemia (AML) cases. It occurs primarily in middle-aged adults, with a slightly higher incidence in men compared to women.

What are common clinical features of this disease?

Patients present with nonspecific symptoms like fatigue and weakness. Patients may also report easy bruising and bleeding (epistaxis, gum bleeding, menorrhagia), with some patients even presenting with severe, life-threatening central nervous system (CNS) or pulmonary hemorrhage and DIC. Thrombotic events are not uncommon, and this can include stroke, pulmonary embolism, and other venous thromboembolic disease. Other patients may present with infectious complaints such as fever, chills, or cough.

CLINICAL PEARL—STEP 2/3

APML is a subtype of AML that often presents with DIC.

In general, what are common hematologic emergencies?

Examples of hematologic and oncologic emergencies include metabolic derangements, such as tumor lysis syndrome, hypercalcemia of malignancy or hyponatremia, or other emergencies such as spinal cord compression or DIC. Early recognition is imperative in order to prevent further morbidity and mortality.

CLINICAL PEARL—STEP 2/3

These hematologic emergencies can occur in any cancer patient at any point in the disease process. These can result from either the cancer itself or as a result of the treatment of the cancer.

What is the next step in management for this disease?
Once APML is suspected, treatment should be started immediately, even without genetic confirmation, as this can be a medical emergency. Death is primarily from complications of bleeding, such as DIC, pulmonary hemorrhage, or intracranial hemorrhage.

The main treatment regimen for this disease involves the use of all-trans retinoic acid (ATRA). ATRA is able to bind to the oncoprotein and lead to its degradation. This results in maturation and differentiation of the immature blast cells.

CLINICAL PEARL—STEP 2/3

In the setting of APML, ATRA is often used with either arsenic trioxide (ATO) or systemic chemotherapy.

CLINICAL PEARL—STEP 2/3

Combination therapy with ATRA and ATO were noted to result in faster times to remission, a lower incidence of relapse disease, and overall improved survival outcomes.

What are some complications to monitor in patients with leukemia?
One should monitor for the presence of coagulopathies and life-threatening bleeding with primary management focused on close monitoring of blood counts and coagulation studies as well as supportive care with blood product transfusions.

CLINICAL PEARL—STEP 2/3

When platelet counts are below 10×10^9/L, there is an increased risk of spontaneous intracranial hemorrhage. Transfusions should be initiated to increase platelet counts above 10×10^9/L, and a computed tomography of the head should be obtained if the patient has altered mental status or focal neurological deficits, especially if platelet counts are less than 10×10^9/L.

CLINICAL PEARL—STEP 2/3

Transfusion goals should be set with a platelet level $\geq 50 \times 10^9$/L, fibrinogen >150 mg/dL, and PT/aPTT near normal in the presence of life-threatening bleeding.

Another concern is infection due to the decreased white blood cell count or the presence of ineffective white blood cells. If infection is suspected and/or the patient develops a fever, a general infectious work-up including blood cultures should be obtained, and the patient should be started empirically on antibiotics.

CLINICAL PEARL—STEP 2/3

In the setting of neutropenic fever, empiric antibiotics with *Pseudomonas aeruginosa* coverage is warranted. If methicillin-resistant *Staphylococcal aureus* (MRSA) infection is suspected, or there is the presence of invasive lines or pneumonia, antibiotic therapy with MRSA coverage should also be initiated.

Antifungal therapy can be considered, especially if patient continues to remain febrile or hemodynamically unstable despite antimicrobial coverage.

What other complication can be seen with leukemia?
Another feared complication is leukostasis. With elevated blood cell counts, the blood viscosity increases, which causes impaired blood flow in the microcirculation, causing hypoxia and ischemia. The two main systems that are affected are usually the pulmonary and neurological system. Prompt recognition and initiation of cytoreduction via medications or leukapheresis is recommended.

The patient is started on therapy with ATRA as well as ATO. The patient is also transfused with platelets and cryoprecipitate. On the next day, the patient's labs are notable for white blood cells (WBC) to 35×10^9/L, sodium of 132 mmol/L, potassium of 5.9 mmol/L, creatinine of 1.34 mg/dL, phosphorus of 7.1 mg/dL, and uric acid of 7.3 mg/dL.

What complications can occur with treatment initiation?
Several complications that can occur after induction therapy for APML include tumor lysis syndrome (TLS) and differentiation syndrome (DS).

DS is a systemic, uncontrolled inflammatory response that can occur after treatment initiation. This entity has a slightly higher incidence in patients receiving ATRA and ATO compared to patients receiving ATRA and chemotherapy. This occurs primarily within the first week of induction therapy. Patients classically present with fever, shortness of breath, and eventually multiorgan failure. This entity requires prompt recognition and management as it holds high morbidity and mortality. Glucocorticoids are the mainstay therapy for this uncontrolled inflammatory response

CLINICAL PEARL—STEP 2/3

If there is suspicion of differentiation syndrome, prompt initiation of glucocorticoids can be life-saving as there is usually a robust response with minimal side effects.

Given the electrolyte derangements, what is the most likely diagnosis in this patient?
This patient most likely has TLS from treatment initiation. TLS occurs when cancer cells release their intracellular contents, such as potassium, phosphorus, nucleic acids, and proteins, into the circulation. This can occur spontaneously due to the high proliferative rate of the tumor or as an effect of chemotherapy causing lysis of the cells. The body then attempts to metabolize these products and eliminate them via the renal system. However, in the case of TLS, the renal system is overwhelmed by the amount of substrate that is filtered. This leads to a toxic build-up of substances, which ultimately can result in end-organ dysfunction or damage.

CLINICAL PEARL—STEP 2/3

The most common organ system that is affected in TLS is the kidney. However, other notable organ systems that are affected include the central nervous system and especially the myocardium, for which cardiac arrhythmias can result given the subsequent electrolyte abnormalities.

Which patients are at risk for TLS?
Risk factors for the development of TLS depend on the type of cancer, the presence of under-lying comorbidities, and the type of therapy involved. Malignancies with rapidly proliferating cells are associated with a higher risk of TLS. Patients with pre-existing renal dysfunction, those who are older, and those taking medications that result in elevated serum uric acid, such as thiazide diuretics, are also at higher risk for the development of TLS. Certain cancer therapies, such as use of corticosteroids, chemotherapy, or radiation, are also associated with a higher risk of TLS.

CLINICAL PEARL—STEP 2/3

TLS is commonly seen in malignancies that involve rapidly proliferating cells. Most notable are the hematologic malignancies such as ALL, AML, and Burkitt's lymphoma.

How does TLS present?
Presentation of TLS is often nonspecific and variable. Patients can present with either clinical symptoms or laboratory abnormalities. Clinical symptoms are a manifestation of the subse-quent metabolic derangements and resultant damage to organ systems in TLS. Metabolic derangements include hyperkalemia, hyperuricemia (secondary to metabolism of purine nucleic acids), hyperphosphatemia, and hypocalcemia. Ultimately, the clinical presentation is nonspecific and patients can present with weakness, nausea/vomiting, signs of dehydration, acute renal failure, arrhythmias, or seizures.

CLINICAL PEARL—STEP 2/3

The onset of TLS is variable, with this clinical entity occurring at any point in the disease process. However, it commonly occurs following the initiation of therapy (chemotherapy, steroids). Thus, the clinician should be aware of the timing of this oncologic emergency and closely monitor clinical and laboratory signs of TLS.

How do you establish a diagnosis of TLS?
Diagnosis of TLS combines clinical and laboratory criteria. A common standardized scoring sys-tem known as the Cairo-Bishop classification, as displayed in the figure below, has been widely used for the diagnosis of TLS. This classification involves evaluating the presence of clinical and/or laboratory TLS within 3 days prior to and 7 days after the initiation of cytotoxic therapy. Laboratory TLS is met if two or more laboratory abnormalities as listed below are present, while clinical TLS is met if one or more of the clinical abnormalities and two or more of the laboratory abnormalities are present.

Cairo-Bishop Classification of TLS

Clinical TLS	Laboratory TLS
• Creatinine ≥1.5 times upper limit of normal • Cardiac arrhythmia, sudden death • Seizure	• Uric acid ≥8.0 mg/dL or a 25% increase from baseline • Potassium ≥6.0 mEq/L or a 25% increase from baseline • Calcium ≤7 mg/dL or a 25% decrease from baseline • Phosphorus ≥6.5 mg/dL or a 25% increase from baseline

What is the treatment for TLS?

Treatment of TLS focuses on preventing and managing complications of TLS in order to limit morbidity and mortality. One of the main treatments for TLS is maintaining adequate hydration and urine output. This involves the use of intravenous fluids (IVFs), usually normal saline, to maintain adequate urine output. Loop diuretics may be used if urine output is below goal.

Treatment also focuses on managing the resulting metabolic derangements with frequent laboratory evaluation. Hyperuricemia is primarily managed with uric-acid lowering agents such as allopurinol and rasburicase.

BASIC SCIENCE PEARL—STEP 1

Allopurinol is a xanthine oxidase inhibitor that competitively inhibits xanthine oxidase from metabolizing xanthine to uric acid, which has poor solubility. Thus, it does not affect existing levels of uric acid.

CLINICAL PEARL—STEP 2/3

Patients of Asian descent (Han-Chinese, Thai, Korean) should undergo evaluation for the presence of HLA-B*5801 allele as allopurinol can cause severe dermatological reactions.

CLINICAL PEARL—STEP 2/3

Febuxostat is another xanthine oxidase inhibitor that does not require dose adjustment in mild to moderate kidney dysfunction as opposed to allopurinol.

Rasburicase is a recombinant urate-oxidase that works by breaking down uric acid into the more soluble metabolite, allantoin. Rasburicase has been noted to significantly lower the levels of uric acid within 4 hours of administration, while it takes several days to see an effect of allopurinol on uric acid levels.

CLINICAL PEARL—STEP 2/3

Rasburicase and allopurinol should not be administered at the same time as there will be less substrate (uric acid) for rasburicase to metabolize. This ultimately limits the effectiveness of rasburicase. Also, this will lead to increased levels of less soluble xanthine and hypoxanthine, which can lead to xanthine crystallopathy and nephropathy.

Hyperkalemia is managed with medical therapy. If medical therapy fails, dialysis may be indicated. In regard to hyperphosphatemia, use of phosphate binders may be indicated. Hypocalcemia generally requires no specific calcium supplementation, especially if patient is asymptomatic. In patients with symptomatic hypocalcemia, a slow infusion of IV calcium gluconate may be given.

CLINICAL PEARL—STEP 2/3

Alkalinization of urine has fallen out of guidelines for treatment of TLS as this may lead to further precipitation and crystallization of calcium-phosphate in the kidneys.

CLINICAL PEARL—STEP 2/3

The mainstay of treatment for TLS involves initiation of IVFs with goal urine output of 80–100 mL/m²/hour. Other metabolic derangements can be managed with medical therapy. Dialysis is an option if the disease is refractory to medical therapy.

The table below summarizes therapies commonly used in TLS.

	Definition	Presentation	Treatment
Hyperuricemia	Uric acid ≥8 mg/dL or 25% increase from baseline	Can occur 3 days before to 7 days after initiation of cytotoxic therapy	• Aggressive IV fluid resuscitation • Allopurinol, Rasburicase
Hyperkalemia	Potassium level ≥6.0 mEq/L or 25% increase from baseline	6–72 hours after initiation of cytotoxic therapy	• Consider short acting IV insulin with dextrose, nebulized albuterol, sodium bicarbonate, or slow infusion calcium gluconate if ECG changes are noted • Dialysis if medical therapy fails
Hyperphosphatemia	Phosphorus level ≥6.5 mg/dL or 25% increase from baseline	24–48 hours after initiation of cytotoxic therapy	• Consider phosphate binders or dialysis depending on severity
Hypocalcemia	Calcium ≤7 mg/dL or a 25% decrease from baseline		• Asymptomatic: monitor; no acute interventions • Symptomatic: IV calcium gluconate repeat as necessary • Treat to control symptoms (tetany, arrhythmia, seizures) rather than normalizing serum calcium levels

Studies have estimated mortality from TLS to be around 15%. Thus, it is integral to rapidly identify risk factors for TLS and promptly manage TLS to prevent life-threatening complications and outcomes.

The patient was immediately started on IVF resuscitation with normal saline. He was also started on rasburicase and his potassium was managed with D50/insulin and potassium binders. The patient's blood work was obtained frequently to monitor the status of his tumor lysis syndrome. Within 48 hours, the patient's labs were notable for potassium of 3.8 mmol/L, creatinine of 0.96 mg/dL, phosphorus of 3.2 mg/dL, and uric acid of 3.2 mg/dL. Subsequently, IVF resuscitation was discontinued, and the patient was encouraged to maintain oral hydration and started on allopurinol. The patient remained hemodynamically stable with resolution of his tumor lysis syndrome and was subsequently transferred from the intensive care unit to the medicine unit for further care.

Case Summary

■ **Complaint/History:** A 48-year-old male with no significant past medical history presents to the emergency department with dyspnea on exertion, weakness, and easy bruising.
■ **Findings:** Visible gum bleeding, ecchymosis on extremities.

■ **Lab Results/Tests:** Pancytopenia, atypical myelocytes, Auer rods present on peripheral smear.

Diagnosis: APML complicated by DIC and TLS.

■ **Treatment:** ATRA and ATO for APML, IVF and rasburicase for TLS.

BEYOND THE PEARLS

- APML accounts for less than 10% of AML cases and is the M3 subtype. It involves the translocation of genes on chromosome 15 and 17. This fusion protein binds to retinoic acid-responsive elements on genes and subsequently blocks further differentiation of promyelocytes.
- Acute coagulopathies, such as DIC and thrombosis, are often complications that can occur in untreated APML. DIC is considered an emergency as patients can develop life-threatening hemorrhage. Prompt initiation of therapy for APML is imperative to prevent further morbidity and mortality.
- APML has an overall excellent prognosis and high remission (>90%) and cure (~80%) rates if treatment is promptly initiated. On the other hand, survival is 1 month or less without treatment of APML.
- ATRA and ATO should be used in those with low-risk disease, such as patients with non-hyperleukocytic disease. ATRA and chemotherapy should be reserved for patients with hyperleukocytosis and high-risk disease.
- One potential side effect of ATRA is the development of pseudotumor cerebri, or idiopathic intracranial hypertension.
- Intracranial hemorrhage and pulmonary hemorrhage are the most common cause of early death in APML.
- Patients considered high risk for the development of TLS or those with laboratory evidence of TLS should receive IVFs and rasburicase. Those with low to intermediate risk can be started on allopurinol.
- Rasburicase is contraindicated in pregnant patients and patients with G6PD deficiency as hydrogen peroxide is a common metabolite during this process and is unable to be metabolized in G6PD deficiency. This can lead to hemolysis and methemoglobinemia.

References

Abedin, S., & Altman, J. K. (2016). Acute promyelocytic leukemia: Preventing early complications and late toxicities. *Hematology. American Society of Hematology Education Program, 2016*(1), 10–15. https://doi.org/10.1182/asheducation-2016.1.1.

Behl, D., Hendrickson, A. W., & Moynihan, T. J. (2010). Oncologic emergencies. *Critical Care Clinics, 26*(1), 181–205.

Belay, Y., Yirdaw, K., & Enawgaw, B. (2017). Tumor lysis syndrome in patients with hematological malignancies. *Journal of Oncology, 2017*, 9684909.

Cairo, M. S., Coiffier, B., Reiter, A., & Younes, A. (2010). Recommendations for the evaluation of risk and prophylaxis of tumour lysis syndrome (TLS) in adults and children with malignant diseases: An expert TLS panel consensus. *British Journal of Haematology, 149*, 578–586. https://doi.org/10.1111/j.1365-2141.2010.08143.

Cicconi, L., & Lo-Coco, F. (2016). Current management of newly diagnosed acute promyelocytic leukemia. *Annals of Oncology, 27*(8), 1474–1481.

Cingam, S. R., & Koshy, N. V. (January 2021). Acute promyelocytic leukemia. [Updated 2021, July 2]. In: *StatPearls [Internet]*. Treasure Island (FL): StatPearls Publishing. Available from. https://www.ncbi.nlm.nih.gov/books/NBK459352/.

Criscuolo, M., Fianchi, L., Dragonetti, G., & Pagano, L. (2016). Tumor lysis syndrome: Review of pathogenesis, risk factors and management of a medical emergency. *Expert Review of Hematology, 9*(2), 197–208.

Halfdanarson, T. R., Hogan, W. J., & Madsen, B. E. (2017). Emergencies in hematology and oncology. *Mayo Clinic Proceedings, 92*(4), 609–641. https://doi.org/10.1016/j.mayocp.2017.02.008.

Jones, G. L., Will, A., Jackson, G. H., Webb, N. J., Rule, S., & British Committee for Standards in Haematology. (2015). Guidelines for the management of tumour lysis syndrome in adults and children with haematological malignancies on behalf of the British Committee for Standards in Haematology. *British Journal of Haematology, 169*(5), 661–671.

Klemencic, S., & Perkins, J. (2019). Diagnosis and management of oncologic emergencies. *The Western Journal of Emergency Medicine, 20*(2), 316–322.

Lewis, M. A., Hendrickson, A. W., & Moynihan, T. J. (2011). Oncologic emergencies: Pathophysiology, presentation, diagnosis, and treatment. *CA: A Cancer Journal for Clinicians, 61*(5), 287–314.

Pi, J., Kang, Y., Smith, M., Earl, M., Norigian, Z., & McBride, A. (2016). A review in the treatment of oncologic emergencies. *Journal of Oncology Pharmacy Practice, 22*(4), 625–638.

Spring, J., & Munshi, L. (2021). Oncologic emergencies: Traditional and contemporary. *Critical Care Clinics, 37*(1), 85–103.

Thandra, K., Salah, Z., & Chawla, S. (2020). Oncologic emergencies-the old, the new, and the deadly. *Journal of Intensive Care Medicine, 35*(1), 3–13.

Wilson, F. P., & Berns, J. S. (2014). Tumor lysis syndrome: New challenges and recent advances. *Advances in Chronic Kidney Disease, 21*(1), 18–26.

Zuckerman, T., Ganzel, C., Tallman, M. S., & Rowe, J. M. (2012). How I treat hematologic emergencies in adults with acute leukemia. *Blood, 120*(10), 1993–2002.

A 28-Year-Old Woman With Fever, Palpitations, Nausea, and Confusion

Nora Bedrossian ■ Braden Barnett

A 28-year-old woman with a history of anxiety presents to the emergency department with 2 months of heart palpitations and 10-pound weight loss and 1 day of fever, nausea, and confusion noted by her family. She was previously evaluated by her primary care provider and referred for cognitive behavioral therapy (CBT) for anxiety management. She has not yet been seen for CBT.

What are some possible etiologies of palpitations in a young woman?

On presentation, she should be evaluated for a broad range of cardiac etiologies, including supraventricular tachycardia, atrial fibrillation, and Wolff-Parkinson-White (WPW) syndrome, with an electrocardiogram (ECG) and a review of personal and family history of cardiac disease. Anemia may lead to tachycardia and palpitations. Anemia may be present for several reasons, including iron deficiency anemia secondary to menorrhagia in a young woman. Pregnancy is a state of increased blood volume which can lead to tachycardia and must be ruled out in a woman of childbearing age. Hypovolemia may lead to tachycardia and palpitations and can be due to a multitude of etiologies—ruling out diabetic ketoacidosis (DKA) and sepsis is essential. Thyrotoxicosis in a patient with uncontrolled hyperthyroidism can lead to sinus tachycardia or several arrhythmias, including atrial fibrillation. Substance use should be considered, including alcohol, cocaine, methamphetamine, nicotine use, and even significant caffeine use. Lastly, it is important to discuss all medications and supplements that the patient may be taking.

This patient's family reports that she does not take any medications. Per chart review from her most recent primary care visit, she is not currently sexually active and does not use any long-acting reversible contraceptive. She has regular menses, which last for about 5 days each month, and she does not have menorrhagia. The last menstrual period was 10 days prior to the presentation. She is a never-smoker. She does not use any illicit drugs. She drinks wine occasionally with her dinner, but never more than two glasses in an evening. She drinks one cup of coffee each morning. The patient's family states there is no family history of cardiac disease. Her maternal grandmother had a thyroidectomy, but they are not sure why.

Physical exam:

Temperature 38.8°C, heart rate (HR) 130 beats per minute, blood pressure (BP) 140/85 mm Hg, respiratory rate (RR) 24 breaths per minute, oxygen saturation (SaO2) 98% on room air.

General: Patient appears anxious and slightly diaphoretic.

Eyes: Bilateral conjunctival chemosis, mild bilateral periorbital edema, extraocular movements intact.

Ear, Nose, Throat: Moist mucous membranes. No oropharyngeal erythema or exudates.

Neck: Enlarged thyroid gland with audible bruit bilaterally. No distinct thyroid nodules palpated. No tenderness to palpation. No lymphadenopathy.

Respiratory: Increased work of breathing on room air. Lungs clear to auscultation bilaterally.

Cardiac: Tachycardic with regular rhythm. Normal S1 and S2. No murmurs, rubs, or gallops.

Abdomen: Soft. Nondistended. No tenderness to palpation. Normal bowel sounds in all 4 quadrants.

Back: Right-sided costovertebral angle tenderness.

Extremities: No edema of bilateral lower extremities.

Skin: Warm, moist.

Neuro: Lethargic, oriented to self only. States she is at home and does not know the date. Tremor of bilateral upper extremities with arms outstretched.

What tests should you order to evaluate her 1-day history of fever, nausea, and confusion?

- Complete blood count (CBC)—to evaluate for leukocytosis, hemoglobin/hematocrit.
- Comprehensive metabolic panel (CMP)—to evaluate blood glucose, anion gap, renal function, liver enzymes.
- Urinalysis—to assess for positive ketones or urinary tract infection.
- Urine culture—to assess for urinary tract infection.
- Blood cultures—to assess for bacteremia.
- Serum beta-hCG—to rule out pregnancy.
- Thyroid function tests—to evaluate for thyrotoxicosis.
- Urine toxicology—to rule out substance use.
- Serum ethanol (EtOH) level—to evaluate for recent alcohol use.

Patient's lab results are as follows:

Laboratory Study	Result	Reference range	Laboratory Study	Result	Reference Range
Complete blood count			Serum beta-hCG	<1 mIU/mL	
White blood cell (WBC)	15.8 K/mm³	4.5–10.0	Troponin	<0.01 ng/mL	
Absolute neutrophils	9.5 K/mm³	1.8–8.0	Serum EtOH	Negative	
Absolute lymphocytes	0.6 K/mm³	1.2–3.3	Urine toxicology		
Absolute monocytes	0.2 K/mm³	0.3–1.0	Amphetamines	Negative	
Absolute eosinophils	<10 K/mm³	0.0–0.4	Barbiturates	Negative	
Red blood cell (RBC)	5.34 K/mm³	3.90–5.10	Benzodiazepines	Negative	
Hgb	15.0 g/dL	12.0–14.6	Cannabis	Negative	
Hct	47.0%	36.0–44.0	Cocaine	Negative	
MCV	87.9 fL	82.0–97.0	Opiates	Negative	
RDW	15.0%	12.0–15.0	Methadone	Negative	
Platelets	223 K/mm³	160–360	Oxycodone	Negative	
Chemistry panel			**Urinalysis**		
Na	141 mmol/L	135–145	Color	Straw	Straw
K	3.7 mmol/L	3.5–5.1	Clarity	Cloudy	Clear
Cl	101 mmol/L	100–110	Specific gravity	1.013	1.005–1.030
CO₂	14 mmol/L	20–30	pH	6.5	5.0–8.0
BUN	12 mg/dL	7–18	Protein	>300 mg/dL	Negative
Cr	0.73 mg/dL	0.5–1.0	Glucose	100 mg/dL	Negative
Glucose	140 mg/dL	65–99	Ketones	Negative	Negative
Ca	8.8 mg/dL	8.5–10.3	Bilirubin	Negative	Negative
Albumin	3.9 g/dL	3.5–5.0	Blood	Large	Negative
Alk Phos	229 U/L	35–104	Urobilinogen	Negative	Negative
Aspartate transaminase (AST)	87 U/L	10–35	Leukocyte esterase	Positive	Negative

continued

Laboratory Study	Result	Reference range	Laboratory Study	Result	Reference Range
Alanine transaminase (ALT)	68 U/L	10–35	Nitrites	Positive	Negative
Total bilirubin	0.6 mg/dL	≤1.0	RBC	6–10/HPF	0–3
Direct bilirubin	0.2 mg/dL	≤3.0	WBC	11–30/HPF	0–3
Lipase	42 U/L	13–60	Bacteria	Moderate	None
Total protein	6.7 g/dL	6.0–8.0	Squamous epithelial cells	4–15/LPF	0–3
Lactate	12.0 mmol/L	0.5–2.2	Hyaline casts	0–4/LPF	0–4
Thyroid function tests			Hyaline casts with granules	1–4/LPF	None
Thyroid stimulating hormone (TSH)	<0.01 μIU/mL	0.27–4.20			
Free T4 (FT4)	4.23 ng/dL	0.93–1.70			

What diagnosis is highest on the differential?

This patient's clinical history of 2 months of heart palpitations and weight loss, bilateral upper extremity tremor, and her thyroid function tests shown above are all consistent with hyperthyroidism. The current presentation with a large, symmetric goiter and findings of Graves' ophthalmopathy strongly suggest Graves' disease as the underlying etiology.

CLINICAL PEARL—STEP 2/3

Graves' disease occurs more frequently in women, with the female to male ratio reported to be in the range of 4:1–10:1. The peak incidence has been reported in women ages 20–39 in some studies, but 40–60 years old in others (Hammerstad & Tomer, 2015). The elderly may not present with typical symptoms of thyrotoxicosis and instead may present with what has been termed "apathetic hyperthyroidism," with symptoms of weight loss, failure to thrive, weakness, fatigue, and memory loss. If these patients are already taking beta blockers, palpitations, tremor, or agitation may not be apparent (Lechner & Angell, 2020).

Decompensated hyperthyroidism leading to thyroid storm is highest on the differential. Thyroid storm is a state of maximal vasodilation to eliminate excess heat produced by increased basal metabolic rate due to the activity of excess thyroid hormone. An inability of left ventricular function to compensate for this increased workload can lead to cardiovascular collapse (Braverman & Cooper, 2012). Thyroid storm occurs in patients with uncontrolled hyperthyroidism triggered by a precipitating event, which will be discussed later.

What metabolic changes occur in patients with hyperthyroidism, and how does this lead to their clinical presentation (Braverman & Cooper, 2012)?

Increased triiodothyronine (T3) increases the basal metabolic rate via a direct effect on beta-3 receptors, increasing tissue thermogenesis and oxygen consumption. To get rid of this excess heat, peripheral vasodilation, via the effect of T3 on the endothelium and beta-2 receptors, and decreased systemic vascular resistance occur. As a result, patients become diaphoretic and, in more severe cases, may become febrile. With this acute vasodilation, effective vascular volume decreases, leading to decreased renal blood flow and activation of the renin-angiotensin system. Sodium reabsorption increases, leading to water retention and increased total blood volume. Thus, increased cardiac output is needed to maintain circulation. To increase cardiac output, T3 takes effect on the beta-1 receptors in the heart, increasing cardiac inotropy and chronotropy. Due to these changes, patients with thyrotoxicosis develop tachycardia and experience palpitations.

The above mechanisms lead to changes in several cardiac parameters as summarized below (Braverman & Cooper, 2012):

Changes in Cardiac Physiology in Hyperthyroidism

Parameter	Changes in Hyperthyroidism	Mechanism
Heart rate	Elevated, 90–100 beats/min in stable patients	T3 effect on beta-1 receptors
Blood pressure	Higher systolic BP Lower diastolic BP Widened pulse pressure	SBP increased due to increased cardiac output DBP decreased due to vasodilation
Cardiac output	Increased	T3 effect on beta-1 receptors
Ejection fraction	Increased if the patient is stable	Increased cardiac output
Systemic vascular resistance	Decreased	T3 effect on endothelium and beta-2 receptors
Blood volume	Increased	Increased serum erythropoietin and renal sodium absorption
Pulmonary pressures	Increased	Increased cardiac preload due to increased blood volume Increased cardiac output

The patient's ECG on arrival is seen below.

Findings: Sinus tachycardia with ventricular rate 132 beats/min, PR interval 134 ms, QRS duration 77 ms, QTc 445 ms.

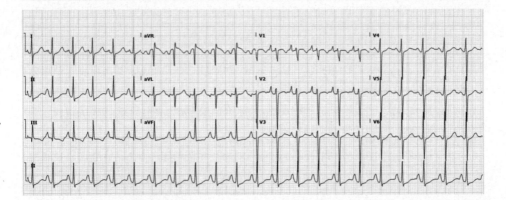

What are some common lab findings in hyperthyroid patients, and why? (Reyes-Castano &
Burman, 2013)

Laboratory Findings Associated with Hyperthyroidism

Lab Parameter	Change in Hyperthyroidism	Mechanism
Hematocrit (Gianoukakis, et al., 2009)	35%–40%	Dilutional secondary to increased blood volume Possible effects of inflammation on erythropoiesis
WBC	Relative neutropenia and lymphocytosis	Abnormal granulopoiesis
Platelets	May be low	Increased clearance Platelets coated with TSH receptor antibodies and sequestered in the spleen
Calcium	Elevated	Increased thyroid hormone-mediated bone resorption
Creatinine	Low	Decreased conversion of creatine to creatinine
Blood glucose	Hyperglycemia	Catecholamine-induced inhibition of insulin release Increased glycogenolysis
Alkaline phosphatase	Elevated	Increased bone turnover Hypermetabolic liver
Aspartate transaminase, Alanine transaminase	Elevated	Relative hypoxia in perivenular regions due to increased hepatic oxygen demand without an increase in hepatic blood flow
Total bilirubin	Elevated	As serum thyroxine levels rise, some more is shunted into bile as a conjugate and competes with the bile for conjugation, leading to indirect hyperbilirubinemia
Prothrombin time/ International normalized ratio (INR)	Prolonged	Increased metabolism of vitamin K

What are the diagnostic criteria for thyroid storm?

The diagnosis of thyroid storm requires biochemical evidence of hyperthyroidism along with severe and life-threatening symptoms of hyperthyroidism. The Burch-Wartofsky scoring system, published in 1993, is a common diagnostic tool used to assess for thyroid storm (Ross, et al., 2016). This scoring system, detailed in the chart below, uses the severity of thermoregulatory, central nervous, gastrointestinal-hepatic, and cardiovascular system dysfunction to predict the likelihood of thyroid storm. A score ≥45 is highly suspicious and very sensitive for thyroid storm.

Burch-Wartofsky Scoring System for Thyroid Storm

Temperature (F)		Cardiovascular Dysfunction	
99–99.9	5 pts	Tachycardia (beats/min)	
100–100.9	10	99–109	5
101–101.9	15	110–119	10
102–102.9	20	120–120	15
103–103.9	25	130–139	20
≥104.0	30	≥140	25
Central nervous system effects		Atrial fibrillation	10
Absent	0	**Heart failure**	
Mild (agitation)	10	Mild (pedal edema)	5
Moderate (delirium, psychosis, extreme lethargy)	20	Moderate (bibasilar rales)	10
Severe (seizure, coma)	30	Severe (pulmonary edema)	15
Gastrointestinal-hepatic dysfunction		**Precipitant history**	
Moderate (diarrhea, nausea/vomiting, abdominal pain)	10	Absent	0
		Present	10
Severe (unexplained jaundice)	20		
Total: <25 storm unlikely; 25–45 impending storm; >45 thyroid storm			

Our patient's score: 15 for temperature + 20 for CNS effects + 10 for GI dysfunction + 20 for tachycardia + 10 for a precipitant history = 75 points, which is concerning for thyroid storm

CLINICAL PEARL — STEP 2/3

Despite the expectation that serum thyroid hormone levels would be higher in thyroid storm as opposed to cases of compensated thyrotoxicosis, statistically significant differences have not been consistently observed. Therefore, the degree of thyroid hormone elevation should not be used to rule in or rule out thyroid storm (Reyes-Castano & Burman, 2013).

One potential downside of the Burch-Wartofsky scoring system is its complexity. The following are a set of four basic diagnostic criteria (Angell, et al., 2015), if all present would be highly suggestive of thyroid storm, that may more easily be committed to memory:
- Chronic uncontrolled hyperthyroidism.
- Altered mental status.
- Fever.
- Precipitating event.

What causes patients with compensated thyrotoxicosis to develop thyroid storm?
There are a multitude of precipitating illnesses or triggers that may lead to decompensated hyperthyroidism, summarized in the table below (Matfin, 2018).

Triggers for Decompensated Hyperthyroidism

Associated with rapid rise in thyroid hormone levels
- Withdrawal of antithyroid drugs
- Radioiodine therapy
- Thyroxine overdose (rare)
- Vigorous thyroid palpation (rare)
- Iodinated contrast dyes
- Thyroid surgery
- Thyroid bed trauma

Associated with acute or subacute nonthyroidal illness
- Nonthyroidal surgery
- Infection
- Cerebrovascular accident
- Myocardial infarction
- Pulmonary thromboembolism
- Diabetic ketoacidosis
- Parturition
- Emotional stress

If the cardiovascular system under its new compensated steady state is challenged with any of the stressors above, it may not be able to compensate for the further adrenergic stimulation. This can lead to poor peripheral perfusion, heat retention and hyperthermia, and encephalopathy.

With regard to a precipitating event for this patient, anemia, pregnancy, substance use, myocardial infarction, and DKA have all been ruled out with labs and history taken thus far. Given the lack of a known history of thyroid disease in the patient, any of the etiologies associated with a rapid rise in thyroid hormone levels are also unlikely. This patient does have evidence of a bacterial infection with leukocytosis with elevated neutrophil count, urinalysis with positive leukocyte esterase and nitrites, and a concern for sepsis secondary to pyelonephritis given fever, tachycardia, tachypnea, CVA tenderness, and elevated lactate. Infection was the trigger for thyroid storm in this patient with previously compensated thyrotoxicosis.

What is the approach to management of patients with thyroid storm? (Braverman & Cooper, 2012;Ylli, et al., 2019)

The management of patients in thyroid storm should be aimed at the following four main goals:
1. Decrease generation and release of thyroid hormone with antithyroid therapy.
2. Decrease tissue effects of high serum T3 and T4 via beta blockade.
3. Diagnose and treat the underlying precipitating factor.
4. Supportive and symptomatic therapy for systemic decompensation.

Given high mortality rates and the need for close monitoring of body temperature, cardiac function, fluid status, and electrolyte derangements, this should all be done in an intensive care unit.

Antithyroid therapy is aimed at decreasing the release of thyroid hormone and reducing the generation of T3. Decreasing synthesis of T4 and T3 can be achieved with an antithyroid drug, either propylthiouracil (PTU) or methimazole (MMI). PTU is preferred as it has the potential advantage of also inhibiting the extrathyroidal conversion of T4–T3, although there are no rigorous studies to prove this effect makes it clinically superior to methimazole for the treatment of thyrotoxicosis, decompensated or otherwise. Release of T4 and T3 from the thyroid follicular cells can be reduced using Lugol's solution or saturated solution of potassium iodide (SSKI).

CLINICAL PEARL—STEP 2/3

It is important to start thionamide therapy at least 1 hour prior to iodine therapy (Lugol's solution or SSKI) to prevent the iodine from potentially being used as a substrate for new thyroid hormone synthesis after the gland takes up iodine (Reyes-Castano & Burman, 2013).

Glucocorticoids are utilized to decrease conversion of T4–T3. Given the activation of the renin-angiotensin-aldosterone system and its negative effects as described above, dexamethasone is often the glucocorticoid of choice in the treatment of thyroid storm since it lacks mineralocorticoid effects compared to other glucocorticoids, although hydrocortisone has also been frequently used with similar success.

Nonselective beta blockers are the treatment of choice for relief of hyperthyroid symptoms and signs due to increased adrenergic tone. Propranolol is preferred, as at high doses it will also block peripheral conversion of T4–T3. Goal heart rate with beta blockade should be 90–100 beats/min to prevent cardiovascular collapse.

Given that one of the most common precipitating factors of thyroid storm is infection, it is imperative to perform a thorough evaluation for any potential source of infection and initiate broad spectrum antibiotics if there is any suspicion of infection based on the patient's presentation or diagnostic testing. Treatment for other apparent precipitating factors should also be started immediately upon diagnosis.

To treat fever/hyperthermia, some guidelines and expert opinions recommend using external cooling sources, such as cooling blankets, despite the lack of any robust evidence supporting their use. Furthermore, there is theoretical concern that using an external cooling source will cause peripheral vasoconstriction (which will inhibit further heat shedding) and shivering (which would generate additional unwanted heat). A commonly used alternative tactic to avoid the use of external cooling sources is to give one-time IV doses of chlorpromazine and meperidine (typical dose of 25 mg of each). The chlorpromazine appears to inhibit hypothalamic factors that contribute to fever, and the meperidine effectively prevents or resolves shivering.

STEP 1 PEARL

Avoid salicylates as an antipyretic as they can decrease thyroid protein binding to serum proteins and disproportionately increase levels of free thyroid hormone (Reyes-Castano & Burman, 2013).

Therapies, dosing, and the mechanism of action are detailed in the table below (Braverman & Cooper, 2012; Ross, et al. 2016; Matfin, 2018):

Management of Hyperthyroidism

Therapy	Dosing	Mechanism of Action
Antithyroid drugs		
Propylthiouracil (PTU)	200–400 mg by mouth (PO) every 6–8 hours (hr)	Inhibits synthesis of T4 and T3 Reduces peripheral conversion of T4–T3
Methimazole (MMI)	20–30 mg PO every 6 hr	Inhibits synthesis of T4 and T3
Saturated solution of potassium iodide	5 drops PO every 6 hr or 5–10 drops per rectum every 6–8 hr	Inhibits release of T4 and T3 from thyroid gland
Lugol's solution	4–8 drops PO every 6–8 hr or 5–10 drops per rectum every 6–8 hr	Inhibits release of T4 and T3 from thyroid gland
Alternative therapies		
Lithium	300 mg PO every 6 hr	Reduces release of T4 and T3 from thyroid gland
Levocarnitine	990 mg three times daily with meals	Blocks T3 receptor to reduce end-organ effects of thyroid hormone
Cholestyramine	4 g PO daily	Decreases reabsorption of thyroid hormone from the enterohepatic circulation
Treatment of peripheral effects of thyroid hormone		
Beta blockers		
Propranolol preferred	60–80 mg PO every 4 hr	At high doses, blocks peripheral conversion of T4–T3
Steroids		
Dexamethasone	2 mg IV every 6 hr	Reduces peripheral conversion of T4–T3
Hydrocortisone	Load with 300 mg IV, then continue 100 mg IV every 8 hr	Reduces peripheral conversion of T4–T3
Antipyretic		
Acetaminophen	325–650 mg PO or per rectum every 4–6 hr as needed (prn)	

This patient was started on propranolol 60 mg PO every 4 hours, SSKI drops, PTU 200 mg PO every 8 hours, dexamethasone 2 mg IV every 6 hours, and acetaminophen 650 mg PO PRN every 6 hours. She was also started on broad spectrum antibiotics to treat pyelonephritis. Over the course of 24 hours, she became normothermic, her mentation returned to baseline, and her heart rate decreased to 90–100 beats per minute. Propranolol dose was reduced, and her steroids were tapered slowly. Once results of her urine culture became available, antibiotics were narrowed to an oral option. She was discharged home with a course of antibiotics to complete, methimazole 30 mg daily, propranolol 20 mg every 8 hours as needed for HR greater than 110, and endocrinology follow-up in 6 weeks.

What are the risks of using antithyroid drugs? (Reyes-Castano & Burman, 2013)
The main serious side effects to be aware of for MMI and PTU include agranulocytosis and hepatotoxicity. Agranulocytosis can occur at any time during therapy with either medication and will resolve with discontinuation of the medication. Hepatotoxicity can occur in 0.1%–0.2% of patients using MMI or PTU and leads to hepatocellular injury pattern with the use of PTU and a cholestatic pattern of injury with the use of MMI. Hepatotoxicity secondary to PTU can be potentially life-threatening.

How should we approach long-term management after a patient has been treated for thyroid storm?

Once the patient has been treated for thyroid storm, definitive management of hyperthyroidism should be discussed in those patients with persistent causes of thyrotoxicosis to prevent future recurrence of this life-threatening event. The two options for definitive management include radioactive iodine ablation therapy and thyroidectomy. After treatment of thyroid storm using iodine, radioactive iodine therapy would have to be delayed for several weeks to months until the thyroid gland is able to take up iodine once again. Thyroidectomy must also be delayed until the patient is euthyroid to avoid the risk of thyroid storm precipitated by surgery (Reyes-Castano & Burman, 2013). Patients should have close follow-up to discuss and implement these therapies.

At her 6-week follow-up, the patient reported compliance with MMI and stated that although she initially required propranolol three times a day, she is now only taking it about twice a week. Blood work was completed, and she was found to have a TSH of 0.01 μIU/mL and FT4 of 1.62 ng/dL, now within normal limits. After discussing the risks and benefits of radioactive iodine ablation therapy and thyroidectomy as well as the need for life-long levothyroxine therapy after either treatment, she opted for thyroidectomy. She was referred to endocrine surgery for definitive management of her Graves' disease.

Case Summary

- **Complaint/History:** A 28-year-old woman with fever, palpitations, nausea, and confusion.
- **Findings:** Tachycardia, prooptosis, tremors.
- **Lab Results/Test:** Elevated FT4, low TSH, elevated WBC, positive UA.

Diagnosis: Thyroid storm precipitated by urinary tract infection.

- **Treatment:** Beta blocker, SSKI, antithyroid medication, steroids, and intravenous antibiotics.

BEYOND THE PEARLS

- Atrial fibrillation secondary to thyrotoxicosis will not respond to cardioversion while the patient is still thyrotoxic. Treat hyperthyroidism to treat atrial fibrillation, and use beta blockers for rate control as necessary (Braverman & Cooper, 2012).
- Patients with decompensated thyrotoxicosis may present with pedal or pulmonary edema from heart failure. Diuretics should be used with caution as these patients are maximally vasodilated with a relative intravascular volume deficit and over-diuresis may lead to cardiovascular collapse.
- If you have high suspicion for but are still unsure about the diagnosis of thyroid storm, it is safer to treat as untreated decompensated thyrotoxicosis can be fatal.
- The combination of an antithyroid drug, SSKI, and dexamethasone can decrease T3 levels by 80% within 48–72 hours.
- In more difficult to manage and critically ill patients, other strategies that have been attempted include lithium to further inhibit the release of thyroid hormone from the thyroid gland, levocarnitine to reduce end-organ effects of thyroid hormone by blocking the T3 receptor, cholestyramine to decrease reabsorption of thyroid hormone from the enterohepatic circulation, and plasmapheresis to remove circulating thyroid hormone by removing thyroid-binding globulin with bound thyroid hormone and using colloid replacement to provide new binding sites for the circulating free thyroid hormone. While all of these options sound theoretically plausible, none of them have any robust clinical outcome evidence to support their use (Braverman & Cooper, 2012).

References

Angell, T. E., Lechner, M. G., Nguyen, C. T., Salvato, V. L., Nicoloff, J. T., & LoPresti, J. S. (2015). Clinical features and hospital outcomes in thyroid storm: A retrospective cohort study. *The Journal of Clinical Endocrinology and Metabolism*, *100*(2), 451–459. https://doi.org/10.1210/jc.2014-2850.

Braverman, L. E., & Cooper, D. (2012). *Werner & Ingbar's the thyroid*. Philadelphia, PA: Wolters Kluwer.

Gianoukakis, A. G., Leigh, M. J., Richards, P., Christenson, P. D., Hakimian, A., Fu, P., et al. (2009). Characterization of the anaemia associated with Graves' disease. *Clinical Endocrinology*, *70*(5), 781–787. https://doi.org/10.1111/j.1365-2265.2008.03382.x.

Hammerstad, S. S., & Tomer, Y. (2015). Epidemiology and genetic factors in Graves' disease and Graves' ophthalmopathy. In R. Bahn (Ed.), *Graves' disease*. New York, NY: Springer. https://doi.org/10.1007/978-1 -4939-2534-6_3.

Lechner, M. G., & Angell, T. E. (2020). Severe thyrotoxicosis and thyroid storm. In R. Garg, J. Hennessey, A. Malabanan, & J. Garber (Eds.) (2018). *Handbook of inpatient endocrinology*. Cham: Springer. https://doi. org/10.1007/978-3-030-38976-5_4.

Matfin, G. (Ed.) (2018). *Endocrine and metabolic medical emergencies: A clinician's guide*. Newark, NJ: John Wiley & Sons, Incorporated.

Reyes-Castano, J. J., & Burman, K. (2013). Thyrotoxic crisis: Thyroid storm: *Endocrine emergencies* (pp. 77–97). Humana Press. https://doi.org/10.1007/978-1-62703-697-9_9.

Ross, D. S., Burch, H. B., Cooper, D. S., Greenlee, M. C., Laurberg, P., Maia, A. L., et al. (2016). 2016 American Thyroid Association Guidelines for Diagnosis and management of hyperthyroidism and other causes of thyrotoxicosis. *Thyroid*, *26*(10), 1343–1421. https://doi.org/10.1089/thy.2016.0229.

Ylli, D., Klubo-Gwiezdzinska, J., & Wartofsky, L. (2019). Thyroid emergencies. *Polish Archives of Internal Medicine*, *129*(7–8), 526–534. https://doi.org/10.20452/pamw.14876.

A 64-Year-Old Female With Altered Mental Status

Sophie Mestman Cannon ■ Braden Barnett

A 64-year-old undomiciled woman with an unknown medical history is brought to the emergency department by emergency medical services for hypothermia and altered mental status (AMS) in December. She was found unresponsive at a nearby bus stop, and the temperature outside is 62 degrees. She is obtunded and oriented to self, but otherwise somnolent.

What is the differential diagnosis of a patient presenting with altered mental status?
The differential diagnosis for altered mental status is quite broad (Table 47.1). Features of the history and physical exam can help to narrow the differential diagnosis. If the information is available from the history, the onset of the change in mentation, history of trauma, past medical history, past surgical history, and medications (over the counter, recreational, and prescription) should be reviewed. Vital signs and a physical exam should be telling.

The patient is somnolent, oriented to self only, and is unable to provide any additional history. Her temperature is 90°F, heart rate is 46 beats per minute, respiratory rate is 10 breaths per minute, blood pressure is 89/56 mm Hg, weight is 70 kg, height is 160 cm (body mass index [BMI] 27), and her oxygen saturation is 91% on room air. Physical exam is notable for a well-healed 6–7 cm transverse surgical scar on the anterior neck, 3 cm above the jugular notch. Facial features are coarse, and the patient is noted to have nonpitting bilateral lower extremity edema to the knees. Skin is dry and she exhibits delayed relaxation of the bilateral patellar reflexes. A computed tomography (CT) scan of the head is unremarkable.

How do we consolidate these findings?
The patient is a 64-year-old female with an unknown past medical history presenting during the winter months with an altered mental status of unclear chronicity. Precipitating factors are unable to be elicited by history, and it is unknown if there is a history of trauma, though a CT scan of the head is unremarkable. She is hypothermic, bradycardic, hypotensive, and with bradypnea and mild hypoxia on exam.

Following initial examination, laboratory studies are obtained and subsequently reveal hyponatremia to 121 mmol/L, hypoglycemia to 62 mg/dL, and an elevated creatinine to 2.67 mg/dL. She remains oriented to self only and lethargic in appearance.

How does this information narrow your differential diagnosis?
While hyponatremia is an etiology of altered mental status, the patient's corresponding hemodynamic instability and hypoglycemia suggest an alternative unifying diagnosis, with hypothyroidism,

TABLE 47.1 ■ Causes of Altered Mental Status

Metabolic	**Uremia**
Hypo/hypernatremia	Chronic kidney disease or acute kidney failure
Hypercalcemia	
Oxygenation	**Psychogenic**
Hypoxia	Depression
	Psychosis
Vascular	
Cerebrovascular accident (ischemic or hemorrhagic)	**Infection**
Myocardial infarction	Meningitis/Encephalitis
Congestive heart failure	Pneumonia
	Skin and soft tissue infection (SSTI)
Endocrine	Genitourinary infection (urinary tract infection,
Hypoglycemia	pyelonephritis, prostatitis)
Hyper/Hypothyroidism	Gastrointestinal infection
	Endocarditis
Seizure	
Post-ictal state	**Drugs**
Trauma	Intoxication
	Withdrawal

Rhee, C. (2010, August 26). *Altered mental status—DDx & management*. Altered Mental Status. Retrieved January 18, 2022, from http://errolozdalga.com/medicine/pages/AlteredMentalStatus.cr.8.26.10.html

infection, and/or adrenal insufficiency towards the top of the differential diagnosis. Clinical features of severe hypothyroidism include course facial features, myxedema, dry skin, and delayed relaxation of deep tendon reflexes, which are noted in our patient. Another clinical clue is the scar on this patient's neck, which indicates she may have had a thyroidectomy. Hypothyroidism, specifically myxedema coma (decompensated hypothyroidism), is now suspected.

CLINICAL PEARL—STEP 2/3

In patients with unexplained altered mental status and an unknown past medical history, thyroid function tests should be obtained to assess for hypothyroidism as an etiology.

What additional tests should be ordered? What lab abnormalities do you expect?

When myxedema coma is suspected, laboratory tests should be obtained, including a basic metabolic panel (to assess for hyponatremia and elevated creatinine), arterial blood gas (to assess for hypercapnia and hypoxemia), thyroid stimulating hormone (TSH), and free T4 (FT4). A broad infectious work-up should also be initiated.

Additional laboratory tests are drawn and are presented in Table 47.2, revealing a markedly elevated thyroid stimulating hormone (TSH) and undetectable FT4. Her labs are consistent with overt biochemical hypothyroidism, and her clinical findings are highly suspicious of myxedema coma.

What is myxedema coma?

Myxedema coma represents severe, life-threatening, decompensated hypothyroidism. Cardinal symptoms of myxedema coma are severe hypothyroidism *in addition to* a precipitating event, hypothermia, decreased mental status, and hypoventilation with risk of pneumonia and hyponatremia (Tables 47.3 and 47.4).

TABLE 47.2 ■ Laboratory Tests

White blood count (4.5–10.0)	7200 K/mm³
Hemoglobin (12.0–16.0)	15.6 g/dL
Hematocrit (35.0–47.0)	45.5%
Platelets (140–440)	230,000 K/mm³
Arterial blood gas	pH 7.25
	pCO₂ 58 mm Hg
	paO₂ 57 mm Hg
	HCO₃ 26 mmol/L
Sodium (135–145)	121 mmol/L
Potassium (3.5-5.1)	4.2 mmol/L
Chloride (100–110)	93 mmol/L
CO₂ (20–30)	57 mmol/L
BUN (8–22)	21 mg/dL
Creatinine (0.5–1.30)	2.67 mg/dL
eGFR (>90)	34 mL/min/1.73 m²
Glucose (65–99)	62 mg/dL
TSH (0.27–4.2)	142 μIU/mL
Free T4 (0.93–1.70)	<0.5 ng/dL
Cortisol (4.8–19.5)	In process
Urinalysis	3+ leukocyte esterase, 2+ Nitrites, >50 WBCs, Spec Grav 1.090.
Blood and urine cultures	In process

TSH, Thyroid stimulating hormone.

TABLE 47.3 ■ Diagnosis of Myxedema Coma

Chronic hypothyroidism
Altered mental status
Hypothermia
Precipitating factor or illness
Older adult (often, but not always)

CLINICAL PEARL—STEP 2/3

When myxedema coma or severe hypothyroidism is suspected, assess for any history of thyroid disease, history of thyroid hormone therapy, and history of head/neck surgery or radioiodine ablation therapy. Assess the neck for any surgical scar or palpable thyroid tissue. Assess for signs and symptoms of severe hypothyroidism: myxedema (nonpitting edema) of hands, feet, and periorbital area, macroglossia, course, dry, scaly skin, delayed relaxation of deep tendon reflexes, low and hoarse voice, and hypothermia.

What differentiates myxedema coma from severe hypothyroidism?

Most patients with myxedema coma have had symptoms of hypothyroidism for many months, followed by a precipitating event tipping them into myxedema coma. Myxedema coma represents a form of decompensated hypothyroidism and is differentiated by the presence of a precipitating event, marked stupor, confusion, or coma and hypothermia in a patient with hypothyroidism. It represents the inability of chronically hypothyroid patients to adapt effectively to a stressor. Characteristic laboratory abnormalities (Table 47.5) can also differentiate severe hypothyroidism from myxedema coma.

TABLE 47.4 ■ Physiology of Myxedema Coma—Basic Science Pearls

System Impacted	Clinical Manifestation
Temperature	**Hypothermia** is present in 75% of patients with myxedema coma.
Respiratory	Decreased hypoxic drive & decreased ventilatory response to **hypercapnia** lead to alveolar hypoventilation, carbon dioxide (CO_2) narcosis, and finally coma.
	Principal factor behind coma is depressed respiratory center response to CO_2.
	Increased risk of **aspiration pneumonia** and **hypoxemic respiratory failure**.
Cardiovascular	**Cardiac enlargement, decreased cardiac contractility, non-specific ECG abnormalities**, and **bradycardia** common.
	Cardiac enlargement can be secondary to ventricular dilation or pericardial effusion which leads to decreased stroke volume and cardiac output.
	Frank heart failure is rare.
Gastrointestinal	**Paralytic ileus, megacolon**, and **ascites** can be seen.
Electrolytes	**Hyponatremia** is often noted secondary to an inability to excrete free water due to decreased delivery of water to the nephron and excess vasopressin production.
	Decreased glomerular filtration rate (GFR) with an **elevated creatinine**, bladder atony, and urinary retention can also be noted.
	Hypoglycemia is likely secondary to decreased gluconeogenesis.
Neuropsychiatric	**Cognitive dysfunction**, depression, slowed mentation, lethargy, and psychosis can be seen.
	Twenty-five percent of patients have **focal or generalized seizures**.
	Altered mental status (AMS) can be secondary to **hypercapnia** and/or **hyponatremia**.
Infection	**Impaired host response to infection** during myxedema coma and/or infection may have been the **precipitating factor** that tips a patient from severe hypothyroidism into myxedema coma.

TABLE 47.5 ■ Common Laboratory Findings in Myxedema Coma

Electrolytes	↓Na
	↓Glucose
Renal function	↑Creatinine
White blood count	Normal or ↓
Liver function	↑AST, ALT, creatine phosphokinase (CPK)
Electrocardiogram (ECG)	Low voltage
	Bradycardia
Arterial blood gas	↑PCO_2, ↓PO_2

Nicoloff, J. T., & LoPresti, J. S. (1993). Myxedema coma. A form of decompensated hypothyroidism. *Endocrinology and Metabolism Clinics of North America, 22*(2), 279–290.

CLINICAL PEARL—STEP 2/3

Patients with central hypothyroidism may have a low or normal TSH with a low fT4. Central hypothyroidism is characterized by a defect of thyroid hormone production due to insufficient TSH with an otherwise normal thyroid gland. It is much less common than primary hypothyroidism.

TABLE 47.6 ■ Management of Myxedema Coma

Endocrine support	Send thyroid function tests (thyroid stimulating hormone [TSH], fT3, fT4)
	Obtain random serum cortisol
	Administer 100 mg IV hydrocortisone
	Treat hypothyroidism with IV 200–500 µg levothyroxine
Infection	Urinalysis, blood cultures, sputum culture, empiric antibiotics
Respiratory support	Low threshold for intubation for hypercapnic or hypoxemic respiratory failure
Cardiovascular support	Fluids
Hypothermia	Passive warming
	Avoid active warming unless temperature <30°C.

Adapted from Braverman, L. E., & Cooper, D. S. (2013). *Werner & Ingbar's the thyroid: A fundamental and clinical text* (10th ed., pp. 600–605).

The patient's breathing is labored, and her pulse oximetry reading is now 89% on 4 L nasal cannula with a respiratory rate of 9 breaths/min. Arterial blood gas (ABG) findings are consistent with a primary respiratory acidosis with corresponding metabolic compensation (see Table 47.2).

What respiratory support is recommended in the management of myxedema coma?

Pulmonary compromise is a common cause of death in patients with myxedema coma, secondary to respiratory depression, pulmonary infection, and airway obstruction from macroglossia or myxedema of the larynx. Endotracheal intubation and mechanical respiratory assistance should be initiated at the first sign of respiratory failure as CO_2 retention or hypoxia may lead to rapid cardiovascular collapse (Table 47.6).

The patient is subsequently intubated in the emergency department and a sputum culture is collected. The patient's initial blood pressure is 89/56 mm Hg and hypotension persists after intubation with a subsequent blood pressure reading of 87/52 mm Hg.

What cardiovascular and electrolyte support is recommended in the management of myxedema coma?

Hyponatremia can contribute to mental status changes, especially in patients with a serum sodium less than 120. Hyponatremia in patients with myxedema coma should be managed per standard guidelines. The hyponatremia seen in myxedema coma can be secondary to a combination of hypovolemic hyponatremia (fluid shifts) and euvolemic hyponatremia (increased vasopressin production). Fluid resuscitation and careful monitoring are advised.

Hypotension in a patient with myxedema coma should be considered an ominous sign. Common causes of volume loss include peripheral vasodilation secondary to loss of centrally mediated vasoconstriction or sepsis; iatrogenic vasodilation secondary to external warming; preexisting hypovolemia; and bleeding secondary to possible gastrointestinal bleed.

The patient is resuscitated with 2 liters of 5% dextrose in half-normal saline (D5-1/2NS) and her blood pressure increases to 114/82 mm Hg. Following this, a serum cortisol is drawn and she receives 100 mg IV hydrocortisone in addition to vancomycin and piperacillin-tazobactam.

Why is the use of empiric antibiotics recommended in treatment of myxedema coma?

Sepsis in a patient with myxedema coma is correlated with high mortality. Bacterial infection likely constitutes the most common precipitating event for myxedema coma and should be assumed to be present in all cases until proven otherwise.

Why are glucocorticoids used in the management of myxedema coma?
Patients in myxedema coma may also have adrenocorticotropic hormone deficiency (and thus adrenal insufficiency), particularly if the cause is central hypothyroidism. Some patients have primary hypothyroidism and primary adrenal insufficiency both due to chronic autoimmune inflammation (thyroiditis and adrenalitis, respectively), a finding known as Schmidt syndrome. The patient receives 100 mg IV hydrocortisone prior to the initiation of thyroid hormone.

If a glucocorticoid is used, why is it given before thyroid hormone replacement?
Unless the cause of hypothyroidism can definitively be attributed to either total thyroidectomy or prior radioiodine ablation, it is imperative to administer glucocorticoids prior to levothyroxine, as in a patient with adrenal insufficiency, thyroid hormone can increase the clearance of cortisol and precipitate adrenal crisis. A serum cortisol level should be drawn prior to administering glucocorticoids, although it is not necessary or advisable to wait for the result. Rather, empiric treatment with glucocorticoids, followed by thyroid hormone (see below) should commence, and glucocorticoids should be withdrawn later if the serum cortisol level and/or subsequent clinical findings argue against concomitant adrenal insufficiency. Typical dosing of hydrocortisone is 50–100 mg every 6–8 hours followed by a taper once adrenal insufficiency is ruled out. If a clear cause of primary hypothyroidism is present and is not known to be associated with adrenal insufficiency (total thyroidectomy or radioiodine ablation), then treatment with glucocorticoids is not necessary or indicated.

The patient is hemodynamically stable with a recheck of blood pressure now at 116/81 mm Hg. Prior to transfer from the emergency department to the intensive care unit, she will need levothyroxine to treat her myxedema coma.

How should thyroid hormone replacement be given in the treatment of myxedema coma?
In a patient without thyroid disease, the thyroid secretes primarily 80% thyroxine (T4) and 20% liothyronine (T3). T4 is a pro-hormone which is activated to T3 by deiodinase enzymes in peripheral tissues; thus T3 is the active form of thyroid hormone in the body. The optimal type of treatment with thyroid hormone is controversial, and there are several methods employed using only T4, only T3, or a mixture of both. The methods are outlined here, and the recommendations of the authors of this case are presented.

The first method is the use of T3 alone. As T3 is the active form of thyroid hormone, the onset is more rapid. Of note, hypothermia and hypoxemia typically improve 2–3 hours after IV administration of T3, and 8–14 hours after administration of T4. However, given rapid onset and offset, serum and tissue concentrations fluctuate more between doses. The administration of high doses of T3 alone can also be associated with a higher risk of adverse cardiovascular events and increased mortality. Therefore, the authors of this case prefer the treatment of T4 alone.

The second method is the use of T4 alone, which is recommended in the 2014 American Thyroid Association guidelines. The authors of this case agree with and prefer this method. The use of T4 alone allows for a steady and smooth (though slower) onset of action as compared to T3 with lower risks of adverse effects. After respiratory and cardiovascular support are established, and after administration of hydrocortisone, a loading dose of 200–500 µg levothyroxine is given, followed by a daily replacement dose of 1.6 µg/kg body weight (100% if given by mouth, and 50%–75% if given IV). For patients with a higher cardiovascular risk, consider a reduced loading dose and daily maintenance dose. Otherwise, a higher loading dose will restore euthyroidism more rapidly than a lower loading dose, and higher doses should generally be utilized. As noted, for younger patients and patients with a known, low risk for cardiac complications (specifically myocardial infarction and arrhythmias), higher doses can be utilized. The third method is the use of combination T4 and T3 therapy.

What is the decision point to administer high-dose LT4 (myxedema coma) vs. Weight-based thyroid hormone replacement (severe hypothyroidism)?

Fatigue and somnolence can occur in patients with severe hypothyroidism; it can be difficult to make a clear clinical distinction. This distinction can be important in elderly patients due to the cardiovascular risks of high-dose thyroid hormone in elderly patients. In a patient who is lethargic or somnolent, assess for the presence of abnormalities associated with myxedema coma (hyponatremia, hypoventilation, hypothermia). If these abnormalities are not present, consider the diagnosis of severe hypothyroidism. In a somnolent patient with these abnormalities, consider high-dose levothyroxine administration and a diagnosis of myxedema coma.

Following administration of hydrocortisone, the patient received a lower loading dose of 300 μg IV levothyroxine given her age and unknown cardiac history, and following this dose, she continued to receive 88 μg IV levothyroxine daily while she remained intubated. She was persistently hypothermic to 90°F –92°F in the hours after intubation.

How is hypothermia managed in myxedema coma?

Thyroid hormone will correct hypothermia, but its onset is slow. Passive rewarming with blankets can be utilized, and active rewarming should be avoided as it carries a risk of vasodilatation and worsening hypotension. Active rewarming may be reasonable for severe hypothermia (less than 82°F), but only with extreme caution, conservative heat settings, and for the shortest amount of time necessary. Normothermia in a myxedematous patient can mean there is an underlying infection, as this can represent a febrile response from the hypothermic state. Likewise, any presence of band cells in the blood is concerning for underlying infection.

The patient was persistently hypothermic to 90°F–92°F in the hours after intubation and underwent passive rewarming with blankets. Her temperature improved to 98°F over the following 24 hours. After 48 hours, her urine culture grew pan-sensitive *E. coli*, and antibiotics were narrowed to ceftriaxone. On hospital day 2, the patient's serum cortisol from admission resulted and was noted to be 24 μg/dL. Hydrocortisone was tapered from 100 mg every 8 hours to 50 mg every 8 hours for 24 hours, then 25 mg every 8 hours for an additional 24 hours, and subsequently discontinued. After 72 hours, her mentation and hyponatremia improved.

After treatment of myxedema coma with levothyroxine, what therapeutic endpoints should be targeted?

Therapeutic endpoints in myxedema coma include improved mental status, cardiac function, and pulmonary function. It is recommended to measure thyroid hormone every 1–2 days to ensure a favorable trajectory. Optimal levels for serum TSH, FT4, and free T3 (FT3) are not well defined. Failure of an elevated TSH to downtrend or failure of thyroid hormone levels to improve could be considered indications to increase levothyroxine therapy or add liothyronine. Likewise, high FT3 measurements could be considered an indication to decrease or stop T3 dosing. In one study of hypothyroid patients, normalization of thyroid hormone levels occurred within 4 days, and improvements in TSH were seen within 1 week.

On hospital day 3, repeat TSH was noted to be 112 uIU/mL and fT4 was noted to be 0.82 ng/dL. The patient was extubated on hospital day 4 and her IV levothyroxine was transitioned to weight-based 112 μg PO levothyroxine daily. She was noted to be alert and oriented to self, place, month, and year, but not the situation and inquired into the events of her hospitalization.

TABLE 47.7 ■ **Common Precipitating Events for Myxedema Coma[a]**

Hypoglycemia	Trauma
Hypothermia	Stroke
Infection	Drug overdose
CO_2 narcosis	Diuretics
CHF	Sedatives

[a]Adapted from Nicoloff, J. T., & LoPresti, J. S. (1993). Myxedema coma. A form of decompensated hypothyroidism. *Endocrinology and Metabolism Clinics of North America, 22*(2), 279–290.

CLINICAL PEARL—STEP 2/3

Myxedema coma is more likely to occur in the winter than in the summer. This suggests that low temperatures may precipitate the syndrome. Other common precipitating factors are CHF (congestive heart failure), infections, trauma, hypothermia, hypoglycemia, cerebrovascular accidents, CO_2 narcosis, and medications (such as sedatives, analgesics, antipsychotics, and amiodarone) (Table 47.7). The general clinical course is several months of lethargy that then progresses to stupor, followed by coma and hypothermia.

Upon interview, the patient confirmed a history of thyroid cancer (status post total thyroidectomy) and noted that she had run out of medication 3 months prior due to loss of health insurance and homelessness. She described symptoms of dysuria and increased urinary frequency in the day prior to her hospitalization, but did not have access to a primary care physician to discuss these symptoms or treatment. She was referred to several shelters as well as to primary care clinic to establish care. Patient presented to her first appointment with compliance with her thyroid medications.

Case Summary

- **Complaint/History**: A 64-year-old undomiciled woman with an unknown medical history is brought to the emergency department for hypothermia and altered mental status.
- **Findings**: The patient is somnolent and oriented to self only, with hypothermia, bradypnea, bradycardia, and hypoxia. She has coarse facial features, myxedema, dry skin, delayed deep tendon reflexes, and a surgical scar on the neck.
- **Labs/Tests**: Hyponatremia, hypoglycemia, elevated creatinine, hypercapnia, hypoxemia, and a markedly elevated thyroid stimulating hormone (TSH).

Diagnosis: Myxedema coma.

- **Treatment:** Respiratory and cardiovascular support (intubation and fluid resuscitation), IV hydrocortisone, IV levothyroxine, supportive management.

BEYOND THE PEARLS

- Myxedema coma represents a form of decompensated hypothyroidism and is differentiated by the presence of a precipitating event, marked stupor, confusion or coma, hyponatremia, and hypothermia in a patient with hypothyroidism.
- Consider this diagnosis in a patient with altered mental status of unclear etiology in the setting of hyponatremia, hypoglycemia, and hypotension.
- If there are no clinical signs of improvement after 24–48 hours following IV levothyroxine replacement, consider an alternative diagnosis as clinical improvement should be seen as early as 24 hours into treatment.

- All patients with myxedema coma should receive stress-dose steroids (50–100 mg hydrocortisone every 8 hours) and broad-spectrum antibiotics until adrenal insufficiency and infection, respectively, are conclusively ruled out.
- A loading dose of 200–500 μg IV levothyroxine should be administered, followed by daily administration of 1.6 μg/kg body weight levothyroxine daily.
- Patients can be transitioned to oral levothyroxine once awake and alert but consider continued IV replacement in patients who are hypervolemic if there is concern for small bowel edema leading to decreased absorption, or for patients who may have impaired oral absorption for any reason.
- Note that an elevated serum creatinine in these patients is thought to represent a decrease in plasma blood flow and glomerular filtration rate (GFR), but increased products of muscle breakdown due to severe hypothyroidism may also contribute. The elevation is reversible with proper treatment of hypothyroidism.
- Severe hypothyroidism can cause proteinuria. If proteinuria is due to hypothyroidism, its presence should resolve after the euthyroid state is achieved.
- Patients can present with a low-pitched voice due to edema of the vocal cords, which likewise resolves after the euthyroid state is achieved.

References

Braverman, L. E., & Cooper, D. S. (2013). *Werner & Ingbar's the thyroid: A fundamental and clinical text* (10th ed., pp. 600–605). Philadelphia, PA: Lippincott Williams & Wilkins.

Jonklaas, J., Bianco, A. C., Bauer, A. J., Burman, K. D., Cappola, A. R., Celi, F. S., et al. (2014). Guidelines for the treatment of hypothyroidism: prepared by the American Thyroid Association Task Force on Thyroid Hormone Replacement. *Thyroid: Official Journal of the American Thyroid Association, 24*(12), 1670–1751.

Ladenson, P. W., Goldenheim, P. D., Cooper, D. S., Miller, M. A., & Ridgway, E. C. (1982). Early peripheral responses to intravenous L-thyroxine in primary hypothyroidism. *The American Journal of Medicine, 73*(4), 467–474.

Nicoloff, J. T., & LoPresti, J. S. (1993). Myxedema coma. A form of decompensated hypothyroidism. *Endocrinology and Metabolism Clinics of North America, 22*(2), 279–290.

Spitzweg, C., Reincke, M., & Gärtner, R. (2017). Thyroid emergencies: Thyroid storm and myxedema coma. *Der Internist, 58*(10), 1011–1019.

Yamamoto, T., Fukuyama, J., & Fujiyoshi, A. (1999). Factors associated with mortality of myxedema coma: report of eight cases and literature survey. *Thyroid, 9*, 1167–1174.

Wiersinga, W. M. (2000). Myxedema and coma (severe hypothyroidism). In K. R. Feingold, B. Anawalt, & A. Boyce, et al. (Eds.), *Endotext [Internet]*. South Dartmouth, MA: MDText. com, Inc. [Updated 2018 Apr 25].

Page numbers followed by "*f*" indicate figures, "*t*" indicate tables, and "*b*" indicate boxes.